Surgical Treatment of Congenital Heart Disease

Springer Nature More Media App

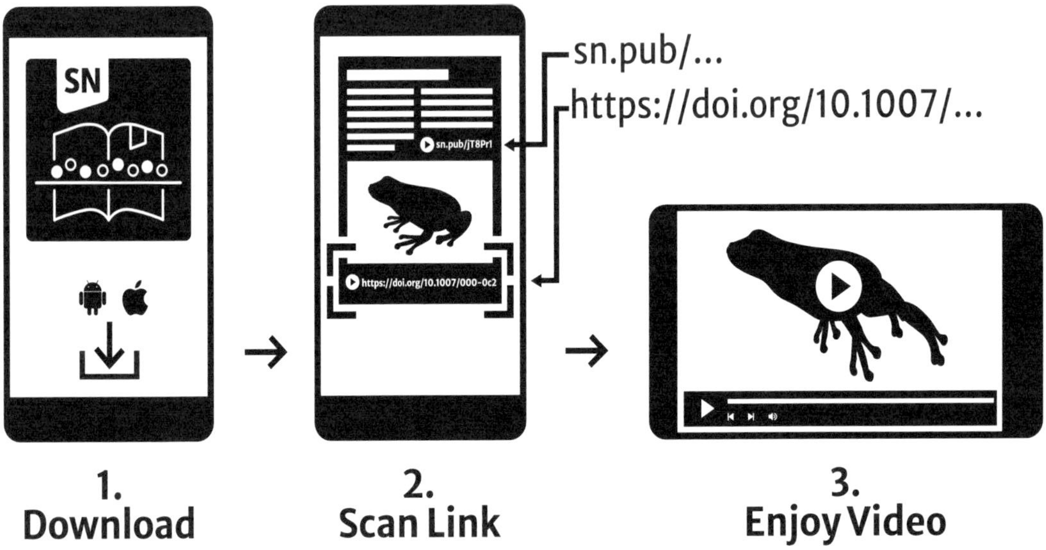

Support: customerservice@springernature.com

Masaaki Yamagishi

Surgical Treatment of Congenital Heart Disease

Understanding Morphology and Ultimate Three-Dimensional Reconstruction

Springer

Masaaki Yamagishi
Department of Pediatric Cardiovascular Surgery
Kyoto Prefectural University of Medicine
Kamigyo-ku, Kyoto, Kyoto, Japan

This work contains media enhancements, which are displayed with a "play" icon. Material in the print book can be viewed on a mobile device by downloading the Springer Nature "More Media" app available in the major app stores. The media enhancements in the online version of the work can be accessed directly by authorized users.

ISBN 978-981-96-6193-0 ISBN 978-981-96-6194-7 (eBook)
https://doi.org/10.1007/978-981-96-6194-7

Translation from the Japanese language edition: "Sentensei Shinshikkan no Geka Chiryo" by Masaaki Yamagishi, © MEDICAL VIEW CO., LTD. 2024. Published by MEDICAL VIEW CO., LTD. All Rights Reserved.

This Springer imprint is published by the registered company Springer Nature Singapore Pte Ltd.
The registered company address is: 152 Beach Road, #21-01/04 Gateway East, Singapore 189721, Singapore

To Kiriko, Marifu, and Miori

Recommendation

This book is a surgical text that is filled with so much content (knowledge and volume) that it would be impossible for a single surgeon to write. At the same time, it is a surgical text that is filled with the actual, detailed surgical techniques (elaboration and quality) that could only be achieved by a single surgeon.

Thank you, Dr. Masaaki Yamagishi, for this inspiring surgical text.

I have known Dr. Masaaki Yamagishi since university. Although we went to different universities, we were fierce rivals on the rugby football team that played across the Kamogawa River, and we would often had open-hearted get-togethers after matches. After graduating from university, he went on to the Heart Institute of Japan, Tokyo Women's Medical University, and I went on to the Department of Cardiovascular Surgery at Kyoto University, but we lost touch for a while. About 10 years later, we realized that we were both presenting at academic conferences as congenital heart surgeons, and since then we have been friends who compete, respect, and drink together while discussing things. I would like to write honestly about what I feel as a sworn friend.

Dr. Yamagishi began his training at Tokyo Women's Medical University, The Heart Institute of Japan, which was founded by Dr. Shigeru Sakakibara, who is revered as the "Father of Cardiac Surgery" for laying the foundation of cardiac surgery in Japan, and Dr. Soji Konno, who developed the Konno operation with his ingenious perspective and creativity (Dr. Konno also graduated from Kyoto Prefectural University of Medicine, the same university as Dr. Yamagishi), and Dr. Yasuharu Imai, who led Japanese pediatric and congenital cardiac surgery with his overwhelming theoretical and surgical skills, and who was mentored by Masahiko Ando, the founder of congenital heart disease and morphology in Japan, and Dr. Hiromi Kurosawa, who developed new surgical techniques based on his research on the conduction system and logical ideas backed by anatomy, and who laid the foundation for pediatric and congenital heart surgery. I feel that the background to his achievements is a wonderful lineage inherited from the great predecessors of The Heart Institute of Japan.

Of course, not everyone will achieve greatness if they are trained by outstanding predecessors. What makes him so great is that he has used the wonderful lineage he inherited from his great predecessors to carefully construct a theory based on his overwhelming anatomical knowledge of the issues he has experienced in real clinical practice, and has then put this into practice in new techniques and surgical strategies. Furthermore, he has taken this surgery and refined it into an art form using his exceptional concentration and surgical skills. It is not difficult to imagine the enormous amount of time and effort that must have been spent, which is unimaginable to most people. This book includes all of this without hiding anything. In particular, the surgical strategy for creating a superior three-dimensional configuration from a fluid dynamics perspective is described in detail in the surgical procedures developed by Dr. Yamagishi himself, and it is clear that he has written this book with the next generation of professionals in mind.

I would like to say a few words to those who will pick up this book.

"It is not easy to reproduce the surgery that can be called the art of Dr. Masaaki Yamagishi. However, I would like to express my gratitude for the intention of Dr. Masaaki Yamagishi, who gave us this irreplaceable gift, and I would like to ask you to read this book carefully, make further efforts, and inherit the high quality surgery that can contribute to children with congenital heart disease. I am sure you can."

Finally,

"Thank you, Dr. Masaaki Yamagishi, for bringing this inspiring and stimulating surgical text to the world."

Shizuoka Children's Hospital
Shizuoka, Japan
January 2024

Kisaburo Sakamoto

Preface to English Version

When I saw a human heart for the first time during my anatomy class at university, I was overwhelmed by the complexity of its form and the almost perfect beauty of its shape, which had been created by nature. This was one of the reasons that led me to choose to go into cardiovascular surgery.

When performing surgery, I made sure to achieve stable surgical results, and I also tried to develop various new techniques and procedures that were not bound by existing treatment methods, in order to achieve better prognoses. This book is a record of my clinical and surgical experiences at Kyoto Prefectural University of Medicine and other institutions over the past quarter of a century.

An understanding of anatomy and hemodynamics is a minimum requirement for a pediatric cardiac surgeon. It is also important to examine the child carefully and formulate the most appropriate medical and surgical treatment strategy for each individual child. On this basis, it is necessary to carry out a three-dimensional reconstruction of the heart that makes sense from a fluid dynamics perspective, while also taking into account the element of growth, so that the best possible hemodynamics can be maintained for many decades after the operation.

In order to achieve these goals, surgical technical skills are an essential requirement. I would like young doctors to continue to accumulate technical training not only to complete ideal surgery but also to reduce surgical invasion. In the near future, surgical treatment will likely undergo major changes through the use of 3D image simulation, robotic surgery, and artificial intelligence technology. However, I believe that in the field of pediatric cardiac surgery, the importance of a surgeon's reconstructive skills and basic techniques to safely complete surgery will remain the same.

With the above in mind, this book differs from the usual textbook format in that it contains a minimum of explanations of general matters and instead consists mainly of my own approach (treatment strategy), basic techniques, surgical innovations, and surgical videos. The surgical videos are not just an introduction to the basics, but have been edited to a longer length so that the techniques can be clearly seen. Explanations are also given for each scene.

Although this book focuses on surgical techniques, it is not just a book about surgery but also includes morphological explanations using illustrations and CT images. We hope that not only cardiothoracic surgeons but also pediatricians and internists will use this book to find the best treatment strategy. I did all the editing of the text, illustrations, CT images, and surgical videos myself. As the illustrations were drawn by the surgeon himself, there may be some parts that are not very good, but I have tried to be as accurate as possible in the details so that you can understand the tricks of the surgery.

I hope that this book will be useful not only in actual surgery, but also in improving treatment and developing new surgical techniques, and that it will give as many children with heart disease a future as possible.

September 2025 Masaaki Yamagishi

Acknowledgments

I would like to express my gratitude to Dr. Hiromi Kurosawa for his guidance at Department of Cardiac Surgery, Tokyo Women's Medical University and Department of Cardiac Surgery, The Jikei University School of Medicine.

I am grateful to Dr. Yuzuru Nakamura, Chief of Department of Cardiovascular Surgery, for giving me the opportunity to operate on patients at the Saitama Children's Medical Center and for teaching me how to be a doctor who is close to patients and their families.

I would also like to thank Dr. Hidefumi Kishimoto, Osaka Maternal and Child Health Center; Dr. Hideaki Kado, Fukuoka Children's Hospital; Dr. Hisataka Yasui, Kyushu University; Dr. Masahiro Yamaguchi, Hyogo Children's Hospital; Dr. Hiroshi Ohkita, Kobe University; Dr. Yuichi Ueda, Nagoya University; Dr. Toshikatsu Yagihara, National Cardiovascular Center; Dr. Kyosuke Nishigaki, Osaka City General Medical Center; Dr. Shunji Sano, Okayama University; Dr. Akira Mishima, Nagoya City University; Dr. Yorikazu Harada, Nagano Children's Hospital; Dr. Yoshitaka Okamura, Wakayama Medical University; Dr. Tetsuya Kitagawa, Tokushima University; and Dr. Hitoshi Yaku, Kyoto Prefectural University of Medicine for their guidance and support since my arrival in Kyoto.

I am grateful to Dr. Shinichiro Oda, Dr. Yoshinobu Maeda, Dr. Hisayuki Hongu, Dr. Shuhei Fujita, Dr. Eijiro Yamashita, Dr. Hiroki Nakatsuji, Dr. Takashi Nagase, Dr. Rie Nakai, and other members of the Department of Pediatric Cardiovascular Surgery, Kyoto Prefectural University of Medicine; Dr. Nobuyasu Kato, Hokkaido University; Dr. Masaaki Koide, Seirei Hamamatsu Hospital; Dr. Masafumi Yashima, Seirei Hamamatsu Hospital; Dr. Koji Nomura, Saitama Children's Medical Center; Dr. Keiichi Itatani, Nagoya City University; Dr. Satoshi Asada, Kinki University; Dr. Yoshie Ochiai, JCHO Kyushu Hospital; Dr. Koichi Nishida, Fukui Cardiovascular Hospital; and Dr. Shintaro Okazaki, Fukui Cardiovascular Hospital, who assisted in surgery, image preparation, fluid analysis, etc.

Contents

Partial Anomalous Pulmonary Venous Return (PAPVR)

1

1 Morphology and Treatment Strategy

1.1 Morphology of Partial Anomalous Pulmonary Venous Return

Partial anomalous pulmonary venous return (PAPVR) is a condition in which one or several pulmonary veins do not connect to the left atrium but to the systemic veins or the right atrium.

The sites of abnormal pulmonary venous return are (1) superior vena cava (SVC), (2) innominate vein, (3) right atrium, and (4) inferior vena cava (IVC), and in rare cases, multiple abnormal return sites may occur. The SVC return type is the most frequent. Most cases are associated with atrial septal defects. In this disease, a large right atrial appendage is often seen along with right atrial and right ventricular enlargement due to the increased preload on the right heart system (Figs. 1.1 and 1.2).

1. SVC Return Type PAPVR

   The most common type of PAPVR. The right superior pulmonary vein returns to the SVC as a single vein, or multiple veins return to the SVC without merging. In addition to the right superior pulmonary vein, the right middle pulmonary vein may anomalously return to the SVC. The pulmonary veins join the right posterior or lateral aspect of the superior vena cava. Abnormal pulmonary veins often return near the junction of the superior vena cava and right atrium, but they may also return cephalic pulmonary vein may return much higher (near the innominate vein junction). In many cases, abnormal pulmonary veins drain into the superior vena cava at a position more caudal than the draining site of the azygos vein. The superior vena cava is dilated by the returning pulmonary vein.

   The superior sinus venous type atrial septal defect (ASD) is often associated near the junction of the superior vena cava and the right atrium.

2. Innominate Vein Return Type PAPVR

   The left superior pulmonary vein or all left pulmonary veins return to the innominate vein.

3. Right Atrium Return Type PAPVR

   One or more right pulmonary veins return to the posterior wall of the right atrium. The inferior venous sinus type ASD is often associated.

4. IVC Return Type PAPVR (Scimitar Syndrome)

   The right inferior pulmonary vein or all right pulmonary veins return to the inferior

Supplementary Information The online version contains supplementary material available at https://doi.org/10.1007/978-981-96-6194-7_1. The videos can be accessed individually by clicking the DOI link in the accompanying figure caption or by scanning this link with the SN More Media App.

M. Yamagishi, *Surgical Treatment of Congenital Heart Disease*,
https://doi.org/10.1007/978-981-96-6194-7_1

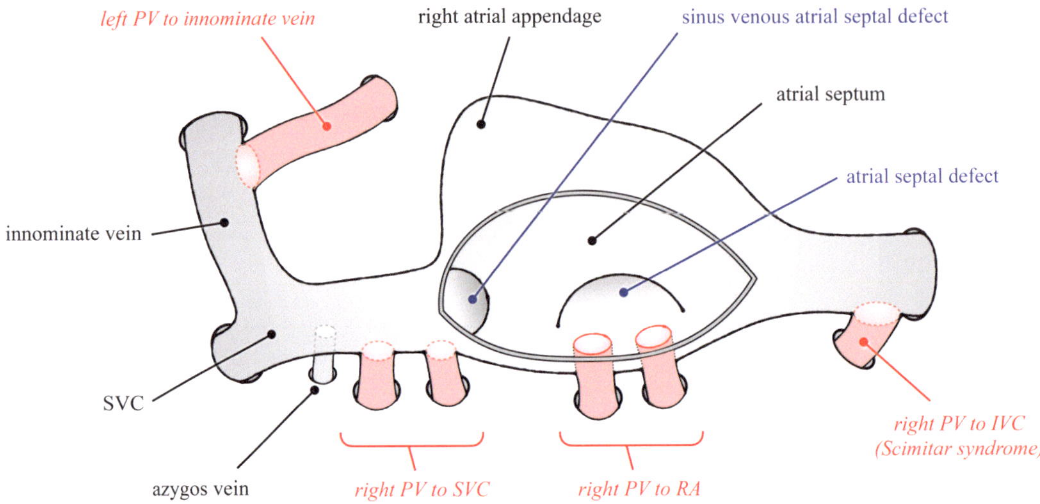

Fig. 1.1 Morphology of PAPVR

vena cava between the inferior vena cava-right atrial junction and the hepatic vein junction.

In some cases, pulmonary hypertension is associated with pulmonary sequestration (a blockage of lung tissue in which blood flow is supplied by an abnormal vessel that connects to the aorta and has no connection to the normal trachea).

5. Mixed Type PAPVR

   It is a rare type. The left superior pulmonary vein often returns to the innominate vein and the right superior pulmonary vein to the superior vena cava.

The sinoatrial node is located on the lateral surface of the right atrium near the sulcus terminalis.

The sinus nodal artery runs anterior to the right atrial junction with the superior vena cava.

The superior vena cava connects to the dorsal side of the crista terminalis on the superior wall of the right atrium.

1.2 Surgery for SVC Type PAPVR

When repairing PAPVR, it is important to choose a technique that allows for a wide superior vena cava and pulmonary venous return and avoids late complications. The following are some of the limitations of PAPVR.

1. *The sinoatrial node and artery must be preserved. Therefore, the superior aspect of the superior vena cava-right atrial junction cannot be incised.*
2. *To avoid atrial arrhythmias, it is important to minimize atrial incisions to a minimum and not incise the sulcus terminalis (epicardial surface) or the crista terminalis (endocardial surface).*
3. *Care must be taken to avoid overstretching of the atrial wall after repair.*
4. *Prosthetic patch enlargement of the superior vena cava and pulmonary veins should be avoided as much as possible because of the possibility of inducing remote stenosis.*

The following repair techniques have been reported:

1. Partitioning of blood flow pathways within the superior vena cava and lateral wall enlargement
2. End-to-end anastomosis of SVC and right atrial appendage (Warden's method)
3. Double-decker technique

Partitioning of blood flow pathways and Warden's method have the concern of narrowing the systemic and pulmonary venous return pathways and/or the risk of arrhythmia.

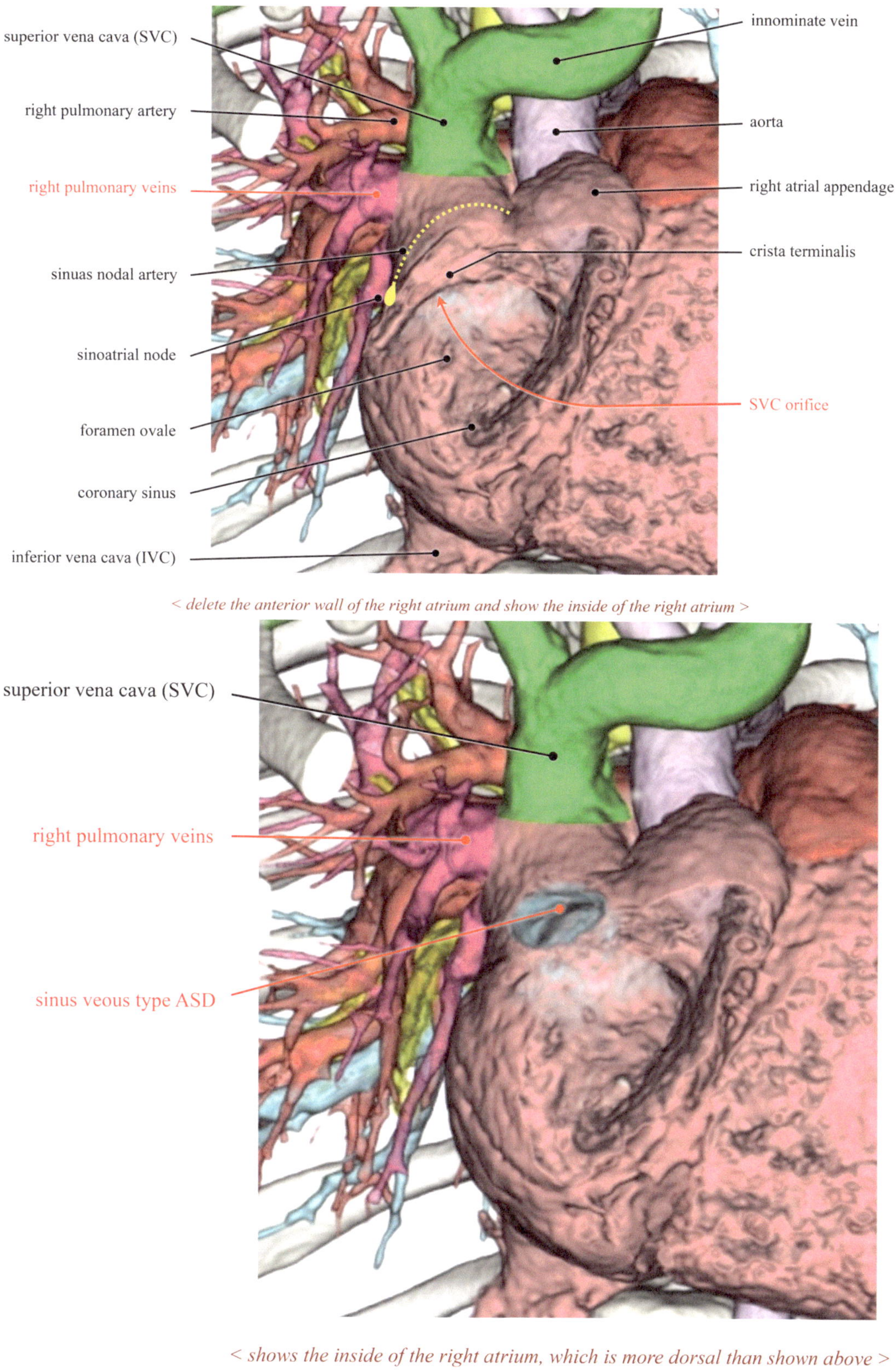

Fig. 1.2 CT images of PAPVR to SVC

On the other hand, the double-decker technique is a useful technique that avoids these complications and is applicable to infants and adults (Figs. 1.3 and 1.4).

1. Partitioning of Blood Flow Pathways Within the Superior Vena Cava and Lateral Wall Enlargement

Procedure

1. Through the atrial incision, divide the SVC lumen vertically using a patch (green line) and create a pulmonary venous pathway from the right pulmonary venous orifice to the sinus venosus type ASD.
2. Make a longitudinal incision in the SVC and right lateral atrial wall dorsal to the sinoatrial node.
3. Autologous pericardium is anastomosed to the incision, and the pulmonary venous pathway is enlarged.

Merit
- Sinoatrial node and sinoatrial artery are preserved.

Demerit
- Requires atrial incision, which raises concerns about late arrhythmias.
- Requires sufficient caliber of superior vena cava to divide the blood flow pathway in the SVC.
- Potential for stenosis of both venous return pathways remains.

2. End-to-end anastomosis of SVC and right atrial appendage (Warden's method)

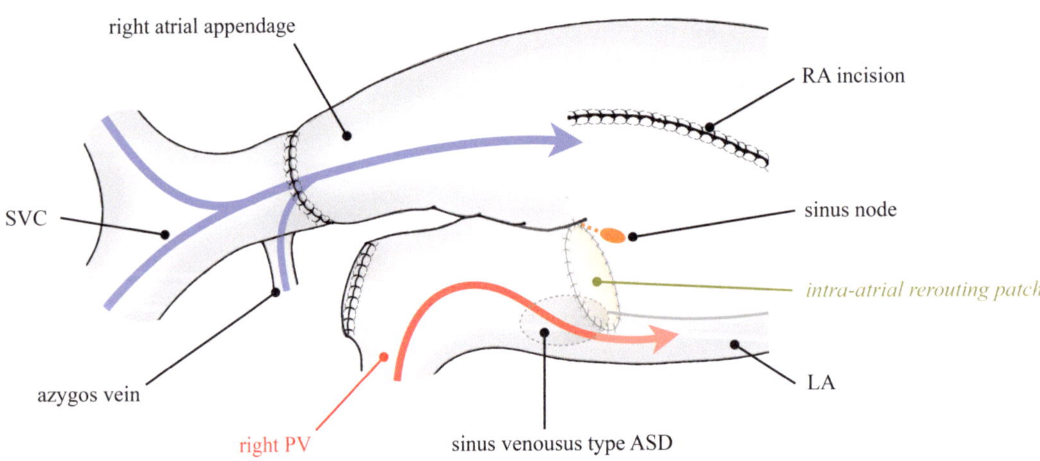

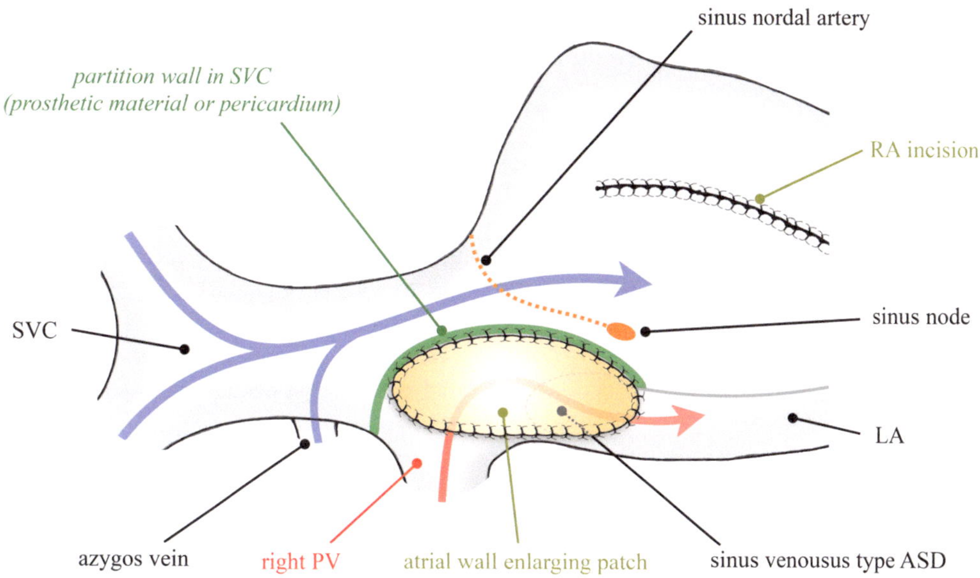

Fig. 1.3 Surgical strategies for SVC type PAPVR

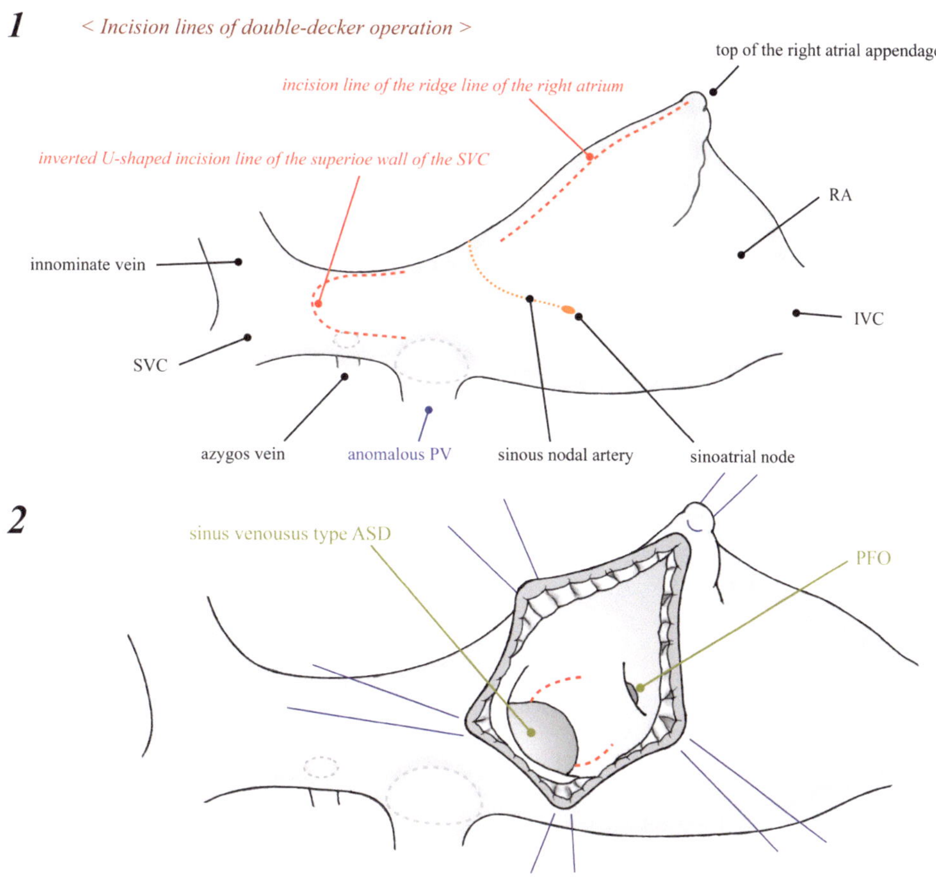

Fig. 1.4 Surgical strategies for SVC type PAPVR

Procedure

1. The SVC is transected cephalad to the site of abnormal pulmonary venous return.
2. The proximal stump of the SVC is sutured closed.
3. Patch closure of the SVC orifice through the atrial incision.
4. End-to-end anastomosis of the distal stump of the SVC and the right atrial appendage.

Merit

- Sinoatrial node and sinoatrial artery are preserved.
- Provide a wide pulmonary venous return pathway.

Demerit

- Requires atrial incision and stretching of the atrial wall, which raises concerns about late arrhythmias.
- The SVC and right atrial appendage must be circumferentially anastomosed, leaving the possibility of anastomotic stenosis.
- Overstretching of the right atrial appendage and possible stenosis within the right atrial appendage remains.

3. Double-decker operation

Procedure

1. Incise the ridge line on the cephalic side of the right atrium and patch closure of the ASD and SVC opening through this incision.
2. The upper wall of the SVC is incised in an inverted U-shape and sutured to the inner floor of the SVC to form the lower part of the double-decker (pulmonary venous pathway).
3. Anastomose the right atrial appendage incision with the upper wall of the SVC and the SVC orifice to form the upper part of the double-decker (systemic venous pathway).

Merit

- Sinoatrial node and sinoatrial artery are preserved.
- No additional atrial incision required.
- No circumferential anastomosis, thus avoiding stenosis of the systemic venous pathway in the late phase.

Demerit

- If the right atrial appendage is too small, a supplement may be needed.

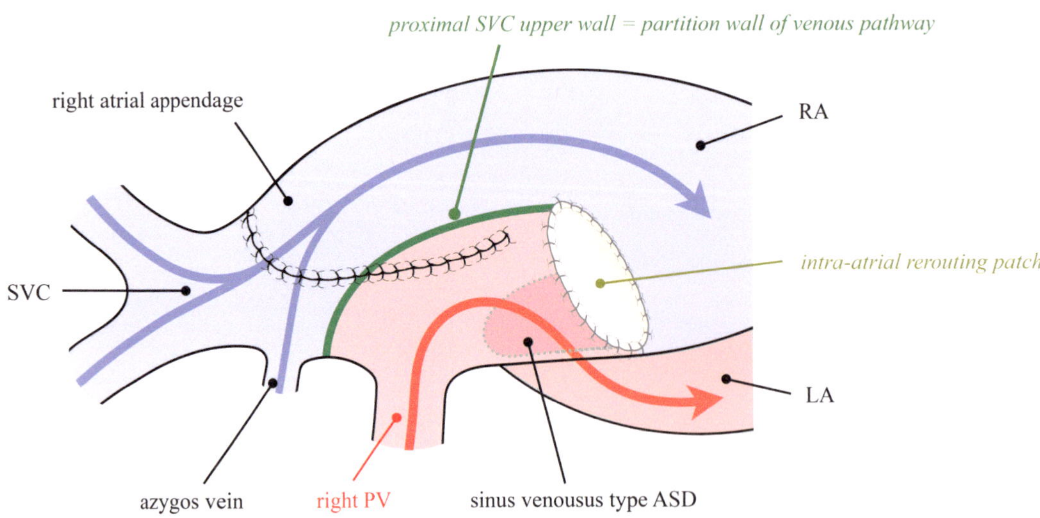

2 Double-Decker Operation for SVC Type PAPVR

2.1 Procedure of Double-Decker Operation

- A linear incision is made at the cephalic ridge line of the right atrium and several traction sutures are placed to allow visualization.
- The SVC opens dorsal to the crista terminalis, and a sinus venosus type ASD is recognized dorsal to the SVC orifice.
- *Red dotted line*: Incision lines from both sides of the inferior border of the sinus venosus type ASD to the caudal side.

3

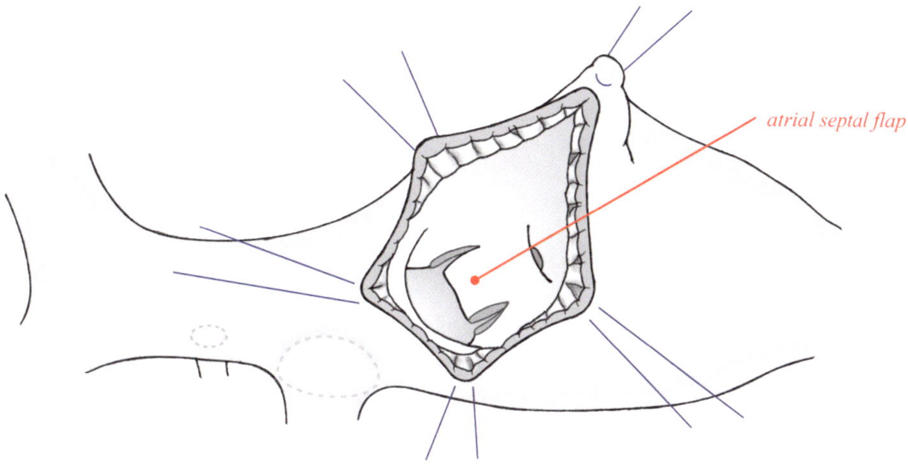

- Incise caudally on both sides of the inferior border of the ASD to create an atrial flap.

4

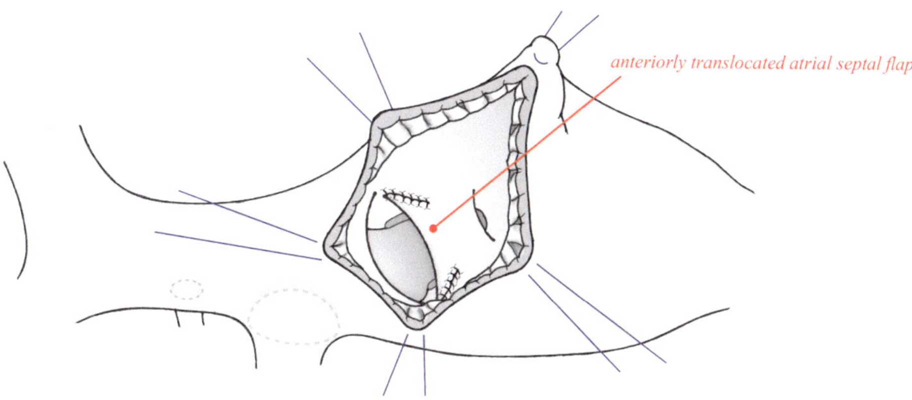

- Anterior translocation of the atrial septal flap and anastomosis to the inner atrial wall.
- This anterior translocation of the atrial septal flap is not necessary, but it is useful to provide a smooth pulmonary venous pathway.
- Anterior transposition of the atrial septal flap should be attempted in cases of small defects where the inferior margin of the defect does not extend much caudally.
- In large defects with caudal extension of the atrial septal defect, anterior translocation is not necessary, and only blood flow diversion with an autologous pericardial patch is required.

5

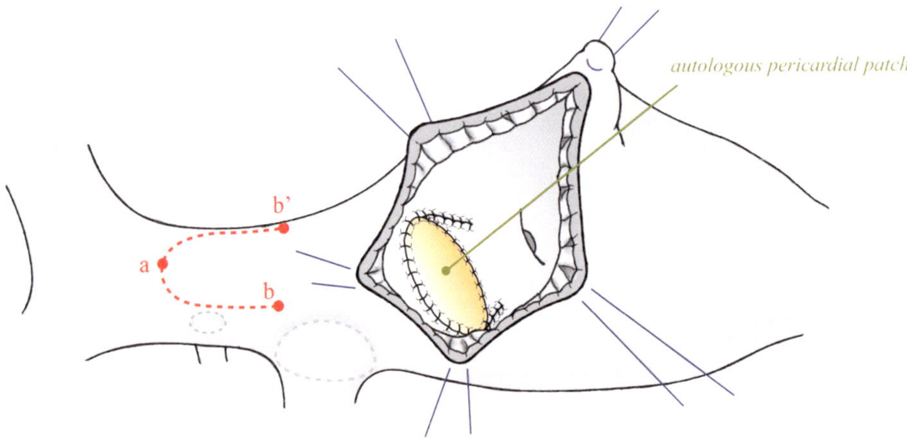

- *Red dotted line*: Inverted U-shaped incision line of the roof of the SVC.
- The uppermost point (a) of the incision line is the point where the apex of the right atrial appendage is displaced and the atrial wall is not overstretched (cephalad of the azygos vein junction).
- The lowermost point (b and contralateral b′) is the cephalic end of the connection of the anomalous pulmonary vein to the lateral wall of the superior vena cava.
- The remaining atrial septal defect and the SVC opening are closed with an autologous pericardial patch. The superior edge of the patch is sutured to the crista terminalis.

6

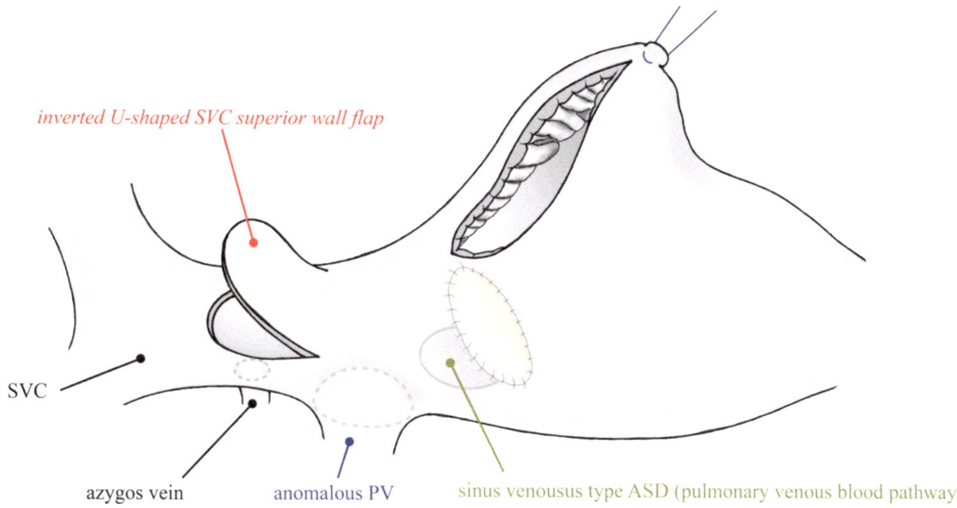

- Incise the superior vena cava wall flap so that the top of the flap is not V-shaped but inverted U-shaped.

7

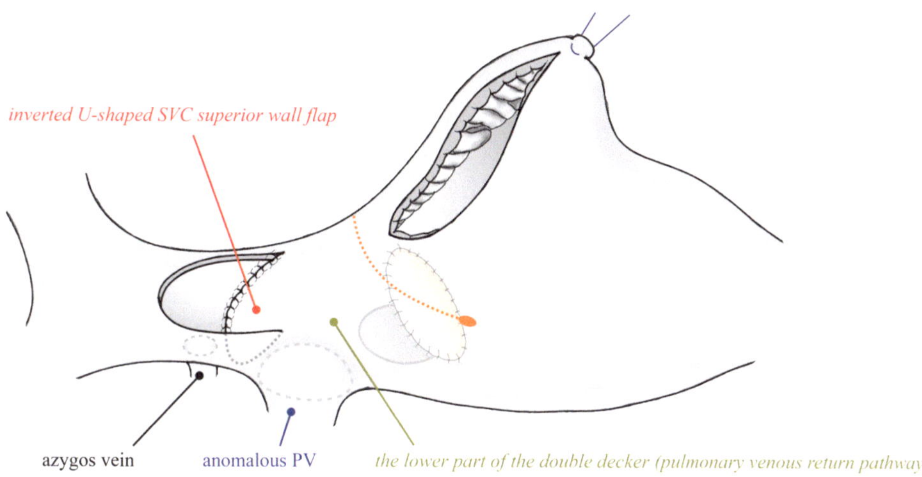

- The SVC superior wall flap is transposed dorsally and anastomosed to the inner wall of the SVC.
- The top of the flap is anastomosed cephalad to the pulmonary vein opening and caudal to the azygos vein opening.
- Once the anastomosis of the SVC superior wall flap is completed, the lower part of the double-decker (pulmonary venous return pathway) is complete.

8

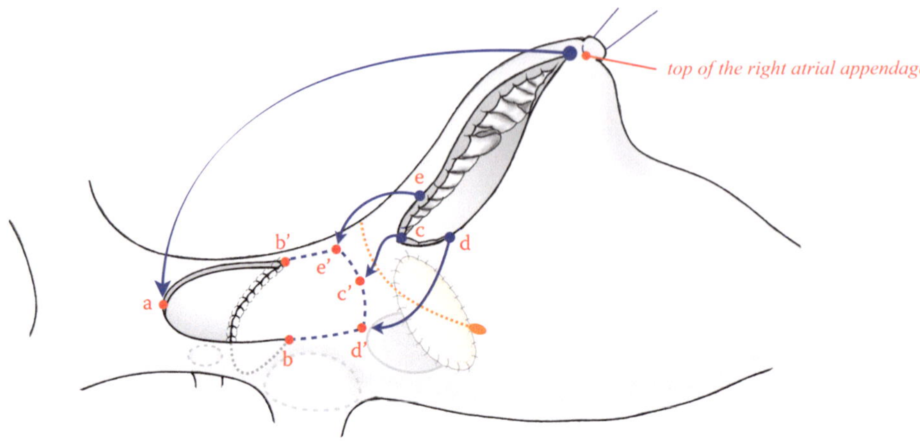

- Anastomose the lowermost atrial incision (c) to the upper wall of the SVC (c′), cephalad to the sinoatrial node artery.
- The top of the right atrial appendage is displaced to the top of the SVC incision (a).
- The atrial wall is anastomosed to the superior lateral wall of the SVC perpendicular to the long axis of the SVC (e → e′, d → d′). By anastomosing the right atrial incision section from the superior SVC wall to the lateral wall (in the direction of the short axis of the SVC), the base of the upper part of the double-decker (systemic venous return pathway) is widely formed.
- The suture line now crosses the SVC-RA junction, preserving the sinus nodal artery.

9

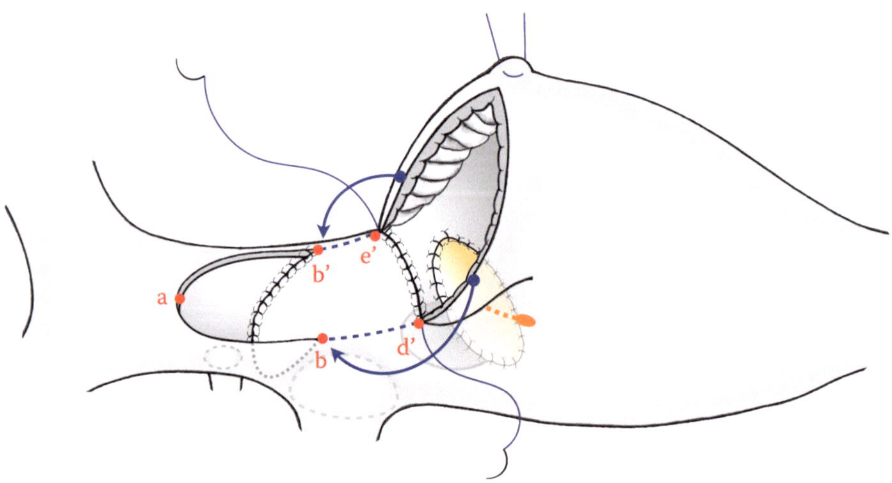

- After suturing the atrial wall to e′ and d′, suture to the superior lateral wall of the SVC parallel to the long axis of the SVC (e′ → b′, d′ → b).

10

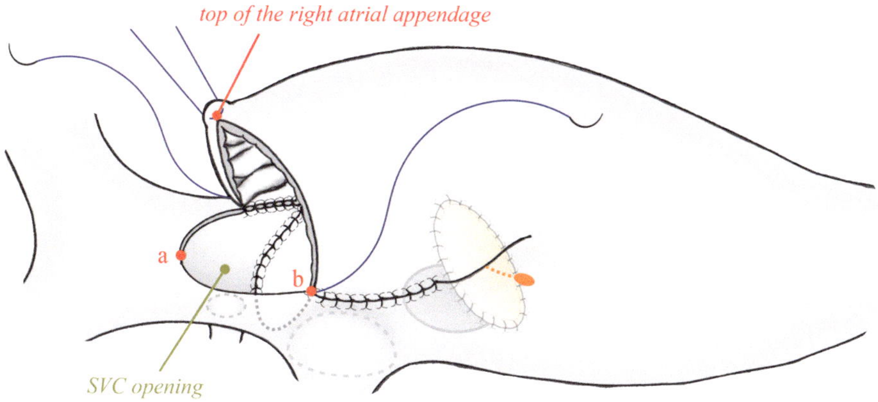

- Anastomose the atrial wall to the SVC opening, taking care to the balance of the left and right atrial wall incisions so that the top of the atrial appendage corresponds to the top of the SVC opening (a).

11

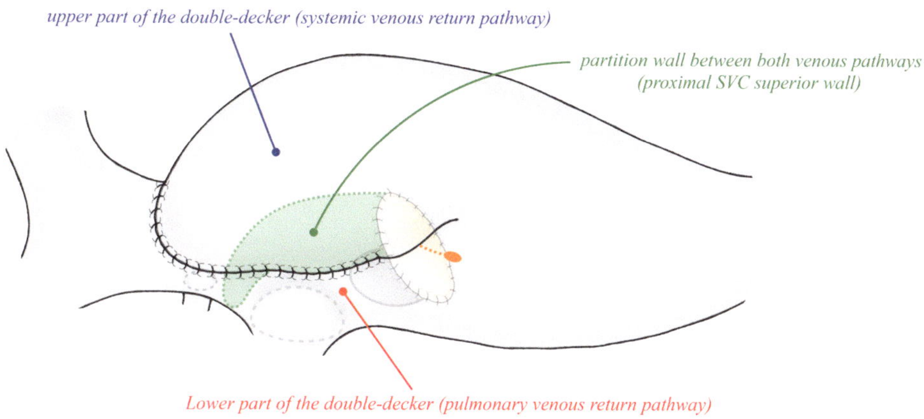

- Completion of the double-decker operation.
- The upper wall of the proximal SVC serves as a septum for both venous return pathways.
- Vascular growth is expected because of double-decker operation using only autologous tissue.
- No circumferential anastomosis in both venous return pathways, thus avoiding late phase both venous stenosis.

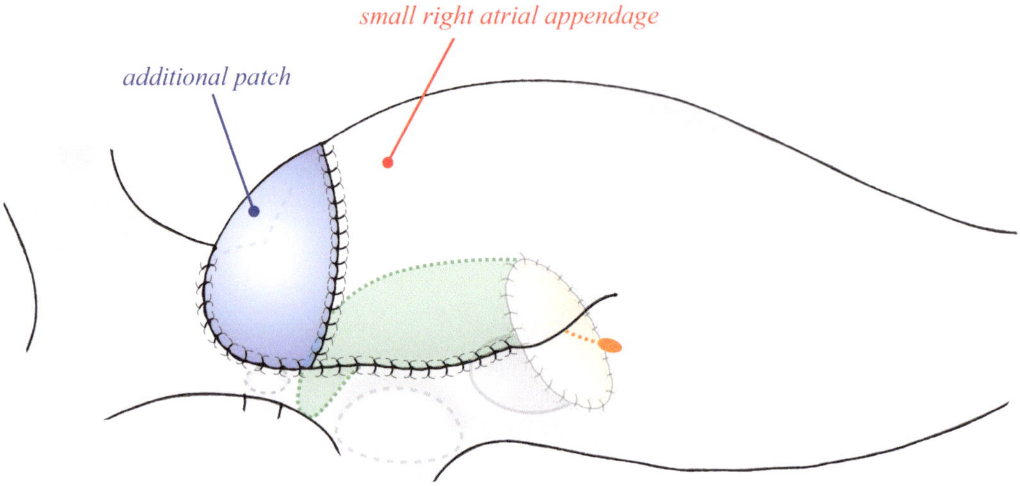

- If the right atrial appendage is small or cannot be stretched in adult cases, the cephalic end of the SVC anastomosis is supplemented with a dome-shaped prosthesis (e.g., autologous pericardium, ePTFE patch, etc.).

2.2 Double-Decker Operation (Surgical Video)

Although a median sternotomy approach is commonly used, this procedure can be performed with a right posterolateral approach and third intercostal thoracotomy in cases with no complications other than SVC type PAPVR and sinus venosus type ASD.

The right lobe of the thymus is completely resected to secure a view of the superior vena cava. The left lobe of the thymus is preserved as much as possible (Scene 1.1).

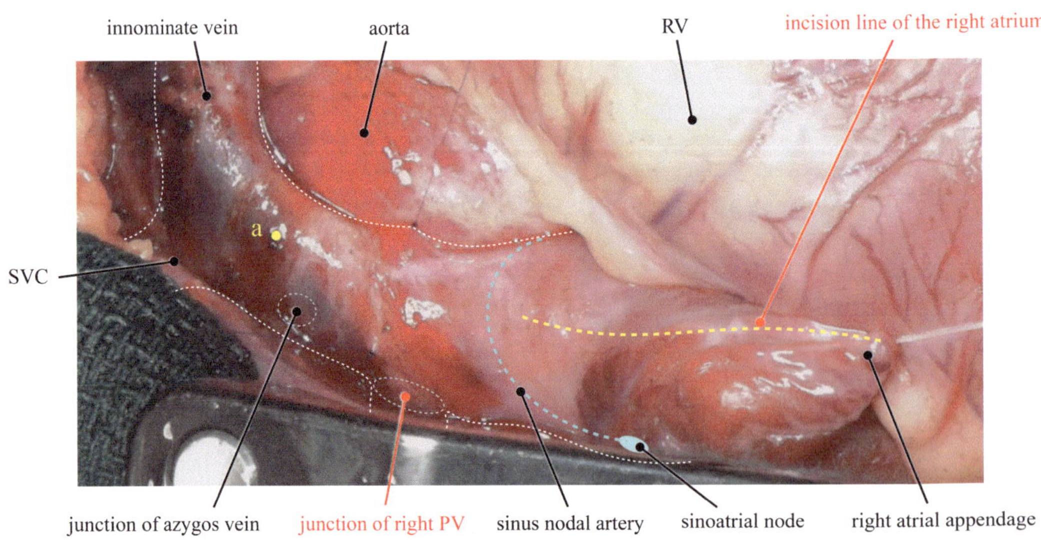

Scene 1.1 SVC, pulmonary vein, and right atrium (Video 00 min 05 s)

- The superior vena cava is dissected cephalad from the innominate vein junction. The proximal portion of the innominate vein should also be dissected.
- The pulmonary vein need not be dissected.
- The superior vena cava cannulae are inserted into the superior SVC and the innominate vein, respectively (Scene 1.2).

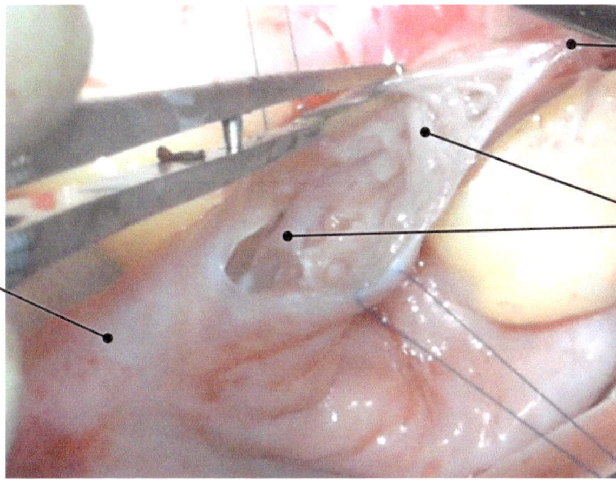

Scene 1.2 Right atriotomy 1 (Video 03 min 00 s)

- A linear incision is made at the cephalic ridge line of the right atrium and several traction sutures are placed to allow visualization.
- Resect the trabeculations in the right atrial appendage as much as possible.
- Be careful not to penetrate the atrial wall when resecting the trabeculations (Scene 1.3).

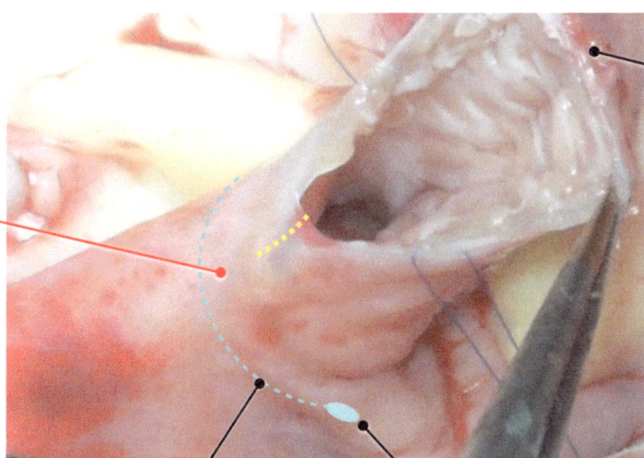

Scene 1.3 Right atriotomy 2 (Video 05 min 00 s)

1. Extend the atrial incision to approximately 5 mm before the SVC-RA junction (*yellow dotted line*).
2. The junction is easily seen from the luminal side (Scene 1.4).

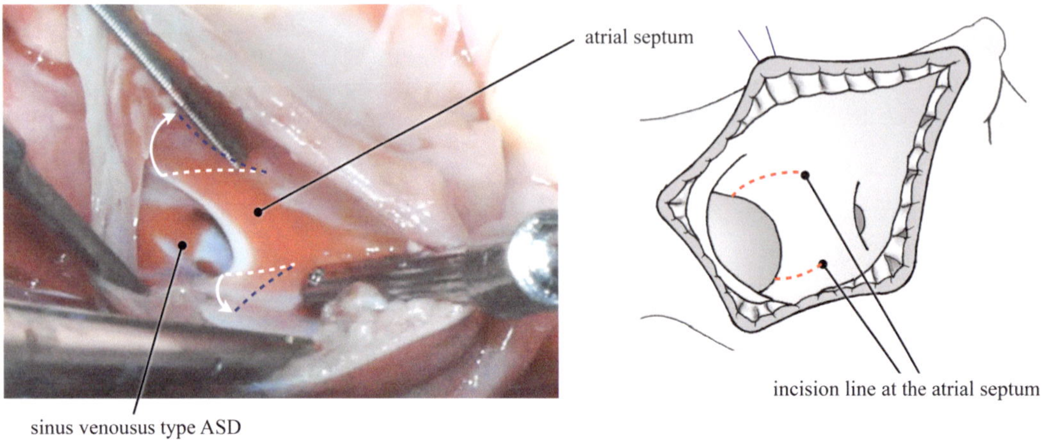

Scene 1.4 Sinus venosus type ASD (Video 05 min 09 s)

1. Make a 10 mm incision caudally on both sides of the inferior margin of the ASD (white dotted line in the left figure, *red dotted line* in the right figure).
2. Dislocate the created atrial septal flap anteriorly to *the blue dotted line* in the left figure (Scene 1.5).

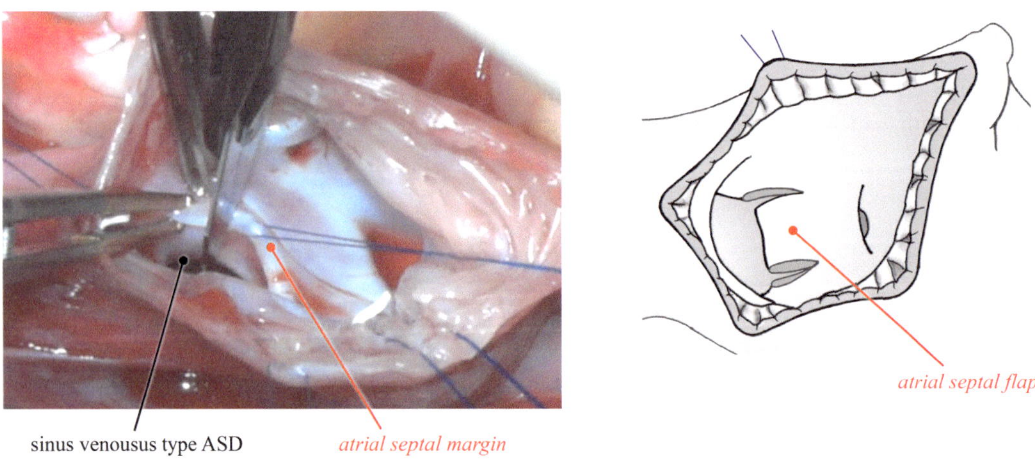

Scene 1.5 Atrial septal flap (Video 05 min 48 s)

1. The atrial septum is incised caudally while pulling traction sutures over the atrial septal margin (Scene 1.6).

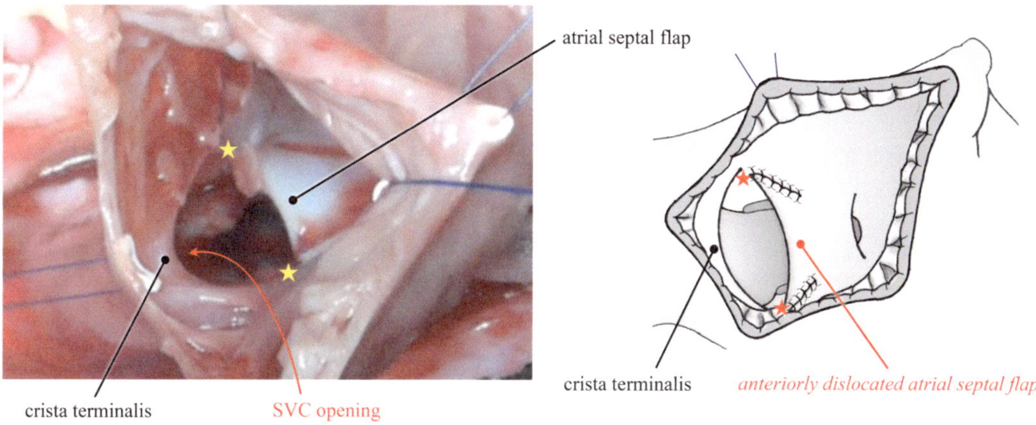

Scene 1.6 Anterior translocation of the atrial septal flap (Video 06 min 13 s)

1. The anteriorly dislocated atrial septal flap is anastomosed to the border of the crista terminalis (*yellow* ★ in the left figure, *red* ★ in the right figure) (Scene 1.7).

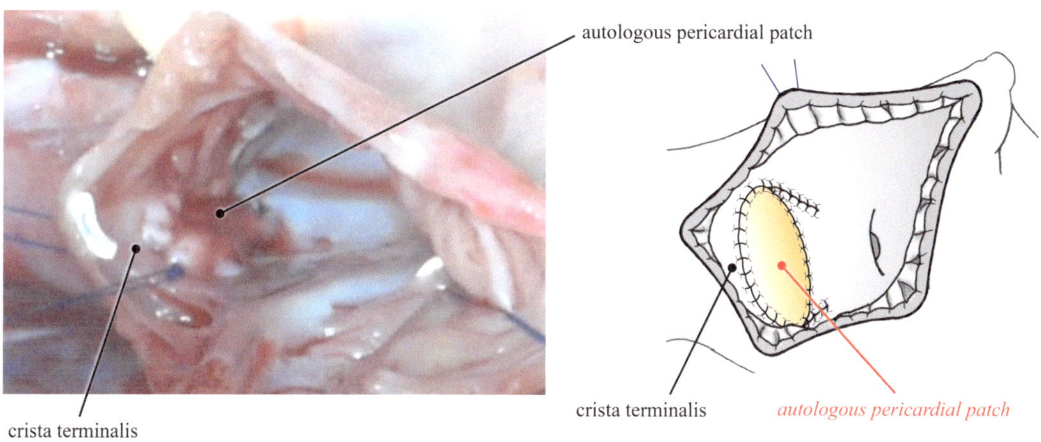

Scene 1.7 Closure of sinus venosus type ASD (Video 08 min 00 s)

1. The remaining atrial septal defect is closed with an autologous pericardial patch.
2. The upper edge of the patch is anastomosed to the crista terminalis.

- All returning pulmonary venous blood from the SVC now passes through the enlarged ASD and flows into the left atrium (Scene 1.8).

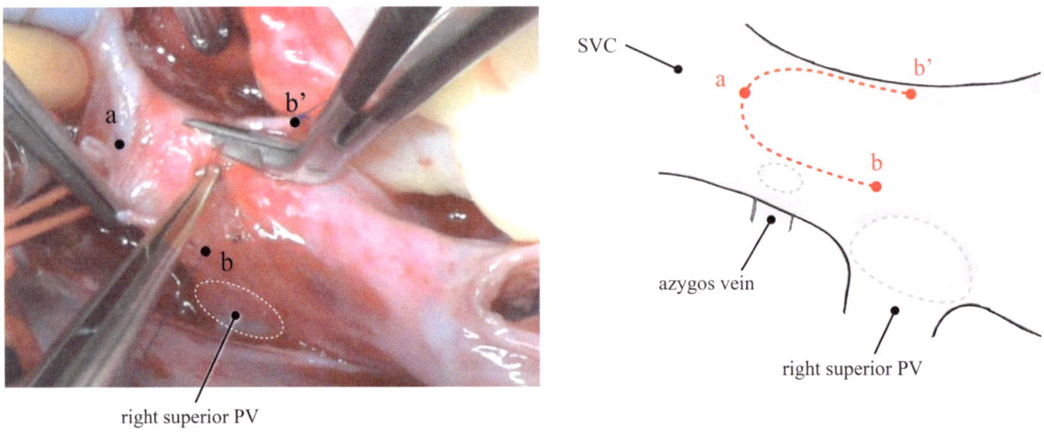

Scene 1.8 Inverted U-shaped incision of the superior vena cava wall (Video 13 min 05 s)

- Incise the superior wall of the superior vena cava in an inverted U-shape.
- The uppermost point (a) of the incision line is the point where the right atrial appendage is dislocated and the atrial wall is not overstretched (cephalad of the azygos vein opening).
- The lowermost point (b and contralateral b') is the cephalic end of the connection of the anomalous pulmonary vein to the lateral wall of the superior vena cava (Scene 1.9).

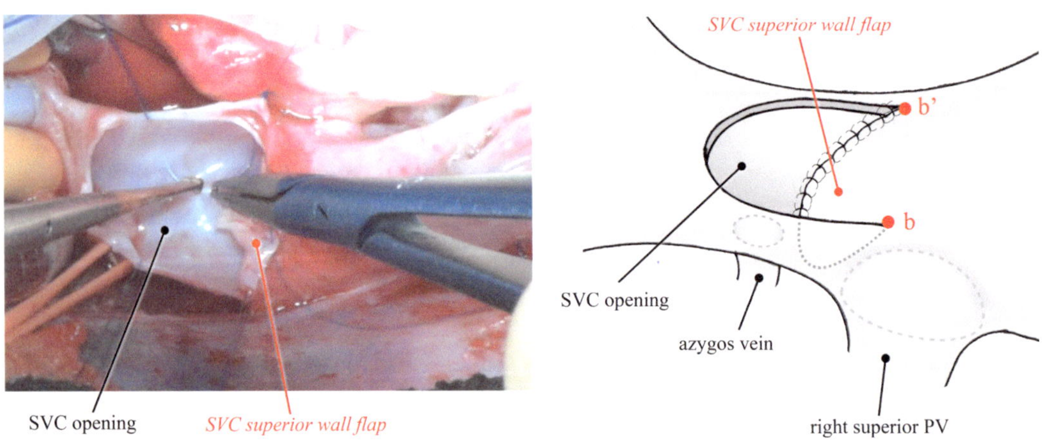

Scene 1.9 Anastomosis of the SVC superior flap (Video 14 min 38 s)

1. The superior wall flap of the SVC is transposed dorsally and sutured to the posterior inner wall of the SVC.
2. The top of the flap is anastomosed cephalad to the pulmonary vein opening (caudal to the azygos vein opening) (Scene 1.10).

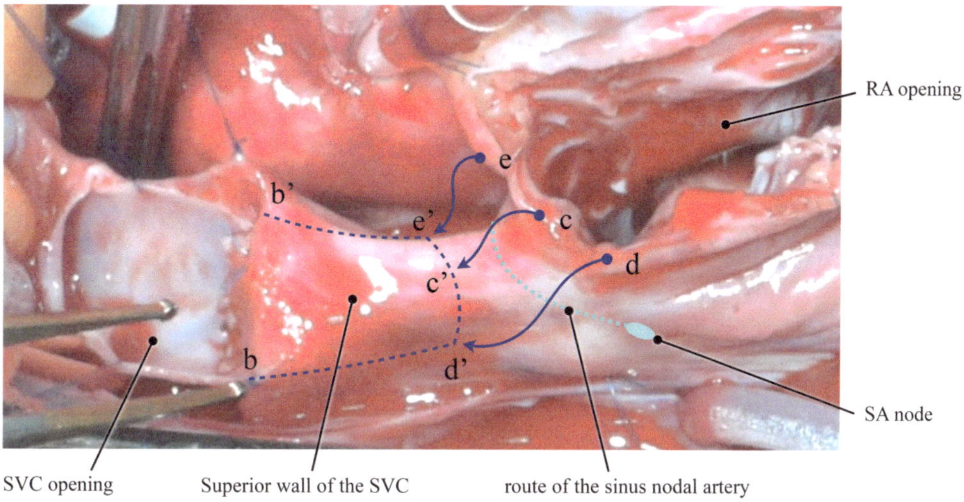

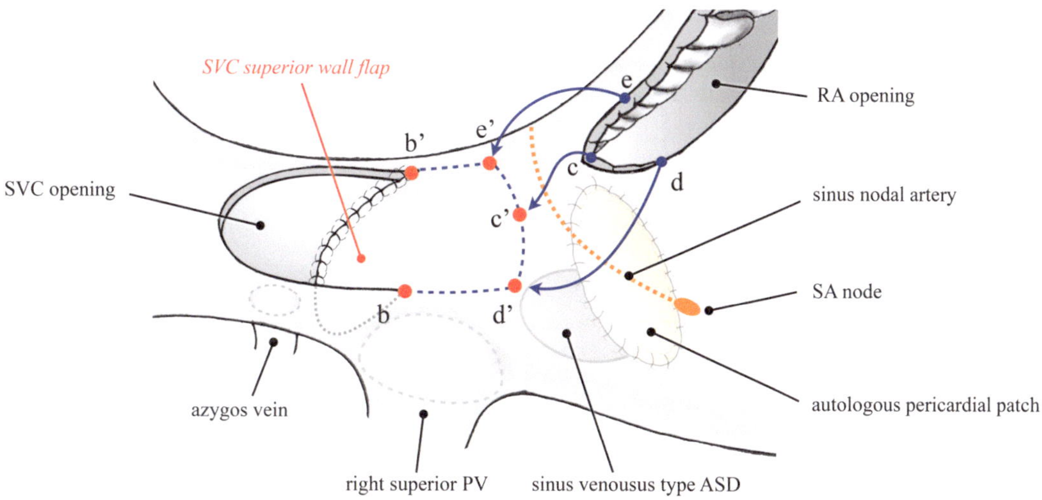

Scene 1.10 Suture line of the atrial opening to the SVC superior wall (Video 18 min 27 s)

1. Anastomose the lowermost atrial incision (c) to the superior wall of the SVC (c′) cephalad to the sinus nodal artery.
2. Anastomose the right atrial wall perpendicular to the long axis of the SVC (e → e′, d → d′). *Blue dotted line*: Suture line of the upper wall of the SVC (Scene 1.11).

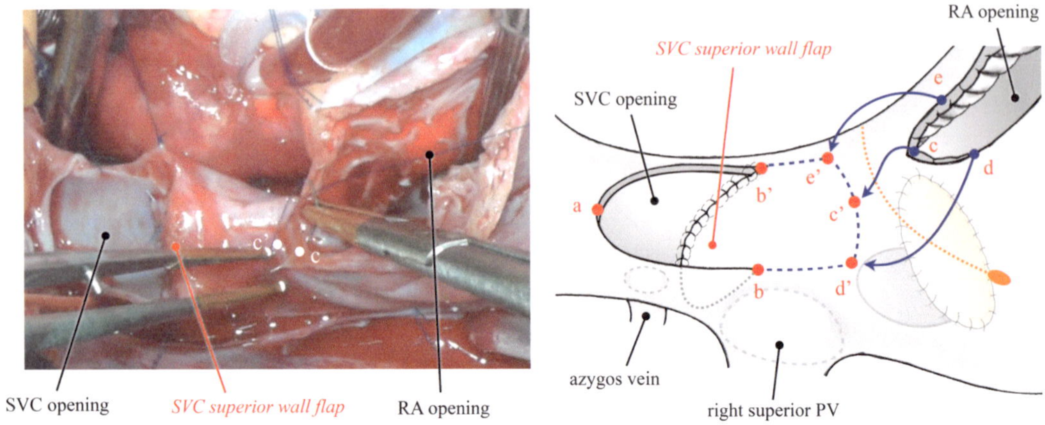

Scene 1.11 Anastomosis of the RA opening to the superior SVC wall 1 (Video 18 min 36 s)

First, anastomose (c) and (c′). The superior vena cava wall does not need to be inserted deeply into all layers (insert into the adventitia and tunica media) (Scene 1.12).

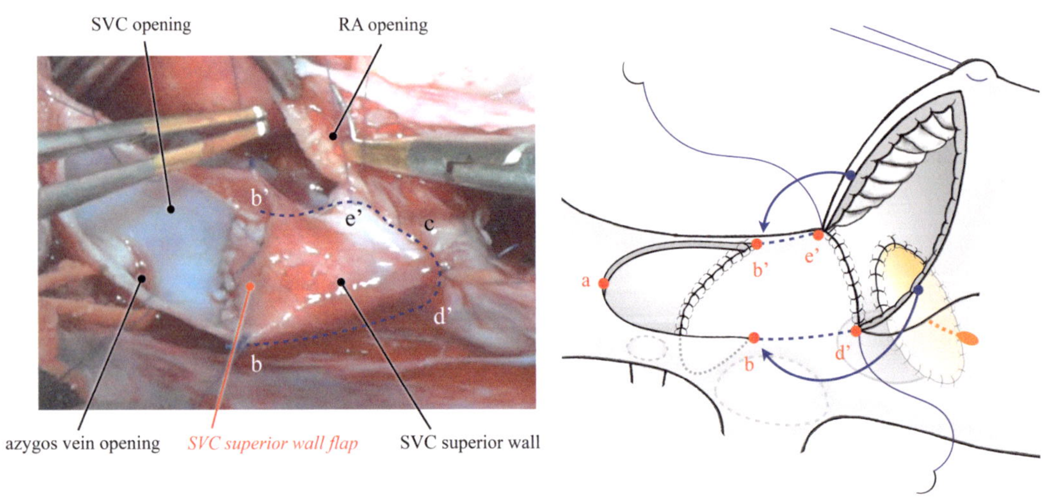

Scene 1.12 Anastomosis of the RA opening to the superior SVC wall 2 (Video 19 min 17 s)

1. After suturing the atrial wall (e) to the lateral wall (e′), suture the atrial wall (left lateral section) in the direction of the SVC long axis to the SVC opening (b′)

Blue dotted line: Suture line of the upper wall of the SVC (Scene 1.13).

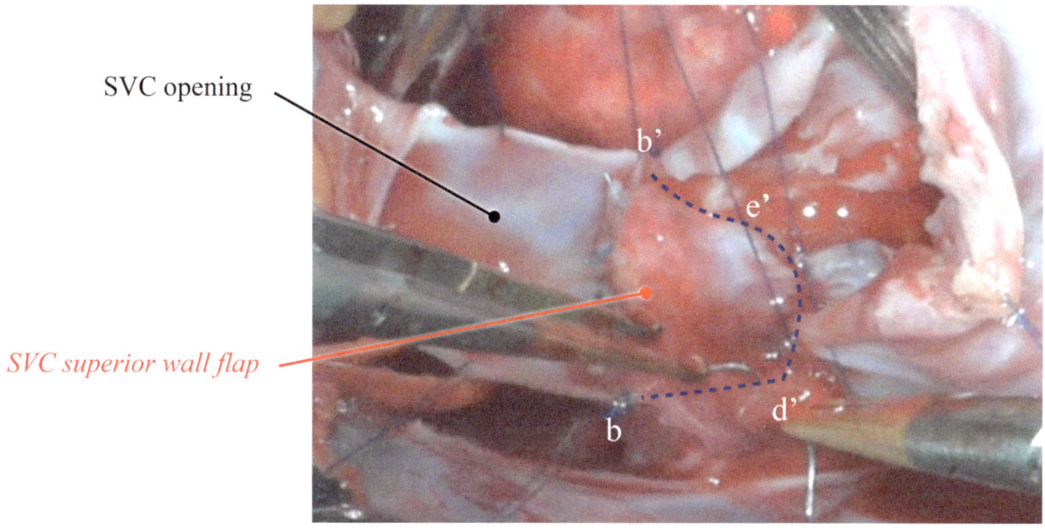

Scene 1.13 Anastomosis of the RA opening to the superior SVC wall 3 (Video 21 min 20 s)

1. Similarly, anastomose the right side of the atrial wall (d) to the lateral wall of the SVC (d′).
2. Anastomose the right side cross section of the right atrium in the direction of the SVC long axis to the SVC orifice (b).

Blue dotted line: Suture line of the upper wall of the SVC (Scene 1.14).

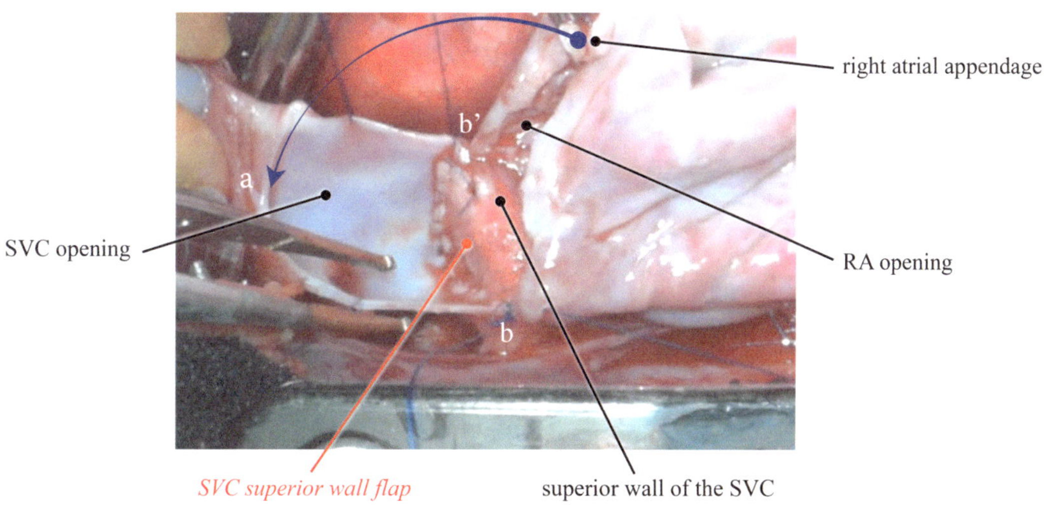

Scene 1.14 Anastomosis of the right atrial appendage to the SVC opening 1 (Video 23 min 20 s)

1. Anastomose the right atrial opening to the lower edge of the SVC opening on the lateral wall of the SVC (b, b′).
2. Then, adjust the top of the right atrial appendage to the uppermost edge of the SVC opening (Scene 1.15).

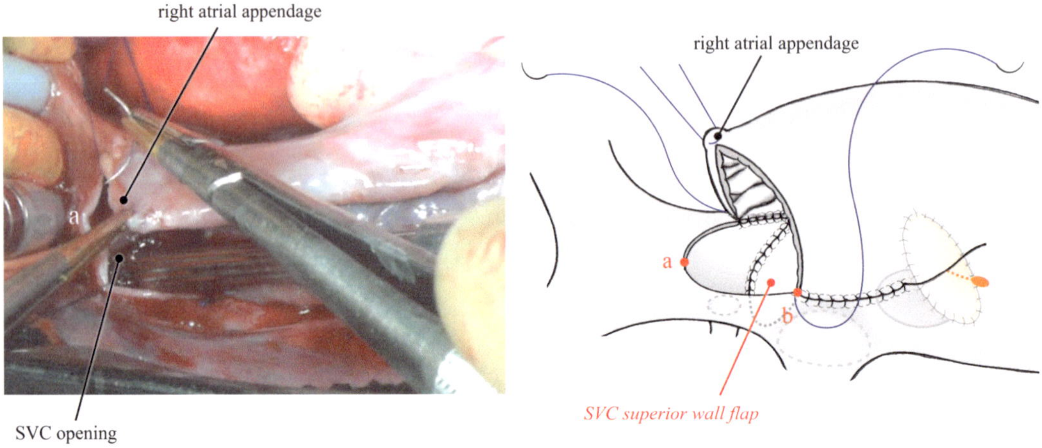

Scene 1.15 Anastomosis of the right atrial appendage to the SVC opening 2 (Video 24 min 40 s)

1. Anastomose the right atrial wall to the SVC opening, taking care to balance the left and right atrial wall incisions so that the top of the right atrial appendage corresponds to the top of the SVC opening (a) (Scene 1.16).

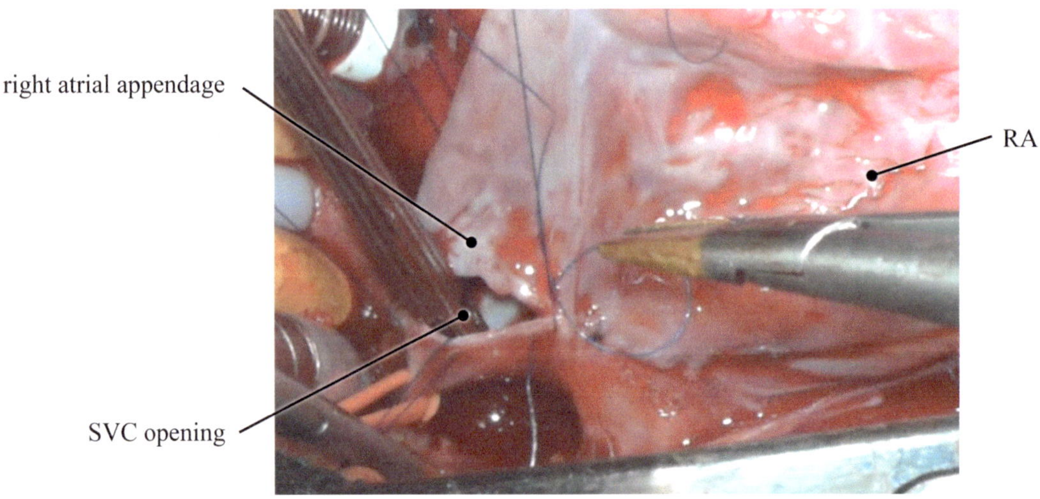

Scene 1.16 Anastomosis of the right atrial appendage to the SVC opening 3 (Video 26 min 05 s)

1. Anastomose the atrial wall to the remaining opening.
   - Be careful not to constrict the SVC opening by continuous anastomosis (Scene 1.17).

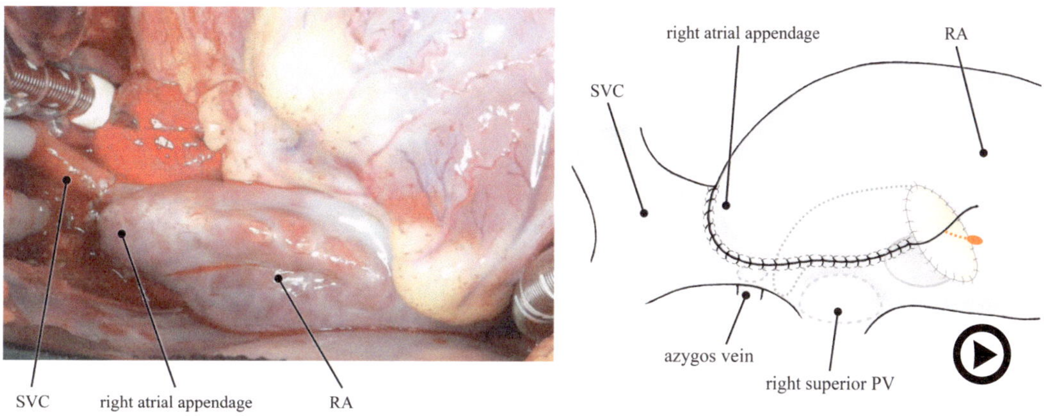

Scene 1.17 Completion of the double-decker operation (Video 27 min 10 s) (▶ https://doi.org/10.1007/000-hk3)

- Completion of the double-decker operation.
- Ensure that the right atrial appendage and atrial wall are not twisted or stretched.

SPOTLIGHT CT Image After the Double-Decker Operation (Right Lateral View)

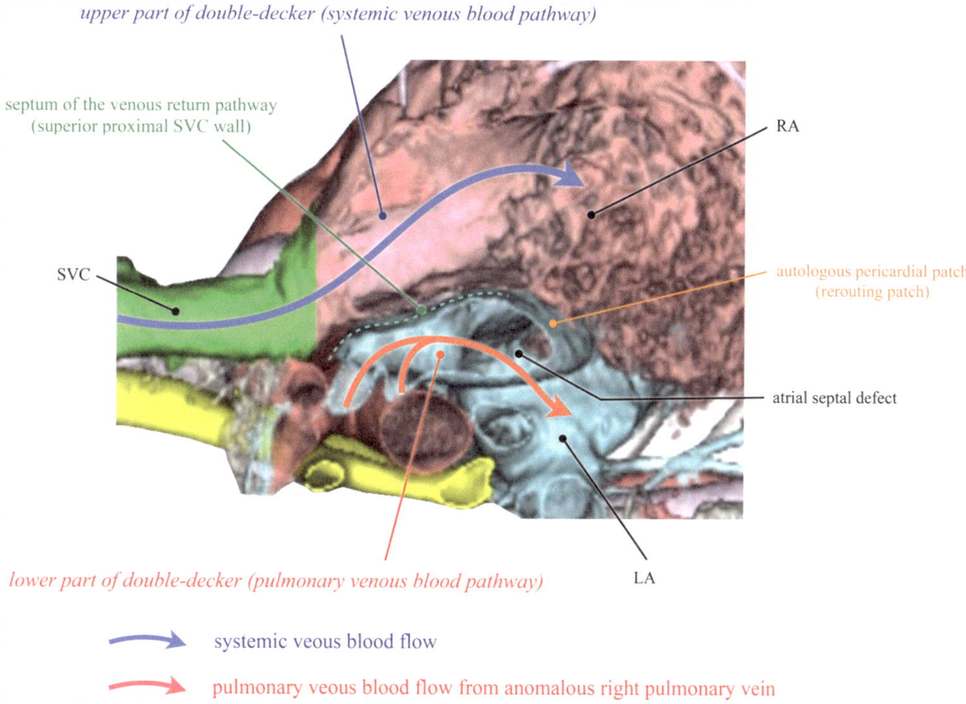

- Wide and smooth superior vena cava and pulmonary venous return pathways are seen without stenosis.
- Both venous return pathways were constructed entirely with autologous tissue and there is no circumferential anastomosis, so there is potential for growth and no concern for late complications of stenosis.

References

Partitioning of Blood Flow Pathways Within the Superior Vena Cava

Stark JF, Tsang VT. Secundum atrial septal defect and partial anomalous pulmonary venous return. In: Stark JF, de Leval MR, Tsang VT, editors. Surgery for congenital heart defects. 3rd ed. London: Wiley; 2006.

End-to-End Anastomosis of SVC and Right Atrial Appendage

Warden HE, Gustafson RA, Tarnay TJ, Neal WA. An alternative method for repair of partial anomalous pulmonary venous connection to the superior vena cava. Ann Thorac Surg. 1984;38:601–5.

Double-Decker Operation

Yamagishi M, Fujiwara K, Yaku H, Wada Y, Kitamura N. Repair of partial anomalous pulmonary venous connection with a minimal atriotomy. Jpn J Thorac Cardivascu Surg. 2000;48:370–2.

Late Results of Double-Decker Operation

Hongu H, Yamagishi M, Maeda Y, Itatani K, Asada S, Fujita A, Yaku H. Double-decker repair of partial anomalous pulmonary venous return into the superior vena cava. J Thorac Cardiovasc Surg. 2019;157:1970–7.

2 Total Anomalous Pulmonary Venous Return (TAPVR)

1 Morphology, Hemodynamics, and Treatment Strategy

Total anomalous pulmonary venous return (TAPVR) is a condition in which all pulmonary veins (PVs) return to a venous system other than the left atrium. Hypoxemia and severe pulmonary hypertension in the neonatal period and early infancy require urgent surgical treatment. It is complicated by a patent foramen ovale (PFO).

1.1 Morphological Check Point for Surgical Repair of TAPVR

The following morphologic and hemodynamic points are important in the surgical management of total anomalous pulmonary venous return (TAPVR) (Fig. 2.1).

Morphological Check Point 1: Pulmonary Vein (PV)

- Morphology and course of the four pulmonary veins (right superior PV, right inferior PV, left superior PV, and left inferior PV).
- Presence of PV stenosis or hypoplasia: If the PVs themselves are stenotic or hypoplastic, there is concern for postoperative PVO.

Morphological Check Point 2: Common Pulmonary Vein (CPV)

- Are all four pulmonary veins connected to the CPV?
- Identify PVs that are not attached to the CPV and the site of attachment.
- Is the CPV large enough for anastomosis: A small CPV may cause anastomotic stenosis?
- Positional relationship to the atrium (left atrium): Is the CPV in close proximity to the left atrium (LA) to be anastomosed?

Morphological Check Point 3: Vertical Vein (VV)

- Pathway of the VV and type of the VV (supracardiac, cardiac, infracardiac, mixed).
- Stenosis of VV: Stenosis of VV causes pulmonary congestion and pulmonary hypertension; stenosis tends to occur at its junction with CPV, at its junction with body veins, at its intersection with pulmonary artery and bronchus, and at its diaphragmatic passage.

Supplementary Information The online version contains supplementary material available at https://doi.org/10.1007/978-981-96-6194-7_2. The videos can be accessed individually by clicking the DOI link in the accompanying figure caption or by scanning this link with the SN More Media App.

M. Yamagishi, *Surgical Treatment of Congenital Heart Disease*,
https://doi.org/10.1007/978-981-96-6194-7_2

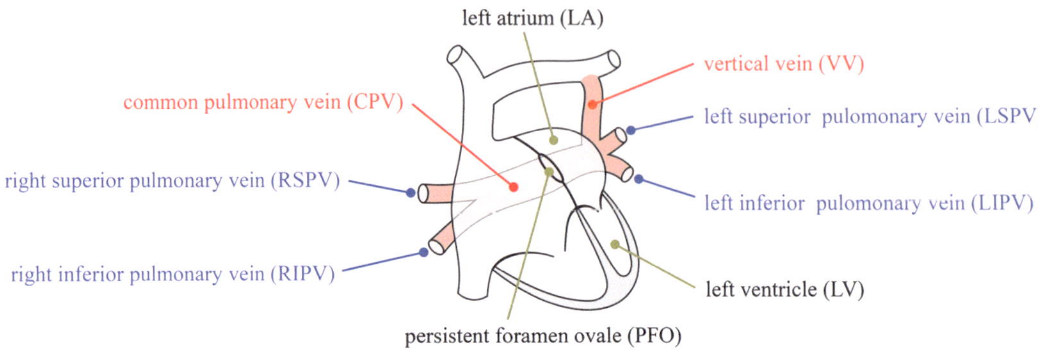

Fig. 2.1 Pulmonary veins of total anomalous pulmonary venous return

Morphological Check Point 4: Ventricle, Atrium (Left Atrium, Single Atrium), and PFO

- Left ventricular hypoplasia due to decreased left ventricular volume load.
- Location of CPV and atrial septum: Is the atrial septum in close proximity to the proposed anastomosis site?
- Left atrial volume: Is there enough volume to create an adequate anastomotic orifice?
- Morphology of the left auricle: If the left atrial appendage is to be used for anastomosis, a trabeculation in the atrial appendage should be resected.
- Size of interatrial communication (PFO): If the PFO is small, there is concern for low cardiac output syndrome due to decreased left ventricular volume load and pulmonary hypertension due to increased pulmonary congestion. In such cases, the oxygen saturation of the arterial blood is also decreased.

Morphological Check Point 5: Presence or Absence of Heterotaxia Syndrome (Asplenia, Polysplenia)

- Patients with this syndrome complicated by heterotaxia syndrome have a high risk of pulmonary hypertensive crisis (PH crisis) due to residual postoperative pulmonary hypertension and a poor prognosis due to pulmonary venous obstructive lesions caused by intrapulmonary venous wall thickening and intimal proliferation. Postoperative pulmonary venous obstruction (PVO) and anastomotic stenosis may occur due to pulmonary vein wall thickening.
- In addition, the development of thick atrial walls and intra-atrial trabeculation in heterotaxia syndrome may complicate postoperative anastomotic stenosis.

1.2 Types of TAPVR, Hemodynamic Characteristics, and Surgical Strategy

The Darling classification, based on the site of pulmonary venous return, is commonly used to classify TAPVR. The timing of surgery depends on the presence or absence of PVO (Fig. 2.2).

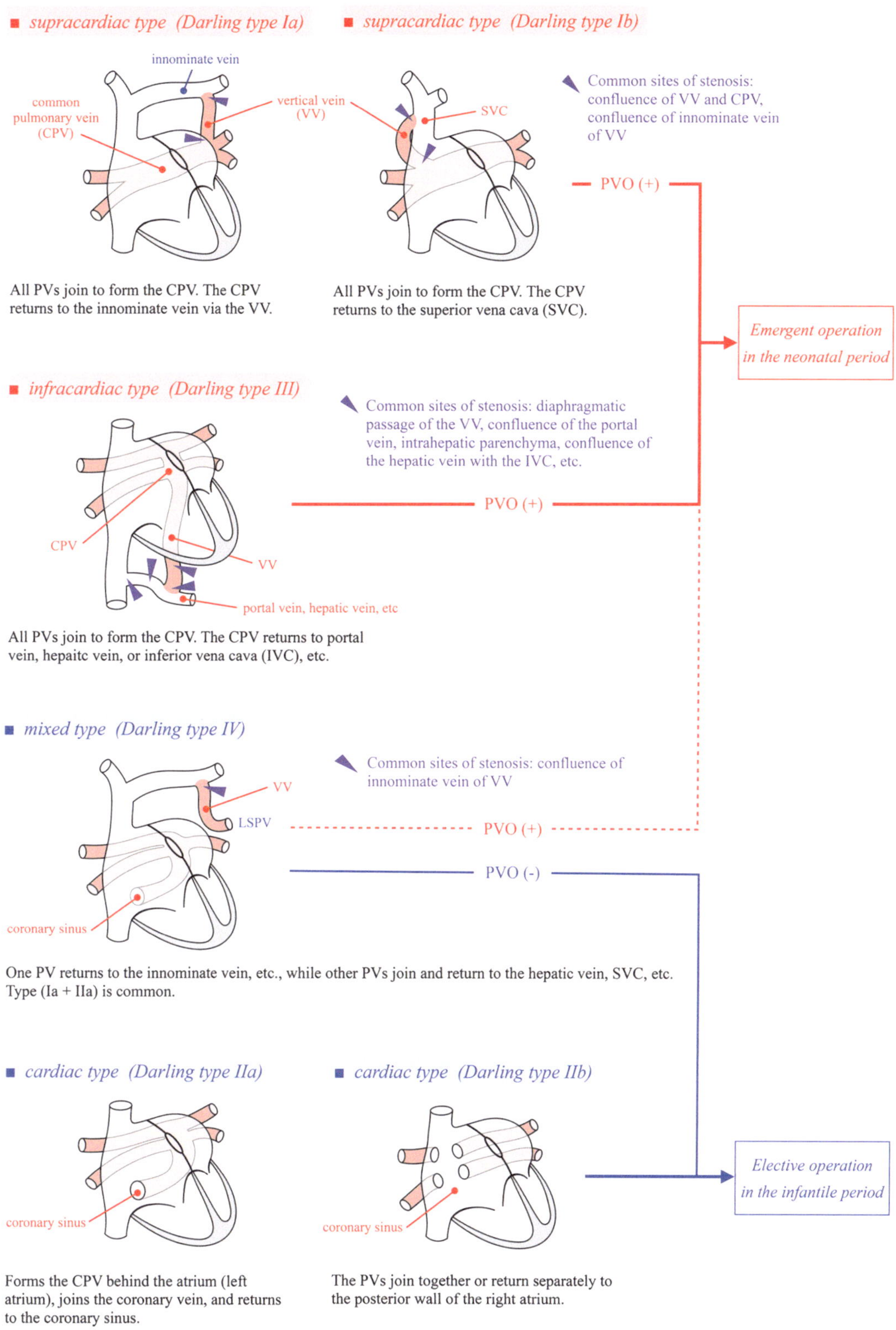

Fig. 2.2 Darling classification of TAPVR and hemodynamic characteristics

1.3 Morphology of Extracardiac Type (Darling Type I, Type III) of TAPVR

The supracardiac (Ia, Ib) and infracardiac (III) types are considered extracardiac, in which the pulmonary vein returns outside the heart. The extracardiac type is often complicated by stenotic lesions at various sites in the return pathway. CT images of each type are shown below (Fig. 2.3).

Vertical vein (VV) returns to the innominate vein (*Darling type Ia*). VV is thick and not stenotic. No stenosis is seen in each pulmonary vein (PV). Left superior pulmonary vein (LSPV) joins the common pulmonary vein (CPV) at a site distant from the other pulmonary veins.

■ *supracardiac type (Darling type Ib)*

< dorsal view >

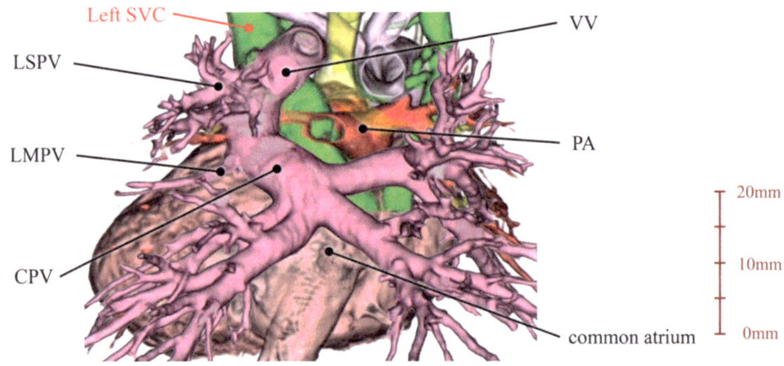

TAPVR associated with asplenia syndrome with VV returning to the left superior vena cava (*Darling type Ib*). No stenosis in VV and each PV. The LSPV and left middle pulmonary venin (LMPV) join the CPV at a site distant from other PVs. In particular, the LSPV joins the VV at a higher level than the left PA. A slight misalignment of the atria (single atrium) relative to the CPV is noted.

■ *supracardiac type (Darling type Ia)*

< dorsal view >

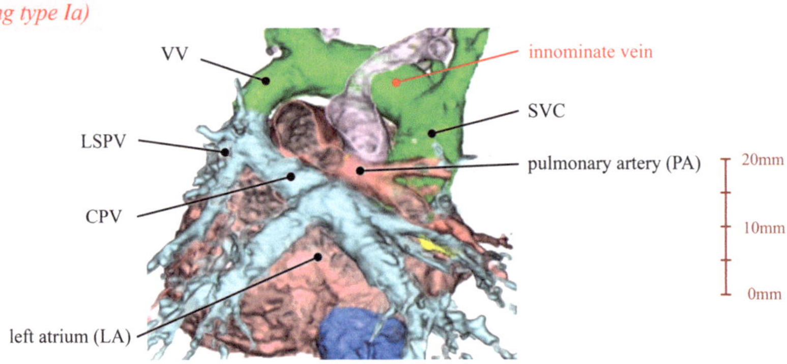

Fig. 2.3 CT images of extracardiac type TAPVR (Darling types I and III)

■ *infracardiac type (Darling type III)*

< dorsal view >

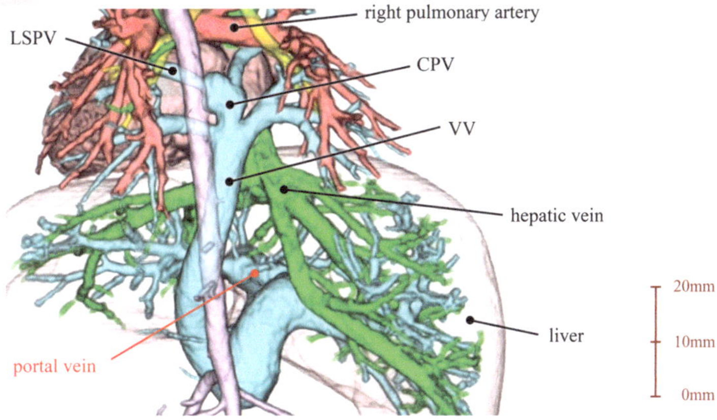

Each pulmonary vein joins to form the CPV. The CPV connects to the VV. The VV passes through the diaphragm and meanders before joining the portal vein (*Darling type III*). There is no stenosis at the confluence of the VV and the portal vein.

The most common late complications of this syndrome are anastomotic stenosis and pulmonary vein stenosis. To avoid these as much as possible, it is important to create as wide an anastomotic opening as possible and to perform the anastomosis without twisting and thickening.

2 Surgical Treatment for Extracardiac Type TAPVR

The repair technique for the extracardiac type consists of common pulmonary vein (CPV)—left atrium (LA) anastomosis and closure of the patent foramen ovale. The following points are important in CPV—LA anastomosis, especially the relative position of the CPV to the left atrium, the method of approach, and the method of anastomosis.

1. Morphology of pulmonary veins and CPV: Stenosis or hypoplasia.
2. Relative position of CPV and LA (atrium): Are they close together or far apart?
3. Method of approach: Superior, posterior, or other?
4. Anastomotic opening: Atrial incision method and CPV (or PV) incision site.
5. Method of anastomosis: CPV-LA direct anastomosis or sutureless method.

2.1 Relative Position of the Pulmonary Veins to the Atrium

It is important to understand the morphology of the CPV, PV, and VV and the relative position of these vascular systems to the LA in order to determine the method of approach and anastomosis (Fig. 2.4).

Supracardiac type (Darling type Ia) < *dorsal view* >.

< Case with good relative position of CPV and LA >

In this case, the LA is relatively large (*yellow dashed line*) and the CPV is close to the upper dorsal surface of the LA, and the relative positional relationship between the CPV and the LA is good.

Direct CPV-LA anastomosis is possible with the *superior approach*.

Infracardiac type (Darling type III) < *dorsal view* >.

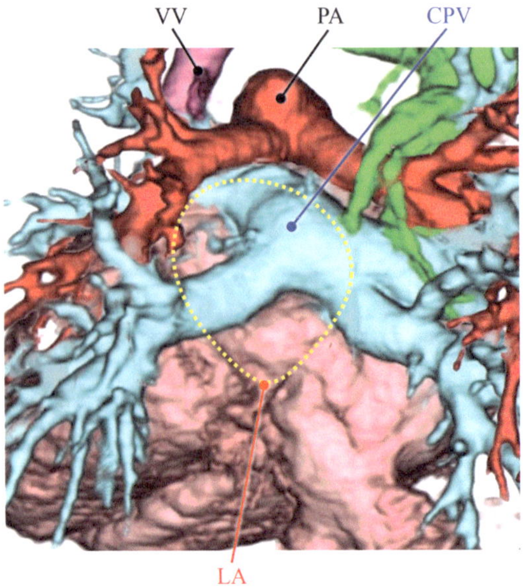

Fig. 2.4 Relative position of VV, CPV, and LA

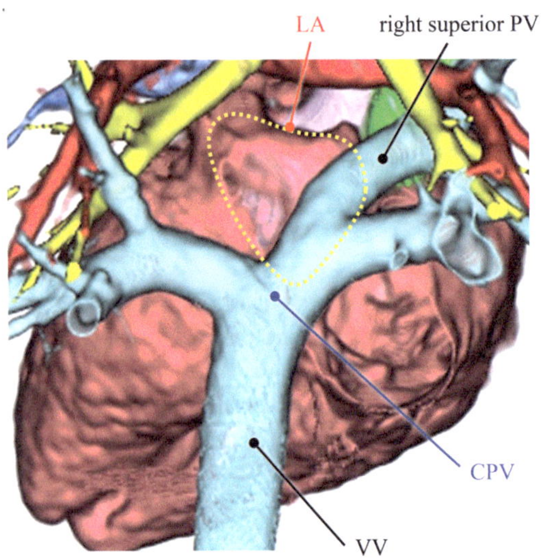

< Case with poor relative position of CPV and LA >

- In this case, the LA (*yellow dashed line*) is small and the CPV is almost nonexistent.
- The LA and PV are relatively far apart (only the right superior PV is close to the LA).
  - It is difficult to reach the LA and incise it optimally with a posterior approach alone, so the *superior approach* should be used in combination with the *posterior approach*.
  - The CPV and LA are relatively far from each other, *so the sutureless or hybrid method (direct and sutureless anastomosis)* is recommended instead of direct anastomosis alone.
  - Anastomosis is performed using the right superior PV and CPV.

Infracardiac type (Darling type III) < *dorsal view* >.

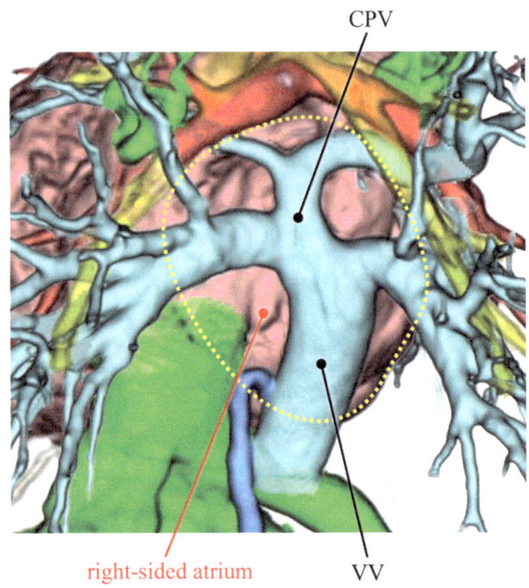

< Case with good relative position of CPV and atrium >

- TAPVR complicated by asplenic syndrome.
- The CPV is thin while the VV is thick.
- The CPV and the VV are located dorsal to the right-sided atrium.
- Relative position of the CPV and the atrium is good.
  - Direct anastomosis of the CPV and right-sided atrium by *right side approach* is preferable.

2.2 Approach Method for CPV to LA (Single Atrium) Anastomosis

The PV and CPV are located on the dorsal side of the heart, making it difficult to obtain a good field of view during the procedure. The choice of approach to the anastomotic site is important to ensure reconstruction of the pulmonary venous blood flow pathway with a good field of view. The optimal method of approaching the anastomotic site should be selected based on the morphology of the CPV and the relative positional relationship between the CPV and the LA or single atrium. The methods of approaching the CPV-LA (single atrium) anastomosis and the advantages of each are shown below (Fig. 2.5).

- The superior approach is a method to reach between the superior vena cava (SVC) and the ascending aorta (AAo) to the posterior mediastinum. It is useful in supracardiac types (types Ia and Ib). It is difficult to reach the caudally deviated CPV or the vertical vein (VV) of the inferior cardiac type (type III).
- The field of view is limited by the SVC and AAo, resulting in a rather narrow field of view, but sufficient field of view can be obtained by applying traction sutures to the AAo and SVC and extending them to the left and right.
- The relative position of the CPV and the posterior wall of the LA in its natural state can be determined, allowing for accurate incision lines and torsion-free suturing.
- Good field of view within the LA, making it easy to avoid damage to the coronary sinus and mitral annulus.

■ *Superior approach*

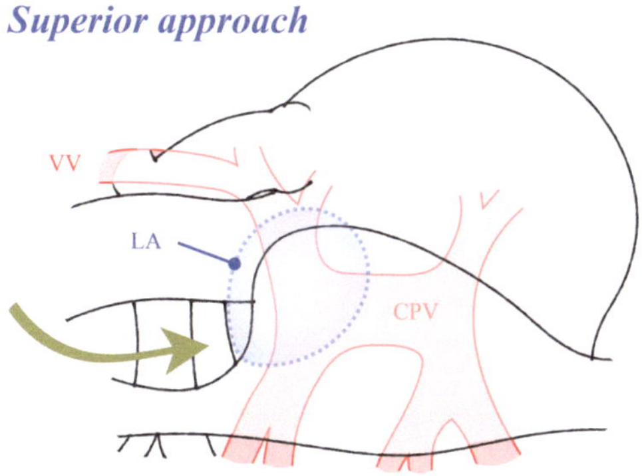

■ *Posterior approach*

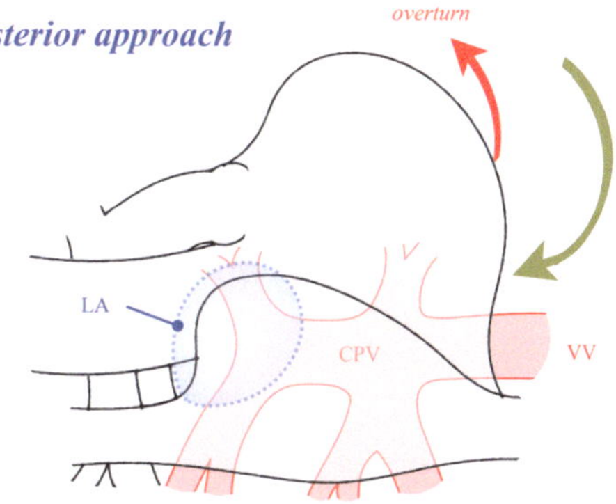

- This is a method of reaching the heart by overturning the apex upward. It is easy to reach the CPV located inferiorly and the VV of the lower cardiac type (type III).
- In the posterior approach, the LA is more difficult to reach.
- Visualization of the superior LA and the cephalic end of the CPV is also poor.
- The natural position of the LA in relation to the CPV is difficult to determine because the heart is overturned, making it difficult to determine the appropriate LA incision line.
- It should be noted that the anastomosis must be performed with the LA incision and CPV opening misaligned, which may cause twisting of the anastomosis.

■ *Right side approach*

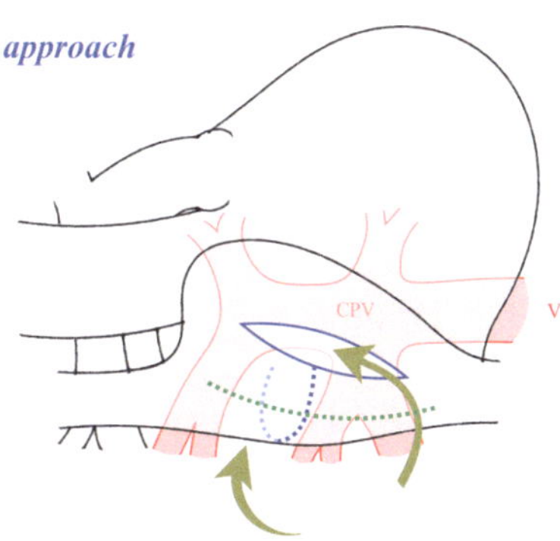

Fig. 2.5 Approach methods

- This is a useful method to reach the CPV on the dorsal side of the right atrium in single atrial cases of asplenia syndrome.
- It can be accessed both from the epicardial side and from the atrial lumen through a transatrial incision (*blue line*).
- Since the atrial wall is thicker in asplenia syndrome, it is useful to identify the intra-atrial trabeculation of the inner atrial wall through a transatrial incision to avoid anastomotic stenosis.
- A horizontal incision (*blue dashed line*) across the crista terminalis (*green dashed line*) should be avoided because of the possibility of inducing postoperative arrhythmias.

■ ***Combined superior and posterior approach***

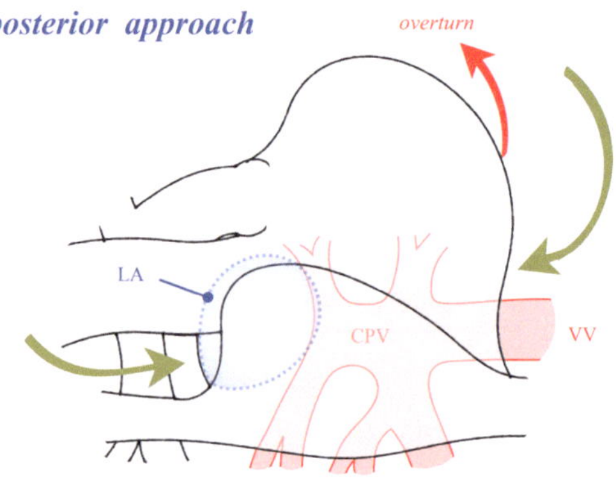

- The dissection and transection process of the inferiorly located CPV and the VV in lower cardiac type (type III) is performed from the posterior approach, and the additional incision of the CPV, LA incision, and anastomosis are performed from the superior approach.
- The inferior anastomosis can also be performed from the posterior approach.
- This combined approach is especially useful in cases where the relative positions of the CPV and the LA are misaligned (the CPV is not close to the LA).

2.3 Creation of Atrial and CPV Openings

The incision of the posterior wall of the left atrium should be made according to the morphology of the CPV and PV. However, in cases where the CPV and LA are misaligned relative to each other or in cases of small left atria due to low preoperative left atrial volume loading, a sufficiently large anastomotic opening may not be obtained through the usual longitudinal or transverse incisions alone. Therefore, it is desirable to obtain as large an anastomotic opening as possible by using a T-shaped incision, an inverted U-shaped incision, or a circular resection in the posterior LA wall as shown in the figure below when creating an atrial opening in this syndrome.

The T-shaped and inverted U-shaped incisions flap the atrial wall, which is expected to reduce CPV and PV distortion even in cases of poor relative positioning. The following LA incision methods can be flexibly adapted to create as large an opening as possible (Fig. 2.6).

- The lower end of the longitudinal incision is made anterior to the mitral annulus.
- Take care not to damage the coronary sinus.

■ ***Inverted U-shaped incision***

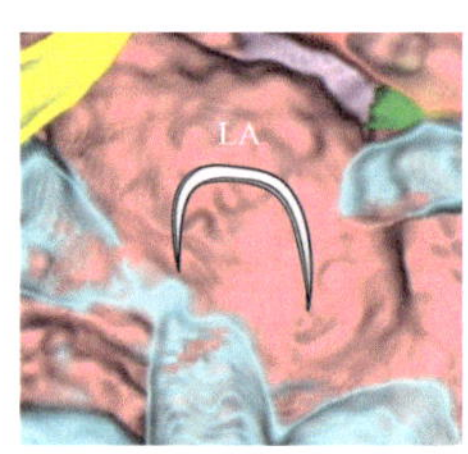

■ *T-shaped incision*

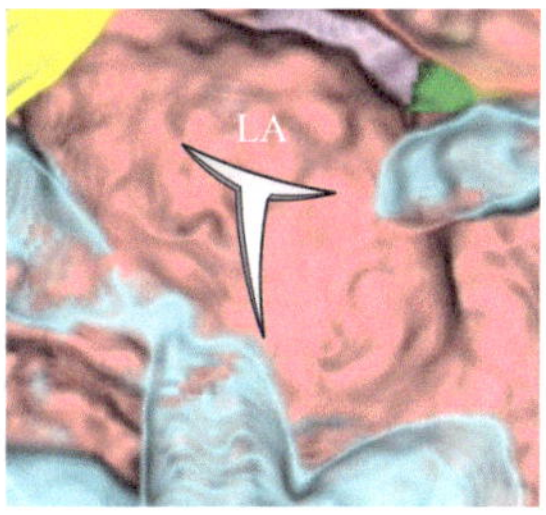

Fig. 2.6 LA incision (dorsal view)

■ *supracardiac type (Darling type Ia, Ib)*

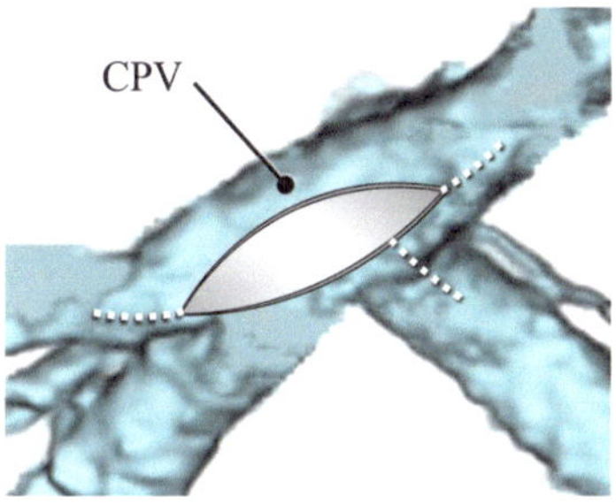

Fig. 2.7 CPV incision (anterior view)

- If the CPV is located slightly below the LA, the posterior wall of the left atrium is incised in an inverted U-shape and dislocated in a flap-like fashion.

■ *Circular incision*

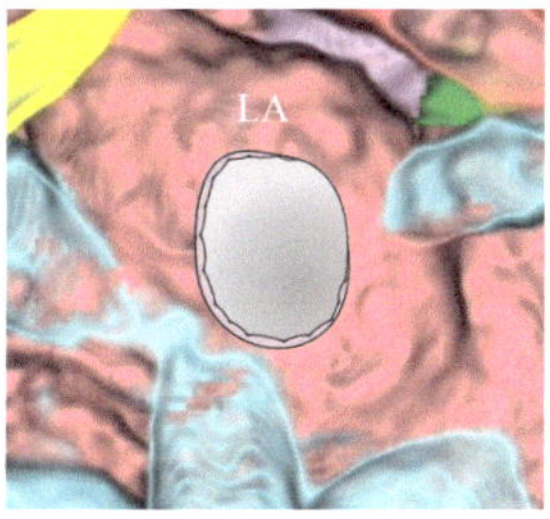

- In cases in which the CPV and the LA are well positioned relative to each other, the posterior wall can be circularly resected (Fig. 2.7).

- Incise the CPV wall longitudinally relative to the LA.
- If the CPV is thick, a piece of the anterior wall may be resected.
- As a rule, do not cut into the PV. If there is a stenotic lesion or the CPV is thin, incise to the PV (*white dashed line*).

■ *infracardiac type (Darling type III)*

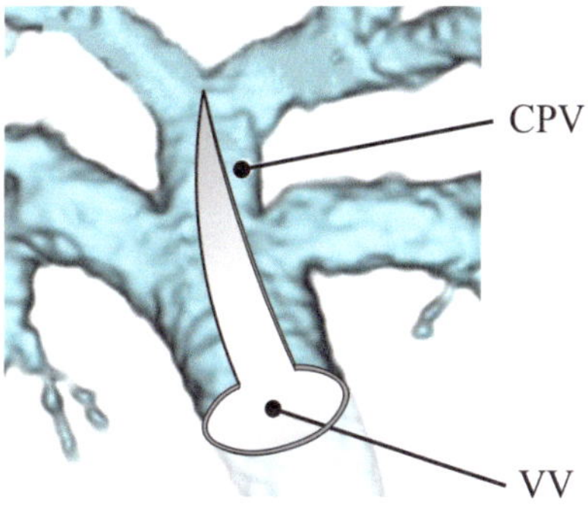

- In the infracardiac type, the VV is transected and a longitudinal incision is made through the CPV.
- The proximal VV stump and the CPV opening are used for anastomosis.

2.4 CPV-LA (Atrium) Anastomosis Method

In cases in which the relative position of the LA (atrium) and the CPV is good, direct CPV-LA (atrium) anastomosis is the first choice.

In the sutureless technique, the LA orifice (LA wall) is anastomosed to the mediastinum around the CPV opening rather than to the CPV opening. Although turbulent pulmonary venous return may occur at the CPV opening, it is a useful anastomosis in cases in which the relative positioning of the LA and CPV is poor. The sutureless technique can also be used in cases of postoperative pulmonary vein stenosis (Fig. 2.8).

- In the case of conventional anastomosis, the anastomosis protrudes into the lumen in a ridge-like shape, which causes turbulent blood flow.
- Turbulent blood flow causes intimal hyperplasia, which leads to anastomotic stenosis.

Fig. 2.8 Direct CPV- LA (atrium) anastomosis method

■ ***Conventional anastomosis***

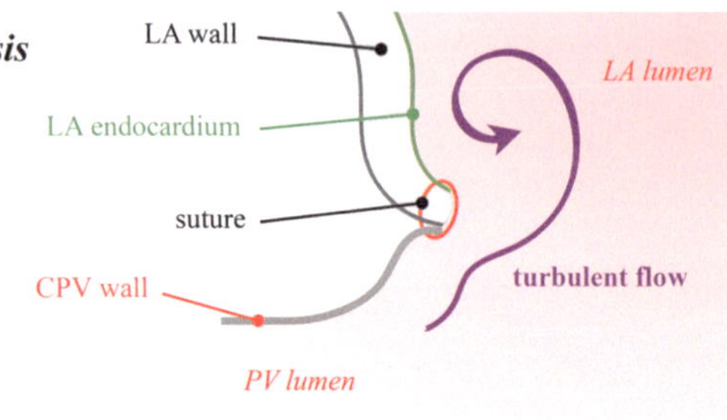

■ ***Endocardium conjugation method***

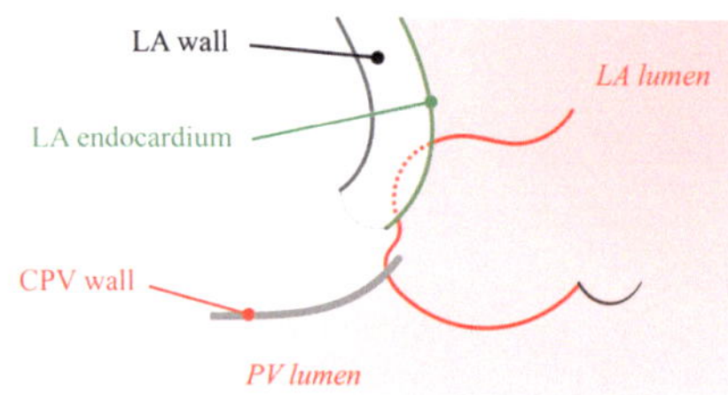

1. Insert into the LA endocardium and stab out through the LA endocardium before the incision line.
2. Insert sutures through the CPV wall from outside to inside.

- In the endocardium conjugation method, in which the CPV wall is sutured to the endocardium rather than to the entire LA wall, the anastomosis does not protrude into the lumen and does not induce turbulent flow.

■ ***Epi and endocardial anastomosis***

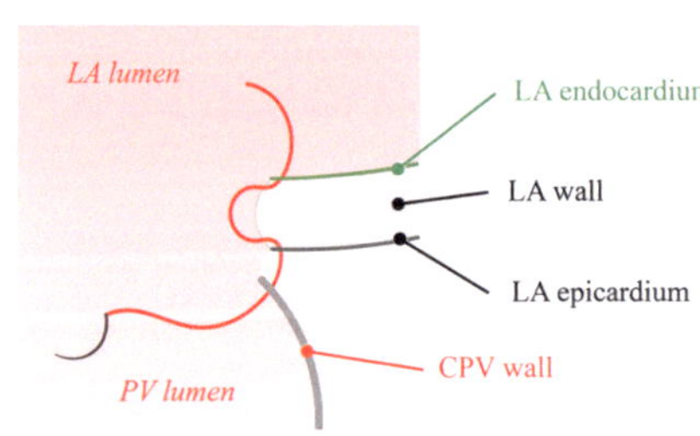

1. Insert into the endocardium of LA and stab out through the incise section and insert into the incise section and stab out the epicardium. Avoid involving much of the atrial muscle in the suture. Insert the suture through the CPV wall from the outside to the inside.
2. With this anastomosis method (epicardial and endocardial anastomosis), the anastomosis is not raised and does not protrude into the lumen.

- When the atrial wall is thick, as in asplenia syndrome, this suturing technique is recommended without involving the LA wall muscle layer in the anastomosis.

3 CPV-LA Anastomosis for Type Ia (Surgical Video)

Case 2.1: CPV-LA Anastomosis for Type Ia (Surgical Video)

< dorsal view >

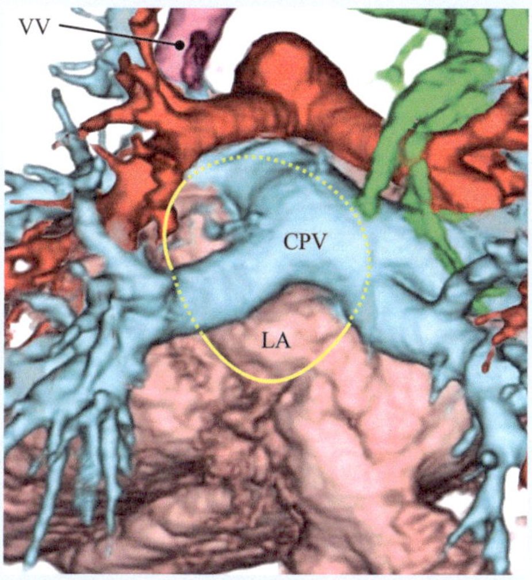

- TAPVR (supracardiac type, Darling type Ia).
- Good relative position of CPV and LA.
- All PVs join together to form a thick CPV.
- Pulmonary venous obstructions are not complicated.
- The CPV is located dorsal to the LA (*yellow line* + *yellow dashed line*) and their relative positions are good.
  - Direct CPV-LA anastomosis with superior approach is selected.
  - The LA wall is resected in a circular fashion to create the largest possible anastomotic opening (Case 2.1, Scene 1).

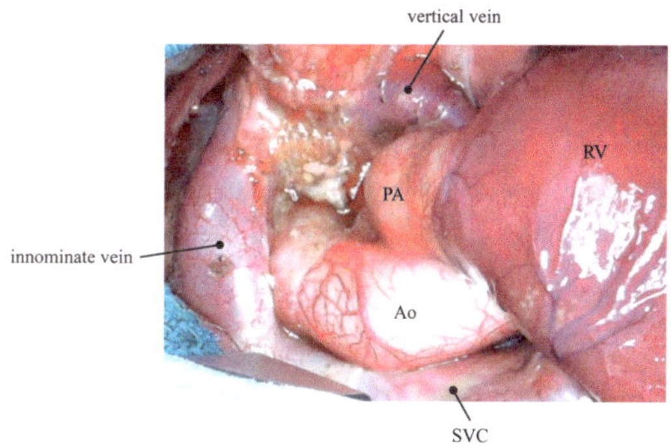

Case 2.1, Scene 1 Vertical vein returning to the innominate vein (Video 00 min 05 s)

1. The thymus is removed subtotally except for a portion to provide visualization and relieve pressure on the VV.
   - An enlarged innominate vein and the superior vena cava (SVC) are noted.
   - Minimize dissection of the VV, innominate vein, and SVC before starting extracorporeal circulation to avoid PVO due to surgical maneuvers.
   - Taping of the VV and SVC should be performed after starting extracorporeal circulation.
2. To avoid pulmonary congestion, start extracorporeal circulation with aortic cannulation and venting from main pulmonary artery first, followed by cannulation in the inferior vena cava (IVC) and then in the SVC (Case 2.1, Scene 2).

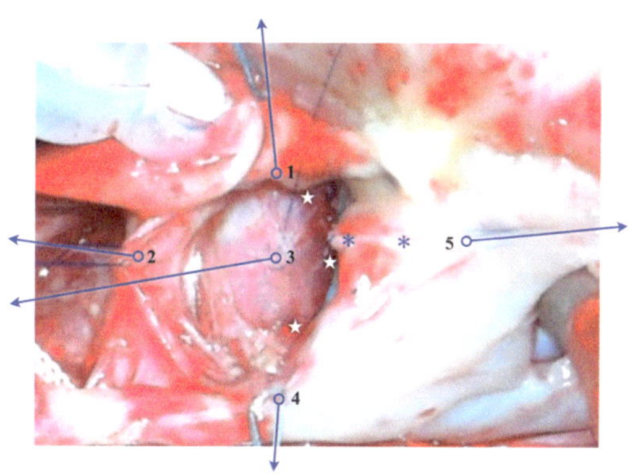

Case 2.1, Scene 2 Traction suture and incise line markers to secure field of view (Video 01 min 55 s). ○⟶ Traction suture and direction of traction. 1: Right-sided wall of the aorta, 2: Right pulmonary artery, 3: Superior wall of CPV, 4: SVC, 5: Superior wall of LA. *LA wall incision line markers (top and bottom). ☆ CPV wall incision line markers (T-shaped incision)

1. Reached by superior approach from between the aorta and the SVC.
2. The CPV is seen on the caudal and dorsal side of the right pulmonary artery.
3. Sew traction sutures to the right lateral wall of the aorta, the anterior wall of the right pulmonary artery, the superior wall of the left atrium, and the anterior wall of the superior vena cava, and apply radial traction to each to provide a clear view.
4. Sew incision line marking sutures (7–0 monofilament suture) to the posterior wall of the left atrium and CPV (Case 2.1, Scene 3).

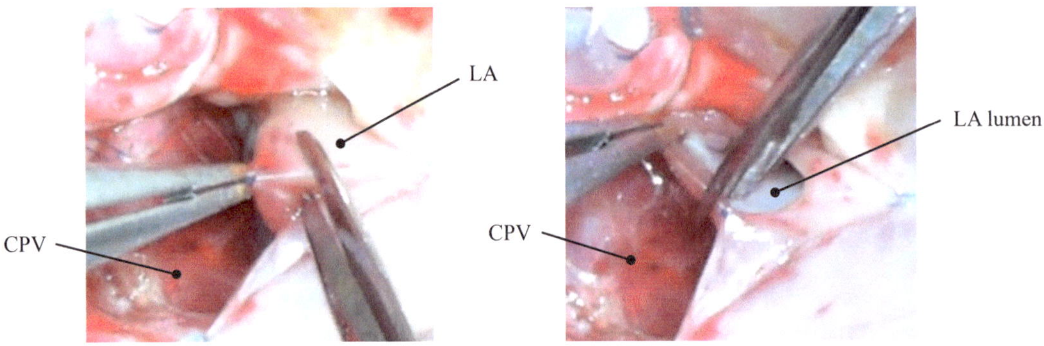

Case 2.1, Scene 3 Incise the posterior wall of the left atrium (Video 02 min 20 s)

1. Incise the posterior wall of the LA while referring to the marking suture.
2. While checking the LA lumen, incise the left atrial wall to avoid damaging the mitral valve annulus and the coronary sinus adjacent to the annulus (Case 2.1, Scene 4).

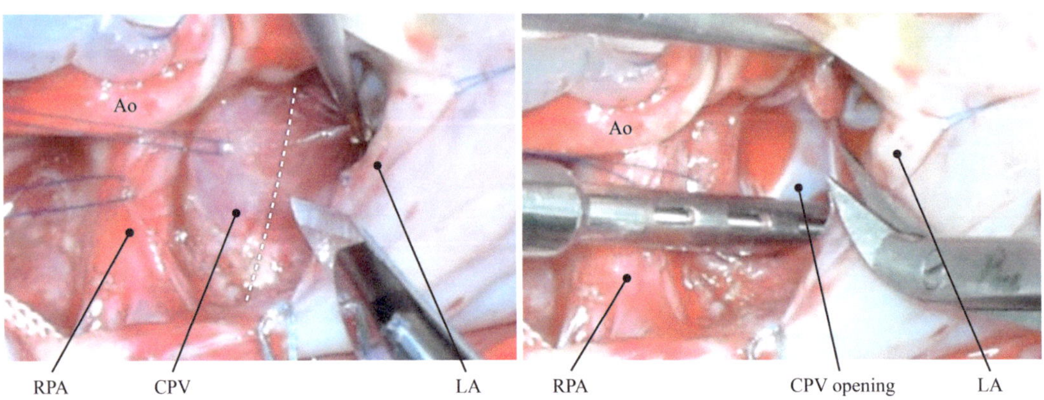

Case 2.1, Scene 4 Incise the common pulmonary vein (Video 02 min 51 s)

1. (*Left figure*) Because it is important to make a precise incision, traction sutures are applied to the CPV walls on both sides of the assumed incision line (*white dashed line*) to secure the CPV before the incision is started.
2. (*Right figure*) In order to create the largest possible incision, a flap incision may be made.

- Although cutting into the branches of the PV should be avoided as much as possible, it may be necessary to cut into the PV in cases where the relative position of the CPV and LA is not good, or in cases where the CPV is small or thin.
- The parietal pleura in the anterior aspect of the CPV around the anastomotic opening should be completely removed (Case 2.1, Scene 5).

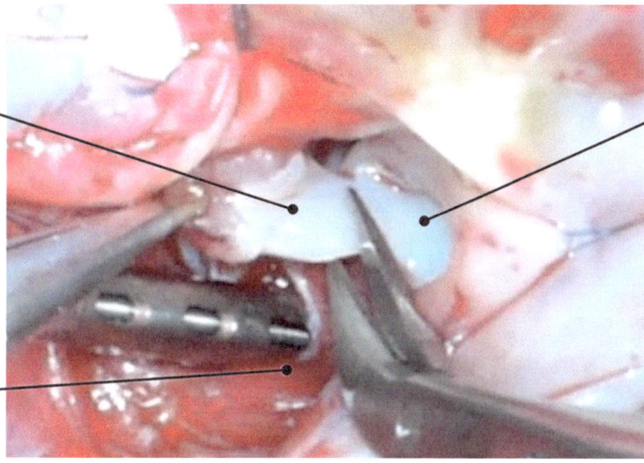

Case 2.1, Scene 5 Circular resection of the LA wall (Video 03 min 36 s)

1. Considering the size of the CPV incision, resect the LA wall in a circular fashion.

- In cases in which the LA and CPV are relatively far apart, the inferior LA wall of the incision may be left as a flap (Case 2.1, Scene 6).

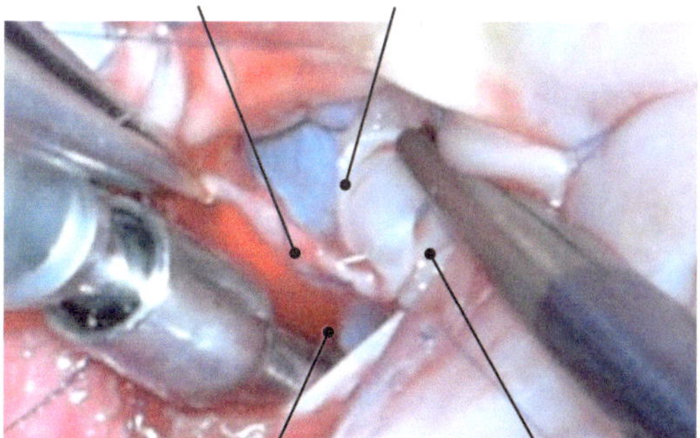

Case 2.1, Scene 6 CPV-LA direct anastomosis 1 (Video 03 min 58 s)

1. First, ligate the lowest point of the CPV and LA openings with a U-shaped suture.
2. Anastomose with a continuous 7–0 monofilament suture.
3. Anastomosis from the luminal side is performed using the "endocardial conjugation method".

< endocardial conjugation method >

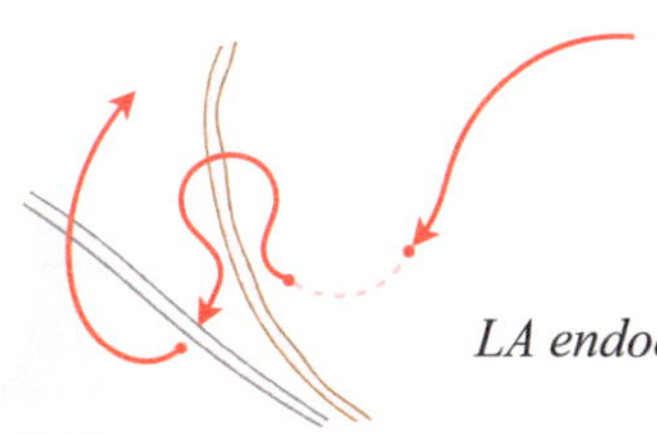

- To avoid that the anastomosis between the CPV and LA does not protrude into the lumen, the suture needle is inserted into the LA endocardium, stab out into endocardium, and the CPV wall penetrates all layers (Case 2.1, Scene 7).

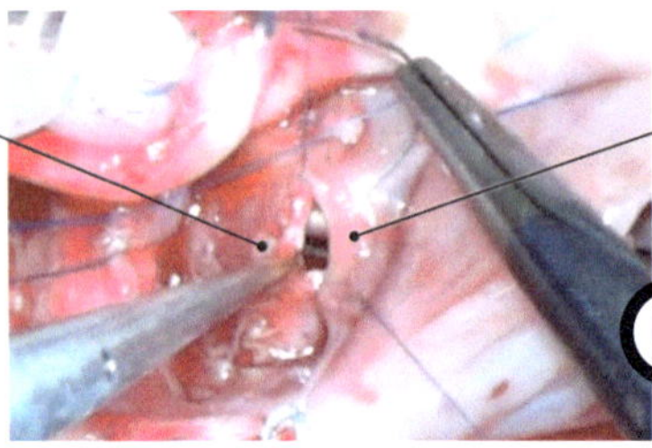

Case 2.1, Scene 7 CPV-LA direct anastomosis 2 (Video 09 min 27 s) (▶ https://doi.org/10.1007/000-hk6)

1. A flexible suction tube from the right atrium into the LA and CPV through the ASD provides a good field of view.
2. Additional incisions are made in the CPV wall or LA wall as needed to adjust for the difference in caliber.
3. Complete the CPV-LA anastomosis.

- Avoid excessive volume overload during withdrawal of extracorporeal circulation, as this is a condition in which the LV is not volume loaded preoperatively. Provide inhaled nitric oxide for residual pulmonary hypertension.

4 Hybrid Method (Direct and Sutureless Anastomosis) for Type III (Surgical Video)

Case 2.2: Infracardiac Type III, Poor Relative Position of CPV and LA
< dorsal view >

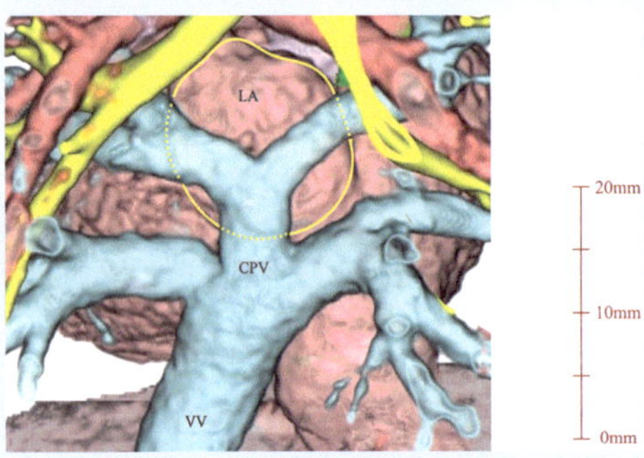

- TAPVR (infracardiac type, Darling type III).
- Poor relative position of CPV and LA.
- All PVs join to form the CPV, but the cephalic CPVs are slightly thinner.
- VV is thicker.
- CPV is located caudally and its relative position to the LA (*yellow line* and *yellow dashed line*) is poor.
- The superior approach allows incision of the LA, but does not provide a good view of the CPV and VV.
- Both superior and posterior approaches should be used.
- In order to obtain a sufficient anastomotic orifice, not only the CPV opening but also the VV stump should be used for the anastomosis.
- Direct anastomosis of CPV-LA over the entire circumference of the anastomotic opening is difficult due to poor relative positioning, so the sutureless method is also used.
- ***Approach method*** < *Anterior view* >.

(continued)

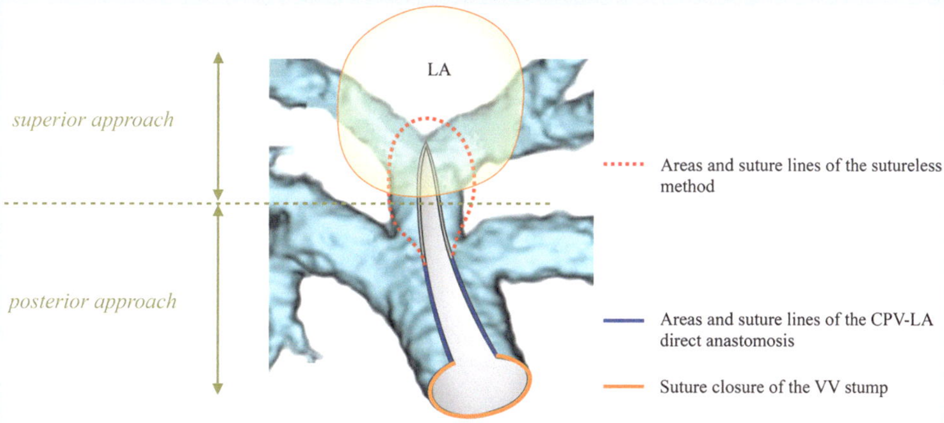

- The VV is transected and a longitudinal incision is made from the VV to the anterior wall of the CPV.
- Sutureless anastomosis between the CPV and the LA opening on the cephalic side is performed via the superior approach.
- Sutureless anastomosis on the caudal side, direct CPV-LA anastomosis, and suture closure of the VV are performed via the posterior approach (Case 2.2, Scene 1).

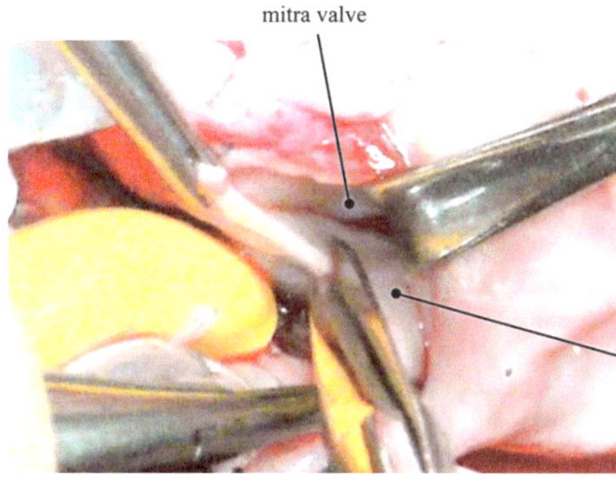

Case 2.2, Scene 1 T-shaped incision of the posterior LA wall from superior approach (Video 00 min 43 s)

1. Make a T-shaped incision in the posterior wall of the LA from the superior approach.
2. Incise straight down as far as possible, taking care not to damage the mitral annulus and coronary sinus by inspecting the lumen (Case 2.2, Scene 2).

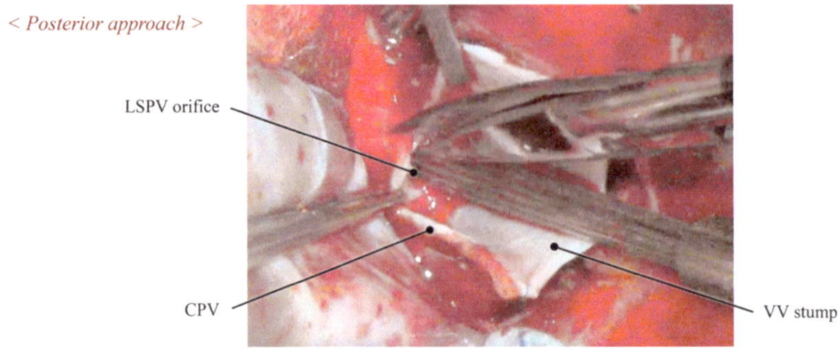

Case 2.2, Scene 2 Transection of the VV and longitudinal incision of the CPV from posterior approach (Video 01 min 10 s)

1. The VV is transected just above the diaphragm using a posterior approach, and the caudal side is ligated and closed.
2. The upper wall of the VV and the CPV are incised straight to the confluence of the right and left superior PVs, confirming the PV openings (Case 2.2, Scene 3).

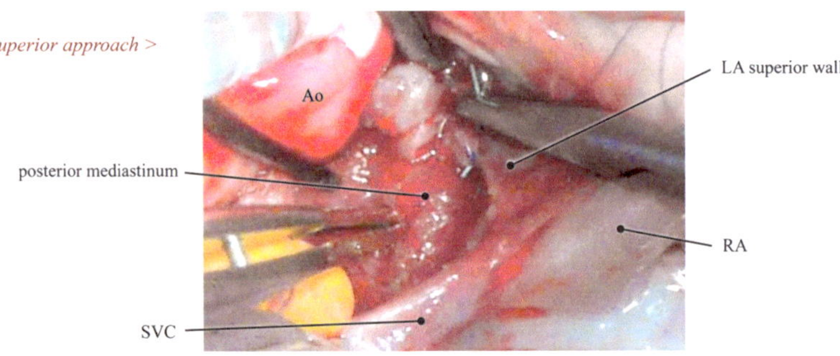

Case 2.2, Scene 3 Sutureless anastomosis from superior approach (Video 03 min 02 s)

1. Return to the superior approach and anastomose the upper part of the LA opening to the dorsal wall (mediastinum) around the CPV opening using sutureless technique.
2. Anastomose from the superior approach as far as possible.
3. On the right side of the LA opening, anastomose to the mediastinum at the posterior aspect of the SVC (Case 2.2, Scene 4).

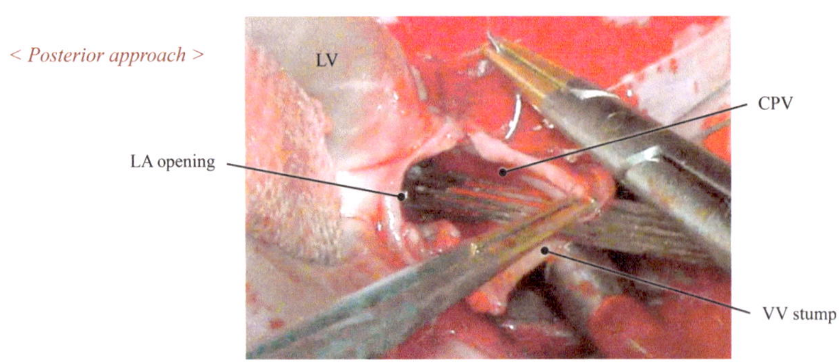

Case 2.2, Scene 4 CPV-LA direct anastomosis from posterior approach (Video 06 min 29 s)

1. Change to posterior approach again.
2. The sutureless anastomosis line is redirected to the CPV opening.
3. The lower part of the CPV opening is anastomosed directly to the LA opening.

- Take care not to damage the coronary sinus during anastomosis (Case 2.2, Scene 5).

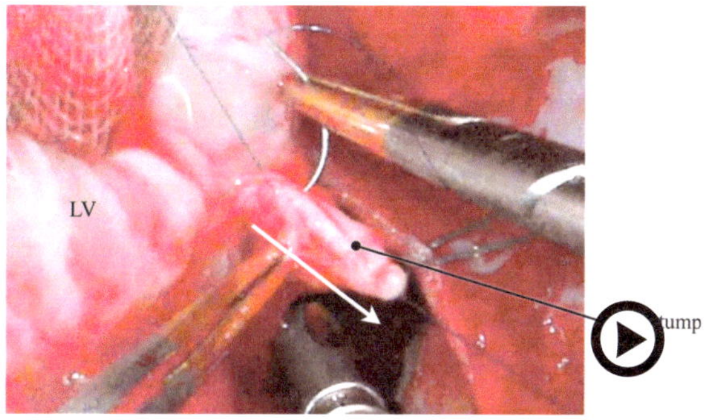

Case 2.2, Scene 5 Suture closure of the VV stump from posterior approach (Video 15 min 25 s) (▶ https://doi.org/10.1007/000-hk5)

1. The remaining VV stump is sutured longitudinally (white arrow) to form a pouch shape.

Case 2.2: Pre and Postoperative CT Images

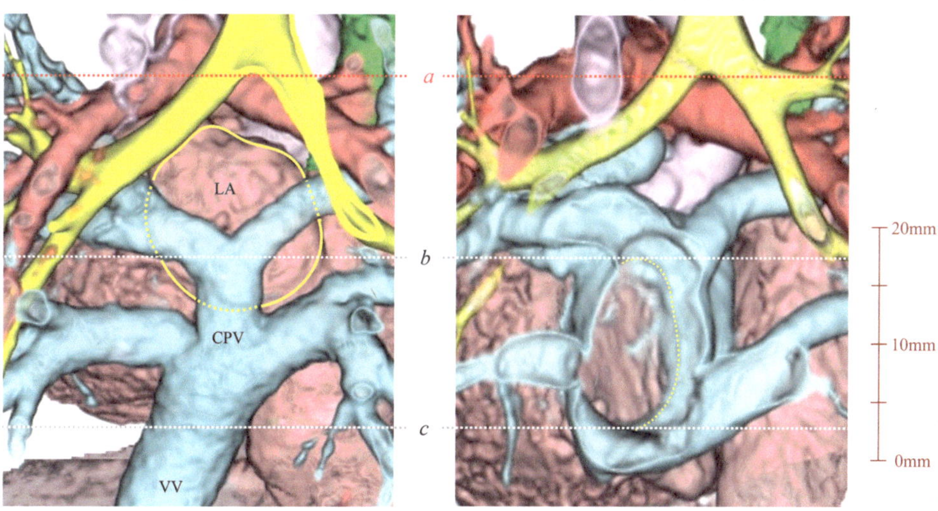

dotted line a: bottom edge of the tracheal bifurcation
dotted line b: top edge of the anastomosis
dotted line c: bottom edge of the anastomosis

(continued)

- A large anastomotic opening (*yellow dashed line*) is ensured.
- No difference between direct and sutureless anastomosis.
- The superior wall of the LA is shifted caudally.
- The right and left superior PVs are slightly displaced cephalad compared to the preoperative position.

Postoperative CT image
< left lateral view, cross-section >

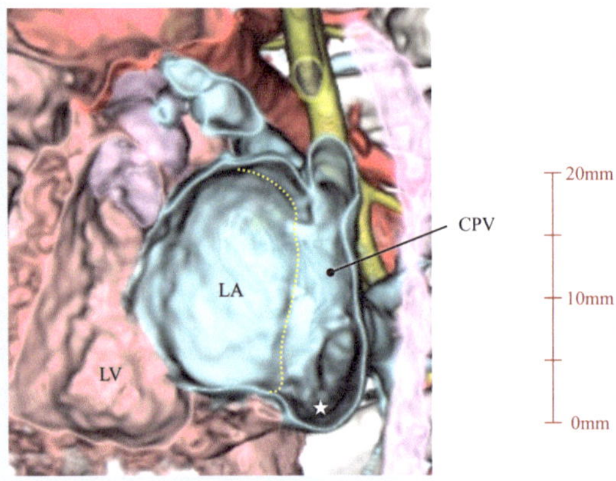

- The anastomosis (*yellow dashed line*) is smooth.
- The caudal side of the CPV (☆) has a wide lumen created by pouch formation.

5 CPV-Right-Sided Atrium Direct Anastomosis for Type III with Heterotaxia Syndrome (Surgical Video)

Case 2.3: Infracardiac Type III, Poor Relative Position of CPV and LA
< dorsal view >

< Dorsal view >

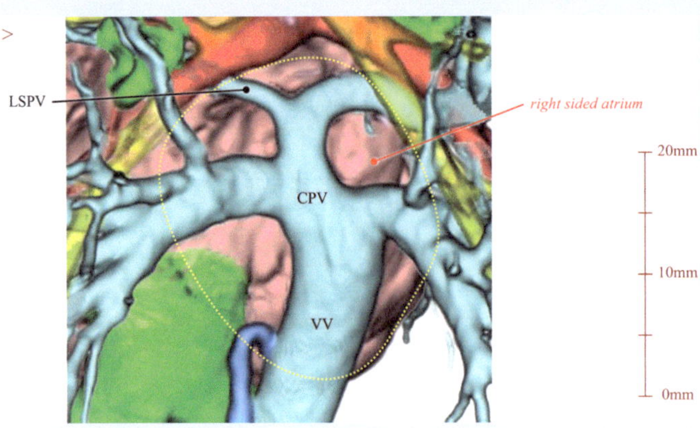

(continued)

- Infracardiac type TAPVR (type III) associated with heterotaxia, single atrium, and single ventricle.
- All PVs join to form CPV. The left superior PV (LSPV) is thin. The VV is thick. No focal stenotic lesions in PVs or VV.
- Relative position of the CPV, the VV, and the right-sided atrium (*yellow dashed line*) is good.
  - Since the CPV and the VV are located on the right dorsal side of the right-sided atrium, the right side approach is selected and anastomosis is performed epicardially and intracardially (Case 2.3, Scene 1).

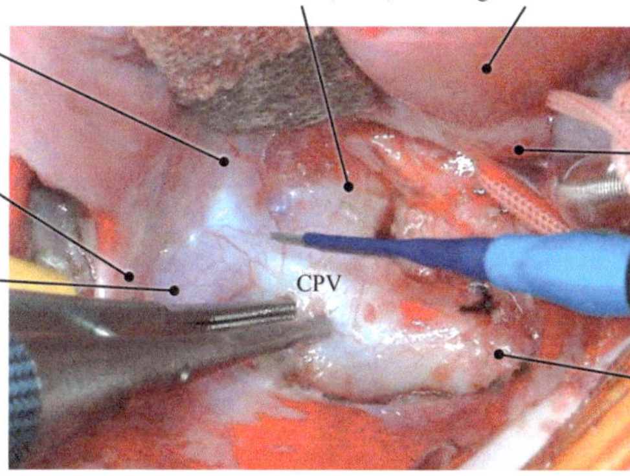

Case 2.3, Scene 1 Dissection of the CPV from right side approach (Video 00 min 05 s)

1. After initiation of extracorporeal circulation, the right atrium is overturned to the left and the dorsal parietal pericardium is incised.
2. The CPV is dissected and the VV is ligated and transected just above the diaphragm.

- Since the pericardium in front of the CPV can cause anastomotic stenosis, as much of the pericardium around the opening as possible is removed.
- The VV is not only ligated, but also transected, because residual cord-like VV tissue may cause tension at the anastomotic site (Case 2.3, Scene 2).

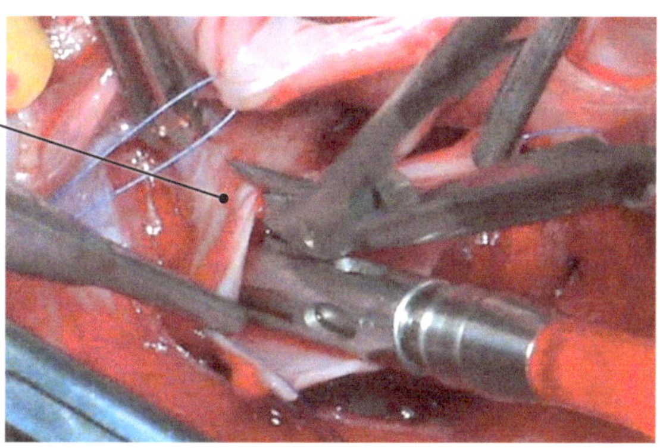

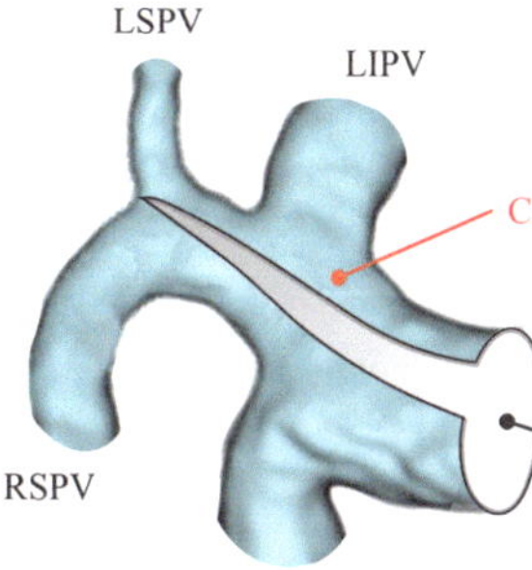

Case 2.3, Scene 2 Longitudinal incision of CPV (Video 01 min 01 s)

1. Incise the center of the anterior surface of the CPV longitudinally from the VV stump to the top edge of the CPV.

- Do not cut into the PV (Case 2.3, Scene 3).

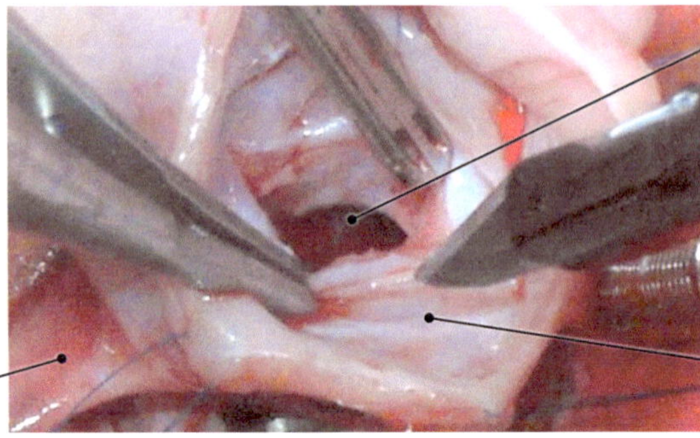

Case 2.3, Scene 3 Incise posterior wall of the right-sided atrium (Video 01 min 12 s)

1. Incise the right atrium and approach through the atrial lumen to make a longitudinal incision in the posterior wall.
2. Make as large a longitudinal incision as possible in the posterior wall of the right atrium relative to the CPV opening.

- In this case, the atrial wall is very thick due to heterotaxia (Case 2.3, Scene 4).

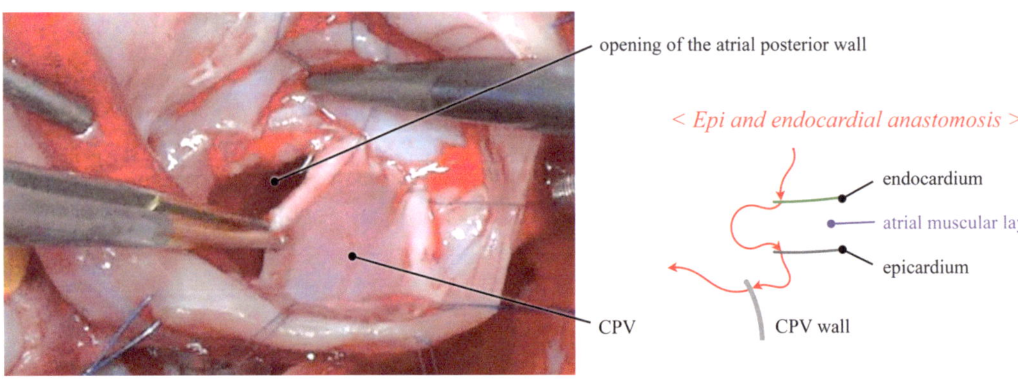

Case 2.3, Scene 4 Atrial wall-CPV direct anastomosis from the atrial lumen (Video 01 min 27 s)

1. The caudal part of the CPV anastomosis to the posterior atrial wall opening directly from the atrial lumen.

- Because the atrial wall is very thick, suture the endocardium, the epicardium, and the CPV wall without including the muscular layer in the atrial anastomosis (epicardial and endocardial anastomosis).
- The endocardium conjugation method can be used, but care should be taken to avoid overstretching of the CPV wall due to the thick atrial wall.
- If the view from the atrial lumen around the cephalic part of the CPV is poor, change to an epicardial approach (Case 2.3, Scene 5).

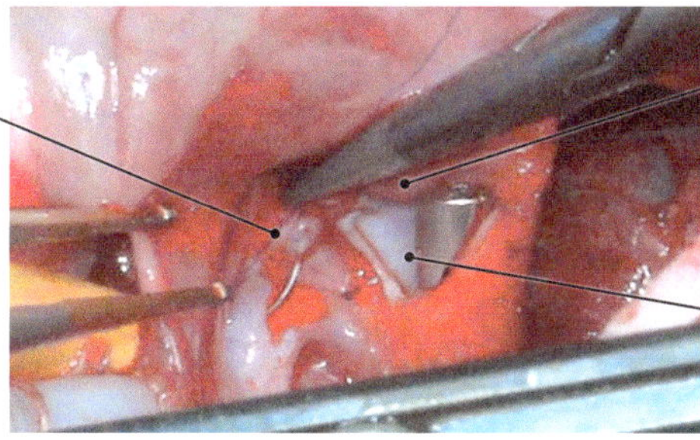

Case 2.3, Scene 5 Sutureless method from epicardial approach (Video 04 min 10 s)

1. Change to the epicardial approach (*right side approach*).
2. Because the atrial wall is very thick, the cephalic anastomosis is performed by anastomosing only the outer layer of the atrial wall to the posterior mediastinal wall (*sutureless method*) (Case 2.3, Scene 6).

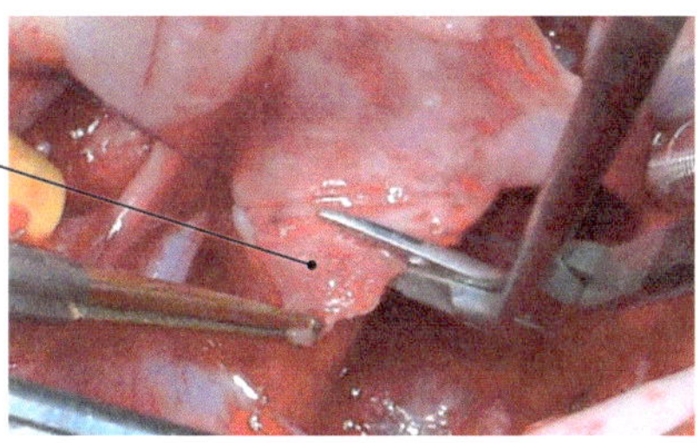

Case 2.3, Scene 6 Resection of excess atrial wall (Video 06 min 38 s)

1. Resection of the remaining atrial wall in the form of a flap and matching the caliber of the opening.

- In this case, the atrial wall was resected because of its thickness.
- In cases where the relative positions of the atrial incision and CPV incision are misaligned, the atrial wall is left as a flap and used for anastomosis (Case 2.3, Scene 7).

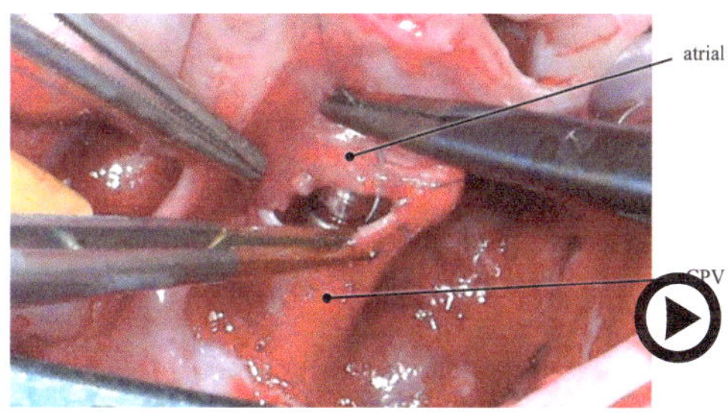

Case 2.3, Scene 7 Completion of direct right-sided atrium-CPV anastomosis (Video 06 min 46 s) (▶ https://doi.org/10.1007/000-hk4)

1. Anastomose the right atrial opening with the CPV opening.

SPOTLIGHT Pre and Postoperative CT Images (Supracardiac Type)

Preoperative CT image
< dorsal view >
CPV cross-section

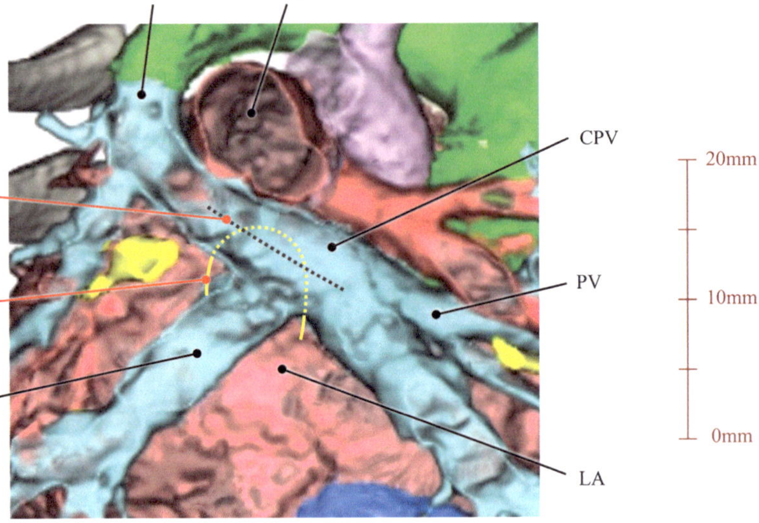

- Supracardiac type (Darling type Ia).
- Good relative position of CPV and LA.

1. The posterior wall of the LA is incised in an inverted U-shape (*yellow solid line* and *yellow dashed line*) to create a large anastomotic opening.
2. The CPV is incised longitudinally (*black dashed line*).
3. The LA incision and inferiorly inverted posterior LA wall are directly anastomosed to the CPV opening.

Postoperative CT image
< dorsal view >

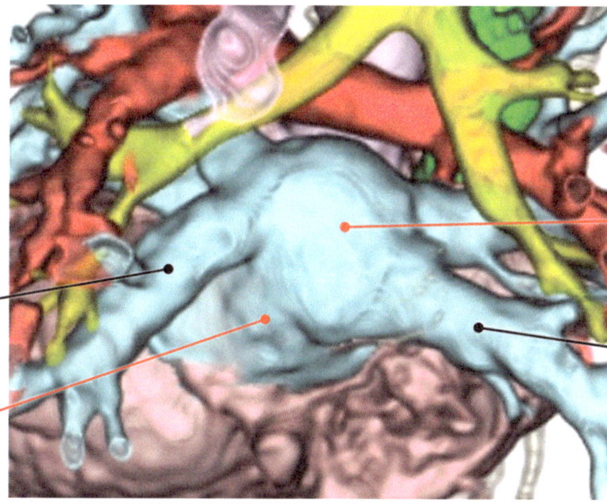

Postoperative CT image
< dorsal view >
neo PV channel cross-section

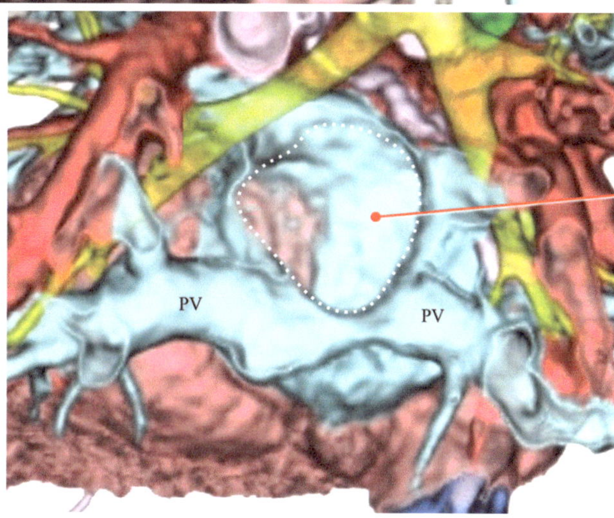

- The posterior wall flap forms the inferior wall of the neo PV channel. A wide opening to the LA has been obtained.
- No stenosis is seen in the PVs.

SPOTLIGHT Pre and Postoperative CT Images (Supracardiac Type)

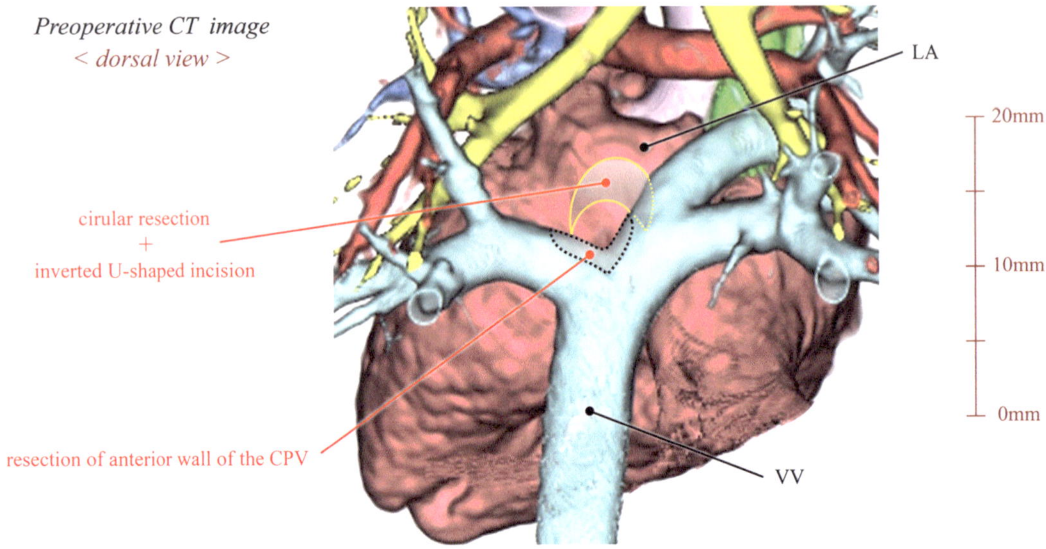

- Supracardiac type (Darling type III).
- Poor relative position of CPV and LA.

1. The posterior wall of the LA is incised in an inverted U-shape (*yellow solid line* and *yellow dashed line*) to create a large anastomotic opening.
2. The CPV is incised longitudinally (*black dashed line*).
3. The LA incision and inferiorly inverted posterior LA wall are directly anastomosed to the CPV opening.

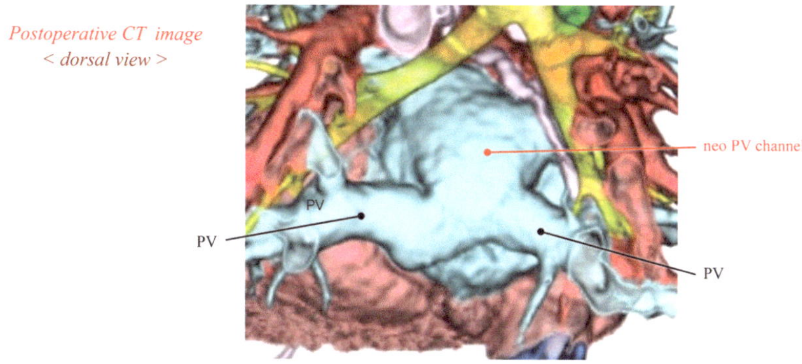

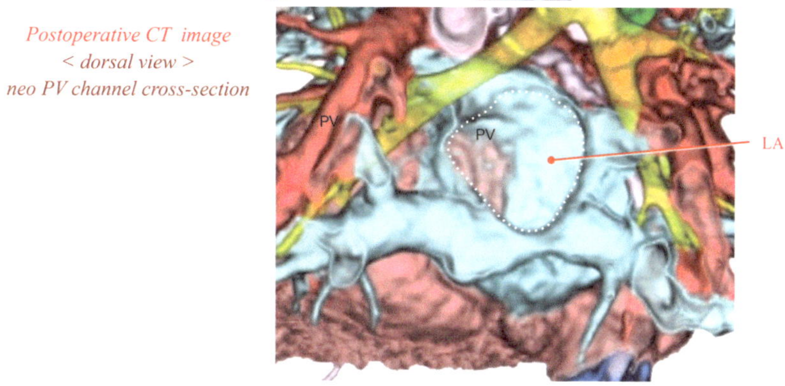

- The posterior wall flap forms the inferior wall of the neo PV channel. A wide opening to the LA has been obtained.
- No stenosis is seen in the PVs.

6 Cardiac Type TAPVR (Darling Type IIa)

6.1 Morphology of Cardiac Type (Darling Type IIa)

Cardiac type TAPVR (Darling type IIa) is a type in which the four PVs join to form the CPV, which runs dorsal to the left atrium and joins the coronary sinus. It is associated with an atrial septal defect. PVO is rare (Fig. 2.9).

- The four PVs join to form the CPV.
- The CPV runs dorsal to the left atrium and joins the coronary sinus.
- The anterior wall of the common pulmonary vein and the posterior wall of the left atrium form a common wall (the area surrounded by *the red dashed line*).

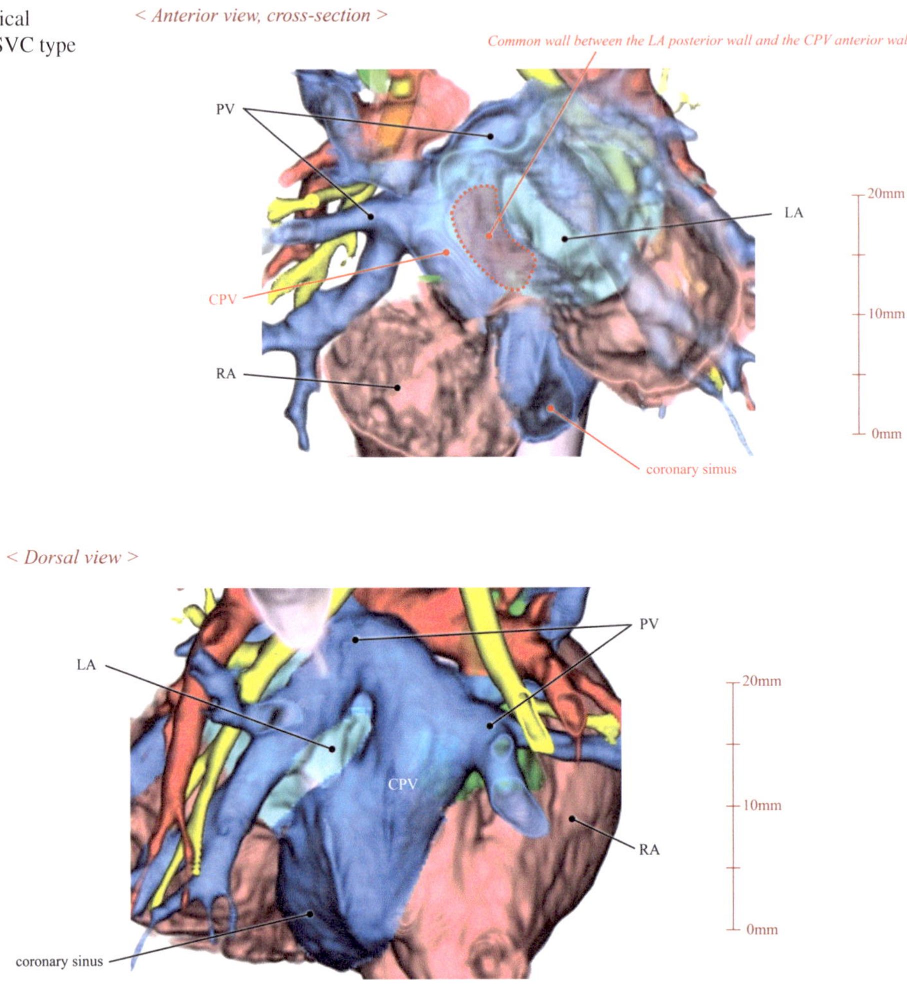

Fig. 2.9 Surgical strategies for SVC type PAPVR

- Thick CPV located longitudinally on the dorsal aspect of the left atrium is present.

< cephalic view, cross-section >

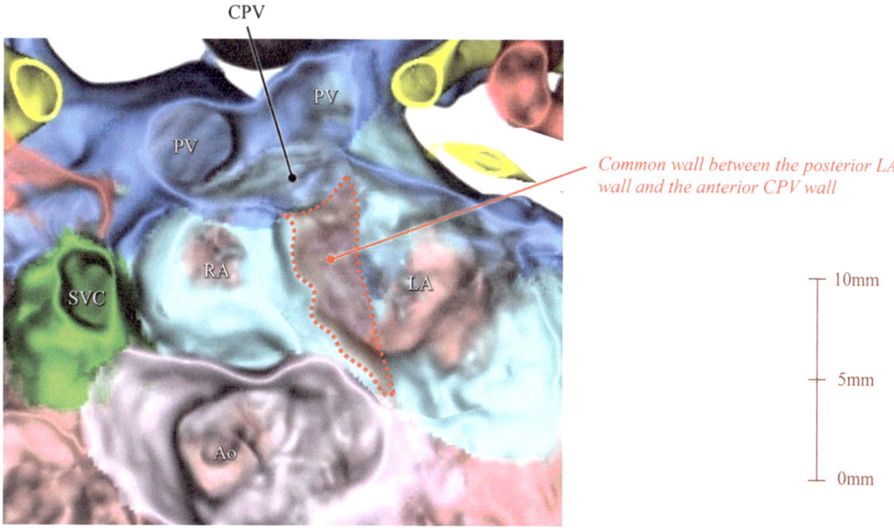

- The area surrounded by *the red dashed line* indicates the common wall between the posterior LA wall and the anterior CPV wall.

6.2 Conventional Surgical Technique for Cardiac Type IIa

The cut back and Van Praagh techniques have been reported as the most commonly used techniques for cardiac type (IIa). Both techniques cannot provide a large enough pulmonary venous return pathway. In addition, there is concern about turbulence and subsequent late stenosis due to the tortuous blood flow pathway in both techniques (Fig. 2.10).

1. Incise the superior wall of the coronary sinus (CS) within the left atrium.
2. The coronary sinus orifice and ASD are closed.

– The size of the pulmonary venous return pathway is limited by the CS incision.

■ *Cut back method*

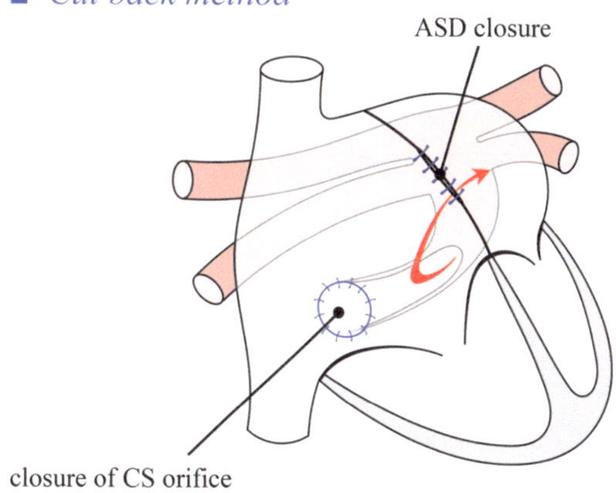

Fig. 2.10 Conventional techniques for cardiac type IIa

■ *Van Praagh's operation*

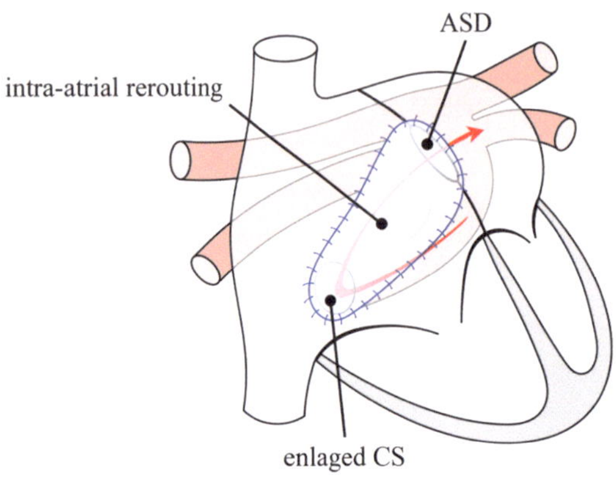

1. Enlarge the CS orifice.

- Intra-atrial blood flow is redirected from the enlarged coronary sinus to the ASD using a supplemental material (e.g., autologous pericardium).
- The size of the pulmonary venous return pathway is limited by the CS orifice, the size of the ASD, and the configuration of the supplemental material.
- Blood flow from the pulmonary vein is significantly tortuous.

7 Surgical Procedure of Transference of the Posterior LA Wall for Cardiac Type IIa

In cardiac type IIa, the CPV is located on the dorsal LA, and the posterior wall of the CPV and the anterior wall of the LA share a common wall. In this procedure, this common wall is incised as a flap, lifted vertically toward the atrial septum, and the edge of the common wall flap is sutured to the limbus of the ASD. The ASD is closed simultaneously with the creation of the pulmonary venous return pathway.

It does not require the use of supplemental material and creates a large, straight pulmonary venous return pathway, thus avoiding a late-stage PVO. However, preoperative CT studies are necessary because this procedure is inappropriate for patients who do not have a large common wall (Fig. 2.11).

1

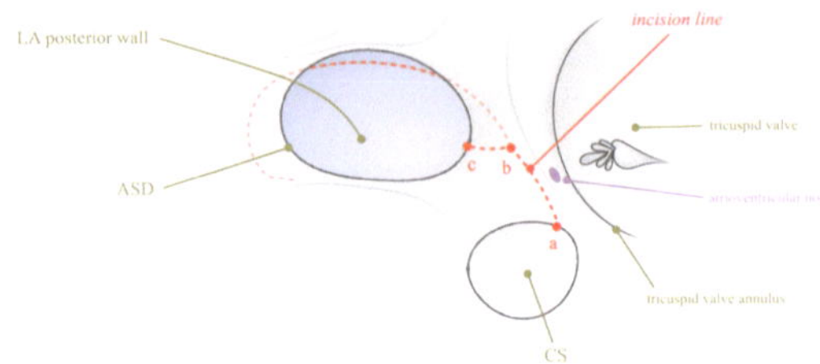

Fig. 2.11 Transference of posterior LA wall for cardiac type IIa

1. Incise from the right edge (a) of the superior wall of the coronary sinus (CS) on the right atrial side to the base of the atrial septum (b).
2. Keep the incision line away from the atrioventricular node.
3. Incise from point (b) to the edge of the atrial septal defect (c).

2

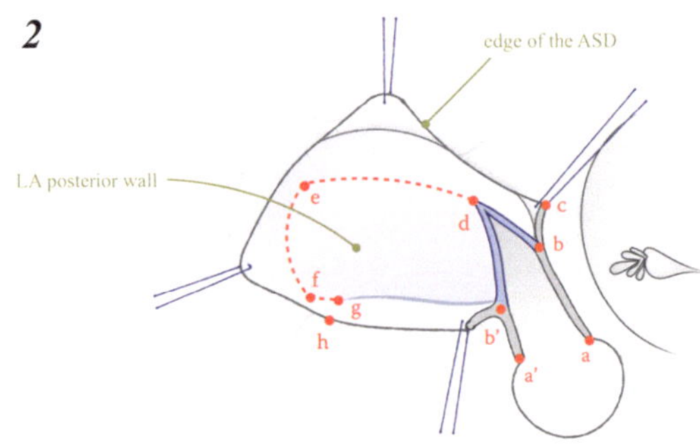

1. Incise the superior wall of the CS on the left atrial side further to the left. Incise while confirming the lumen of the CPV and incise to just before the left margin of the CPV (d).
2. From point (d), incise the posterior wall of the left atrium (common wall) along the left margin of the CPV cranially.
3. After incising to anterior to the opening of the pulmonary vein (e), the incision is shifted to the right.
4. The transverse incision is extended to just before the right margin of the CPV (f).
5. A small incision is made caudally from point (f) to point (g). The distance of the atrial incision from point (f–g) should be equal to the distance from point (g) to the edge of the atrial septal defect (h).

- Be careful not to damage the mitral annulus.
- While checking the pulmonary vein opening, be careful not to cut into the pulmonary vein.

3

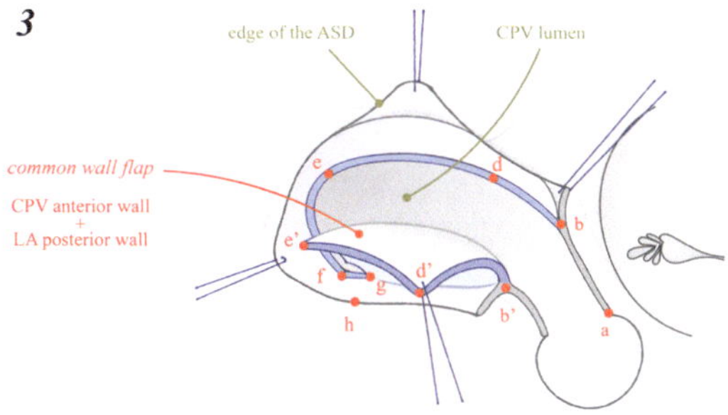

1. Completion of the left atrial posterior wall flap (b' - d' - e' - g) harvesting.
2. Cross section of the left atrial posterior wall (b - d - e - f - g) is repaired with interrupted sutures to align the intima with each other.

4

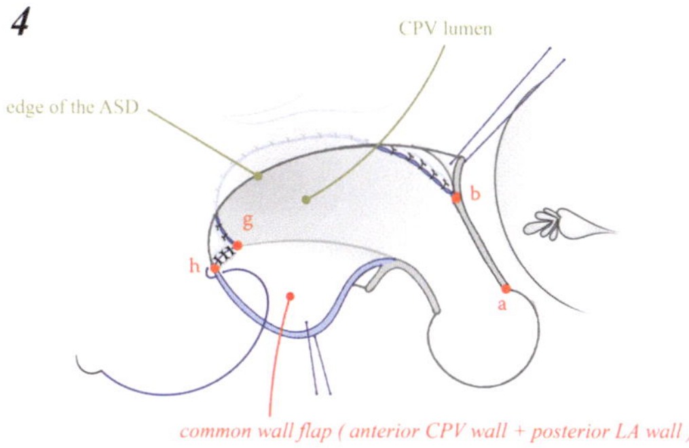

1. Raise the incised common wall flap (left atrial posterior wall flap) toward the atrial septum.
2. First, the flap is sutured to the left atrial inner wall from the edge of the atrial incision (g) to the edge of the atrial septal defect (h).

5

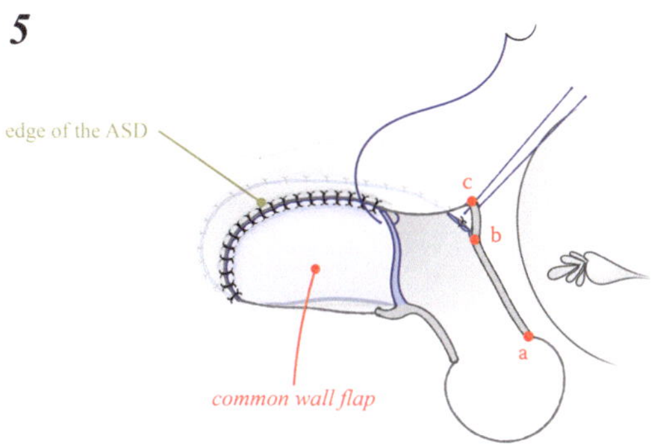

1. The common wall flap (left atrial posterior wall flap) is anastomosed to the edge of the atrial septal defect.

6

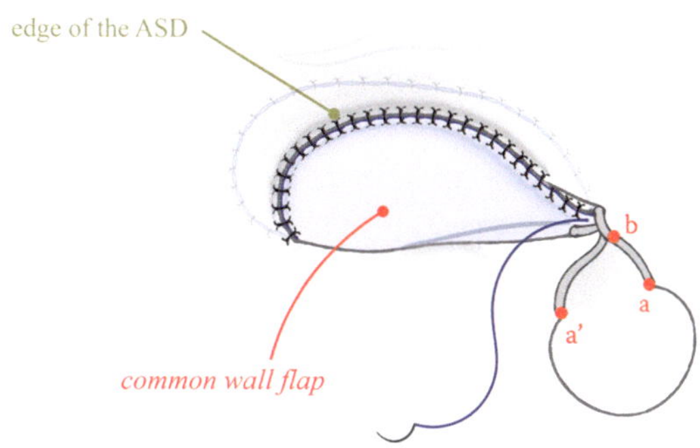

1. After anastomosing the common wall flap (left atrial wall flap) to the anterior edge of the atrial septal defect (b), the suture line is directed toward the left atrial side of the septum.
2. The suture is then directed toward the inner surface of the coronary sinus.

7

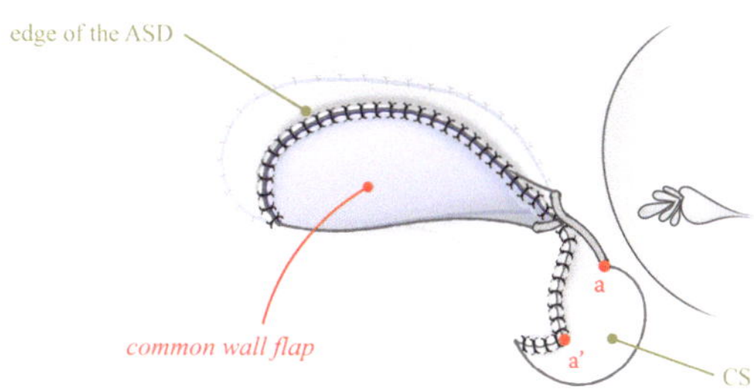

1. Close the coronary sinus orifice by dropping the right atrial upper wall of the coronary sinus to the dorsal side and suturing it to the inner (lower) wall of the coronary sinus.
2. Create a pulmonary venous return pathway and complete closure of the atrial septal defect by transferring the common wall (posterior left atrial wall).

SPOTLIGHT **Pre and Postoperative CT Images (Supracardiac type)**

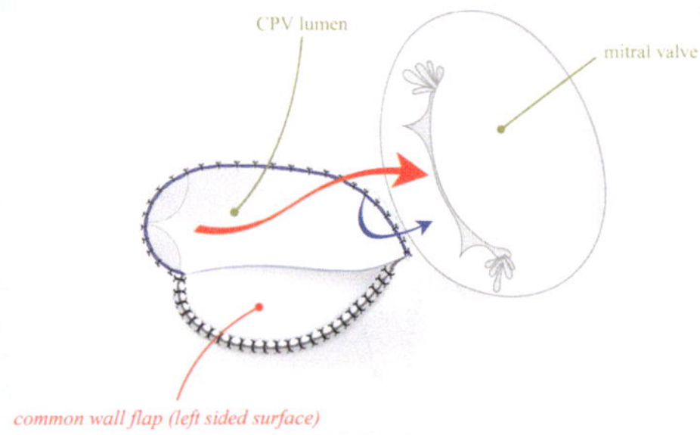

- Viewed from the left atrium, the opening from the CPV is wide, and the venous return pathway (*red arrow*) is straight.
- Blood returning from the coronary sinus also enters into the left atrium (*blue arrow*).

8 Transference of the Posterior LA Wall for Cardiac Type IIa (Surgical Video)

Case 2.4: Cardiac Type (Darling Type IIa)

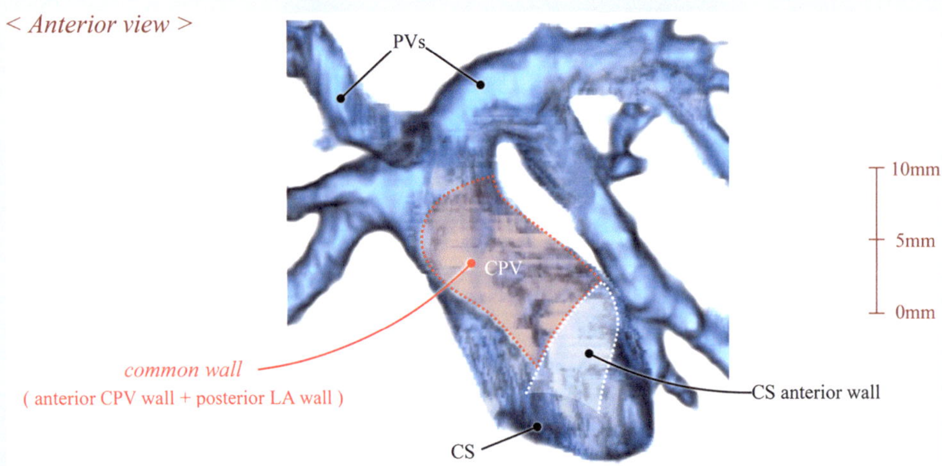

- PVs join to form CPVs, and CPVs join to CS. The CS is enlarged.
- The anterior wall of the CPV forms a broad common wall with the posterior wall of the left atrium (Case 2.4, Scene 1).

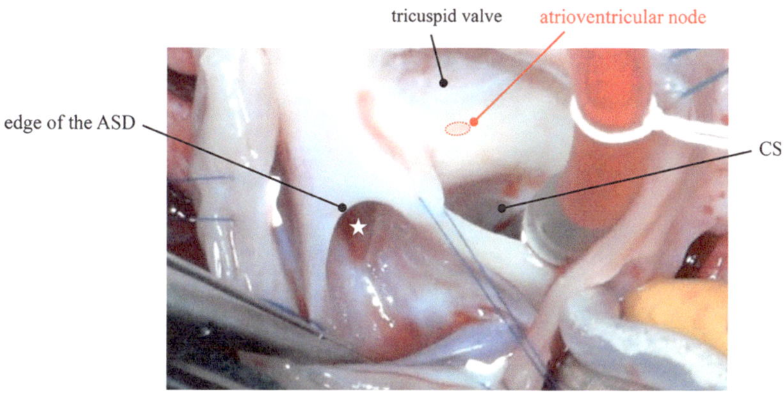

Case 2.4, Scene 1 Confirmation of right atrial morphology (Video 00 min 04 s)

1. Atrial septal defect (ASD: ☆) and enlarged coronary sinus (CS) are noted.
2. Confirm the location of the atrioventricular node.
3. Apply a traction suture anteriorly to the superior wall of the coronary sinus (at the transition with the atrial septum) (Case 2.4, Scene 2).

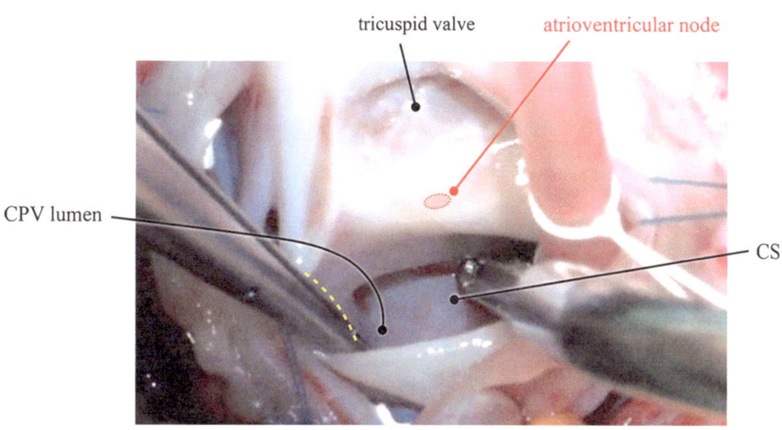

Case 2.4, Scene 2 Confirmation of CS lumen and PV orifices (Video 00 min 30 s)

1. Identify the PV orifices through the lumen of the CS.
2. Set the left margin of the common wall as the presumed incision line (*yellow dashed line*) (Case 2.4, Scene 3).

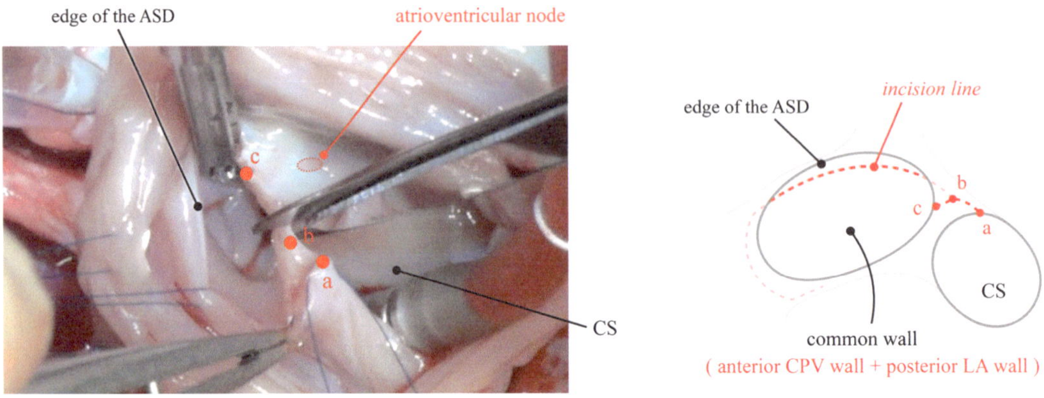

Case 2.4, Scene 3 Incise CS superior wall and atrial septum (right inferior edge of the ASD (Video 00 min 38 s)

1. Start the incision from the upper CS wall near the tricuspid valve annulus (a) toward the left.
2. Keep the incision line (*red dashed line*) away from the AV node.
3. Incise from the intersection of the superior CS wall and the atrial septum (b) to the edge of the ASD (c) (Case 2.4, Scene 4).

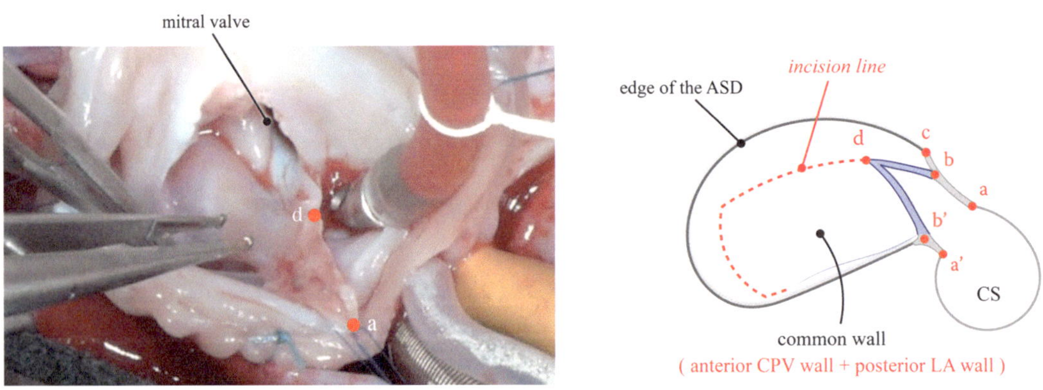

Case 2.4, Scene 4 Incise the left atrial side CS superior wall (Video 01 min 04 s)

1. Incise the upper wall of the CS along the mitral annulus to the left edge of the CPV cavity (d).
   - Be careful not to damage the mitral annulus (Case 2.4, Scene 5).

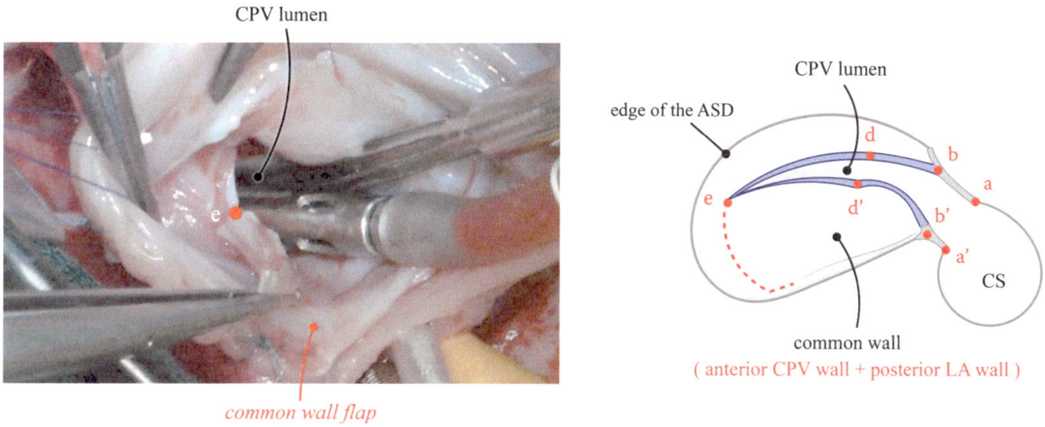

Case 2.4, Scene 5 Incise of the left edge of the common wall (Video 01 min 15 s)

1. Incise the posterior wall of the left atrium along the left edge of the CPV cavity to the cephalic end of the CPV cavity (e) (Case 2.4, Scene 6).

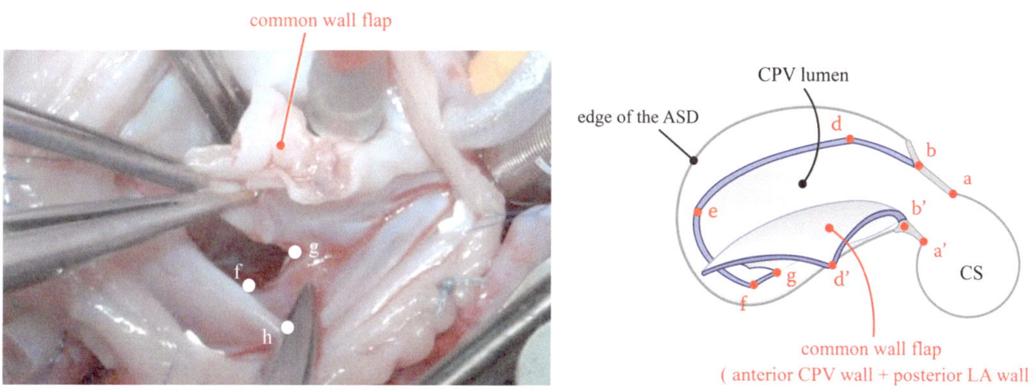

Case 2.4, Scene 6 Incise at the upper edge of the posterior LA wall (Video 01 min 40 s)

1. Incise the superior border of the common wall to the right to the right border of the CPV cavity (f).
2. From point (f), incise caudally to point (g), which is at the level of the cephalic edge of the atrial septal defect (h) (Case 2.4, Scene 7).

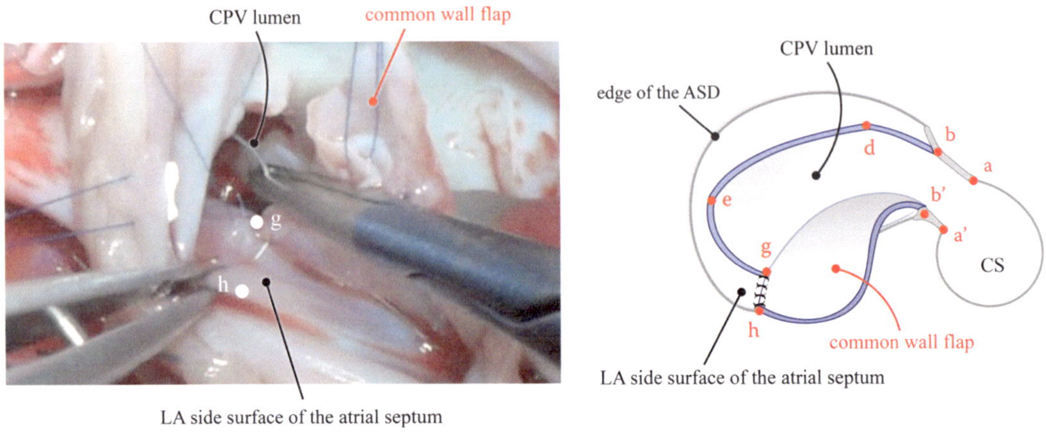

Case 2.4, Scene 7 Anastomose the common wall flap to the atrial septum (Video 01 min 52 s)

1. Raise the common wall flap 90 degrees toward the atrial septum.
2. Anastomose the common flap to the inner surface of the left atrium from the lowest end of the common wall incision (g) to the cephalic edge of the atrial septal defect (h) (Case 2.4, Scene 8).

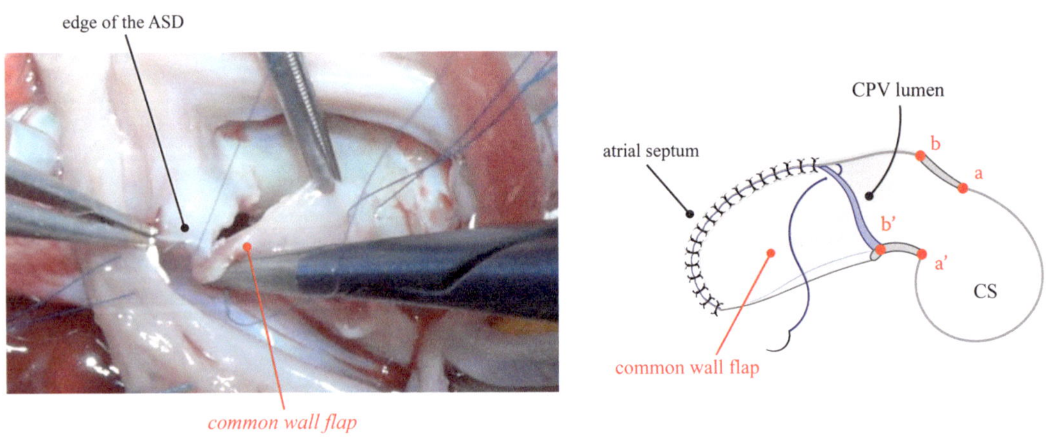

Case 2.4, Scene 8 Anastomose common wall flap to the edge of the ASD 1 (Video 02 min 54 s)

1. Anastomose the raised common wall flap to the edge of the atrial septal defect (Case 2.4, Scene 9).

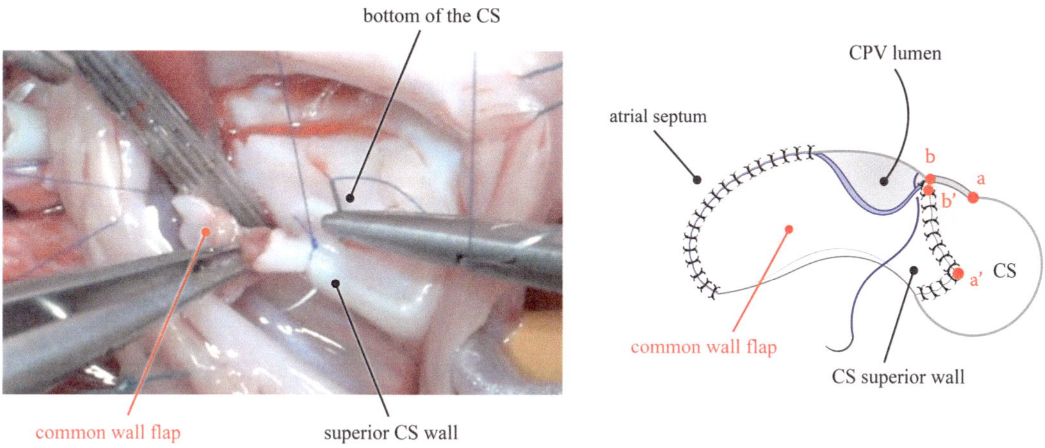

Case 2.4, Scene 9 Anastomose the superior CS superior wall to the bottom of the CS (Video 03 min 29 s)

1. In this case, the superior CS wall on the right atrial side was small, so the superior CS wall was first dropped to the bottom of the CS and anastomosed, and then the CS was closed (Case 2.4, Scene 10).

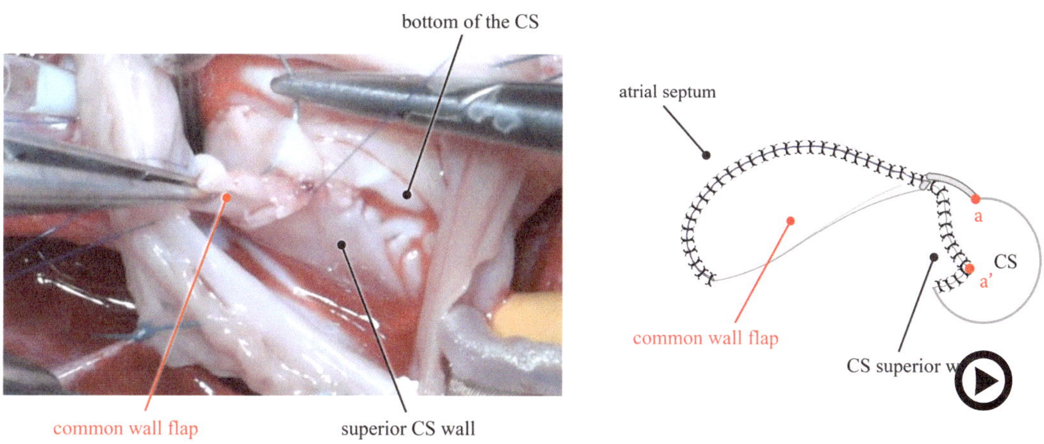

Case 2.4, Scene 10 Anastomose common wall flap to the edge of the ASD 2 (Video 04 min 54 s) (▶ https://doi.org/10.1007/000-hk7)

1. The remaining common wall flap is anastomosed to the edge of the atrial septal defect.

References

Sutureless Technique for Postoperative Pulmonary Venous Obstruction

Viola N, Caldarone CA. Surgical repair of post-repair pulmonary vein stenosis using "sutureless" technique. Oper Tech Thorac Cardiovasc Surg. 2011;16:112–21.

Cut Back Method for Cardiac Type (IIa)

Tsang VT, Stark J. Total anomalous pulmonary venous return and cor triatriatum. In: Stark JF, de Leval MR, Tsang VT, editors. Surgery for congenital. 3rd ed. England: Wiley; 2006.

Van Praagh Operation for Cardiac Type (IIa)

Van Praagh R, Harken AH, De Lisle G, et al. Total anomalous pulmonary venous drainage to the coronary sinus. A revised procedure for its correction. J Thorac Cardiovasc Surg. 1972;64:132–5.

Transference of the Posterior LA Wall for Cardiac Type (IIa)

Yamagishi M, Shuntoh K, Takahashi A, Shinkawa T, Miyazaki T, Kitamura N. Intra-atrial rerouting by transference of the posterior left atrial wall for cardiac-type total anomalous pulmonary venous return. J Thorac Cardiovasc Surg. 2002;123:996–9.

3 Pulmonary Stenosis (PS)

1 Blalock-Taussig Shunt

1.1 Treatment Strategies for Congenital Heart Disease with Decreased

The Blalock-Taussig procedure (BT shunt) is a short-circuiting procedure to increase pulmonary blood flow in patients with cyanotic congenital heart disease with pulmonary artery stenosis as a bridge to radical surgery. Currently, modified BT shunt using ePTFE grafts (Gore-Tex®) is used instead of the original method in which the subclavian artery is directly anastomosed to the pulmonary artery. The BT shunt itself is not a surgically invasive procedure.

Although the BT shunt itself is not very invasive, it increases pulmonary blood flow but also increases ventricular capacitance load, which may lead to heart failure or atrioventricular regurgitation due to high pulmonary blood flow after surgery. On the other hand, postoperative hypoxemia may temporarily occur due to fluctuations (elevations) in pulmonary vascular resistance.

Thus, the BT shunt is a minimally invasive procedure that can cause unstable hemodynamics in the postoperative period, but it is also a procedure with a potentially difficult postoperative course.

- ***Timing of Surgery***

In the neonatal period (especially within the first 2 weeks of life), pulmonary vascular resistance is high and may fluctuate due to physiologic pulmonary hypertension. Therefore, there is concern that if a BT shunt is performed during the neonatal period, the blood flow through the shunt may be unstable, and stable optimal arterial blood oxygen saturation may not be achieved. For this reason, it is desirable to perform the BT shunt around 1 month after birth, when pulmonary vascular resistance has stabilized. Of course, there are cases in which BT shunt must be performed before the first month of life.

Until the optimal timing at 1 month of age, Prostaglandin E1 should be administered to maintain patency of the ductus arteriosus and ensure pulmonary blood flow.

- ***Reference BT Shunt Caliber, Optimal Arterial Blood Oxygen Saturation***

After surgery, an appropriate shunt diameter must be selected, taking into account the conflicting issues of ensuring optimal arterial blood oxygen saturation and avoiding excessive ventricular capacitance load.

Supplementary Information The online version contains supplementary material available at https://doi.org/10.1007/978-981-96-6194-7_3. The videos can be accessed individually by clicking the DOI link in the accompanying figure caption or by scanning this link with the SN More Media App.

M. Yamagishi, *Surgical Treatment of Congenital Heart Disease*,
https://doi.org/10.1007/978-981-96-6194-7_3

A graft with a diameter of 4 mm for a 3000 g patient is the standard graft diameter for BT shunting, based on the weight of the patient. Optimal arterial blood oxygen saturation varies depending on the disease, but should be around 85%.

In addition to body weight, the final determination of the graft diameter is based on various factors such as (1) ventricular and atrioventricular valve morphology, (2) progressive pulmonary blood flow, (3) peripheral pulmonary artery growth, and (4) waiting period before radical surgery (or second-stage surgery).

- ***Ventricular Morphology***

In cases in which biventricular repair can be expected in the future, the graft diameter should be selected as per the standard caliber. In cases with poor peripheral pulmonary vascular growth and poor progressive pulmonary blood flow (blood flow through the pulmonary artery valve), a graft of one size larger in diameter may be selected, and the diameter may be adjusted with a hemoclip.

In Fontan candidates who must proceed to single ventricle repair (especially right ventricular single ventricle cases), there is concern about ventricular dysfunction and exacerbation of atrioventricular regurgitation due to increased volume loading caused by excessive pulmonary blood flow. In such cases, a reference aperture should be selected, and if arterial blood oxygen saturation can be maintained within an acceptable range (SaO_2 around 80%), ventricular capacitance load should be reduced by adjusting the caliber with a hemoclip.

Particularly in Fontan candidates, vigilance should be exercised against atrioventricular regurgitation after BT shunt, and additional BT shunt caliber adjustment should be considered if atrioventricular regurgitation worsens. AV valvuloplasty before second-stage surgery (bilateral cavopulmonary shunt: BCPS) or BCPS should also be considered.

- ***Antegrade Pulmonary Blood Flow***

In cases of moderate pulmonary valve stenosis, the BT shunt may be one size smaller than the reference diameter, as the shunt is intended to supplement the progressive pulmonary blood flow and valve annulus growth can be expected after BT shunt.

On the other hand, in cases of narrow valve annulus or severe funnel stenosis with severe thickening and fish-mouse-like valve morphology, future valve function cannot be expected. In addition, patients with severe funnel stenosis have unstable postoperative progressive pulmonary blood flow.

In such cases in which Rastelli surgery is indicated in the future, stable pulmonary blood flow can be maintained by cutting the main pulmonary artery at its origin during BT shunt and closing the right ventricular outflow tract, making the BT shunt a single source of blood flow.

- ***Peripheral Pulmonary Artery Growth***

In cases with poorly growing peripheral pulmonary arteries, a graft one size larger than the standard caliber may be selected if graft anastomosis to the pulmonary artery is possible. When selecting a larger graft, it is necessary to confirm that the pulmonary artery to be anastomosed has a sufficient caliber. It is also necessary to consider the possibility of volume overload due to excessive blood flow.

- ***Waiting Period Before Radical Surgery (or Second-Stage Surgery)***

In the case of single ventricle repair, the waiting period for second-stage surgery (BCPS) is from 6 months to 1 year, and there is no need to include the waiting period as a condition for caliber selection. In cases of right ventricular outflow tract enlargement and autologous pulmonary valve ring preservation, the waiting period varies from case to case, but generally ranges from 1 to 2 years, again without including the waiting period as a condition for caliber selection.

On the other hand, patients with pulmonary artery occlusion or main pulmonary artery amputation are candidates for the Rastelli operation using a right ventricular-to-pulmonary artery conduit, so it is desirable to wait until they are old enough (around 2–3 years) to use a larger conduit as much as possible. For this reason, it is advisable to select a graft one size larger in diameter at the time of BT shunt, adjust blood flow by hemoclip, and try to remove the hemoclip by balloon catheter when arterial blood oxygen saturation decreases to increase pulmonary blood flow and prolong the time until the radical surgery. An attempt may also be made to prolong the time to radical surgery by increasing pulmonary blood flow.

- ***Pulmonary Artery Morphology (Presence of Stenosis at the Ductus Arteriosus Attachment and/or Bifurcation Stenosis)***

Patients with pulmonary artery stenosis or occlusion and who depend on the ductus arteriosus for pulmonary blood flow frequently have stenosis at the bifurcation of the pulmonary artery to which the ductus arteriosus is attached or proximal to the left and right pulmonary arteries. In order to distribute blood flow evenly to the left and right pulmonary arteries in such cases, (1) complete resection of the ductus arteriosus, (2) enlargement of the stenotic area with a main pulmonary artery flap or autologous pericardial patch should be performed in addition to BT shunt.

- ***Treatment of Ductus Arteriosus***

To stabilize the postoperative management of BT shunt, it is desirable to have a single pulmonary blood flow supply channel. If ductus arteriosus blood flow remains, there are concerns about high pulmonary blood flow immediately after surgery (until spontaneous closure of the ductus arteriosus), hypoxemia after spontaneous closure of the ductus arteriosus, occurrence of stenosis at the ductus arteriosus attachment site, and manifestation of left-right difference in pulmonary blood flow. Therefore, except in special cases, it is recommended that the ductus arteriosus be ligated or cut at the time of BT shunt to maintain stable pulmonary blood flow.

- ***BT Shunt Approach and Pulmonary Artery Lateral Anastomosis Site***

Lateral Thoracotomy Approach To obtain a good view of the cervical artery (subclavian artery), the third intercostal space should be opened. The pulmonary artery anastomosis should be anastomosed more centrally than the bifurcation of the superior pulmonary artery.

If the autologous pericardium is to be used as an angioplasty patch during radical surgery (second-stage surgery), a lateral thoracotomy approach should be chosen to preserve the autologous pericardium. The lateral thoracotomy approach is also used in patients who require unifocalization of the major aortopulmonary collateral arteries (MAPCA) on the dorsal bronchus, which are difficult to treat from the midline.

When pulmonary blood flow on the shunt side is interrupted intraoperatively, it is important that arterial oxygen saturation can be maintained with only one-lung ventilation and blood supply to the contralateral lung by either progressive pulmonary blood flow or the ductus arteriosus. The lateral thoracotomy approach is difficult to handle with the ductus arteriosus.

Median Sternotomy Approach In the median sternotomy approach, the BT shunt is anastomosed near the midline of the central pulmonary artery through the anterior aorta. If there is a left-right difference in the degree of growth of the left and right pulmonary arteries, it may be anastomosed to the pulmonary artery on the slightly hypoplastic side.

The median sternotomy approach allows for treatment of the ductus arteriosus, pulmonary artery bifurcation, and other enlargement and plasty procedures. The median sternotomy approach is also currently recommended for safety when performing BT shunt without the use of an artificial heart lung (off pump), because it can appropriately handle sudden intraoperative hypoxemia. The same skin incision line is used for radical surgery (second-stage surgery), thus requiring only a single wound. On the other hand, postoperative adhesions, including those of the pericardium, cannot be avoided.

When BT shunt is performed through a median sternotomy approach with extracorporeal circulation (on pump), arterial blood oxygen saturation may remain temporarily low immediately after the procedure due to the extracorporeal circulation (it improves over time).

- ***Anastomotic Angle and Length of BT Shunt***

If the anastomotic angle between the brachiocephalic (subclavian) artery and BT shunt is steep (Fig. 3.1a), turbulent flow at the anastomosis may be amplified. In contrast, the graft is cut and anastomosed so that the anastomosis angle is not too steep (Fig. 3.1b), and the BT shunt is not a straight line with the shortest distance, but rather a slightly longer, gentle curve. If a straight BT shunt is used, the possibility of pulmonary artery entrapment cannot be ruled out (Fig. 3.2).

- If the anastomosis with the brachiocephalic artery is steeply angled, turbulent blood flow in the graft may be enhanced.

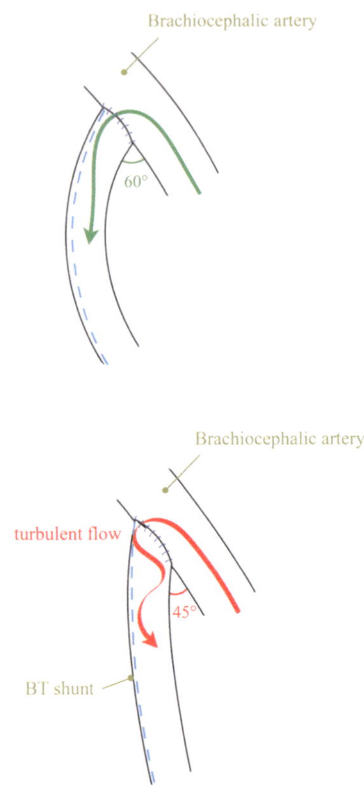

Fig. 3.1 Anastomotic angle of BT shunt

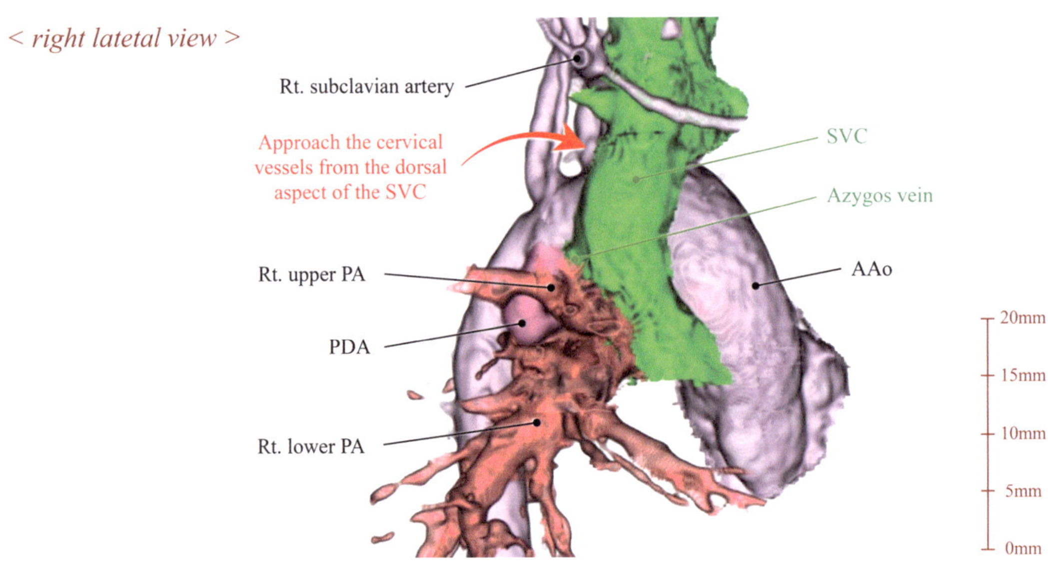

Fig. 3.2 CT images of the vessels via right thoracotomy

- To avoid intimal hyperplasia and anastomotic stenosis due to turbulence, the cut plane of the ePTFE graft should not be less than 60°.
- To keep blood flow in the graft as laminar as possible, the length of the graft should be gently curved, not straight.

SPOTLIGHT CT Images of the Vessels via Right Thoracotomy

1. *Dissection and exposure of cervical vessels*
   - Approach from the dorsal aspect of the superior vena cava to explore the cervical vessels.
   - Dissect between the transverse and recurrent nerves.
   - Be careful not to damage the nerves.
   - Resect surrounding lymph nodes.
2. *Dissect and expose the right pulmonary artery*
   - During dissection, be careful not to incise the pericardium.
   - The superior vena cava is pulled toward the sternum with a traction thread to expand the field of view.
   - Ligate and cut the azygos vein.
   - Approach from the basal (dorsal) aspect of the superior vena cava and dissect the right pulmonary artery toward the central region.

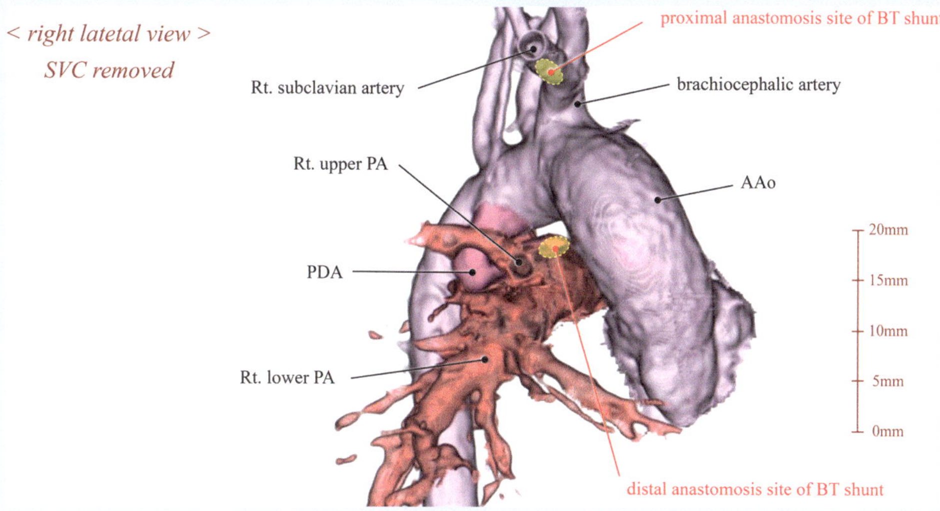

2. *Proximal (subclavian artery side) anastomosis*
   - The proximal anastomosis of the BT shunt should be near the origin of the right subclavian artery.
   - The anastomosis may extend to the brachiocephalic artery in part.
3. *Distal (pulmonary artery side) anastomosis*
   - The anastomosis on the distal side (pulmonary artery side) should be located in the right superior pulmonary artery more centrally than the right superior pulmonary artery origin.
   - The anastomosis should not extend to the right superior pulmonary artery.
   - Because the right lung is collapsed, it is difficult to treat the ductus arteriosus from the right open chest approach.
   - Ensure that arterial blood oxygen saturation can be maintained even if the right pulmonary artery is occluded with vascular forceps.

1.2 Surgical Video of Blalock-Taussig Shunt (Case 3.1: Off Pump)

Even with the median incision approach, it is possible to complete all surgical procedures (BT shunt and division of ductus arteriosus) without using extracorporeal circulation if (1) the main pulmonary artery is large enough to allow anastomosis of the BT shunt and (2) blood flow from the ductus arteriosus to both lungs can be maintained even if the main pulmonary artery is blocked before the pulmonary artery bifurcation. The ductus arteriosus is attached to the pulmonary artery bifurcation.

In cases where the ductus arteriosus is close to the pulmonary artery bifurcation or where the bifurcation is stenosed, intraoperative hypoxemia may occur if the main pulmonary artery is cut off before the pulmonary artery bifurcation. In such cases, BT shunt without extracorporeal circulation should be avoided.

Case 3.1: BT Shunt (Off Pump)

- VSD, PA, PDA, PFO
- 2 months old, 3860 g

In this case, the main pulmonary artery had sufficient diameter and length even though the patient had a closed pulmonary artery. Although the patient was ductus arteriosus-dependent, there was no stenosis at the pulmonary artery bifurcation, and blood flow to both lungs could be maintained even if the main pulmonary artery was closed before the pulmonary artery bifurcation, so an off-pump BT shunt (4 mm diameter) was performed. Because there was a possibility that the occluding clip might dislocate during the procedure, resulting in decreased pulmonary blood flow, and to ensure a clear field of view, the anastomosis was performed from the pulmonary artery side.

preoperative CT (cephalic view)

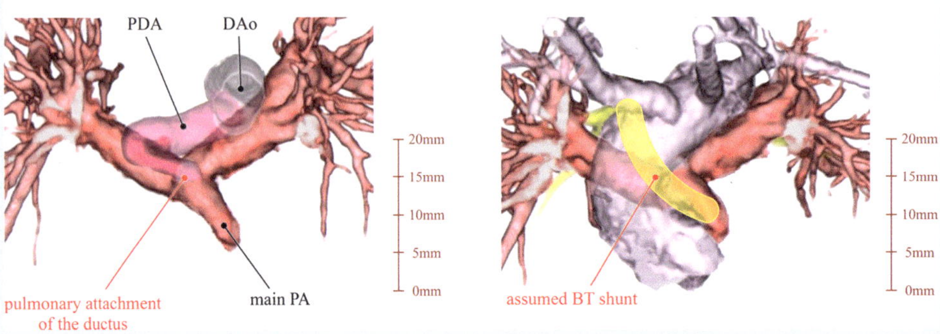

ESSENTIALS Direction of the Traction Suture

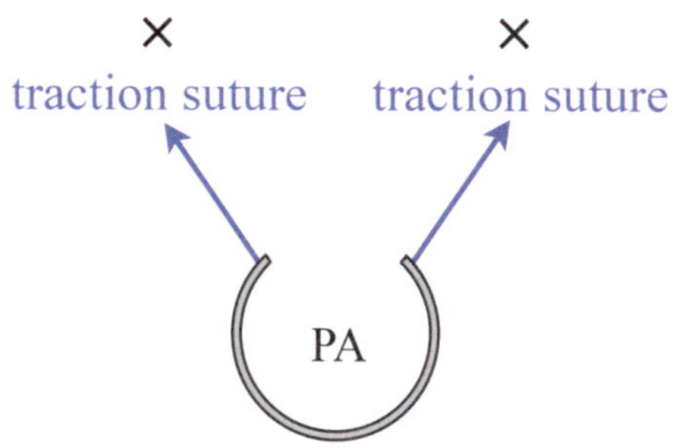

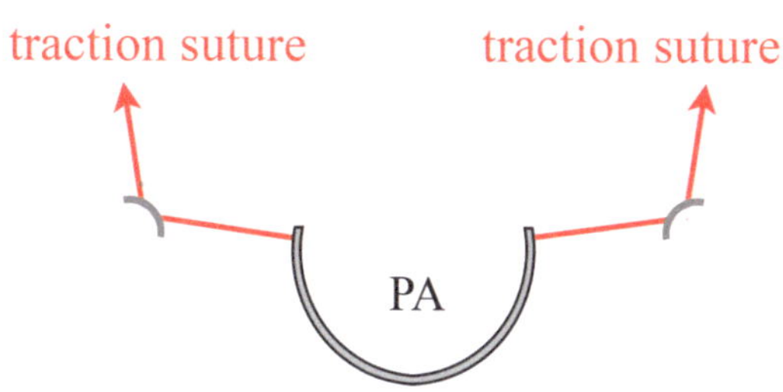

- If the traction suture is pulled up (*blue arrow*) over the edge of the vascular incision (toward the chest opener), the opening is poorly developed and the traction suture also interferes with suturing.
- If the traction suture at the edge of the vascular incision is placed over horizontal tissue (e.g., pericardium) prior to traction (*red arrow*), the orifice will develop well (Case 3.1, Scenes 1 and 2).

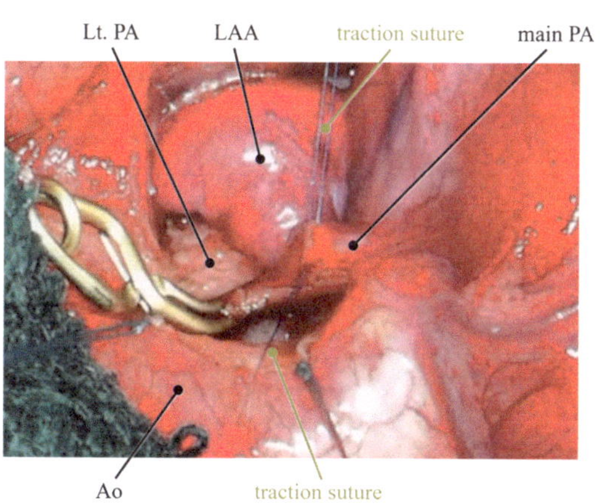

Case 3.1, Scene 1 Clamp at the pulmonary bifurcation, incision of the main PA (Video 01 min 48 s)

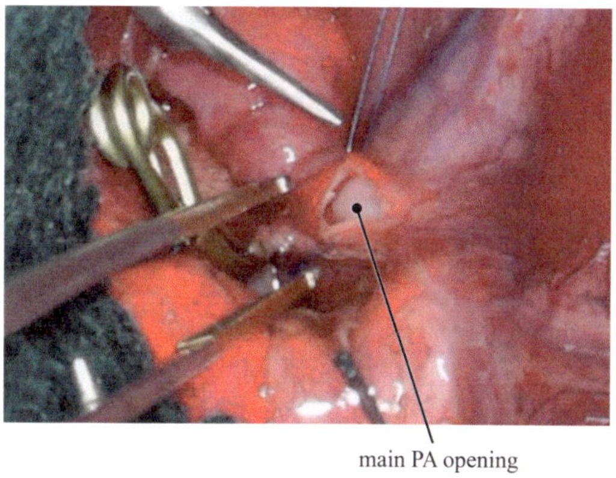

Case 3.1, Scene 2 A longitudinal incision on the anterior surface of the main pulmonary artery (Video 02 min 50 s)

- Since arterial oxygen saturation could be maintained even with the vascular clips placed before the pulmonary artery bifurcation, it was decided to perform a BT shunt without extracorporeal circulation.

1. After dissection around the main artery, two support threads were placed on the anterior surface of the main pulmonary artery, and the artery was pulled horizontally.
2. A longitudinal incision was made on the anterior surface of the main pulmonary artery.
3. The tension of the traction sutures was fine-tuned to develop a sufficient opening (Case 3.1, Scene 3).

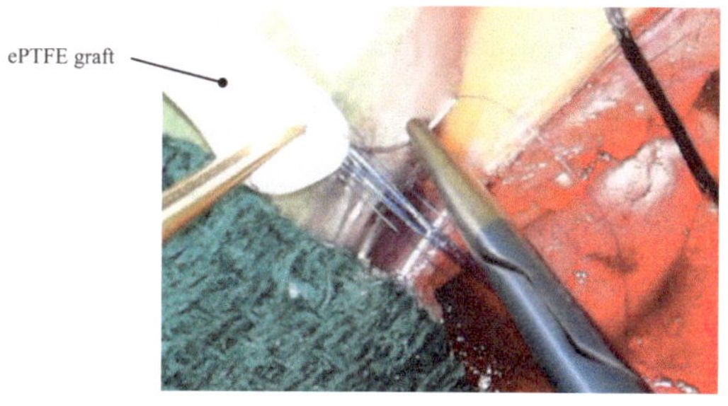

Case 3.1, Scene 3 Main PA-ePTFE graft anastomosis (Video 03 min 12 s)

1. Anastomose the cut end of the ePTFE graft with a continuous 7-0 monofilament suture from the cephalic end of the main pulmonary artery incision.

- Approximately 1/4 of the circumference of the anastomotic opening is sutured before the ePTFE graft is brought to the pulmonary artery using the parachute technique.

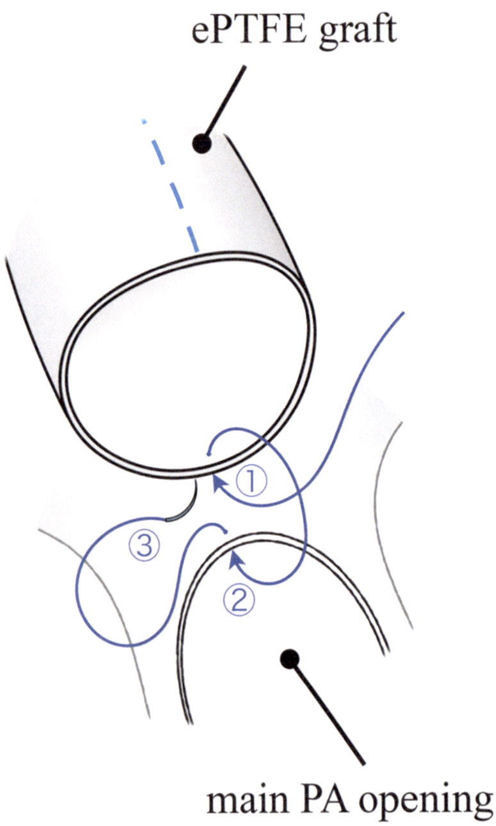

Anastomosis of ePTFE graft to the main PA (1)

First, a few stitches are made with one suture needle (blue).

① ePTFE graft wall: outside→inside
② Main PA wall: inside→outside
③ ePTFE graft wall: outside→inside

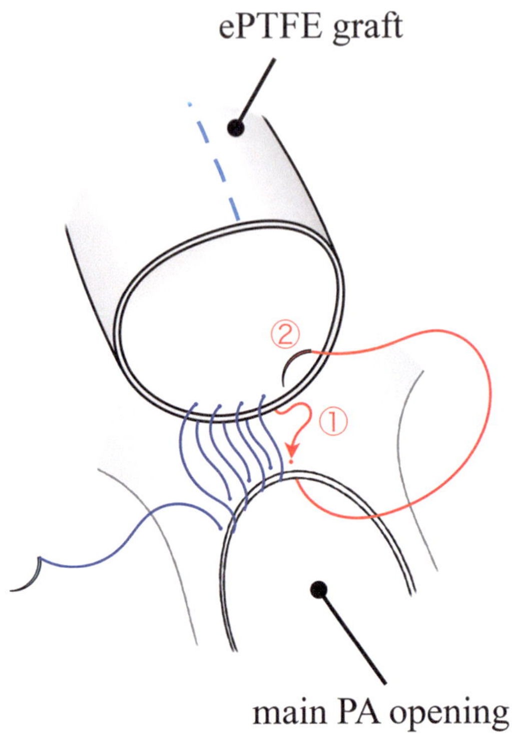

Anastomosis of ePTFE graft to the main PA (2)

Then, several stitches are made with the other suture needle (red).

① Main PA wall: outside→inside
② ePTFE graft wall: inside→outside (Case 3.1, Scene 4)

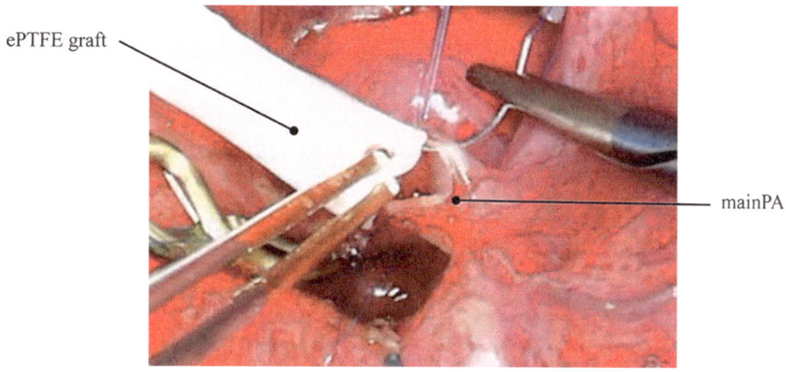

Case 3.1, Scene 4 Main PA – ePTFE graft anastomosis (Video 06 min 06 s)

2. Drop the ePTFE graft and anastomose it to the pulmonary artery orifice with a continuous 7-0 monofilament suture.

- The suture step should be the same width on the graft side and the pulmonary artery orifice side.
- The bite width from the end to the puncture point should be larger on the pulmonary artery than on the ePTFE graft.
- To avoid anastomotic stenosis, it is important to minimize the bite width of the cut end of the ePTFE graft.
- To avoid damage to the vessel wall, the suture needle should be inserted as perpendicular to the vessel wall as possible (Case 3.1, Scene 5).

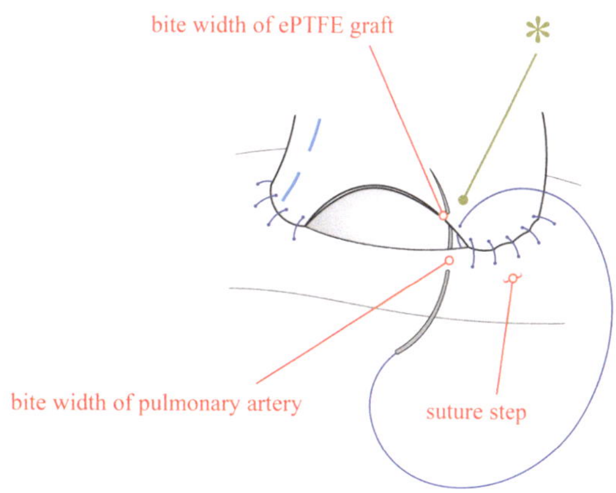

* It is recommended that the suture needle be grasped with a needle holder on the reversed fashion for anastomosis on the surgeon's side to ensure perpendicular penetration into the vessel wall (Case 3.1, Scene 6).

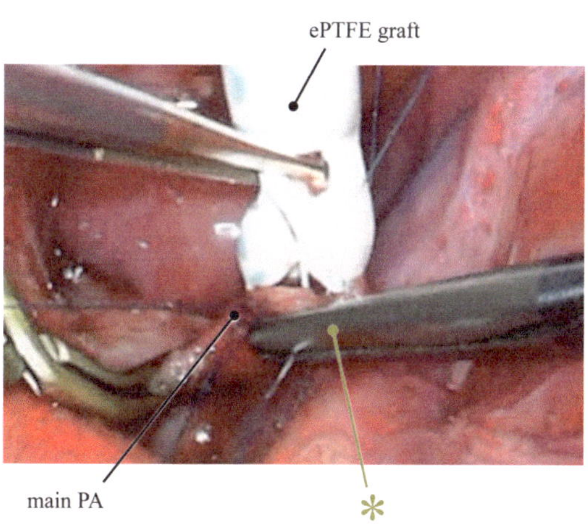

Case 3.1, Scene 5 Main PA – ePTFE graft anastomosis (Video 08 min 02 s)

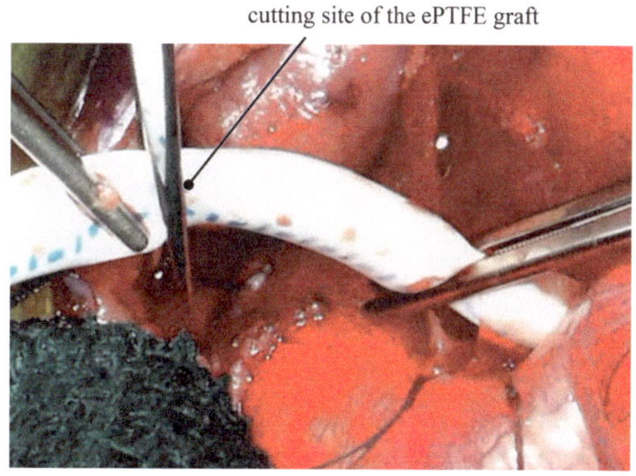

Case 3.1, Scene 6 Cut the ePTFE graft (Video 09 min 49 s)

1. Determine the length of the graft from the assumed anastomosis site of the brachiocephalic artery and cut the ePTFE graft.

- Cut the graft at a length with a gentle curve with a little room to spare.
- The cutting angle is determined by considering the length of the greater curvature side and the length of the lesser curvature side.

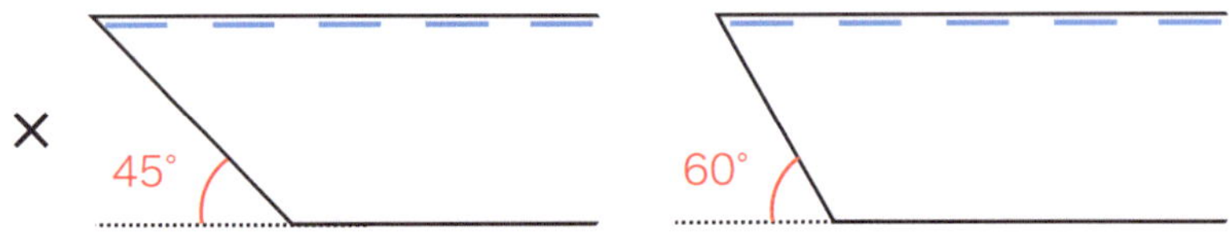

- The angle of the graft should not be less than 60°.
- If the cutting angle is less than 60°, the angle of blood flow at the anastomosis with the brachiocephalic artery becomes steeper, which may cause a high degree of turbulence in the graft and induce intimal hyperplasia (Case 3.1, Scene 7).

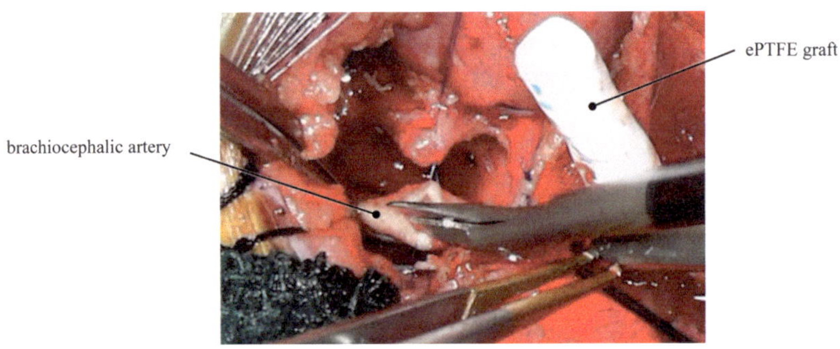

Case 3.1, Scene 7 Incise the brachiocephaic artery (Video 10 min 58 s)

1. Make a longitudinal incision in the brachiocephalic artery equal to the length of the graft incision.

- The anastomosis is made on the distal side of the brachiocephalic artery (just before the subclavian artery bifurcation).
- If the anastomosis is over a branch of the subclavian vein, take care not to damage the posterior wall during the vascular incision.
- Stretch the vessel wall horizontally with a traction suture (Case 3.1, Scene 8).

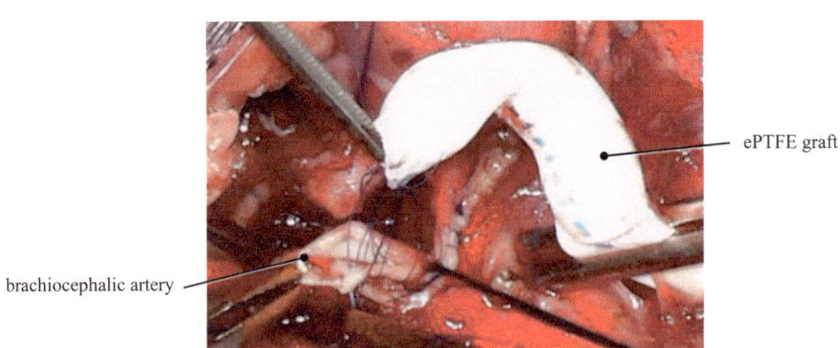

Case 3.1, Scene 8 Brachiochephalic artery-ePTFE graft anastomosis 1 (Video 11 min 20 s)

1. Start suturing from the section on the surgeon's side of the lesser curvature (heel side) of the graft.

- Perform 1/4 circumference using the parachute technique.
- To insert the suture needle perpendicularly into the vessel wall, the suture needle is grasped with a needle holder on the reversed fashion when anastomosing on the surgeon's side (Case 3.1, Scene 9).

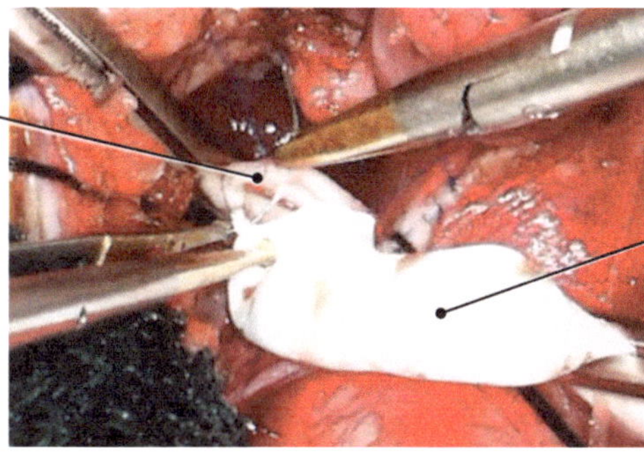

Case 3.1, Scene 9 Brachiochephalic artery-ePTFE graft anastomosis 2 (Video 15 min 42 s) (▶ https://doi.org/10.1007/000-hk9)

1. Once the tip of the graft (toe side) is crossed, the contralateral wall is sutured in the forward fashion.

- When inserting the suture needle, have the assistant relax the suture tension slightly to determine the entry point (it is difficult to identify the exact entry point if the suture tension remains taut).

2. Once the anastomosis is completed, the BT shunt is unblocked and the ductus arteriosus is ligated and cut.

Case 3.1: Postoperative CT

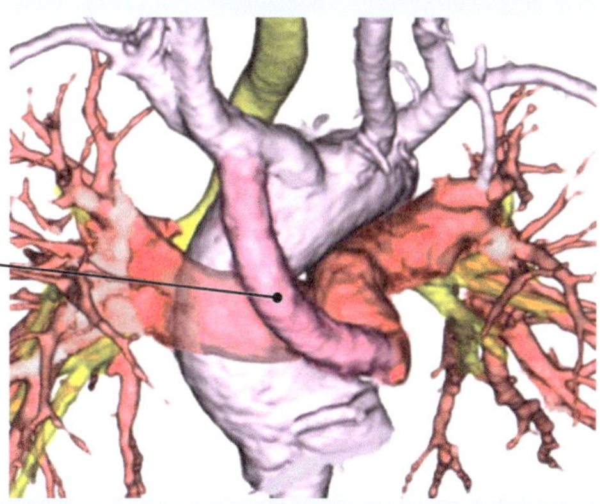

- The graft is anastomosed to the main pulmonary artery in a gentle curve.
- There is no stenosis at the anastomosis or in the graft.
- After BT shunt, there is no stenosis of the central pulmonary artery and the pulmonary artery growth is good.

1.3 Surgical Video of Pulmonary Artery Plasty and Blalock-Taussig Shunt (Case 2: On Pump)

Patients who depend on the ductus arteriosus for pulmonary blood flow are frequently complicated by stenotic lesions at sites where the ductus arteriosus attaches to the pulmonary artery (e.g., pulmonary artery bifurcation, left pulmonary artery). In such cases, it is necessary to dissect the ductus arteriosus and form the central pulmonary artery under extracorporeal circulation in order to ensure equal pulmonary blood flow to both lungs.

Case 3.2: PA plasty and BT shunt (on pump)

- Tetralogy of Fallot, severe pulmonary valvular and subvalvular stenosis, PDA
- 2 months old, 5620 g

In this case, there was a stenotic lesion (marked with white stars) at the pulmonary artery bifurcation where the ductus arteriosus attaches (left pulmonary artery origin), so it was decided to perform a complete resection of the ductus arteriosus tissue and an enlargement and formation of the central pulmonary artery along with dissection of the ductus arteriosus under extracorporeal circulation.

The surgical procedure consisted of (1) anastomosis of an ePTFE graft to the brachiocephalic artery prior to extracorporeal circulation. (2) After extracorporeal circulation was started, the ductus arteriosus was dissected and the ductus arteriosus tissue was completely resected from the pulmonary artery. In this case, (3) the main pulmonary artery was dissected to form a flap, and the left pulmonary artery was enlarged and formed. The ePTFE graft was anastomosed through the anterior part of the aorta to the enlarged and formed central pulmonary artery.

Considering the patient's weight and the waiting period before the Rastelli procedure, a 5-mm diameter ePTFE graft was anastomosed and blood flow was regulated with a hemoclip (Scene 1).

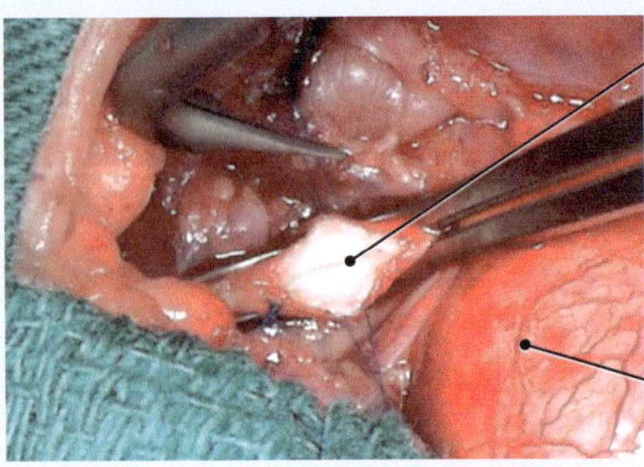

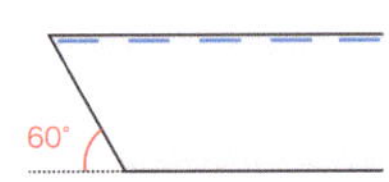

The angle of the graft should not be less than 60°.

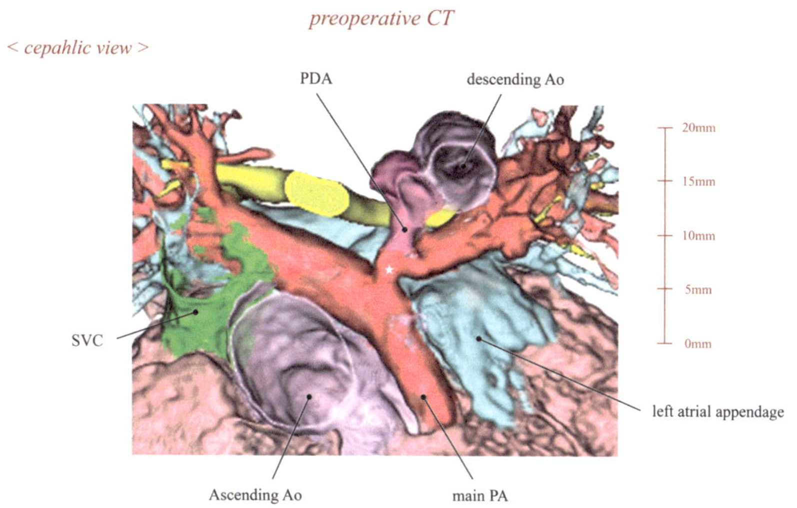

Case 3.2, Scene 1 Clamp and incise the brachiocephalic artery (Video 01 min 25 s)

- ePTFE graft anastomosis to the brachiocephalic artery is performed before starting extracorporeal circulation.
- The right lobe of the thymus is partially or completely resected to secure the visual field.

1. The brachiocephalic artery is dissected and pulled horizontally with a support thread on its superior surface.
2. The ePTFE graft is cut.
3. Make a longitudinal incision on the superior surface of the brachiocephalic artery according to the circumference of the ePTFE graft cut surface (Case 3.2, Scene 2).

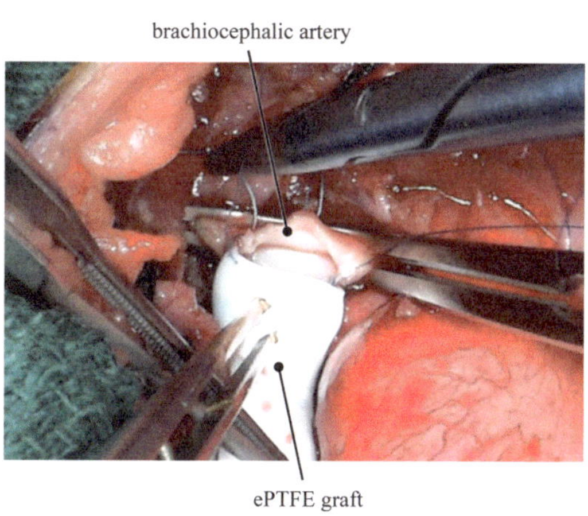

Case 3.2, Scene 2 Brachiochephalic artery-ePTFE graft anastomosis (Video 02 min 10 s)

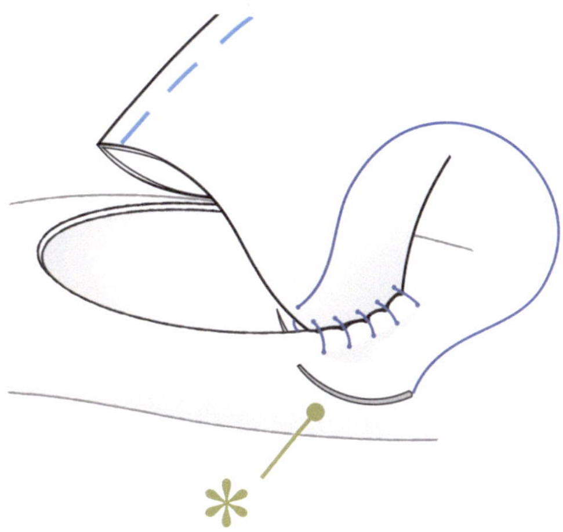

1. ePTFE graft is anastomosed end-to-side at the brachiocephalic artery orifice with continuous 7-0 monofilament suture.

   * The suture needle is grasped with a needle holder on the reversed fashion when anastomosing on the surgeon's side (Case 3.2, Scene 3).

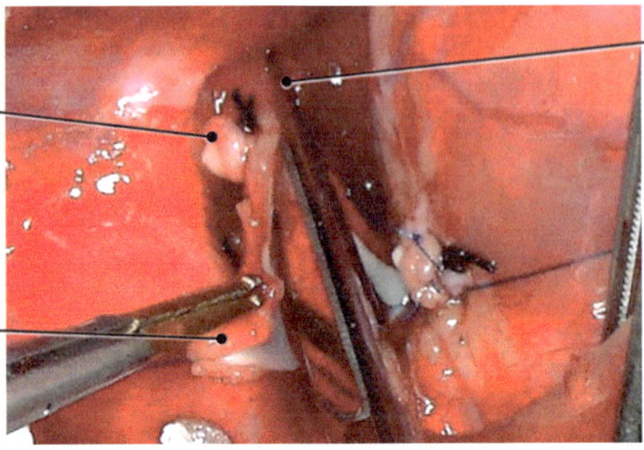

Case 3.2, Scene 3 Divide main PA, incise left PA, resect ductal tissue (Video 10 min 08 s)

1. Ligate and cut the proximal end of the main pulmonary artery and cut the distal end into a flap.
2. Ligate and divide the ductus arteriosus.
3. Incise the left pulmonary artery beyond the attachment of the ductus arteriosus to the right pulmonary artery in front of the upper lobe of the right pulmonary artery.
4. Completely resect the ductus arteriosus tissue.

- The transected end of the duct is pulled in the appropriate direction with 7-0 monofilament to maintain the three-dimensional shape of the duct (Case 3.2, Scene 4).

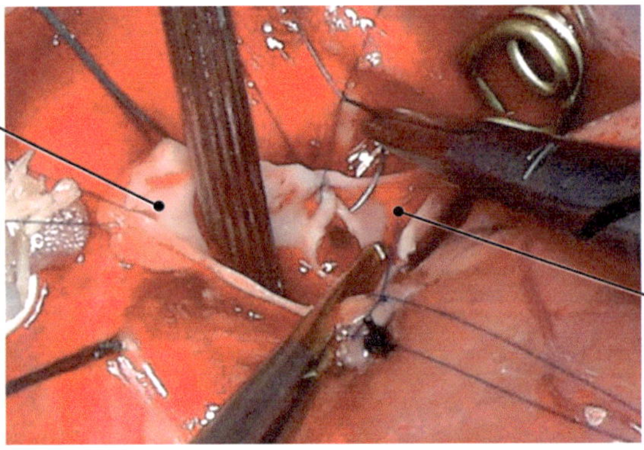

Case 3.2, Scene 4 Left PA plasty 1 (Video 12 min 19 s)

1. Resect the ductus arteriosus tissue and anastomose the dorsal (basal) side of the severed left pulmonary artery with a continuous 7-0 monofilament suture.

- The ends of the vessel to be sutured are firmly pulled in a 90° direction with a traction thread.
- Suture as far outward as possible to avoid excessive ridge in the lumen (Case 3.2, Scene 5).

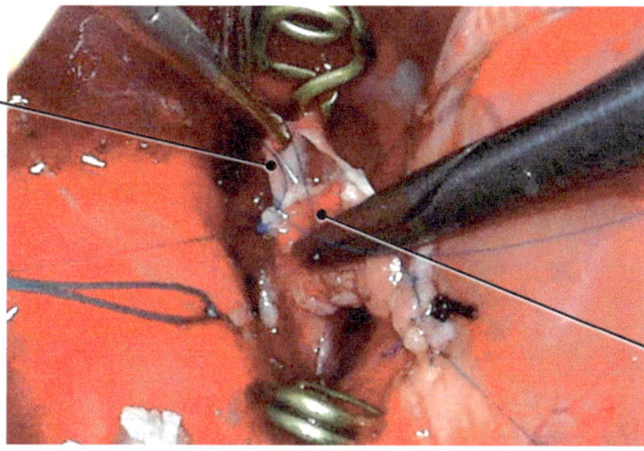

Case 3.2, Scene 5 Left PA plasty 2 (Video 17 min 11 s)

1. Cover the left pulmonary artery incision with the flap-shaped main pulmonary artery.
2. Anastomose with a continuous 7-0 monofilament suture and expand the left pulmonary artery incision.

- If the main pulmonary artery flap alone is not sufficient to expand the incision, an autologous pericardial patch is used to supplement the flap.
- The central pulmonary artery is formed into a larger patch because it will be used as a conduit anastomosis in the Rastelli procedure (Case 3.2, Scene 6).

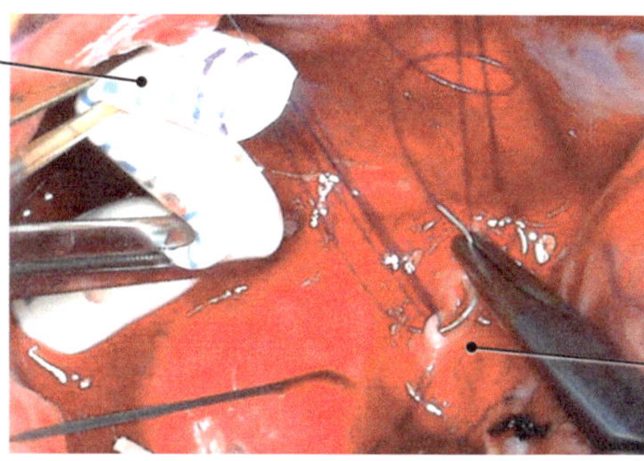

Case 3.2, Scene 6 Central PA-ePTFE graft anastomosis 1 (Video 27 min 08 s)

1. Cut the ePTFE graft in a gently curved length, leaving some space in front of the aorta.
   - Cut the graft (on the central pulmonary artery side) at an angle of approximately 90°.
2. Cut open the pouch-shaped central pulmonary artery (main pulmonary artery flap).
3. First, anastomose the graft using the parachute technique with continuous 7-0 monofilament suture, and when approximately 1/4 of the circumference is anastomosed, bring the ePTFE graft to the central PA (Case 3.2, Scene 7).

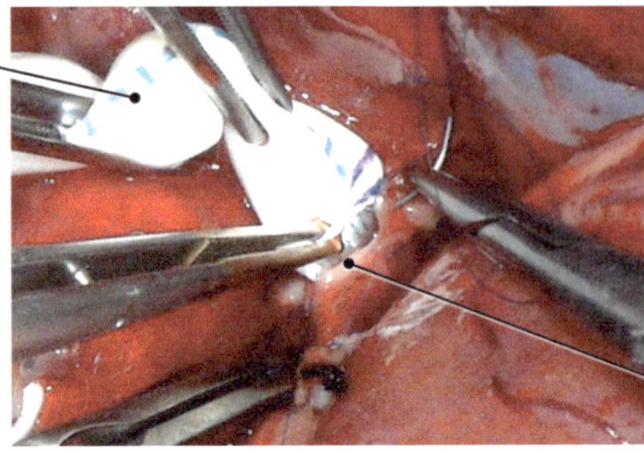

Case 3.2, Scene 7 Central PA-ePTFE graft anastomosis 2 (Video 30 min 29 s)

1. After the ePTFE graft is brought to the pulmonary artery, the surgeon's contralateral wall is sutured with the forward fashion and the anastomosis on the surgeon's side is sutured with the reversed fashion (Case 3.2, Scene 8).

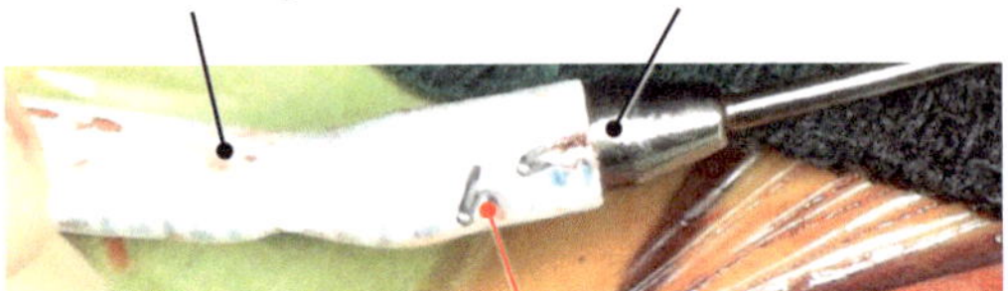

Case 3.2, Scene 8 Caliver of the ePTFE graft adjustment (Video 33 min 32 s)

1. Insert a 4.5-mm diameter sizer into a 5-mm ePTFE graft and bite the graft outer wall with a hemoclip so that the inner diameter is 4.5 mm.
2. This hemoclip bite is used as a reference (sample) when adjusting the bore diameter (Case 3.2, Scene 9).

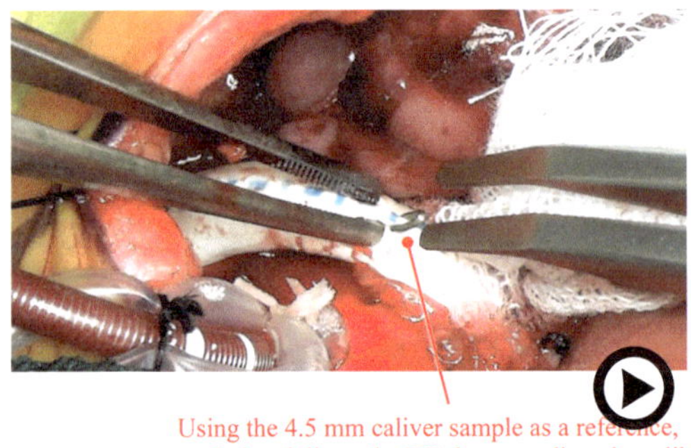

Case 3.2, Scene 9 Apply hemiclip to the BT shunt (Video 33 min 42 s) (▶ https://doi.org/10.1007/000-hk8)

3. Using the sample as a reference, apply hemoclip to the BT shunt to adjust the caliber (flow adjustment).

- The hemoclip is applied near the center of the BT shunt (because there is a concern of endomembrane growth at the anastomosis due to turbulent flow of the clip near the anastomosis).
- (Because there is a possibility of the hemoclip coming off if only one hemoclip is used.)

Case 3.2: Postoperative CT

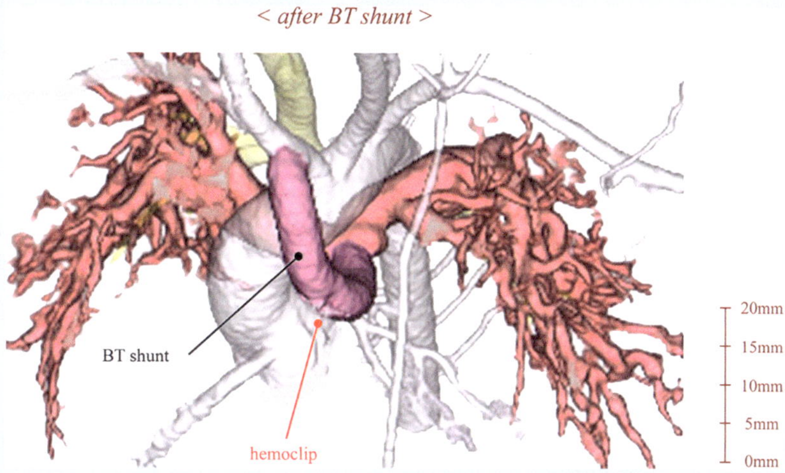

- The BT shunt is gently curved and anastomosed to the central pulmonary artery, and the stenosis at the pulmonary artery bifurcation has been released.
- There is no evidence of hyperextension of the PA pulled by the BT shunt.
- No stenosis at the anastomosis on the pulmonary artery side is observed.
- The intrapulmonary artery morphology is a bit high because of the immediate postoperative CT, but it is expected to adapt to the remote stage as the patient gains weight.

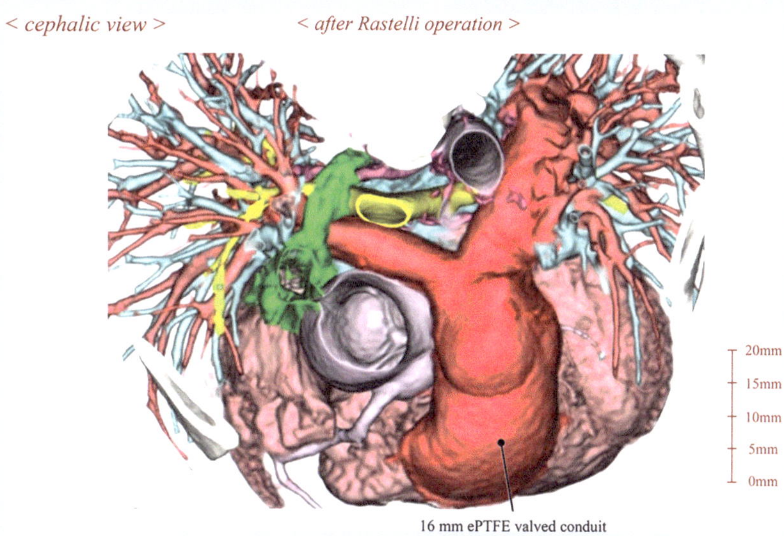

- Rastelli operation (16 mm ePTFE valved conduit) performed 8 months (body weight: 8.7 kg) after BT shunt.
- There was no stenosis in either the right or left pulmonary artery.
- Pulmonary vascular bed was in good condition (BT shunt blood flow was considered to have adapted with weight gain).

4 Ventricular Septal Defect (VSD)

1 Morphology of Ventricular Septal Defect

1.1 Morphological Check Point for Surgical Repair of TAPVR

The ventricular septum is consisted of an inlet septum, a trabecular septum, and an outlet septum. The outlet septum is connected to the infundibular septum between the great arteries. In addition, there is a membranous septum in the inflow segment.

Ventricular septal defects (VSDs) can be found at any location and are morphologically characterized by surrounding structures (Fig. 4.1).

Perimembranous VSD

- The VSD opens into the inlet septum on the outflow side of the membranous septum.
- The VSD lies below (right ventricular side) the anterior and septal leaflets of the tricuspid valve.
- The superior border of the VSD is composed of the ventriculo-infundibular fold (VIF), the anterior border is composed of the anterior limb of the trabecular septomarginalis (TSM), the inferior border is composed of the posterior limb of the TSM or the inlet septum, and the posterior border is composed of the tricuspid valve annulus, the central fibrous body, and the membranous septum (ventricular part).
- The wall of the inferior margin of the VSD is thicker when the posterior limb of the TSM is present, and thinner when the posterior limb of the TSM is almost absent.
- A fibrous membranous flap is present at the postero-inferior margin of the VSD.
- The medial papillary muscle (MPM), accessory papillary muscle, and tricuspid chordae tendineae are attached to the VSD margin.

Muscular Outlet VSD

- The VSD opens into the outflow septum and the margins are composed of muscular tissue.
- Noncoronary or right coronary cusp of the aortic valve may prolapse into the VSD.

Subarterial VSD

- The VSD is located at the infundibular septum just below both semilunar valves (aortic and pulmonary valves).
- Right coronary cusp of the aortic valve prolapses into the VSD.

Supplementary Information The online version contains supplementary material available at https://doi.org/10.1007/978-981-96-6194-7_4. The videos can be accessed individually by clicking the DOI link in the accompanying figure caption or by scanning this link with the SN More Media App.

M. Yamagishi, *Surgical Treatment of Congenital Heart Disease*,
https://doi.org/10.1007/978-981-96-6194-7_4

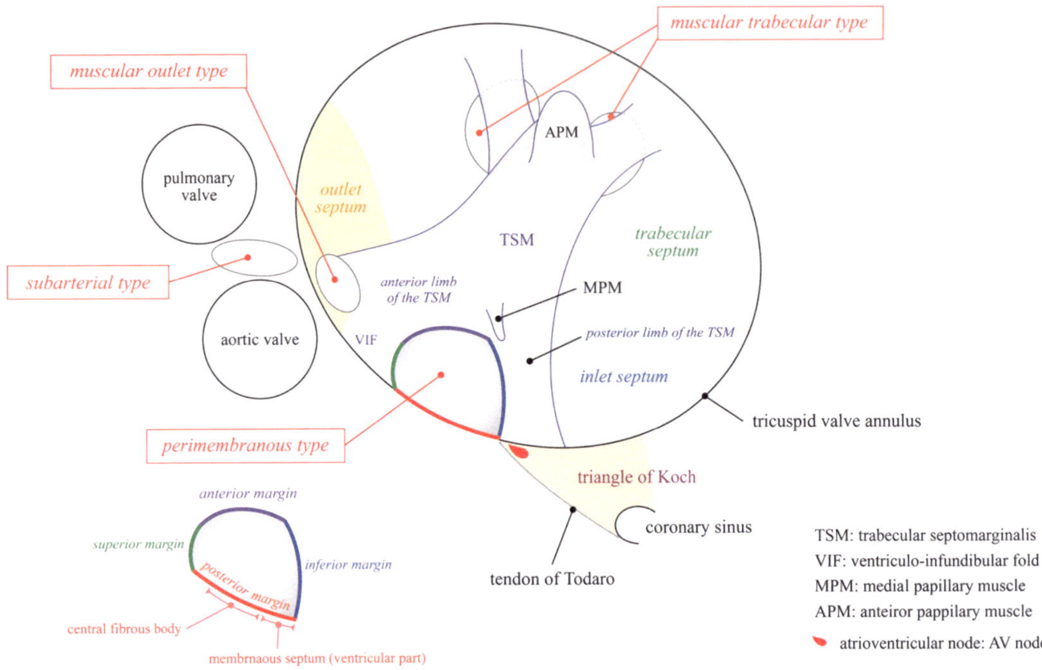

Fig. 4.1 VSD and surrounding structures (trans right atrium overhead view)

Muscular Trabecular VSD

- VSDs often have multiple openings closer to the apex of the trabecular septum (Swiss cheese VSD).
- The openings of the VSD are located behind the TSM muscle bundle.

1.2 Conduction System

The atrioventricular (AV) node is located subendocardially at the apex of Koch's triangle, which is composed of the tricuspid valve annulus, the coronary sinus, and the tendon of Todaro. The conduction system from the AV node runs along the postero-inferior margins of the perimembranous VSD toward the apex. Note that the conduction system is highly variable and may not be typical.

In other types (muscular outlet type, subarterial type, muscular trabecular type), the VSD and the conduction system are not in close proximity (Fig 4.2).

SPOTLIGHT

Non-penetrating non-branching bundle (NPNBB), branching bundle (BB)

- Cases with thick posterior limb of the TSM at the inferior margin of the VSD (e.g., perimembranous outlet type VSD): Both NPNBB and BB are covered by the thick posterior limb of the TSM and run away from the right ventricular endocardial surface.
- Cases with absent or thin posterior limb of the TSM (perimembranous inlet type VSD): Both NPNBB and BB run under the left ventricular endocardium, but at a depth closer to the right ventricular endocardial surface.

Medial papillary muscle (MPM)

- When the MPM attaches to the anterior inferior border of the VSD, the right bun-

(continued)

dle branch often runs near the base of the MPM.

- When the MPM attaches near the anterior or anterior superior margin of the VSD, it is not an indicator of the location of the bundle branch.

1.3 Perimembranous VSD and Conduction System

Perimembranous type VSD (inlet type or outlet type) has a characteristic conduction system. The morphology of the posterior inferior border of the VSD adjacent to the AV node is an important point of the conduction system (Fig. 4.3).

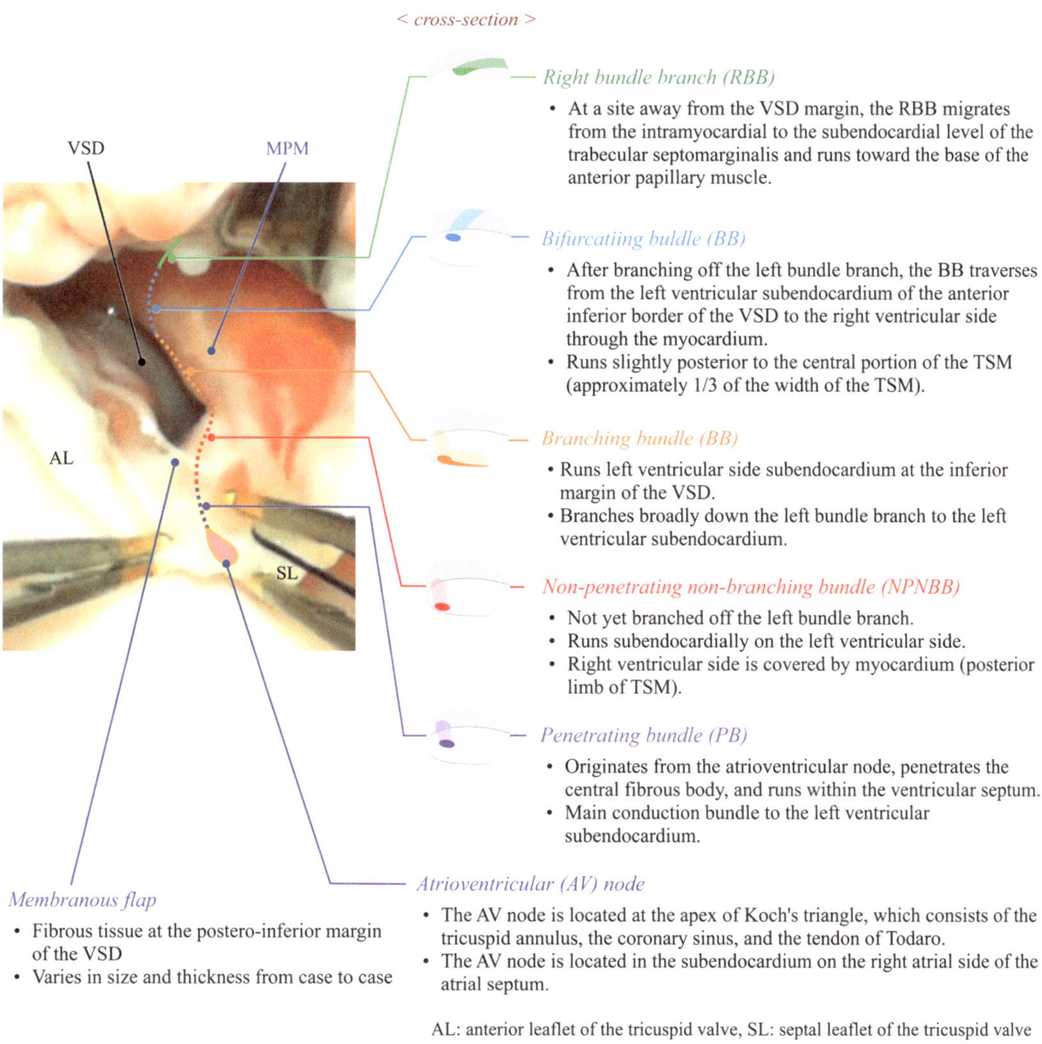

Fig. 4.2 Perimembranous VSD and conduction system (typical configuration)

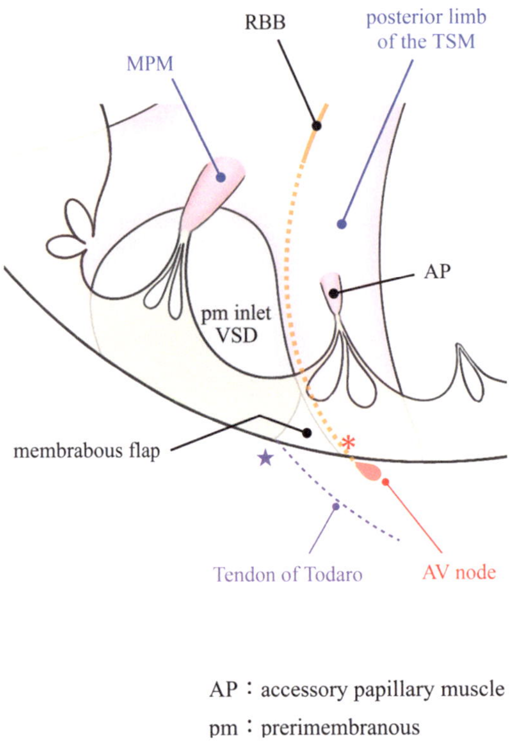

Fig. 4.3 Perimembranous inlet VSD and conduction system

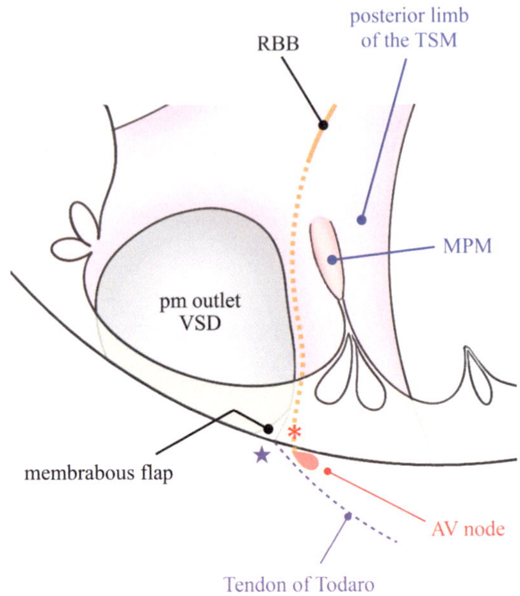

Fig. 4.4 Perimembranous outlet VSD and conduction system

1. Identify the apex of the Koch's triangle (★) where the tendon of Todaro intersects the tricuspid annulus.
2. Identify the posterior inferior margin of the VSD (✱).

- The posterior inferior margin of the VSD (✱) is located on the inflow side of the apex of Koch's triangle (★).
- The AV node is located in the right atrial endocardium just above the posterior inferior border of the VSD (deviated to the right from the apex of Koch's triangle).
- The conduction system descends from the posterior inferior border of the VSD and runs along the VSD limbus to the left ventricular subendocardium (base of the membranous flap).
- The posterior limb of the trabecular septomarginals (TSM) are often absent or thin (thin ventricular wall at the inferior margin of the VSD).
- Thus, the conduction system is located close to the right ventricular endocardium.
- A relatively large membranous flap is often present.
- The madial papillary muscle (MPM) attaches to the anterior or antero-superior border of the VSD.
- The right bundle branch does not pass through the base of the MPM.
- The accessory papillary muscle may be present at the inferior margin of the VSD but is not an indicator of the location of the conduction system (Fig. 4.4).

1. Identify the apex of the Koch's triangle (⋆) where the tendon of Todaro intersects the tricuspid annulus.
2. Identify the posterior inferior margin of the VSD (*).

- The posterior inferior margin of the VSD (*) is located almost coincident with the apex of Koch's triangle (⋆) or slightly to the outflow tract.
- The AV node is located in the right atrial subendocardium just above the postero-inferior margin of the VSD (located at the apex of Koch's triangle).
- The conduction system descends from the postero-inferior border of the VSD and runs along the VSD margin to the subendocardium on the left ventricular side.
- Membranous flap is often small.
- Medial papillary muscle attaches to antero-inferior margin of the VSD.
- The right bundle branch passes the outflow tract side of the base of the medial papillary muscle.

2 Closure of Perimembranous Ventricular Septal Defect

In perimembranous VSDs, the conduction system runs in close proximity to the inferior border of the VSD. In order to avoid the occurrence of conduction disturbances, it is especially important to suture (1) the postero-inferior margin (avoiding the AV node and main conduction system) and (2) the antero-inferior margin (avoiding the right bundle branch) (Fig. 4.5).

2.1 Suture at the Postero-Inferior Margin Avoiding the AV Node and Main Conduction System

VSD Closure Using the Membranous Flap

①-ⓐ Place the suture at the edge (point (a)) of the membranous flap, slightly away from the muscular septum (this should be a location that does not touch the muscular septum when the pledget is dropped onto it).

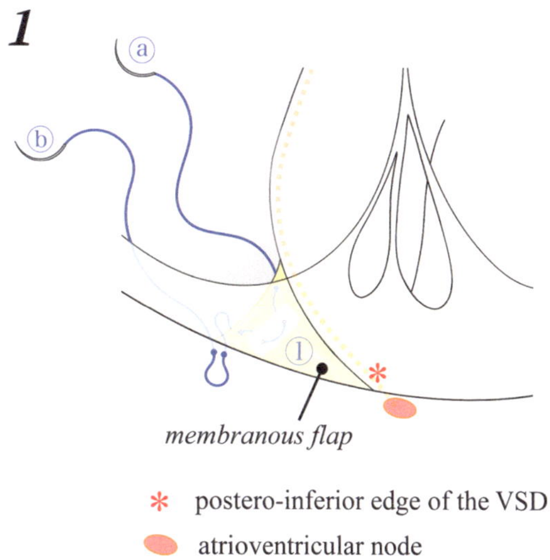

Fig. 4.5 Suture at the postero-inferior margin using the membranous flap

①-ⓑ Suture over the membranous flap just below the tricuspid valve annulus (point (b)), penetrate through the valve annulus, and then again through the valve annulus to the ventricular side.

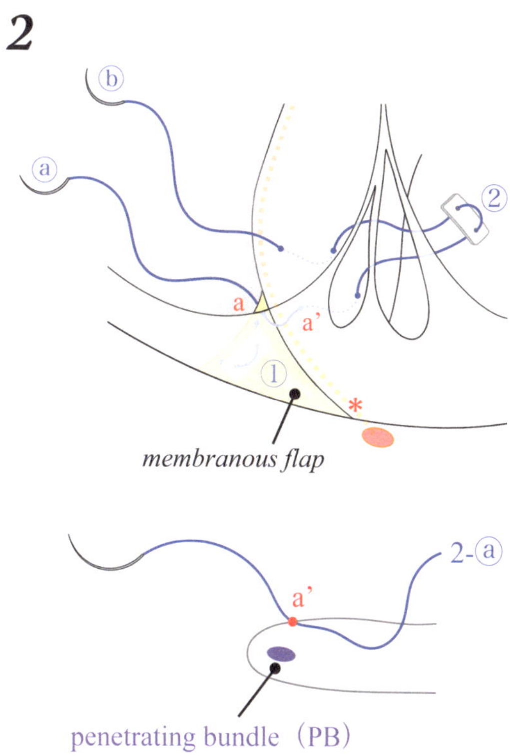

②-ⓐ Insert the suture needle slightly deeper at a point far enough away from the VSD margins. Proceed with the suture needle so that it becomes shallower as it approaches the VSD margin, and then stitch out the suture needle at a point at least 2 mm from the muscular septal margin (point (a')). In addition, the suture needle is inserted across the point (a') of the membranous flap.

②-ⓑ As in ②-ⓐ, a slightly deeper needle is inserted at a point well away from the VSD margin, the needle is advanced so that it becomes shallower as it approaches the margin, and then the suture needle is stitch out at a point at least 2 mm away from the muscular septal margin.

VSD Closure Without Use of the Membranous Flap

If the membranous flap is large and does not compress the conduction system when the suture pledget is dropped onto it, it can be used for VSD closure. It must also have sufficient thickness (strength), and thin membranous flaps, even if large enough, should not be used for VSD closure (Fig. 4.6).

①-ⓐ Insertion the suture needle 2 mm away from the tricuspid valve annulus at the postero-inferior margin of the VSD (*) from the atrial side of the septal leaflet (point (a)) and pull out the ventricular side of the septal leaflet.

The next stitch (transitional stitch) can be done either way (**2-a, b** or **3-a, b**).

1

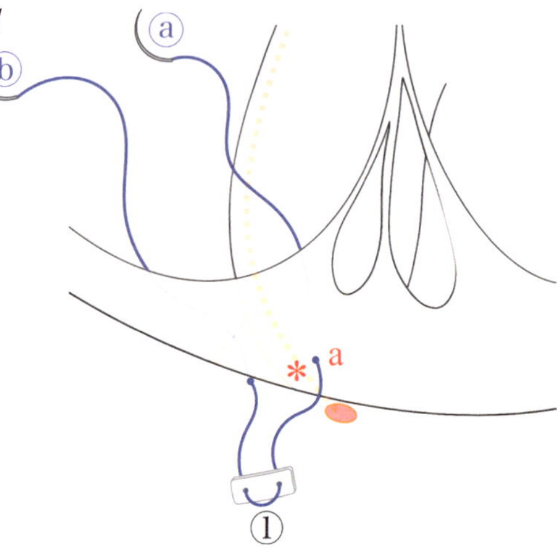

Fig. 4.6 Suture at the postero-inferior margin without use of the membranous flap

Transitional Stitch from Ventricular Side

2a

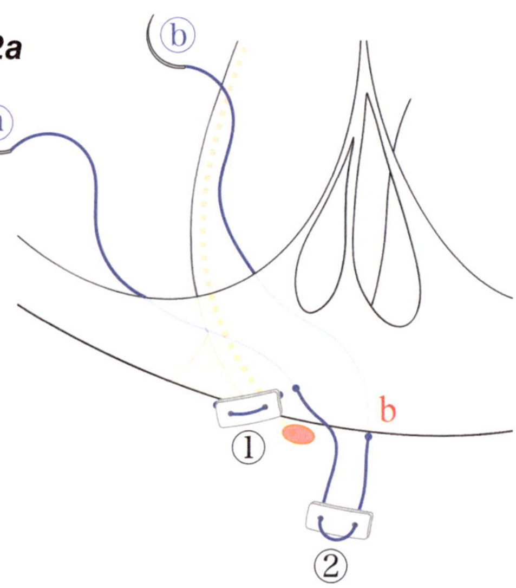

②-ⓐ Insert into the septal leaflet at a site adjacent to ①-ⓐ from the atrial side, and stitch out from the ventricular side of the septal leaflet.

②-ⓑ Insert into the tricuspid annulus from the atrial side, away from the AV node, and stitch out the ventricular side of the leaflet (insertion point (b)).

2b

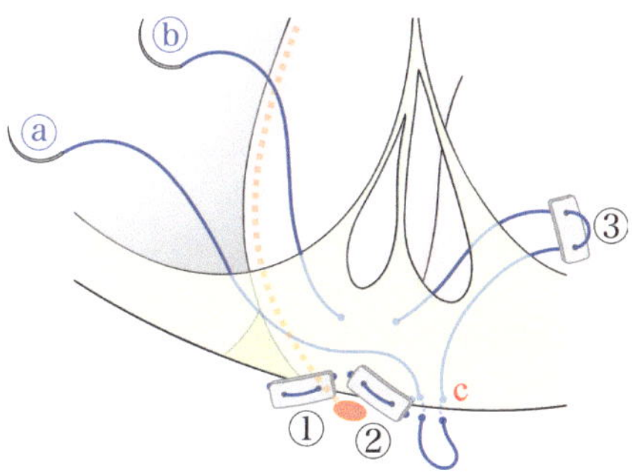

③-ⓐ Insert into the valve annulus just below the ventricular side of the valve annulus (insertion point (c)), and then stitch out from the atrial side of the valve annulus.

Insert into the tricuspid valve annulus adjacent to the insertion point of suture ② from the atrial side and stitch out from the ventricular side of the valve annulus.

③-ⓑ Stitch out at a site away from the VSD margin.

Transitional Stitch from Atrial Side

3a

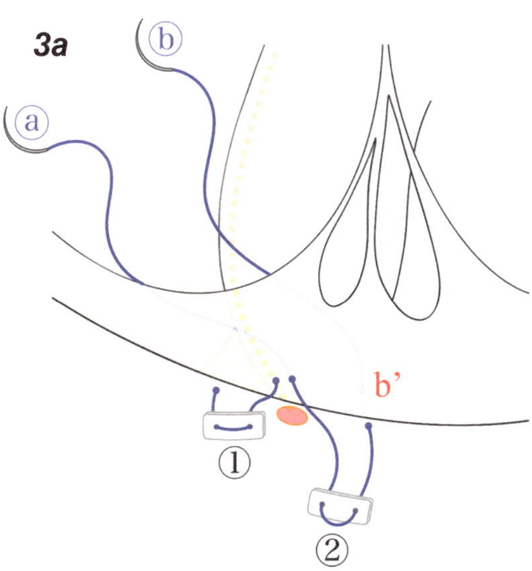

②-ⓐ Insert into the septal leaflet at a site adjacent to ①-ⓐ from the atrial side, and stitch out from the ventricular side of the septal leaflet.

②-ⓑ Insert into the tricuspid annulus from the atrial side, away from the AV node, and stitch out at the ventricular septum (point (b')) a few mm away from the valve annulus.

3b

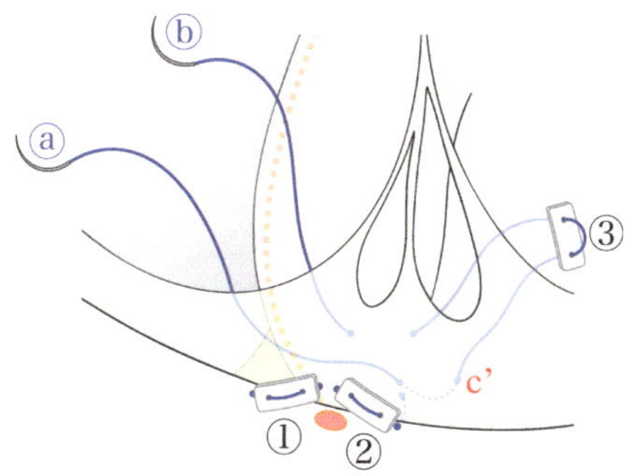

③-ⓐ Insert into a site slightly away from the tricuspid valve annulus (point (c')) and the stitch-out point of the suture ② adjacent to the stitch-out point of the suture.

③-ⓑ Stitch out at a site away from the VSD margin.

SPOTLIGHT Suture Near the Penetrating Bundle

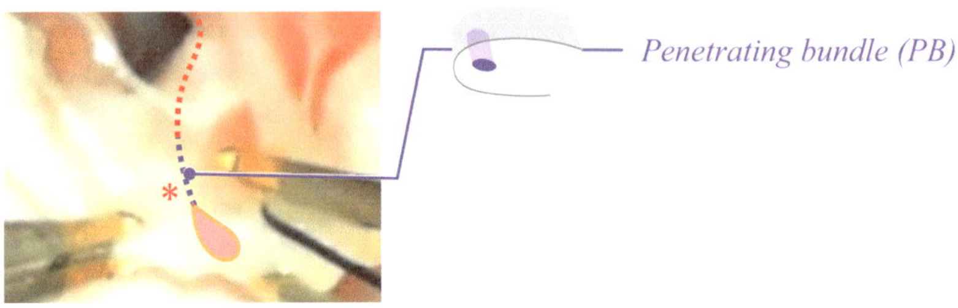

- The PB from the atrioventricular node (subendocardial right atrial side of the atrial septum) penetrates the central fibrous body and runs to the subendocardial left ventricular side.
- Near the postero-inferior margin of the VSD (*), the PB lies in a shallow area of the right ventricular endocardium.
- Insertion point (②-ⓐ) should be away from the valve annulus, not close to the AV node.
- The point (ⓐ) near the valve annulus is closer to the atrioventricular node, making the insertion and exertion points parallel to the stimulation conduction system.
- Therefore, suture ligation may induce a conduction disturbance.

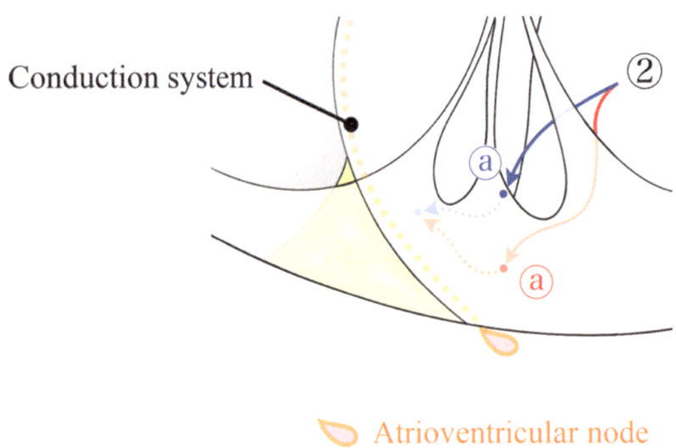

2.2 Suture at the Antero-Inferior Margin Avoiding the Right Bundle Branch (Fig. 4.7)

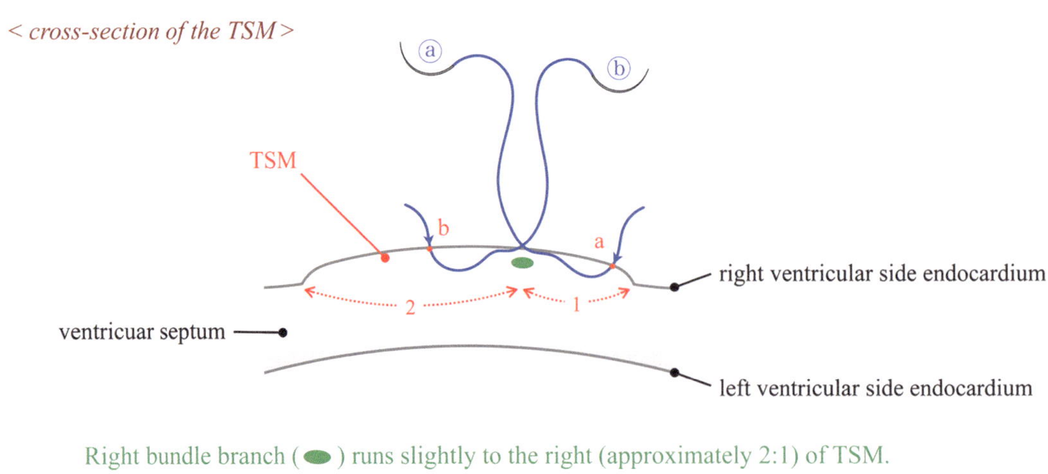

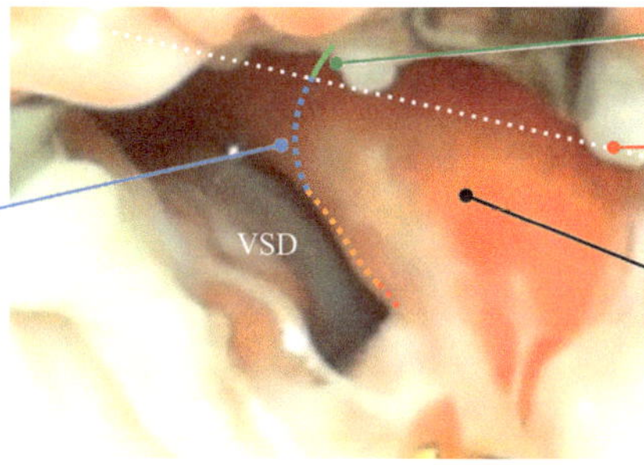

Fig. 4.7 Suture at the antero-inferior margin

ⓐ Insert a slightly deeper insertion point (point (a)) far enough away from the assumed site of the right bundle branch pathway. As the needle approaches the right bundle branch, it is advanced more shallowly, and near the right bundle branch, the needle is advanced as if it were sliding under the endocardium, and then stitched out.

ⓑ Insert the needle into the site (point (b)) contralateral to point (a), and move the needle in the same way as for point (ⓐ).

3 Closure of Perimembranous VSD (Surgical Video)

Perimembranous Outlet VSD Closure Without Use of the Membranous Flap (Scene 4.1)

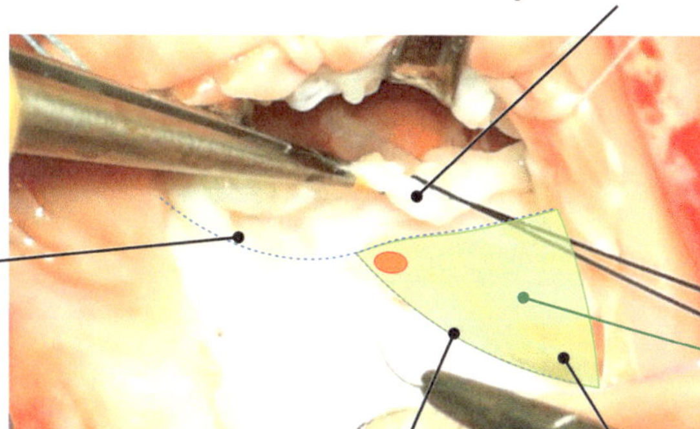

Scene 4.1 Confirmation of VSD morphology and surrounding structures 1 (Video 00 min 18 s)

1 Identify the atrioventricular node (apex of Koch's triangle) from the atrial side.

- Identify the tendon of Tadaro, coronary sinus, and tricuspid valve ring.
- Confirmation of Koch's triangle (Scene 4.2).

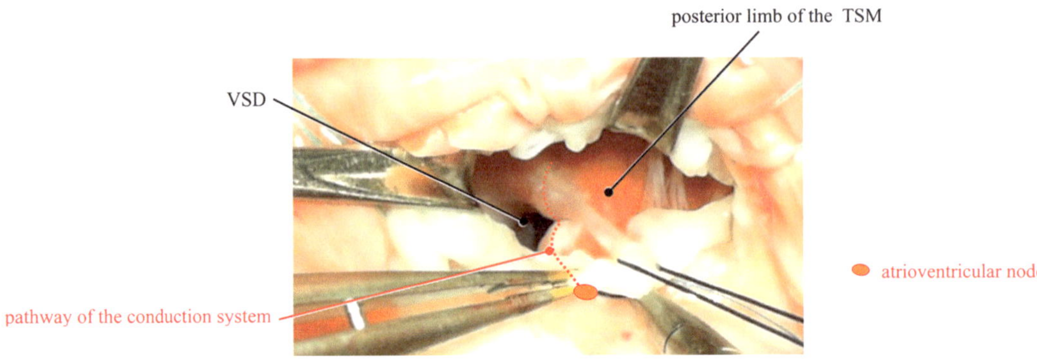

Scene 4.2 Confirmation of VSD morphology and surrounding structures 2 (Video 00 min 30 s)

1. Invert the tricuspid valve septal leaflet to check the morphology of the postero-inferior margin of the VSD.

- *Thickness of the posterior limb of the trabecular septomarginalis (TSM)*: In this case, the posterior limb of the TSM is thick and covers the inferior margin of the VSD.
- *Configuration of the postero-inferior margin of the VSD*: The postero-inferior margin of the VSD is classified as outlet type because it is located on the outflow channel side (left side of the screen) rather than Koch's triangle (if it is located on the inflow side rather than Koch's triangle apex, it is classified as inlet type).
- *Size of the membranous flap*: The membranous flap is present but too small to be used for VSD closure (Scene 4.3).

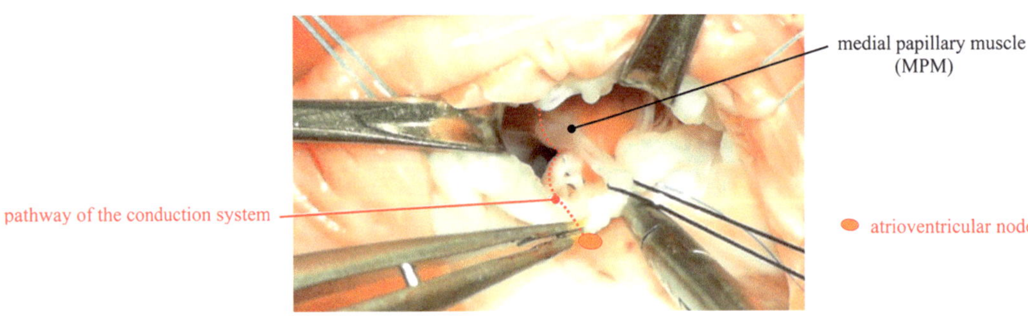

Scene 4.3 VSD closure 1 (Video 00 min 56 s)

1. In this case, the membranous flap is small, so sutures are placed from the atrial side of the septal leaflet to the inferior edge of the membranous flap.

- The suture is a 6-0 monofilament suture with an ePTFE tip.
- The insertion point on the atrial side is approximately 2 mm from the valve annulus (if it is too close to the annulus, the pledget may press on the AV node after ligation) (Scene 4.4).

Scene 4.4 VSD closure 2 (Video 01 min 28 s)

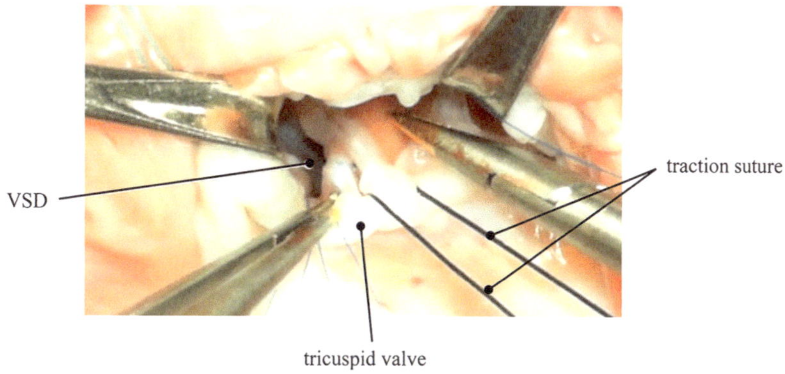

1 The traction suture over the chordae tendineae (black suture) and the sutures placed over the tricuspid valve annulus are pulled anteriorly to secure the field of view of the VSD.
2 The suture is placed so that the puncture point is approximately 2 mm away from the VSD margin.

- Because the posterior limb of the TSM thickly covers the inferior margin of the VSD, the conduction system is far from the right ventricular side endocardium.
- Therefore, even if the suture is placed close to the VSD margin, damage to the conduction system can be avoided (however, the suture needle should not be inserted too deeply) (Scene 4.5).

Scene 4.5 VSD closure 3 (Video 02 min 10 s)

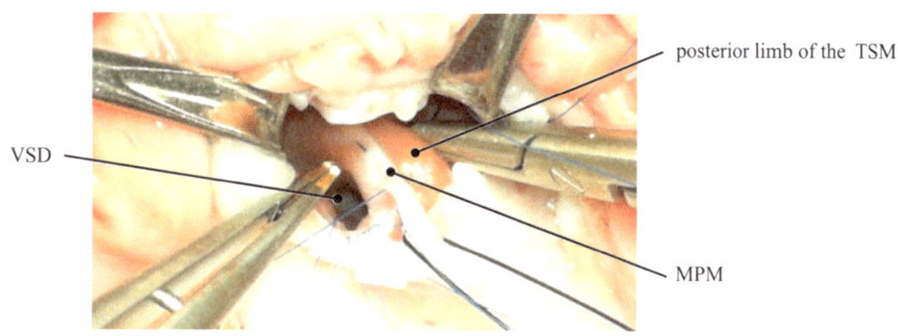

1 Insert the suture needle deeply into the posterior limb of the TSM and stitch out from the lower part of the medial papillary muscle (MPM).

- The lower part of the MPM can be used for suturing, since the medial papillary muscle does not contain the conduction system.
- The stitch-out point should be no closer to the VSD margin than the base of the papillary muscle (Scene 4.6).

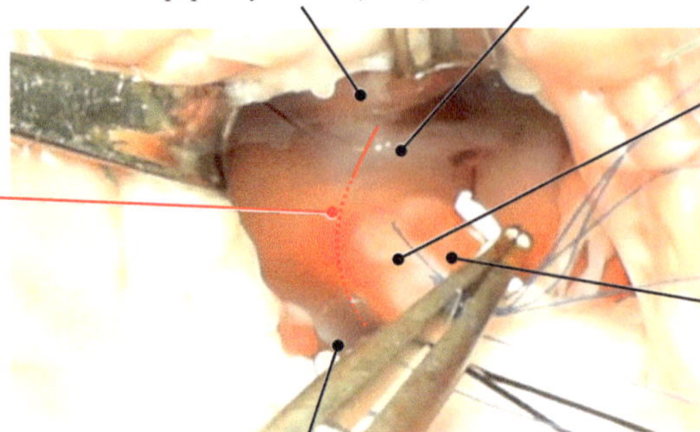

Scene 4.6 Confirmation of pathway of the conduction system (Video 02 min 25 s)

- The presumed course of the right bundle branch (RBB) is shown.
- The RBB runs slightly deeper within the muscular layer near the base of the middle papillary muscle (*red dotted line*).
- The RBB runs from the antero-inferior margin of the VSD to the base of the anterior papillary muscle, slightly to the right of the center of the trabecular septomarginalis (TSM).
- The RBB runs away from the VSD margin and the RBB becomes shallowly subendocardial (*solid red line*) (Scene 4.7).

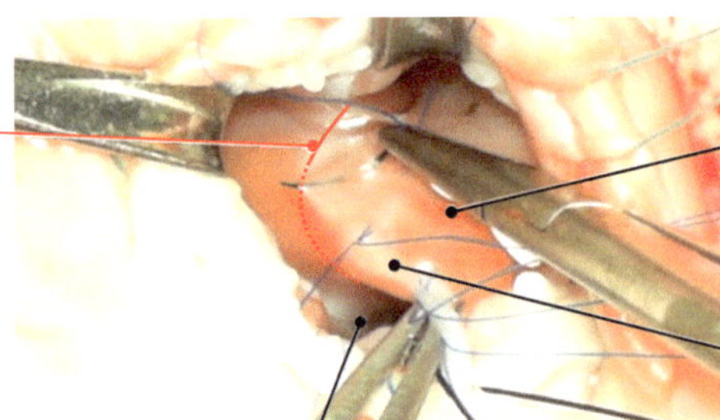

Scene 4.7 VSD closure 4 (Video 02 min 46 s)

- Perform suture on the inflow side across the RBB.

1 After inserting into the TSM, the needle is advanced shallowly as it approaches the RBB, and then slid under the endocardium before stitching into the lumen.

- Directly above the RBB, the suture needle is placed on the endocardium only (Scene 4.8).

Scene 4.8 VSD closure 5 (Video 02 min 57 s)

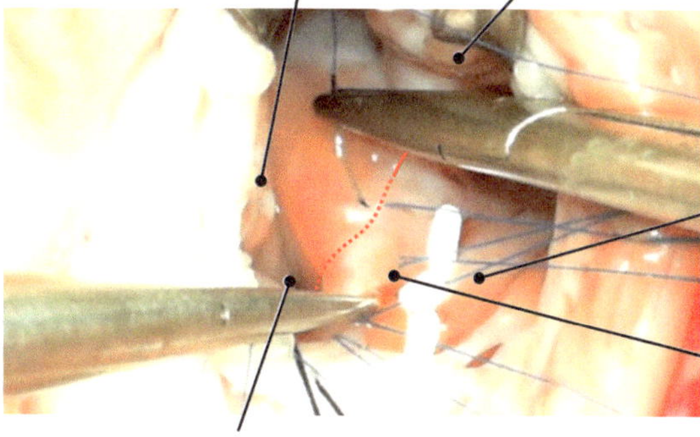

1 The first suture needle movement on the outflow tract side across the RBB is also inserted into the anterior limb of the TSM, then the suture needle is advanced shallowly as it approaches the RBB and advanced to slide under the endocardium before suturing out of the endocardium (Scene 4.9).

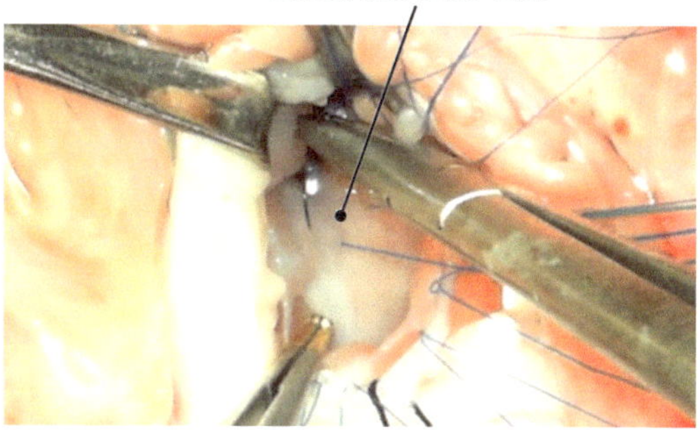

Scene 4.9 VSD closure 6 (Video 03 min 25 s)

1 The anterior margin of the VSD is firmly inserted into the VSD margin.

- If the field of view from the anterior to the superior margin of the VSD is poor, the suture placed in front of the VSD margin is tractioned toward the right side (inflow side) to bring the VSD margin forward and secure the visual field.
- The aortic valve is located on the left ventricular side of the superior margin of the VSD. To avoid damaging the aortic valve, the suture is placed anterior to the aortic valve annulus (Scene 4.10).

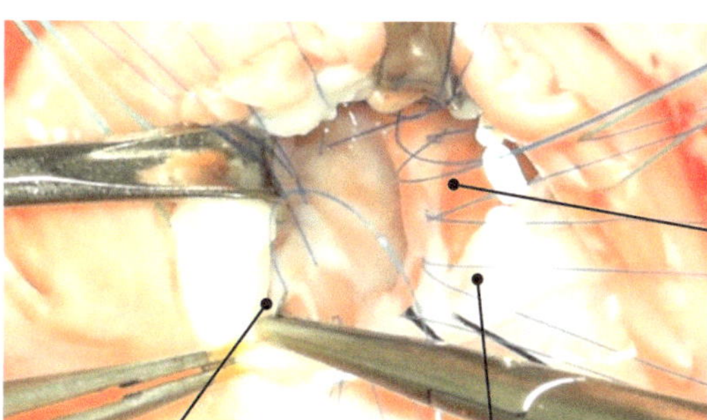

Scene 4.10 VSD closure 7 (Video 04 min 49 s)

1 Place the suture on the ventriculo-infundibular fold (VIF) of the postero-superior margin of the VSD.

- If it is difficult to place the suture only on the muscle bundle of the VIF, the suture may be placed through the valve annulus from the right atrial side (Scene 4.11).

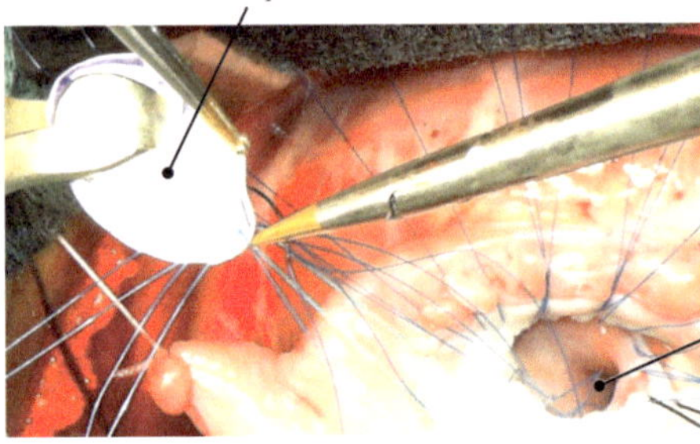

Scene 4.11 VSD closure 8 (Video 05 min 20 s)

1 Place the suture counterclockwise on a 0.4-mm thick ePTFE patch that has been trimmed to a slightly larger size, including the seam allowance.

- It is easier for the first assistant to assist (prepare the next suture) if you proceed in a counterclockwise direction (Scene 4.12).

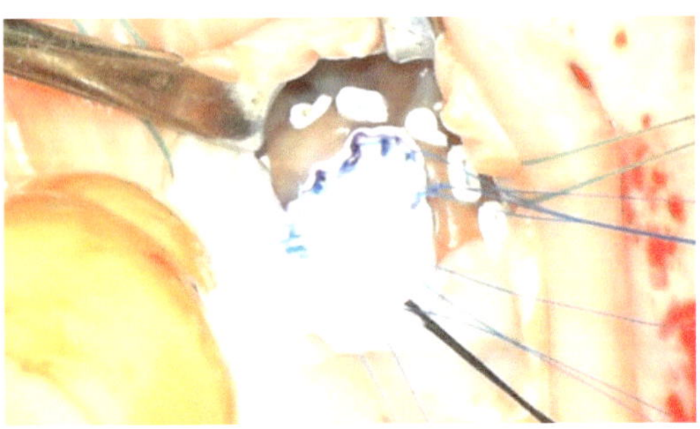

Scene 4.12 VSD closure 9 (Video 05 min 31 s)

1 Starting from the suture at the postero-superior margin of the VSD, ligate the sutures in a clockwise direction.

- The next suture is traction sutured toward the operator to expand the field of view, making it easier to ligate in a clockwise direction (Scene 4.13).

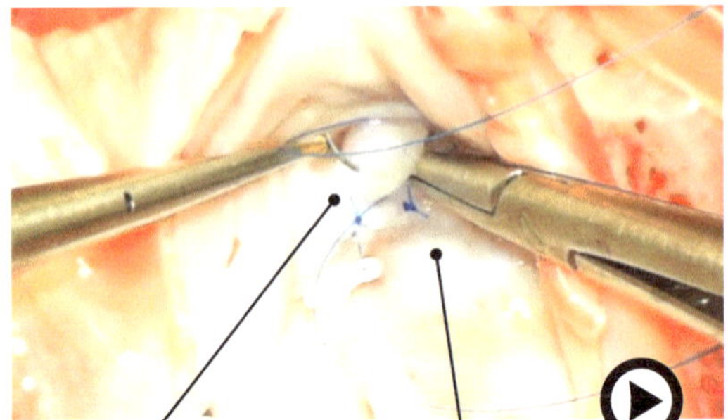

Scene 4.13 Tricuspid valvuloplasty (Video 06 min 25 s) (▶ https://doi.org/10.1007/000-hka)

1 Perform a water test and close the tricuspid valve antero-septal leaflet commissure located above the VSD patch is closed with interrupted 6-0 monofilament sutures.

- Failure to suture closure of the tricuspid valve antero-septal leaflet commissure and deep leaflet indentation may result in regurgitation in the remote phase.

References

Classification of the VSD and Conduction System

Anderson RH, Becker AE. In: Stark J, de Leval M, Tsang VT, editors. The anatomy of ventricular septal defects and their conduction tissues. In Surgery for congenital heart defects. 3rd ed. England: Wiley; 2006. p. 121–43.

Kurosawa H. Conduction system and cardiac surgery. Toyo: Igaku Shoin; 2013.

Atrioventricular Septal Defect (AVSD)

5

1 Atrioventricular Septal Defect

1.1 Morphology of Atrioventricular Septal Defect

An atrioventricular septal defect (AVSD) is a condition in which the ventricular septal inlet (inlet septum) is defective as a result of defective fusion or dysplasia of the endocardial cushion during cardiac development. This results in the following morphological features (Figs. 5.1 and 5.2).

1. Scooping of the upper edge of the ventricular septum due to a defect in the inflow portion of the ventricular septum.
2. Regardless of the disease type, scooping results in a narrowing of the left ventricular outflow tract (goose-neck sign).
3. The aortic valve is deviated anteriorly (non-wedged position) and is not in the normal position between the two atrioventricular valves (wedged position).
4. The atrioventricular valve is classified into incomplete type, intermediate type, and complete type according to its morphology.
5. The incomplete type has an atrial septal defect (primary foramen), while the intermediate and complete types have both an atrial septal defect (primary foramen) and a ventricular septal defect.
6. The atrioventricular valve has five valve leaflets and five papillary muscles (two on the left ventricular side and three on the right ventricular side).
7. Abnormal position of the left ventricular papillary muscles (anterior papillary muscle deviated to the right: closer to the left ventricular outflow tract, posterior papillary muscle deviated to the left: the distance between the two papillary muscles is also closer).
8. The AV node is deviated posteriorly and located above the inferior end of the ventricular septum.

Aortic Valve

- Aortic valve is anteriorly deviated because of the common atrioventricular valve ring.
- Aortic valve is not wedged (unwedged position) between both atrioventricular valves as in the normal heart.

Left-Sided Papillary Muscle

- Anterior papillary muscle deviated to the right ( ) and posterior papillary muscle deviated to the left ( ).

Supplementary Information The online version contains supplementary material available at https://doi.org/10.1007/978-981-96-6194-7_5. The videos can be accessed individually by clicking the DOI link in the accompanying figure caption or by scanning this link with the SN More Media App.

M. Yamagishi, *Surgical Treatment of Congenital Heart Disease*,
https://doi.org/10.1007/978-981-96-6194-7_5

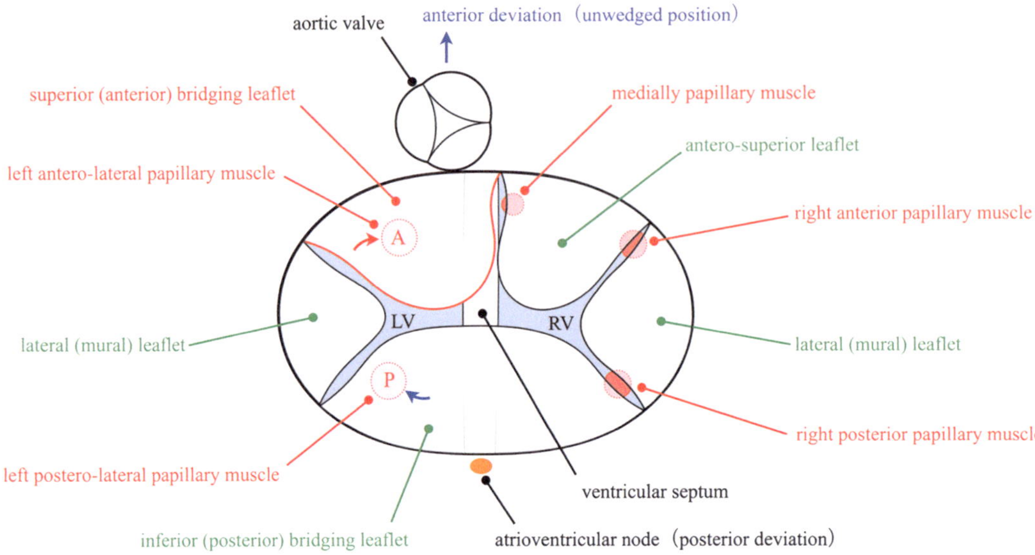

Fig. 5.1 Morphology of AVSD

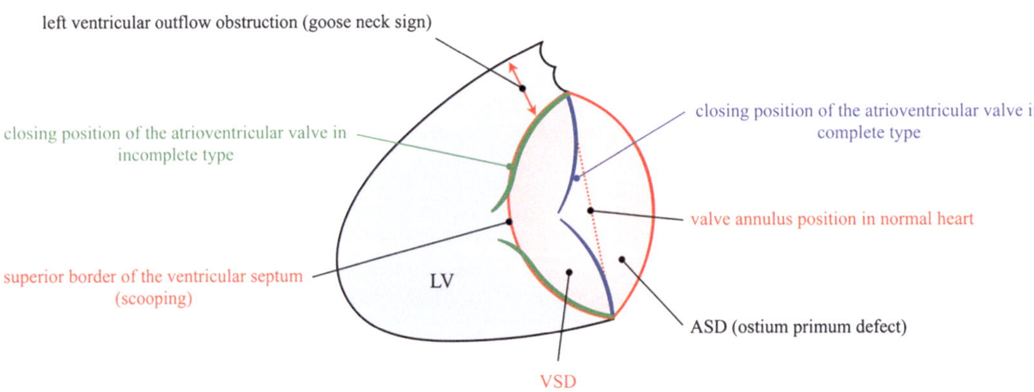

Fig. 5.2 Morphology of AVSD (left ventricular aspect)

- Rightward deviation of the anterior papillary muscle (↗) may induce left ventricular outflow tract obstruction.
- Distance between papillary muscles is also closer.

Atrioventricular Node

- Deviated posteriorly, located at the junction of the posterior inferior margin of the ventricular septum and the atrioventricular valve ring.
- In the complete type, the atrioventricular valve is located above the septum, whereas in the incomplete type, the valve ring is attached to the superior border of the ventricular septum.
- This can cause significant left ventricular outflow tract stenosis in the incomplete and intermediate types.
- In the "modified one patch" procedure for the complete type, the atrioventricular valve is dropped onto the superior border of the ventricular septum, which may result in left ventricular outflow tract stenosis as in the partial type.

1.2 Conduction System of Atrioventricular Septal Defect

The stimulus conduction system of atrioventricular septal defects is characterized by (1) the atrioventricular node being deviated posteriorly from the normal heart and located at the posterior inferior margin of the ventricular septum and (2) the ventricular conduction tract running long at the ridge of the ventricular septum (Fig. 5.3).

1.3 Classification of Complete Type AVSD

Complete atrioventricular septal defect consists of a single valve annulus and a common atrioventricular valve. The type of complete atrioventricular septal defect is classified according to the morphology of the common anterior leaflet (superior bridging leaflet) (Rastelli classification) (Fig. 5.4).

- Most frequent type (approx. 60%).
- Most non-21-trisomy cases are type A.
- 40% of 21-trisomy cases are type A.
- The superior bridging leaflet is divided just above the ventricular septum and the tendon cords attach to the ventricular septum.
- The divided right ventricular side leaflet is antero-superior leaflet.
- The common posterior leaflet (inferior bridging leaflet) is also divided in some cases.
- The left ventricular side leaflet of the common posterior leaflet often has a deep indentation.
- Left ventricular outflow tract stenosis is common.

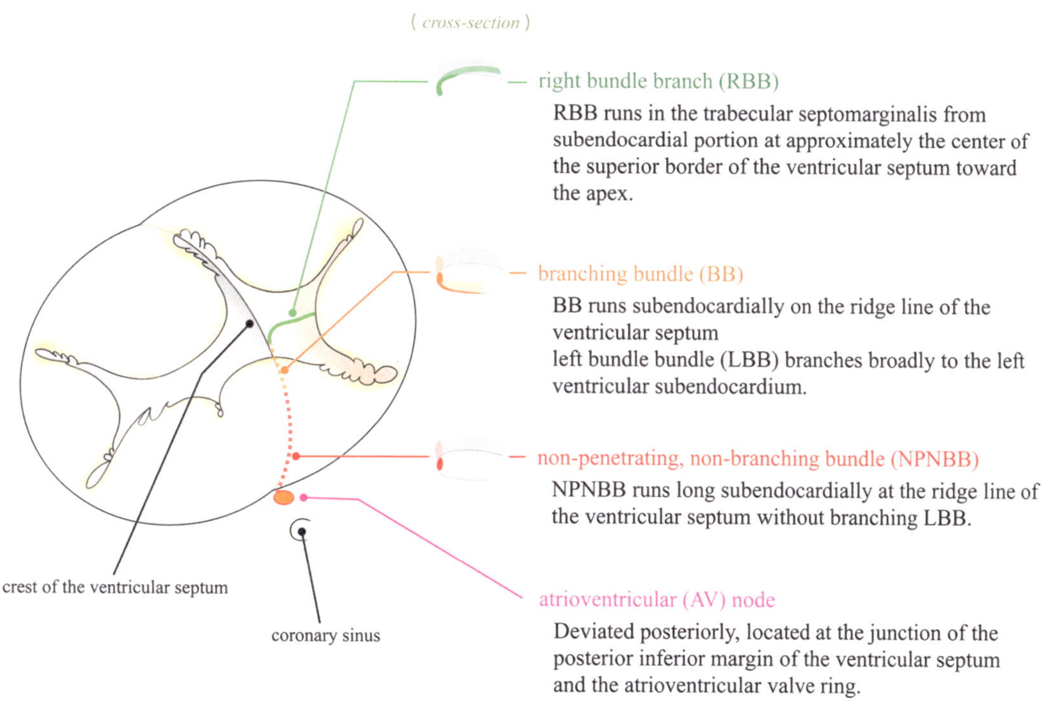

Fig. 5.3 Conduction system of AVSD

Rastelli type A

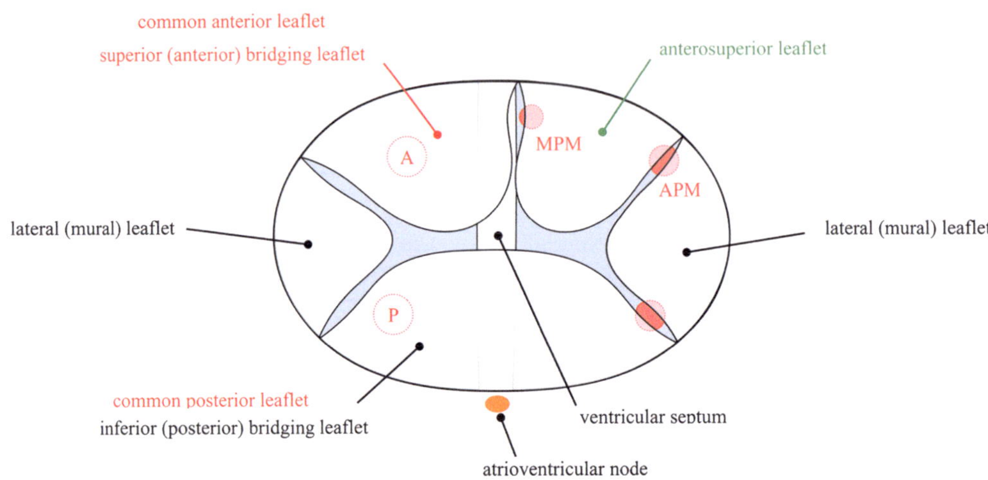

Fig. 5.4 Morphological characteristics of complete type AVSD

Rastelli type B

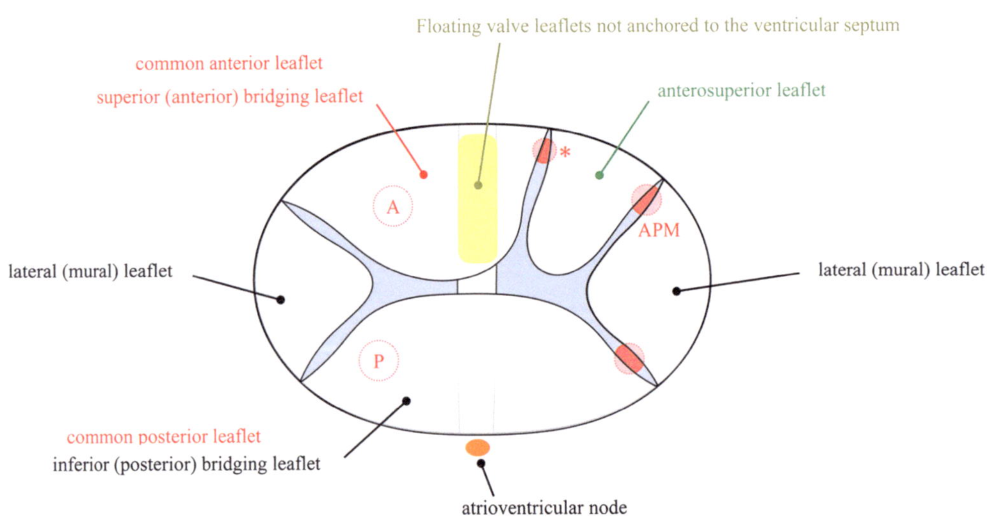

- Rare type (approx. 5%).
- The right ventricular side common anterior leaflet is divided into antero-superior leaflet.
- Antero-superior leaflet is smaller than that of type A.
- Fused papillary muscles (*) are seen below divided part of the right ventricular side common anterior leaflet.
- The common anterior leaflet is not fixed with the superior border of the ventricular septum by chordae (floating leaflet).

■ *Rastelli type C*

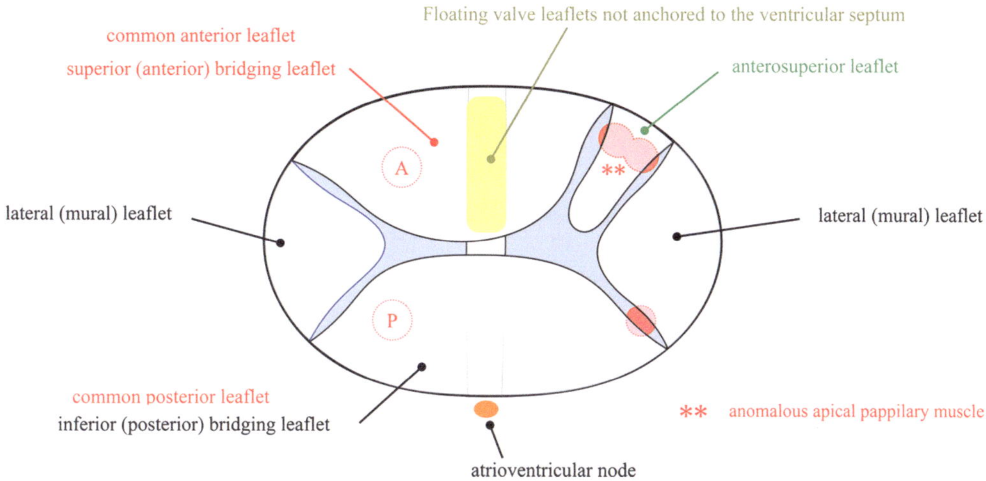

- Second most common type (approx. 35%).
- 60% of 21-trisomy cases are type C (remaining 40% are type A).
- The common anterior leaflet is not fixed with the superior border of the ventricular septum by chordae (floating leaflet).
- The right ventricular side common anterior leaflet is divided into fairly small anterosuperior leaflets.
- Fused papillary muscles (* *) are seen below divided part of the right ventricular side common anterior leaflet.

1.4 Morphology of Partial (Incomplete) Type AVSD and Intermediate Type AVSD (Fig. 5.5)

- Two valve annulus and two valve orifices.
- Cleft in the anterior leaflet of the left atrioventricular valve (mitral valve).
- Complicated by ostium primum defect.
- Uncomplicated ventricular septal defect.

Fig. 5.5 Morphological characteristics of partial and intermediate type AVSD

■ *partial type AVSD*

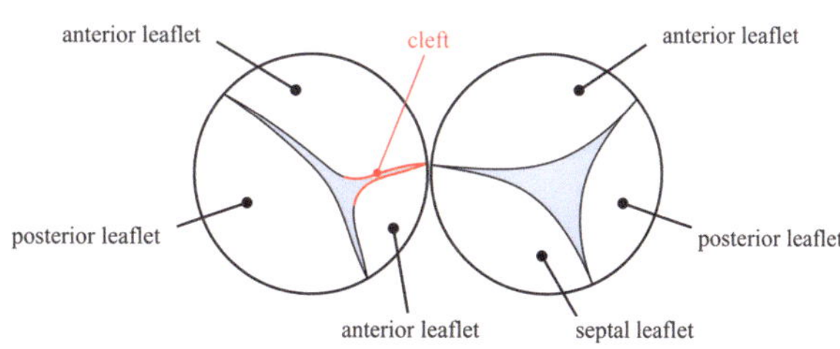

■ *intermediate type AVSD*

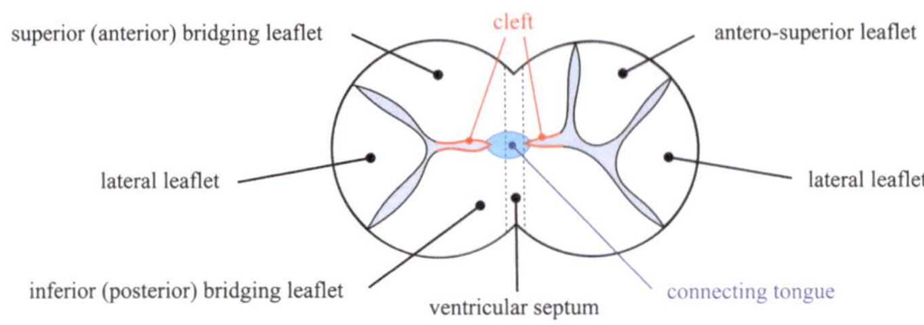

- One valve annulus and two valve orifices.
- Superior bridging leaflet and inferior bridging leaflet are continuous just above the ventricular septum (connecting tongue).
- Complicated by ostium primum defect and small ventricular septal defect.

2 Surgery for Complete Type Atrioventricular Septal Defect

Surgical techniques for complete AVSD include (1) the two patch technique (closure of the ASD and VSD with separate patches), (2) the one patch technique (incising the atrioventricular valve and closing the ASD and VSD with a single patch), and (3) the modified one patch technique (dropping the atrioventricular valve into the ventricular septum and closing the remaining ASD with a single patch).

The two patch method (coronary sinus returns to the right atrial side), which is the most common and least likely to cause postoperative complications, will be discussed in detail (Fig. 5.6).

2.1 Two Patch Repair

- The water test is performed, and a 6-0 monofilament suture is applied to the point just above the ventricular septum where the superior bridging leaflet and the inferior bridging leaflet touch (dividing point).
- The atrioventricular valve is divided into right and left at this point.
- The dividing point should be slightly toward the right ventricle so that more mitral component remains.

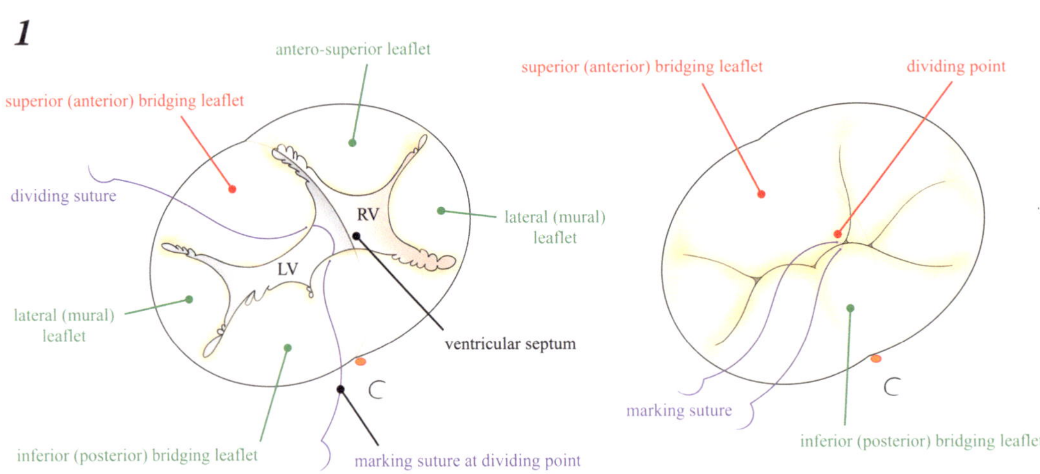

Fig. 5.6 Two patch technique for complete type AVSD

2

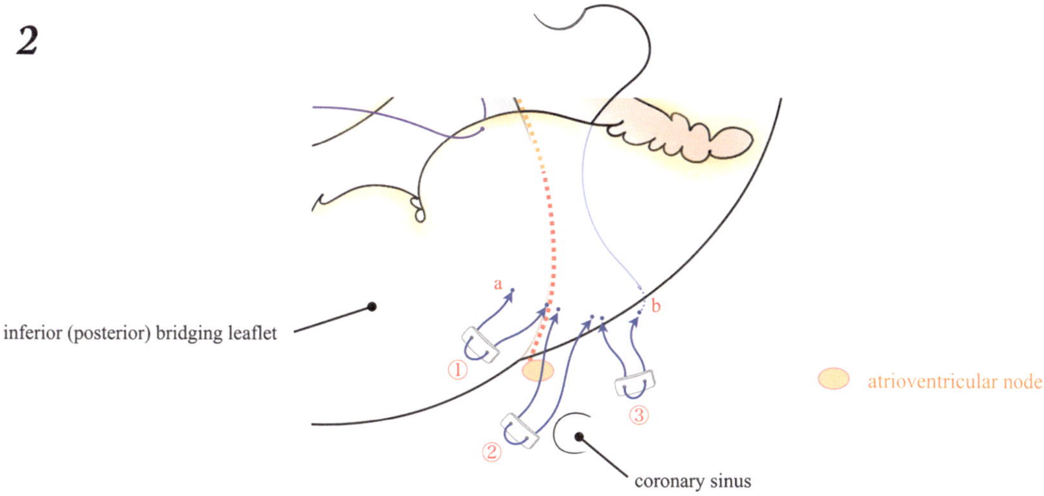

- Start the suture from the posterior edge of the VSD.
- Apply a 6-0 monofilament suture with pledget from the atrial side to the ventricular side of the inferior bridging leaflet approximately 5 mm from the valve annulus to avoid the AV node (②).
- The suture needle ①a is inserted into the inferior bridging leaflet and stitched out from the ventricular side of the leaflet, slightly closer to the valve annulus.
- The suture needle ③b is inserted through the valve annulus and stitched-out from top of the ventricular septum slightly away from the valve annulus (transitional stich).

3

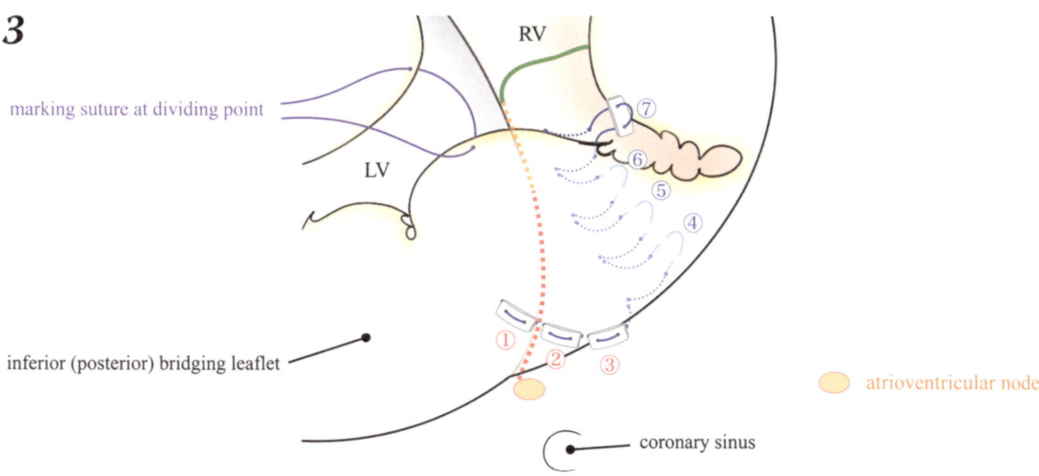

- Start suture from the posterior edge of the VSD.
- The first stitch ④ is placed at the same site as the stitched-out point of ③b.
- The stitches ④ to ⑦ on the right ventricular side of the ventricular septum (below the inferior bridging leaflet) are gradually brought closer to the edge of the ventricular septal defect.
- Since the conduction system runs along the upper edge of the ventricular septum (crest of the defect), the stitched-out points of sutures ⑥ and ⑦ should be placed about 3 mm away from the limbus.
- The chordae tendineae below the inferior bridging leaflet should be preserved as much as possible.
- The sutures ④ to ⑦ should be passed through the chordae tendineae of the inferior bridging leaflet.

4

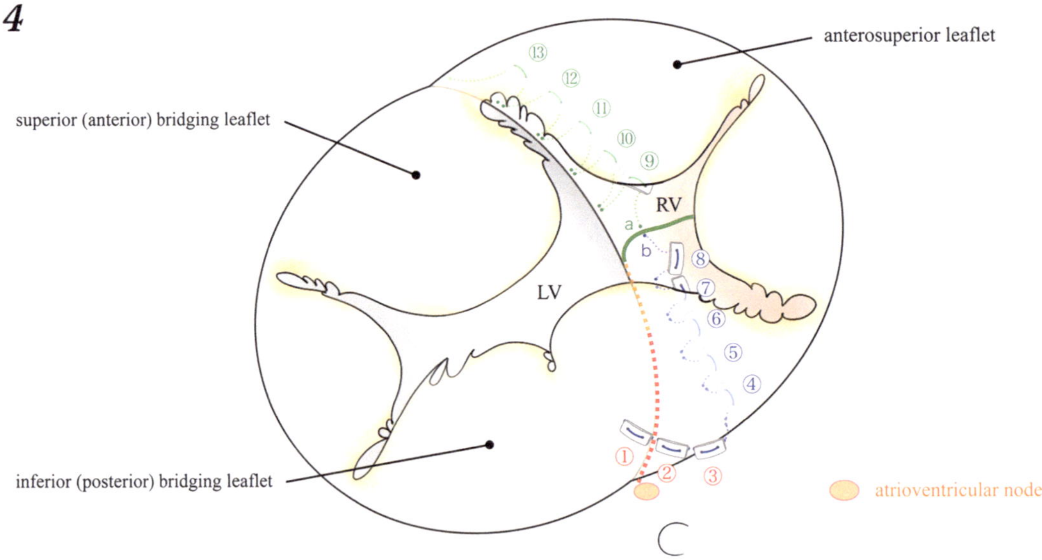

- The thick endocardium at the base of the chordae tendineae around RBB can be used as a stitched-out point.
- The puncture point for ⑩ through ⑬ should be the crest of the ventricular septal defect.
- Be careful to suture out the right ventricular side of the septal defect and not the chordae tendineae, which remain on the mitral side.

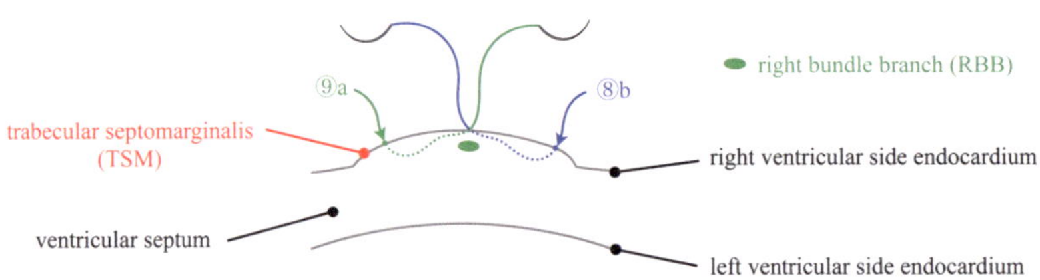

- Cross the RBB between ⑧b and ⑨a.
- The suture needle, inserted slightly deeper into the right ventricular endocardium, becomes shallower as it approaches the RBB and is advanced by sliding beneath the endocardium and stitched out.

5

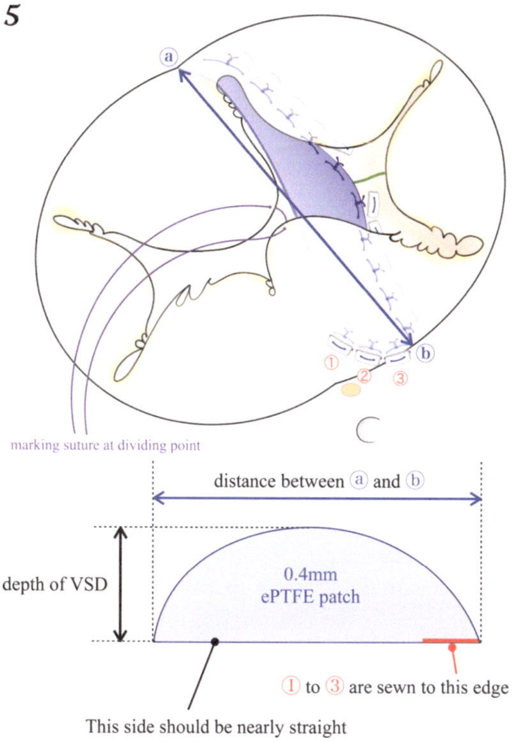

- Cut a 0.4-mm thick ePTFE patch in a semi-elliptical shape.
- The width of the patch is the distance from the anterior edge of the VSD (ⓐ) to the stitch-out point of the suture (ⓑ) at the posterior edge of the VSD (not the width of the AV valve).
- The width of the patch need not be less than the anterior-posterior diameter to reduce the annulus.
- The height of the ePTFE patch is the depth between the position of the dividing suture and the VSD apex when a water test is performed.

6

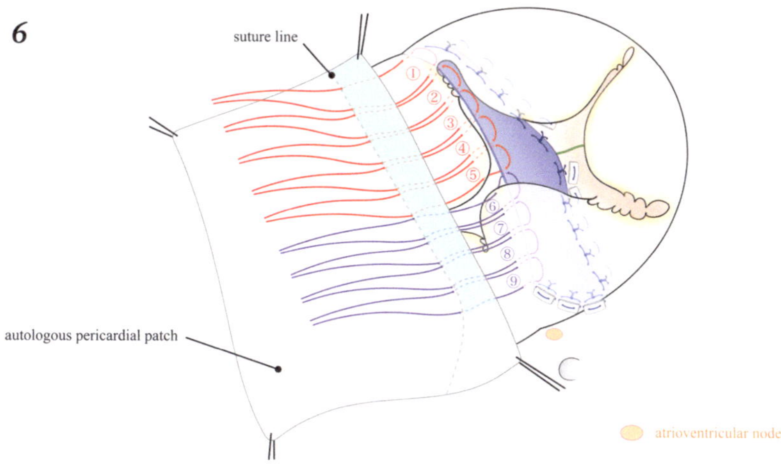

- Apply 6-0 monofilament sutures in the following order: VSD patch → atrioventricular valve → autologous pericardial patch (① - ⑨).
- In the case of type C (floating superior bridging leaflet), the suture is placed to the right of the superior bridging leaflet so that the mitral valve component is increased as much as possible.
- The suture ⑤ of the superior bridging leaflet and the suture ⑥ of the inferior bridging leaflet should be placed at the site of the dividing suture.

- In type A, the suture line of the autologous pericardium should be 5–7 mm from the edge.
- The autologous pericardium closer to the edge than the suture line (light blue area) is used to form the right ventricular side of the atrioventricular valve (especially the superior bridging leaflet).
- The junction of the superior and inferior bridging leaflets should be formed using the edge of the autologous pericardium, even in type C.

8

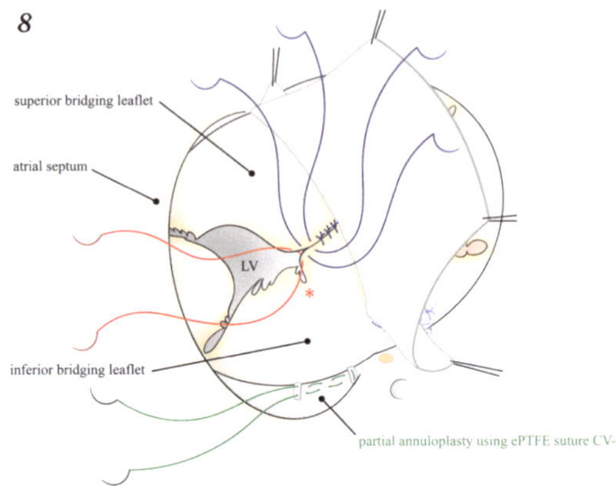

7

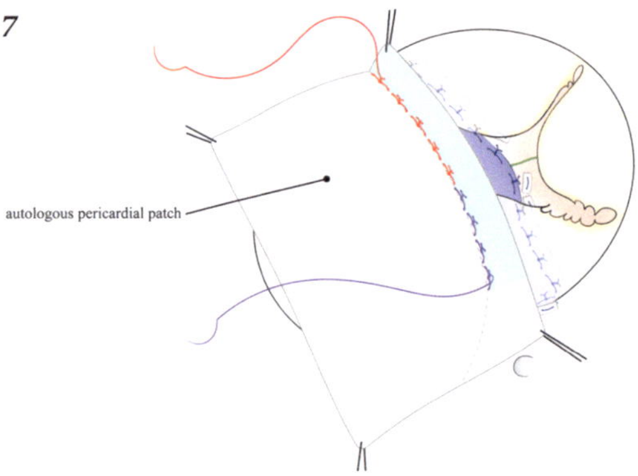

- Ligate the suture over the atrial septal patch.
- The sutures at both ends are left uncut for anastomosis to the atrial septum.

- Flip the autologous pericardium to the right atrial side.
- The remaining cleft between the superior bridging leaflet and inferior bridging leaflet is completely closed with a 6-0 monofilament suture.
- Suture closure of the cleft results in widening of the indentation (✱) of the inferior bridging leaflet, which may result in regurgitation from the indentation site.
- If regurgitation is observed after cleft closure, the valve annulus of the left-side atrioventricular valve corresponding to the indentation is sutured using a suture with autologous pericardial pledget (e.g., ePTFE suture CV-6).

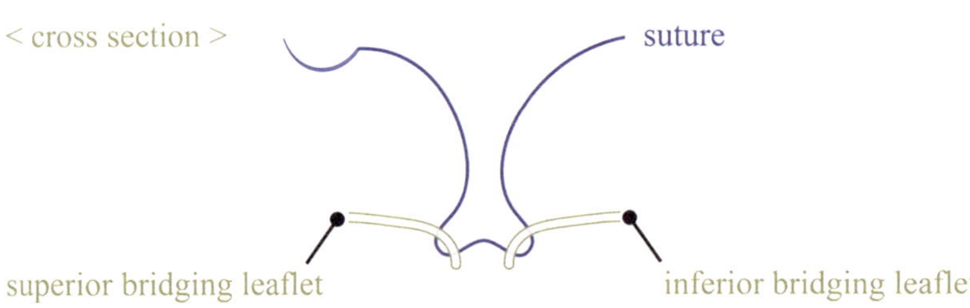

- Suture the valve leaflets so that the valve leaflets are flipped ventrally (valve leaflets stitched in from the atrial side → stitched out from the atrial side).

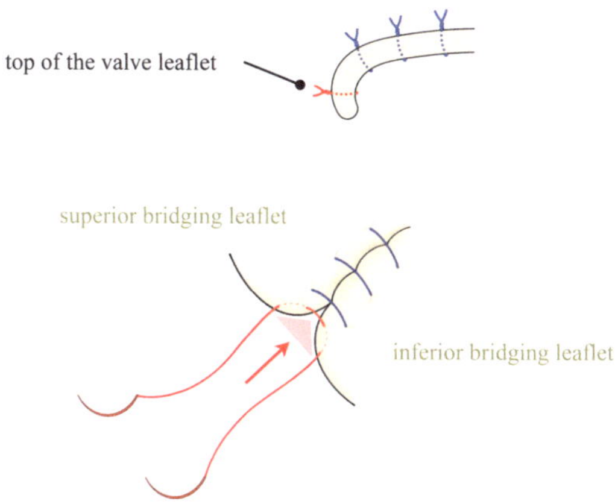

- Suture closure up to the coaptation zone at the top of the valve leaflet.
- If a triangular gap remains at the top of the cleft suture, regurgitation occurs and the possibility of reoperation remains.
- Avoid leaving a triangular gap (*red arrow*) at the apex of the valve leaflet.

9

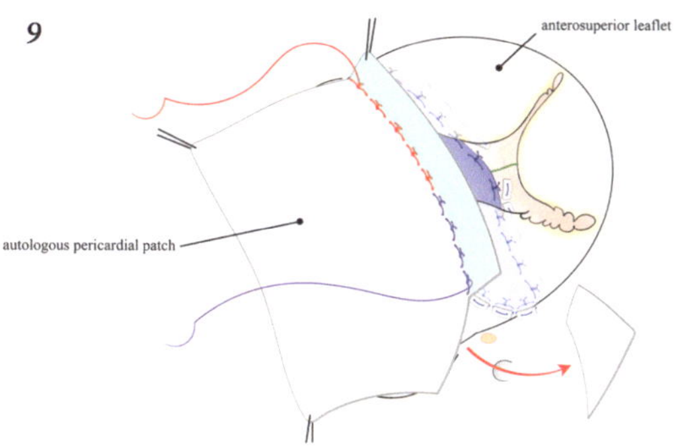

- Trim the posterior inferior margin of the autologous pericardial patch obliquely toward the posterior margin of the atrial septal defect.

10

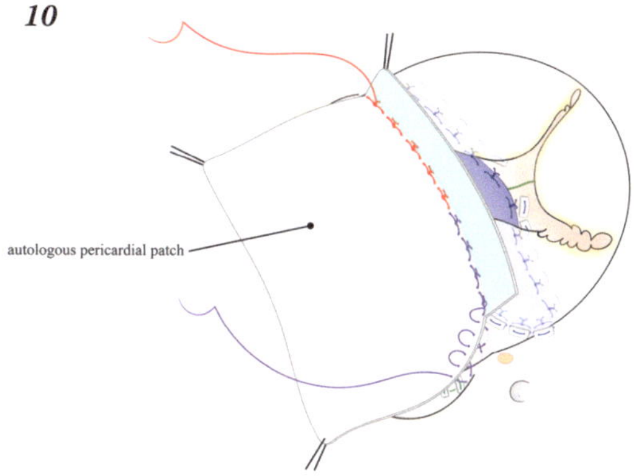

- Sew an autologous pericardial patch to the base of the inferior bridging leaflet, avoiding the AV node.
- The atrioventricular valve leaflet and autologous pericardial patch are sewn together with 6-0 monofilament mattress suture (the autologous pericardial side is half-backstitched to keep them close together).

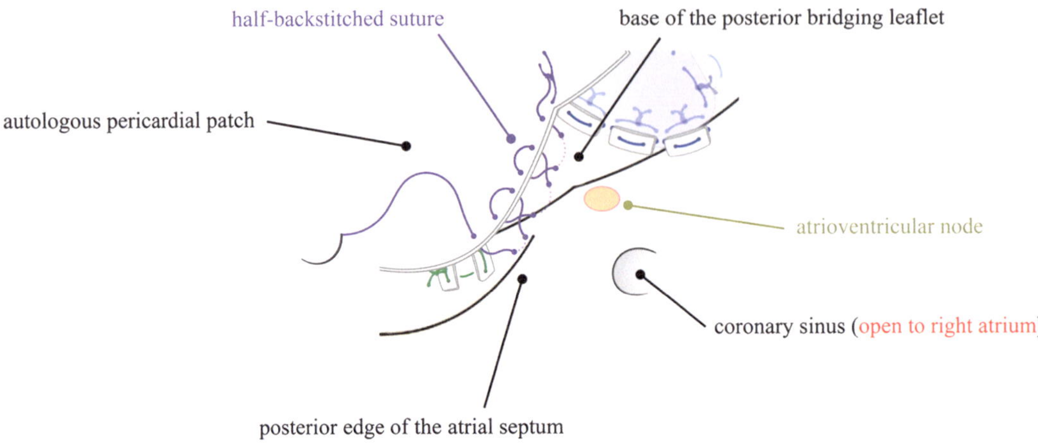

- Perform this half-backstitched suture across the atrial septum to the left ventricular side of the atrioventricular valve annulus, and when the left atrial side of the atrial septum is reached, continue with sutures to the edge of the atrial septum.
- The anastomosis to the atrial septum can be made with continuous sutures.

11

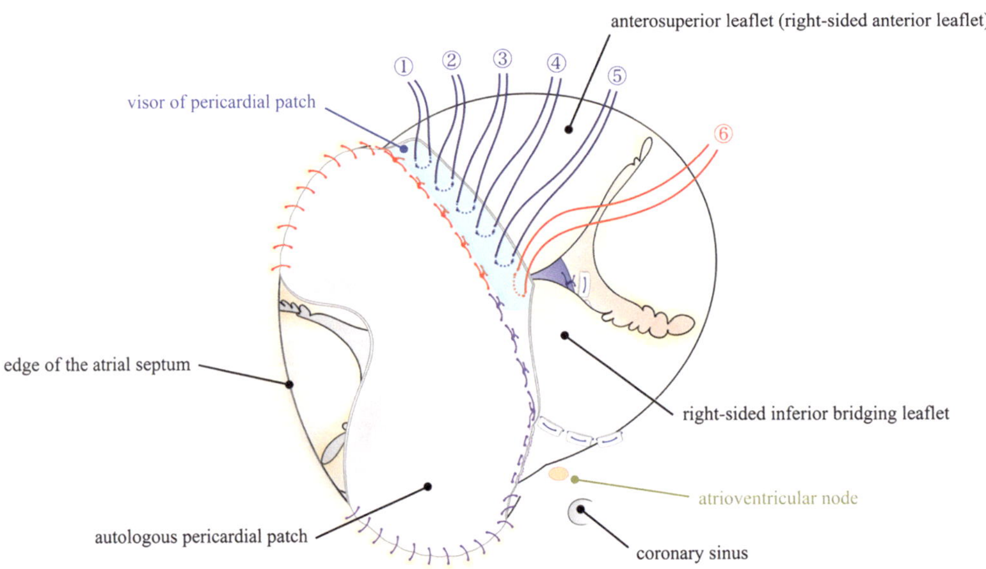

- The anterosuperior leaflet on the tricuspid valve side is sutured to the edge of the autologous pericardial patch left in the form of a bridge with interrupted 6-0 monofilament sutures (①: anterosuperior leaflet → autologous pericardial patch).
- The junction of the anterosuperior leaflet and the inferior bridging leaflet is also sutured to the edge of the autologous pericardial patch (⑤: autologous pericardial patch → anterosuperior leaflet → inferior bridging leaflet → autologous pericardial patch).

- The anterosuperior leaflet on the tricuspid valve side is now fixed to the atrial septum (new tricuspid valve ring).
- The top edge of the autologous pericardial patch is trimmed to match the shape of the ostium primum defect.
- The autologous pericardial patch is sutured to the edge of the atrial septum with a continuous 6-0 monofilament suture.

3 Repair of Type A Complete AVSD (Surgical Video) (Scene 5.1)

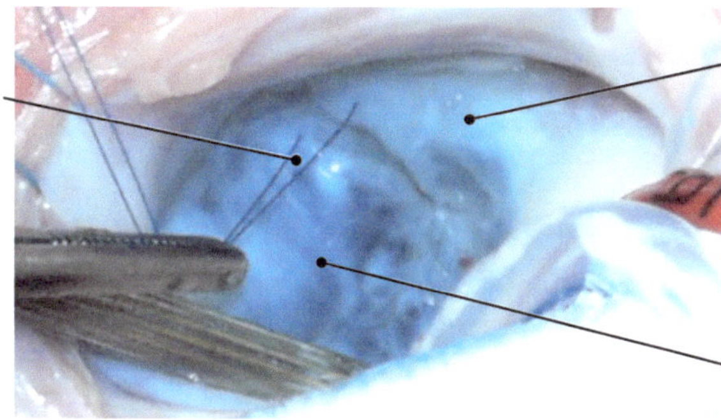

Scene 5.1 Marking suture at dividing point of the both bridging leaflet (Video 00 min 06 s)

1. After the atrioventricular valve is inflated with a water test, a 6-0 monofilament suture is placed just above the ventricular septum at the point where the superior bridging leaflet and inferior bridging leaflet meet (dividing suture).

- Apply slightly to the right so that more of the left-sided atrioventricular valve (mitral valve) component remains.
- Repeat the water test and reapply to obtain the best diving point (Scene 5.2).

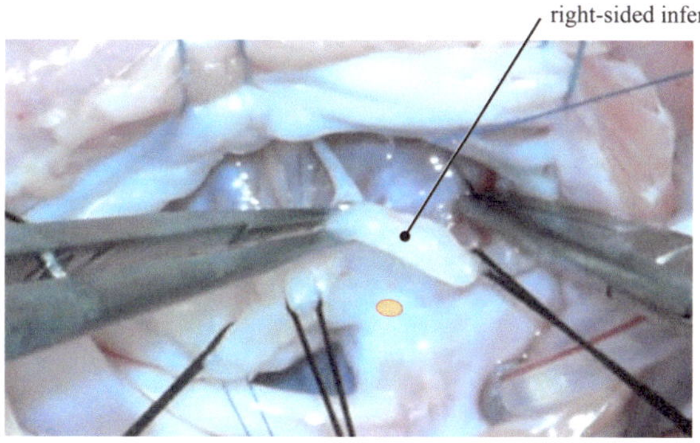

Scene 5.2 VSD closure 1 (Video 01 min 20 s)

1. A 6-0 monofilament suture with pledget for closure of a ventricular septal defect is inserted from the top of the ventricular septum and stitched-out just below the valve annulus away from the AV node.

- The suture can be started from the atrioventricular valve side (Scene 5.3).

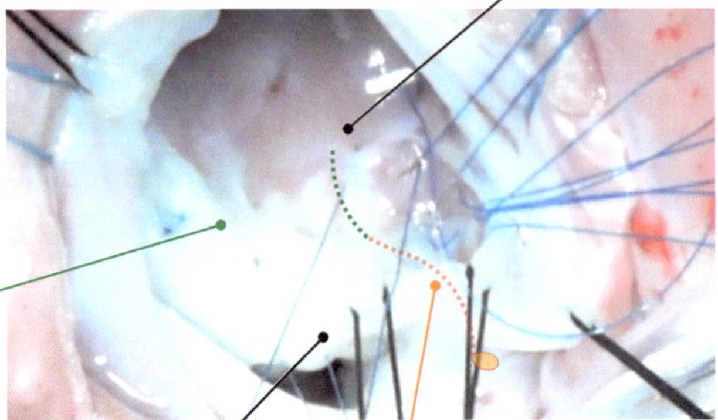

Scene 5.3 VSD closure 2 (Video 01 min 56 s)

1. The stitch-out point of the suture over the posterior ventricular septum (below the inferior bridging leaflet) is gradually brought closer to the edge of the ventricular septal defect.

- The stitch-out point should be approximately 3 mm from the edge of the septal defect because the conduction system runs along the edge of the septal defect.
- In the proximity of the right bundle branch, insert the suture needle only in the endocardium at the base of the chordae tendineae (Scene 5.4).

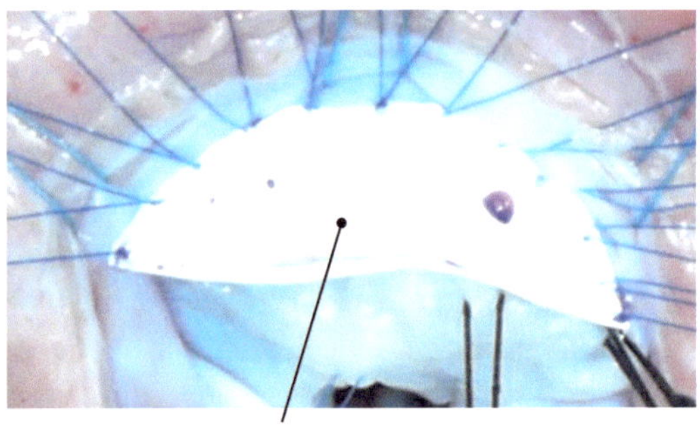

Scene 5.4 VSD closure 3 (Video 05 min 40 s)

1. The VSD is closed by passing a suture through the inferior edge of a 0.4-mm thick ePTFE patch cut in a semi-elliptical shape.

- The transverse diameter of the patch is the distance from the anterior edge of the AV valve annulus to the point of the suture at the posterior edge of the VSD.
- The height of the patch is the depth between the dividing suture and the apex of the VSD during the water test (Scene 5.5).

Scene 5.5 VSD closure 4 (Video 06 min 18 s)

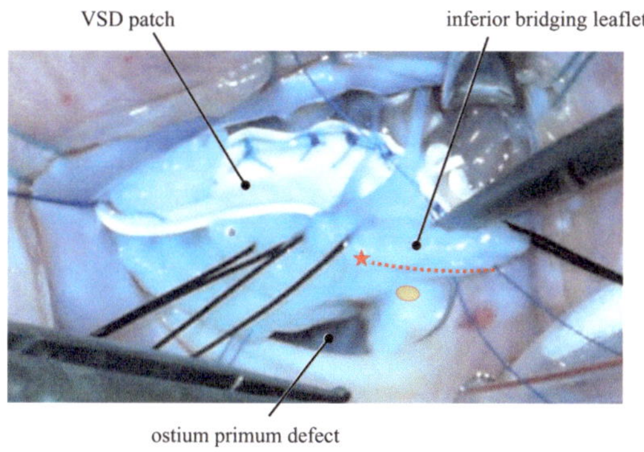

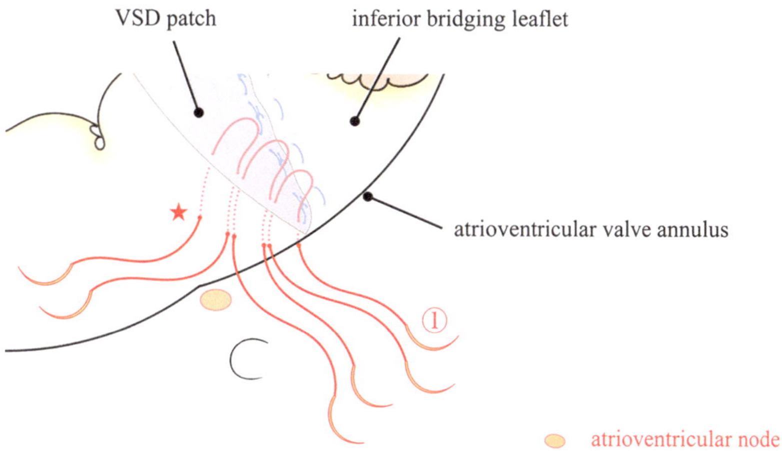

1. After threading 6-0 monofilament mattress sutures through the posterior-superior edge of the VSD patch, pierce them through from the ventricular side of the inferior bridging leaflet to the atrial side.

- Apply 2 or 3 sutures to the inferior bridging leaflet along the suture line (*red dotted line* in the figure above) going just above the ventricular septal defect (⑥).
- Use the inferior bridging leaflet as the suture line, keeping it away from the AV node.
- A suture with a pledgeted suture can be applied from the atrial side (Scene 5.6).

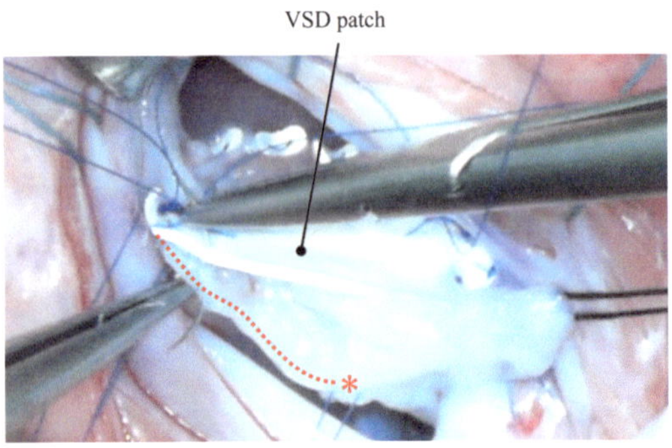

Scene 5.6 Anastomosis of superior edge of VSD patch and ASD closure 1 (Video 07 min 04 s)

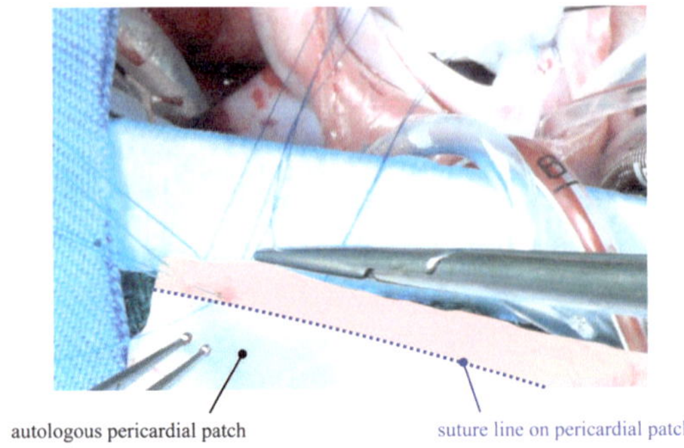

Scene 5.7 The suture line on the autologous pericardium (Video 07 min 50 sec)

1. Apply 6-0 monofilament sutures in the following order: superior edge of VSD patch → superior bridging leaflet → autologous pericardial patch.

- The needle of the 6-0 monofilament mattress suture is inserted at the point of the apex side of the coaptation zone of the superior bridging leaflet and stitched out on the suture line (*red dotted line*) toward the dividing suture (★) (Scene 5.7).

1. The suture line on the autologous pericardium (*blue dotted line*) should be located 5–7 mm from the edge.

- The autologous pericardium closer to the edge than the suture line (*light red area*) is used to form the right ventricular side of the atrioventricular valve (especially the superior bridging leaflet) (Scene 5.8).

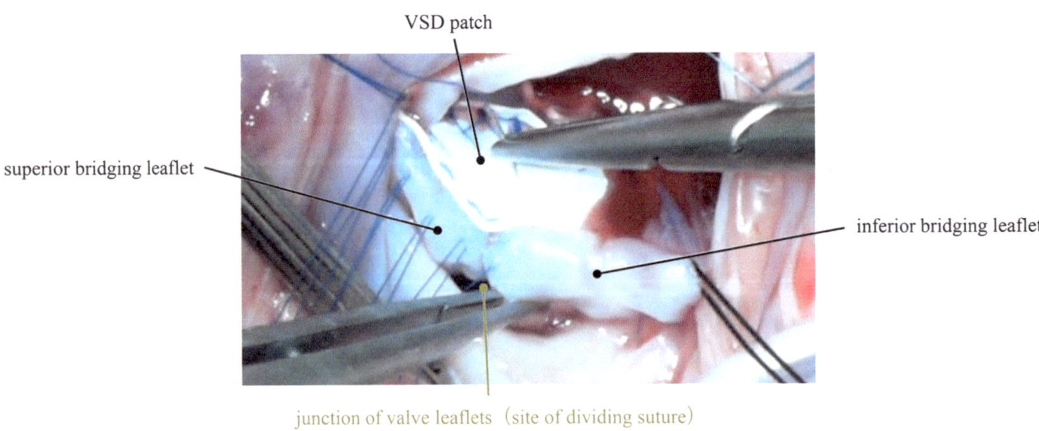

Scene 5.8 Anastomosis of superior edge of VSD patch and ASD closure 2 (Video 08 min 36 s)

1. At the dividing suture site, a mattress suture is applied from the upper edge of the VSD patch to the atrioventricular valve across the margins of both valve leaflets so that the anterior leaflet and common posterior leaflet are joined (Scene 5.9).

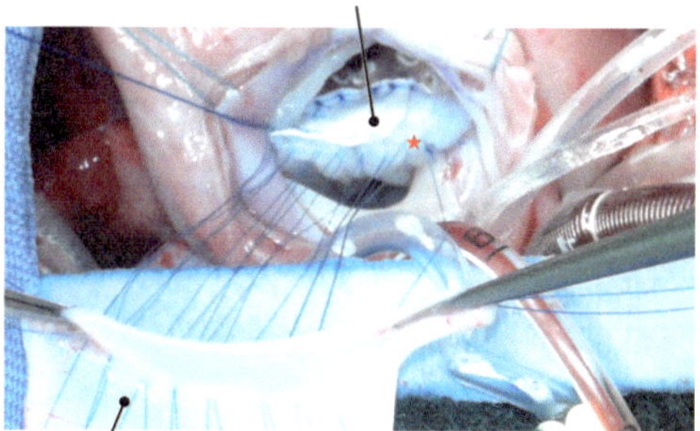

Scene 5.9 Anastomosis of superior edge of VSD patch and ASD closure 3 (Video 10 min 35 s)

1. Apply sutures to the site where the VSD patch and inferior bridging leaflet were anastomosed in Scene 5.5 (*) (apply sutures to the entire superior margin of the VSD patch).
2. Drop the autologous pericardial patch onto the new valve ring (superior edge of the ventricular septum) (Scene 5.10).

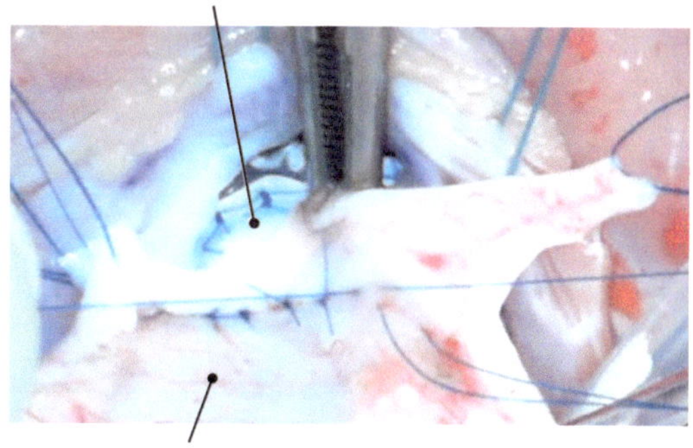

Scene 5.10 Anastomosis of superior edge of VSD patch and ASD closure 4 (Video 11 min 00 s)

1. Ligate sutures to fasten the autologous pericardial patch to the new valve ring and the upper edge of the VSD patch (Scene 5.11).

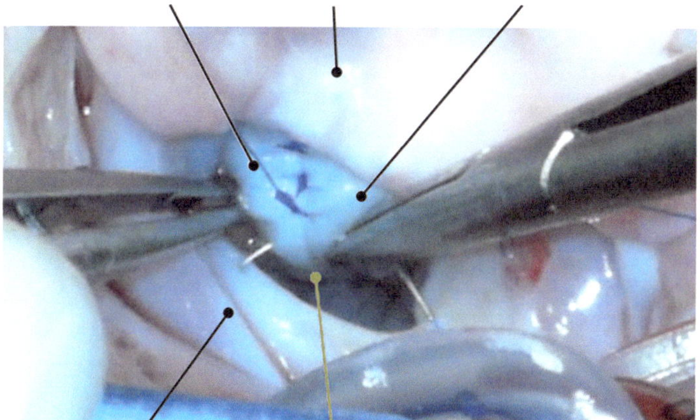

Scene 5.11 Left-sided AV valve cleft closure (Video 11 min 15 s)

1. The remaining cleft between the superior and inferior bridging leaflets on the left ventricular side is completely closed with interrupted suture of 6-0 monofilament sutures to the apex of the leaflets (Scene 5.12).

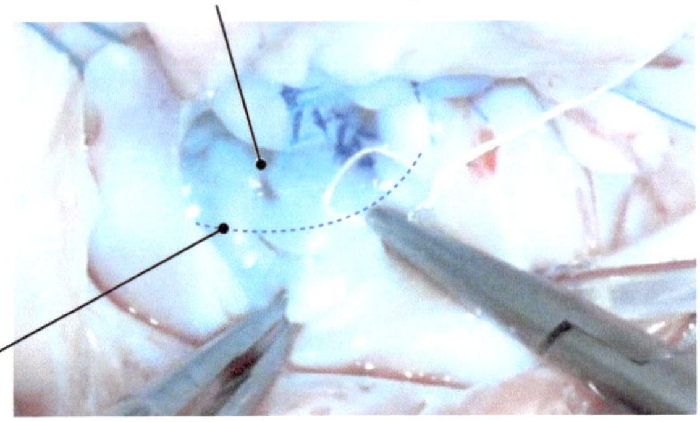

Scene 5.12 Left-sided AV valve annuloplasty (Video 15 min 02 s)

1. For residual regurgitation due to small indentation in the left-sided inferior bridging leaflet, an annuloplasty corresponding to the indentation is performed using ePTFE suture CV-6 with autologous pericardial pledget (Scene 5.13).

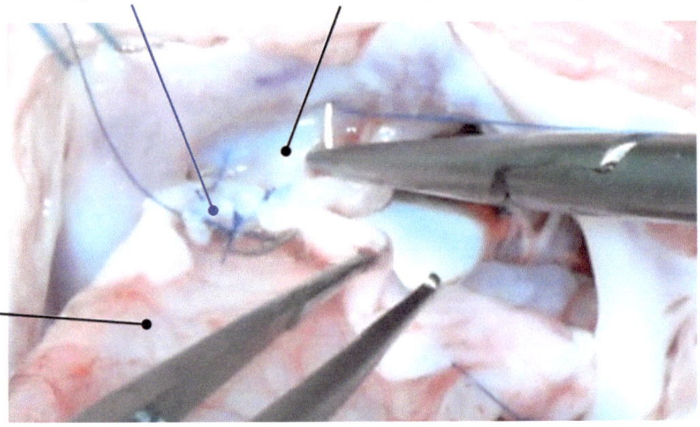

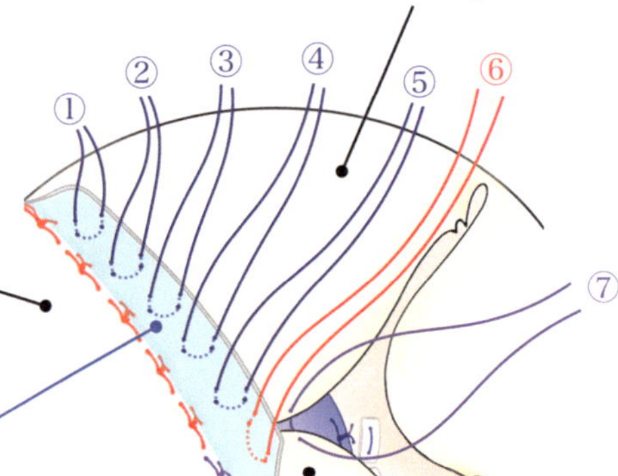

Scene 5.13 Right-sided AV valve annuloplasty (Video 16 min 20 s)

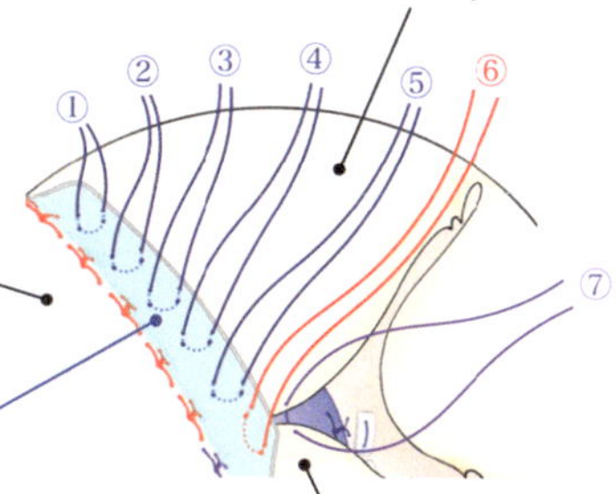

1. Antero-superior leaflet is sutured to the edge of the left visor-shaped autologous pericardial patch with interrupted 6-0 monofilament sutures (Scene 5.14).

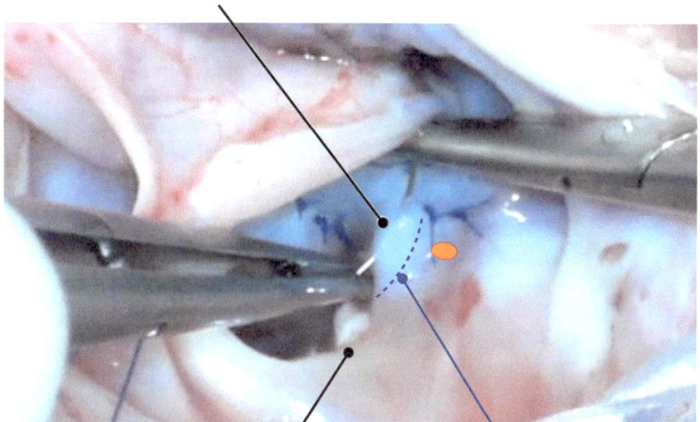

Scene 5.14 Anastomosis of pericardial patch to AV valve annulus (Video 20 min 05 s)

1. Sew an autologous pericardial patch to the base of the inferior bridging leaflet, avoiding the AV node.

- The atrioventricular valve leaflet and autologous pericardial patch are sewn together with 6-0 monofilament mattress suture (the autologous pericardial side is half-backstitched to keep them close together).

2. Perform this half-backstitched suture across the atrial septum to the left ventricular side of the atrioventricular valve annulus, and when the left atrial side of the atrial septum is reached, continue with sutures to the edge of the atrial septum.

- The anastomosis to the atrial septum can be made with continuous sutures (Scene 5.15).

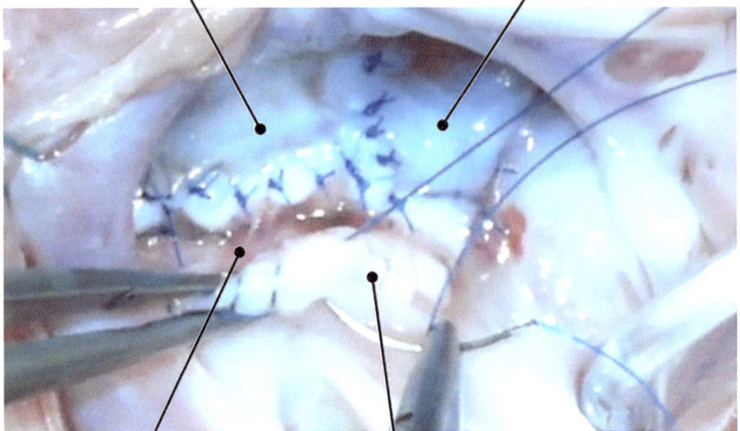

Scene 5.15 Patch closure of ostium primum defect (Video 22 min 10 s) (▶ https://doi.org/10.1007/000-hkb)

1. The top edge of the autologous pericardial patch is trimmed to match the shape of the ostium primum defect.
2. The autologous pericardial patch is sutured to the edge of the atrial septum with a continuous 6-0 monofilament suture.

References

Morphology and Classification of AVSD

Anderson RH, Spicer DE, Hlavacek AM, Cook AC, Backer CL. Lesions with normal surgical connections. In: Wilcox's Surgical Anatomy of the Heart. 4th ed. United Kingdom: Cambridge University Press; 2013. p. 166–85.

Cetta F, Minich LL, Edwards WD, Dearani JA, Puga FJ. Atrioventricular Septal Defects. In: Allen HD, Driscoll DJ, Shaddy RE, Feltes TF, editors. Moss and Adams' heart disease in infants, children, and adolescents. 7th ed. Philadelphia: Lippincott Williams & Wilkins; 2008. p. 646–66.

Conduction System of AVSD

Kurosawa H, Becker AE. Atrioventricular conduction in congenital heart disease. Tokyo: Springer; 1987.

6 Tetralogy of Fallot (TOF)

1 Morphology and Hemodynamics of Tetralogy of Fallot

1.1 Morphology of Tetralogy of Fallot

According to the malseptation theory by Van Mierop, Tetralogy of Fallot (TOF) is caused by a defect in the deviation (shift) of the great arteries during cardiogenesis (Fig. 6.1).

In the normal heart, the aorta is completely left ventricular in origin due to the leftward shift of the aorta, a posterior great artery. The aortic and mitral valves are adjacent in fibrous continuity.

■ *Tetralogy of Fallot*

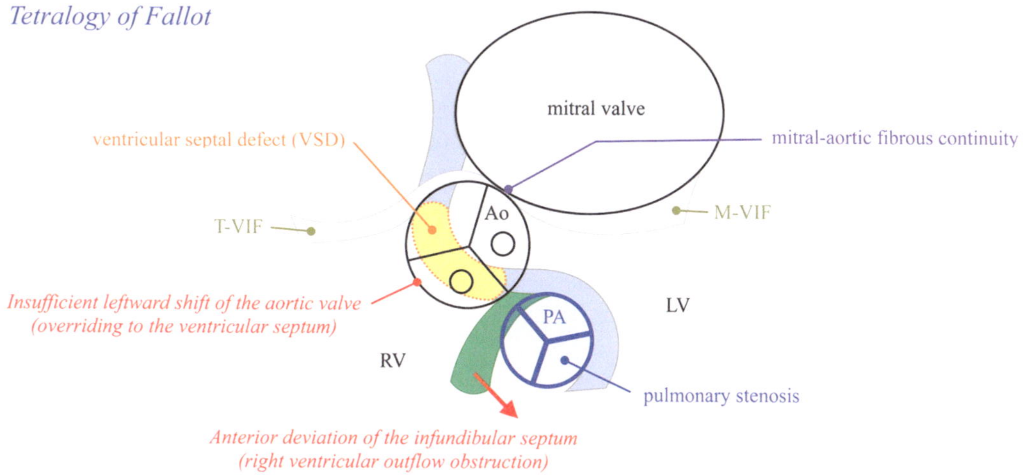

Supplementary Information The online version contains supplementary material available at https://doi.org/10.1007/978-981-96-6194-7_6. The videos can be accessed individually by clicking the DOI link in the accompanying figure caption or by scanning this link with the SN More Media App.

M. Yamagishi, *Surgical Treatment of Congenital Heart Disease*,
https://doi.org/10.1007/978-981-96-6194-7_6

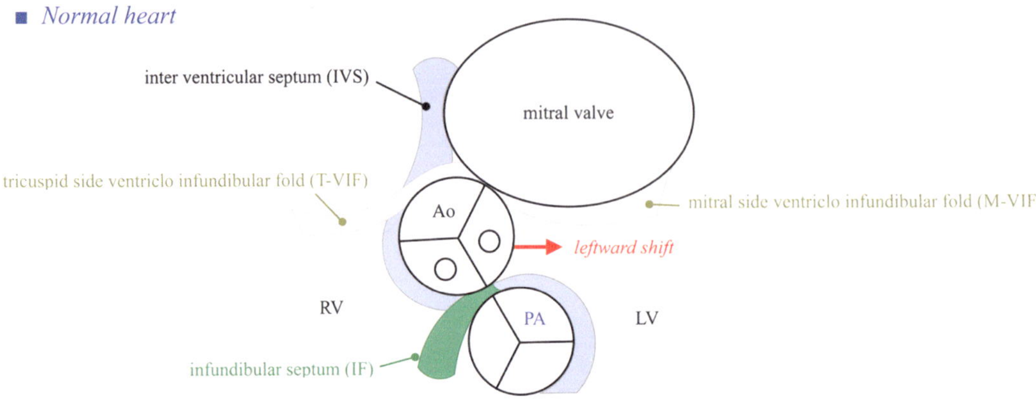

Fig. 6.1 Normal heart and tetralogy of Fallot

In tetralogy of Fallot, the posterior great arteries, the aorta, do not complete leftward deviation (shift) and stop in the process, so that the aorta does not completely originate in the left ventricle but is positioned over the ventricular septum (aortic overriding). The degree of overriding is variable. The leftward deviation (shift) is defective, but the mitral and aortic valve annuli are in contact (mitral-aortic fibrous continuity). The aortic overriding results in a defect beneath the aortic valve (subaortic VSD). The posterior margin of the VSD may extend into the membranous septum, but there is no anterior extension.

The infundibular septum is displaced anteriorly with insufficient leftward diviation of the aortic valve. Anterior dislocation of the infundibular septum results in narrowing of the right ventricular outflow tract (pulmonary artery stenosis, subvalvular stenosis, supravalvular stenosis). In cases of total conus defects, the degree of stenosis is less severe, but the right ventricular outflow tract is tortuous, resulting in subvalvular stenosis. The pulmonary valve is often bicuspid with thickened valve cusps. Unicuspid valves (fish-mouth shape) may also be present.

Pulmonary artery stenosis is accompanied by varying degrees of hypoplasia of the right and left pulmonary arteries. Stenosis of the pulmonary artery bifurcation at the ductus arteriosus attachment site may also be present.

These developmental abnormalities result in (1) aortic overriding, (2) VSD, and (3) pulmonary artery stenosis (Fig. 6.2).

- The aortic valve overrides the ventricular septum.
- The VSD is located beneath the aortic valve. The VSD does not extend anteriorly in tetralogy of Fallot.
- The posterior margin of the VSD consists of the posterior limb of the TSM and the anterior margin of the VSD consists of the anterior limb of the TSM.
- If the posterior inferior margin of the VSD is muscular tissue, it is of the muscular outlet type; if it is membranous septum, it is of the perimembranous outlet type.
- The IF is attached to the anterior border of the TSM (★). The IF obstructs blood flow from the right ventricular inflow to the outflow and results in right ventricular outflow obstruction.
- Anteriorly deviated IF and thickened right ventricular anterior wall cause RVOT muscular stenosis. Balloon dilatation is not effective due to muscular stenosis.

< Coronal cross-section >

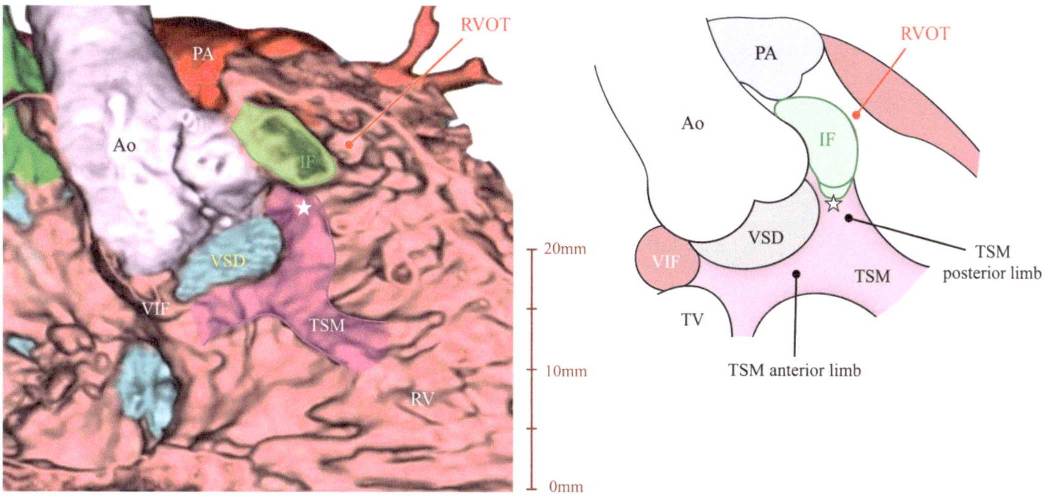

Fig. 6.2 CT images of tetralogy of Fallot. *Ao* aorta, *PA* pulmonary artery, *VSD* ventricular septal defect, *TV* tricuspid valve, *VIF* ventriculo infundibular fold, *IF* infundibular septum, *TSM* trabecular septomarginalis

< Horizontal cross-section ① >

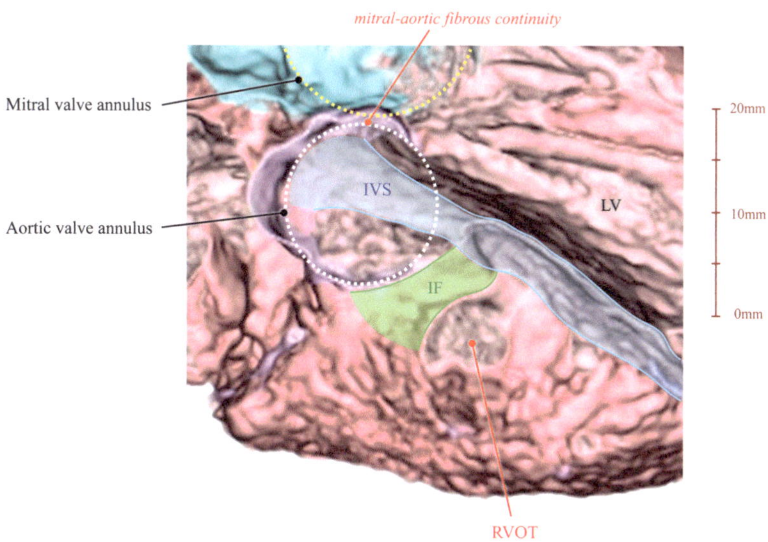

- Aortic valve is overriding the ventricular septum (IVS: *blue zone*).
- Aortic valve and mitral valve are in contact (fibrous continuity).
- In this case, more than 50% of the aortic valve annulus overrides on the IVS, but the diagnosis is TOF and not DORV because of the presence of mitral-aortic fibrous continuity.
- The RVOT is narrow due to anterior deviation of the IF (*green zone*) (subvalvular muscular stenosis).

< Horizontal cross-section ② >

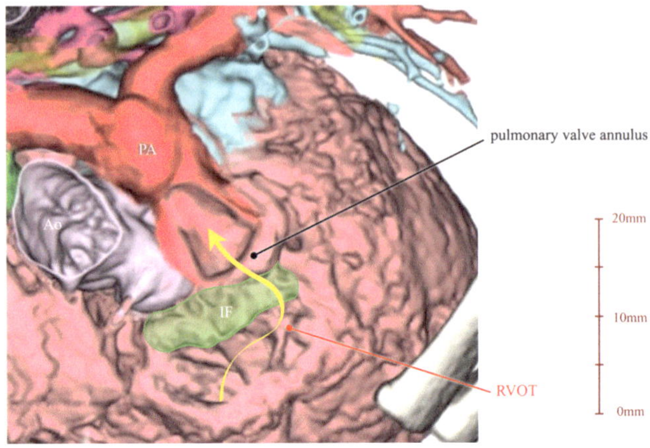

- Subvalvular muscular stenosis (right ventricular outflow tract stenosis) results from an anteriorly deviated IF (*green zone)*.
- Blood flow from the right ventricular inflow portion (*yellow arrow*) is turbulent at this site.

1.2 Morphology of Tetralogy of Fallot (Fig. 6.3)

- Due to the morphological feature of the aortic overriding the ventricular septum, blood is ejected simultaneously from both ventricles into the aorta, and the systolic pressures in both ventricles inevitably become equal (elevated right ventricular pressure).
- The increased right ventricular pressure results in right ventricular hypertrophy.
- Arterial blood oxygen saturation is decreased in tetralogy of Fallot, but it is not a right-left short circuit between the ventricles, but a direct short circuit from the right ventricle to the aorta (a slight right-left short circuit is observed in the early diastolic phase).
- Pulmonary artery stenosis reduces pulmonary blood flow and decreases left ventricular preload; there is also no right-to-left ventricular

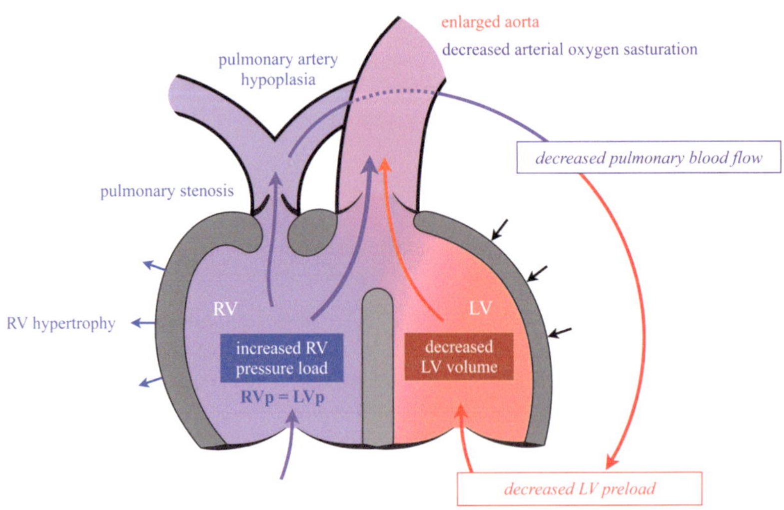

Fig. 6.3 Hemodynamics of tetralogy of Fallot

short-circuit in VSD, so left ventricular preload is decreased.
- Therefore, a decrease in left ventricular volume is observed in tetralogy of Fallot, resulting in a boot-shaped heart.

2 Treatment Strategies for Tetralogy of Fallot

Treatment of this syndrome should aim not only to close the VSD and relieve the right ventricular outflow tract stenosis, but also to develop a well-defined pulmonary artery without left-to-right differences. The treatment strategy is largely determined by the morphology of the pulmonary arteries and the degree of stenosis.

Medical management and appropriately timed surgical intervention should be planned taking into account the severity of the pulmonary artery stenosis.

2.1 Treatment in the Neonatal Period

Medical management is the mainstay of treatment in the neonatal period. In cases of severe pulmonary artery stenosis and severe cyanosis, prostaglandin (PG)E1 is administered to attempt to maintain patency of the PDA. Patients with significant subvalvular muscular stenosis of the pulmonary artery are treated with beta-blockers and may require neonatal surgical intervention (Blalock-Tsussig shunt: BT shunt). BT shunt should wait until after 2 weeks of age, when pulmonary vascular resistance is reduced.

SPOTLIGHT The Pros and Cons of Catheter Intervention in the Neonatal Period and Early Infancy

Pulmonary Artery Valve Balloon Enlargement

The pulmonary artery valve morphology in this syndrome is characterized by the presence of unicuspid and bicuspid valves and thickening of the valve leaflets. Catheter intervention (balloon enlargement) of such valves reduces stenosis, but does not prevent regurgitation because the most vulnerable valve leaflet is torn open at the center of the valve leaflet. Therefore, balloon dilatation should be avoided as much as possible, especially in cases where valve annulus preservation is desired.

Pulmonary Ductal Artery (PDA) Stenting

Because the PDA is connected to the pulmonary artery bifurcation or proximal left pulmonary artery, stenosis of the pulmonary artery bifurcation or left pulmonary artery stenosis is inevitable when a PDA stent is implanted. Because BT shunt can be performed in early infancy, management with PGE1 in the first month of life is not difficult, and PDA stenting for tetralogy of Fallot is contraindicated except in special cases such as inoperable cases.

2.2 Pulmonary Artery Morphology and Degree of Stenosis

- Valve Cusp

Cusp thickening is common in unicuspid (fish-mouth) and bicuspid valves, and cusp thickening is also seen in tricuspid valves.

- Valve Annular Diameter

Various degrees of stenosis or hypoplasia of the valve annulus are seen. In general, when the pulmonary valve annular diameter is less than 60% of normal, valve cusp preservation is not possible even if pulmonary blood flow is increased by BT shunt surgery because of cusp thickening and valve cusp abnormalities.

In cases with annular diameters of 60–70% of normal and mild cusp abnormalities (tricuspid valves and some bicuspid valves), valve ring growth and preservation of the valve annulus may be possible after BT shunt. In cases with severe abnormal valve morphology, preservation of the valve annulus is difficult.

In cases with a 70% of normal value or greater, valve annular preservation should attempted whenever possible.

- Subvalvular Stenosis

Subvalvular stenosis involves the following muscle bundles: (1) the anteriorly deviated infundibular septum (IF), (2) the muscle bundle connecting the IF to the ventricular infundibular fold (VIF), and (3) the muscle bundle connecting the anterior limb of the trabecular septomarginalis (TSM) to the right ventricular free wall. Because the stenosis is caused by muscular tissue, balloon dilatation is not effective, and there is a risk of anoxic spells during balloon dilatation.

- Supravalvular Stenosis, Bifurcation Stenosis, Peripheral Pulmonary Artery Stenosis

Hypoplasia of the main pulmonary artery, stenosis of the pulmonary artery bifurcation, and stenosis of the left pulmonary artery at the site of PDA attachment may occur.

Hypoplasia (stunting) of the left and right pulmonary arteries is seen with decreased pulmonary blood flow. Stenosis of the left pulmonary artery may also be associated with closure of the PDA.

2.3 Palliative Operation in Early Infancy (Blalock-Taussig Shunt)

- BT Shunt and PDA Treatment

The BT shunt should be performed in early infancy (approximately 1 month of age). The standard diameter of the ePTFE vascular graft is 4.0 mm ePTFE graft for a body weight of 3 kg. In cases where progressive pulmonary blood flow remains, a hemoclip is used to adjust blood flow to a 3.5-mm diameter ePTFE graft or a 4.0-mm diameter ePTFE graft. To maintain constant pulmonary blood flow, the PDA should be ligated or amputated.

Patients scheduled for future Rastelli operation may have a longer waiting period in anticipation of weight gain so that a larger diameter conduit can be selected at the time of definitive surgery. For this reason, a large ePTFE graft is selected and a hemoclip is used to regulate blood flow. If oxygen saturation is reduced by the time of radical surgery, the hemoclip is removed by a catheter balloon dilatation.

- BT Shunt Approach and Assisted Extracorporeal Circulation

If a BT shunt is performed on the contralateral pulmonary artery at the PDA attachment site in the lateral thoracotomy, the PDA cannot be treated. In addition, there is concern about hemodynamic deterioration due to hypoxia during surgery, so in principle, BT shunt (+ PDA treatment) under partial extracorporeal circulation through a median sternotomy approach is safer.

- Anastomotic Site

In the case of a median sternotomy, the aortic side is anastomosed to the brachiocephalic artery (just before the beginning of the right common carotid artery). In cases where the PDA originates from the brachiocephalic artery in the right aortic arch, the PDA is amputated under extracorporeal circulation and the PDA tissue is removed from the brachiocephalic artery. A BT shunt is anastomosed to this resection site.

On the pulmonary artery side, anastomosis is performed to the main pulmonary artery, the pulmonary artery bifurcation, and proximal portions of the right and left pulmonary arteries, depending on the configuration of the pulmonary artery. In order to provide equal pulmonary blood flow to the left and right pulmonary arteries, anastomosis to the main pulmonary artery and pulmonary artery bifurcation is preferable.

• Pulmonary Artery Angioplasty

If stenosis is found at the pulmonary artery bifurcation to which the PDA is attached site or at the left pulmonary artery, the stenotic area should be enlarged and formed with an autologous pericardial patch along with PDA amputation. If the stenosis is localized, the stenosis is resected and the pulmonary artery is reconstructed by end-to-end anastomosis.

• Treatment of the Main Pulmonary Artery

In cases of hypoplastic pulmonary valve annulus in which preservation of the pulmonary valve annulus is difficult and progressive pulmonary blood flow is unstable due to subvalvular muscular stenosis, it is necessary to maintain stable pulmonary blood flow and avoid left heart failure caused by temporary increase in pulmonary blood flow. For this reason, the pulmonary blood flow pathway should be a single blood flow pathway from the BT shunt and the main pulmonary artery should be ligated (or cut).

2.4 Definitive Operation

• Optimal Timing for Definitive Operation

In patients who have not undergone prior surgery, definitive operation should be performed around the age of 1 year of age, when cyanosis does not become severe (arterial blood oxygen saturation of less than 70%).

In cases of BT shunt, the standard age for definitive operation is between 1 and 2 years of age, taking into consideration arterial blood oxygen saturation and pulmonary artery growth, if the pulmonary valve annulus can be preserved or if a transannular patch is used to enlarge the valve annulus. In patients with hypoplastic pulmonary valve annulus who are candidates for the Rastelli operation, it is advisable to wait until approximately 2 years of age (8–10 kg) in order to use the largest possible right ventricular-pulmonary artery conduit.

• Pulmonary Valve Annulus Preservation

In cases with a mildly abnormal valvular morphology and a valve annular diameter of more than 70% of the normal ratio, valve annular preservation should be performed as much as possible by the commissurotomy. Again, an autologous pericardial patch is used to eliminate the supravalvular stenosis (main pulmonary artery and pulmonary artery bifurcation augmentation).

The right ventricular outflow tract under the pulmonary artery valve is incised longitudinally to resect the thickened myocardial bundle beneath the pulmonary valve as much as possible, and the right ventricular outflow tract incision is enlarged with an oval patch cut through an ePTFE vascular graft (thin wall graft of approximately 8 mm diameter).

• Transannular Patch (ePTFE Patch with ePTFE Monocusp)

In cases where the valve morphology is moderately abnormal and mobility is preserved, a longitudinal incision is made across the anterior commissure of the pulmonary artery to the main pulmonary artery (before the bifurcation). From the incision of the commissure, an incision is also made anterior to the right ventricular outflow tract toward the right ventricular apex. The right ventricular outflow tract incision should not be too long. The thickened muscular bundle of the right ventricular outflow tract below the pulmonary valve should be resected as much as possible.

The distal main pulmonary artery incision is enlarged by filling in an autologous pericardial patch, and an ePTFE patch with an ePTFE monocusp is sutured from the right ventricular outflow tract incision to the proximal main pulmonary artery.

The ePTFE valve of the transannular patch should be placed slightly more cranially than the autologous pulmonary valve to minimize pulmonary regurgitation.

- Rastelli Procedure

In cases where the valve morphology is severely abnormal and the valve annulus and main pulmonary artery are hypoplastic, a conduit is used to create a right ventricular-pulmonary artery blood flow pathway (Rastelli operation).

In patients with valve annular diameter greater than 60% of normal but with severe abnormal valve morphology, right ventricular dysfunction due to pulmonary valve regurgitation is a concern, because autologous valve function cannot be expected. In such patients with severe valve abnormalities, the Rastelli operation using a small-sized conduit (12–16 mm) may be performed in early infancy to preserve right ventricular function, rather than a transannular patch. Although replacement with a larger conduit (redo surgery) is required as weight increases, good preservation of right ventricular function can be expected.

If the diameter of the pulmonary artery bifurcation where the conduit is to be anastomosed is small, an autologous pericardial patch or ePTFE graft patch is used to enlarge the right and left pulmonary arteries simultaneously.

- Conduit Diameter Selection Criteria for the Rastelli Operation

Based on the results of a Japanese multicenter study, the following table shows the guideline for conduit diameter based on body weight at the time of surgery (see table below). Because an oversized conduit may cause stenosis of the pulmonary artery bifurcation, it is important to select an appropriate conduit size (Tables 6.1 and 6.2).

Table 6.1 Conduit diameter selection criteria

Body weight	8 kg	10 kg	12 kg	30 kg	40 kg	50 kg
Conduit diameter	14 mm	16 mm	18 mm	20 mm	22 mm	24 mm

Table 6.2 Freedom from ePTFE valved conduit exchange (Japanese multicenter study, 2002–2020)

14 mm conduit

1.2 ± 1.1 yo   7.7 ± 2.3 kg

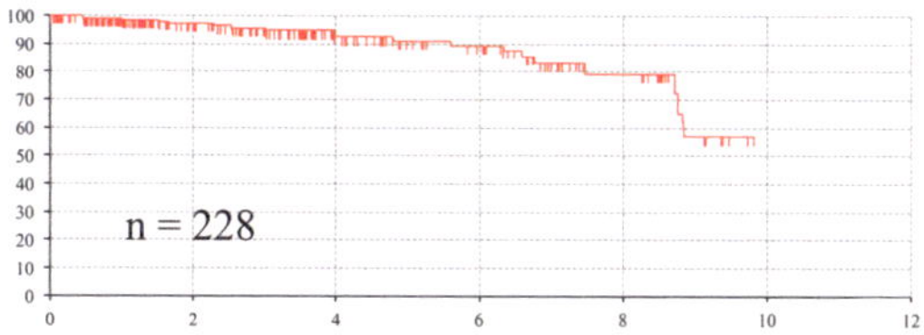

3 year 95.6%
5 year 91.0%
7 year 83.0%

16 mm conduit

2.1 ± 3.0 yo   9.8 ± 7.2 kg

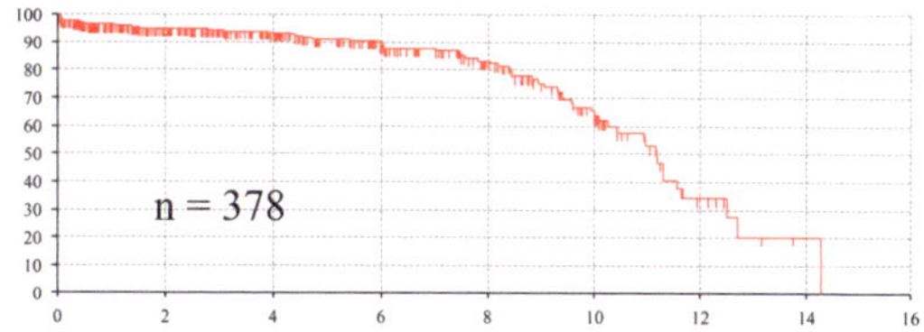

3 year 94.3%
5 year 91.1%
7 year 87.7%
10 year 63.6%

18 mm conduit

4.0 ± 4.5 yo   12.8 ± 9.5 kg

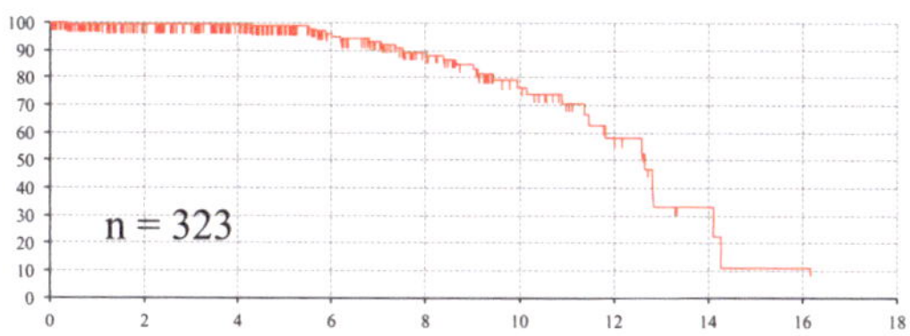

3 year 99.3%
5 year 98.6%
7 year 93.2%
10 year 76.4%

20 mm conduit

10.9 ± 8.2 yo   28.5 ± 14.0 kg

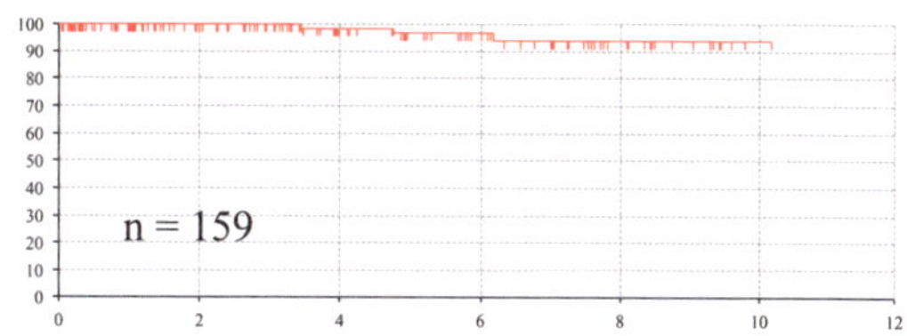

3 year 100.0%
5 year 96.7%
7 year 93.9%
10 year 93.9%

22 mm conduit

14.2 ± 9.6 y   40.9 ± 15.1 kg

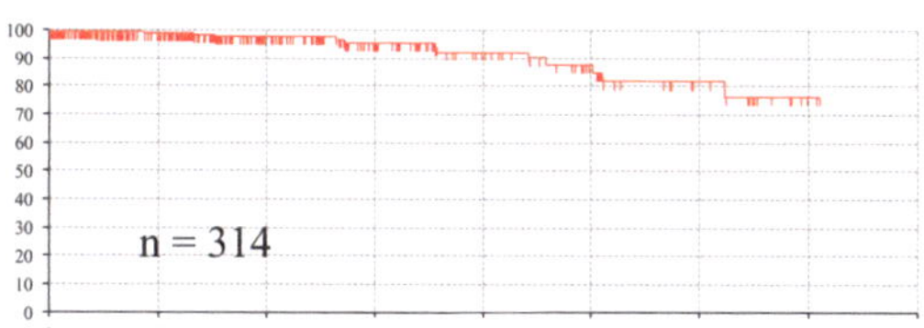

3 year 98.2%
5 year 97.6%
7 year 95.6%
10 year 87.8%

24 mm conduit

17.4 ± 9.9 y   51.0 ± 15.2 kg

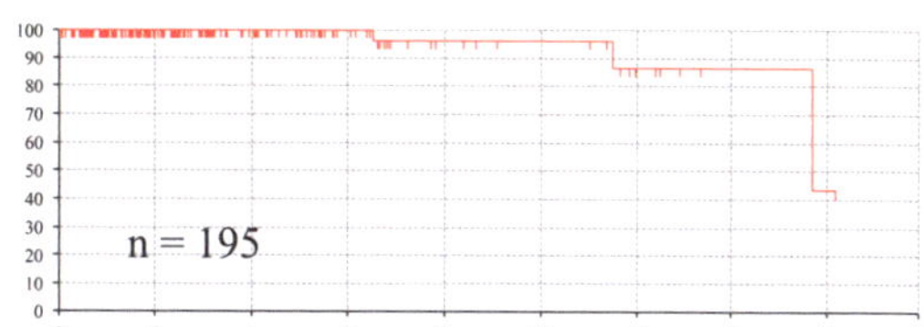

3 year 100.0%
5 year 100.0%
7 year 96.0%
10 year 96.0%

3 Right Ventricular Outflow Reconstruction (Surgical Video)

Case 6.1

- Tetralogy of Fallot, valvular and subvalvular stenosis, bicuspid pulmonary valve
- 10 months old, body weight 6100 g, body surface area 0.32 m^2
- Pulmonary valve annular diameter = 6.6 mm (69% of normal value)
- RV-PA pressure gradient = 80 mmHg
- Pulmonary artery index = 294 mm^2/m^2
- Right ventricular end-diastolic volume = 89% of normal value
- Left ventricular end-diastolic volume = 101% of normal value

This case was complicated by subvalvular and valvular stenosis (bicuspid valve). The left pulmonary artery was bifurcated at a right angle, and stenosis at the bifurcation and hypoplasia of the left pulmonary artery were observed.

Therefore, it was determined that valve annulus preservation was not possible, and the patient underwent an autologous pericardium patch from the left pulmonary artery to the main pulmonary artery, a transannular patch (with ePTFE monocuspid valve) to enlarge the right ventricular outflow tract, and a ventricular septal defect closure.

This case presents only the scene of left pulmonary artery enlargement and right ventricular outflow tract enlargement.

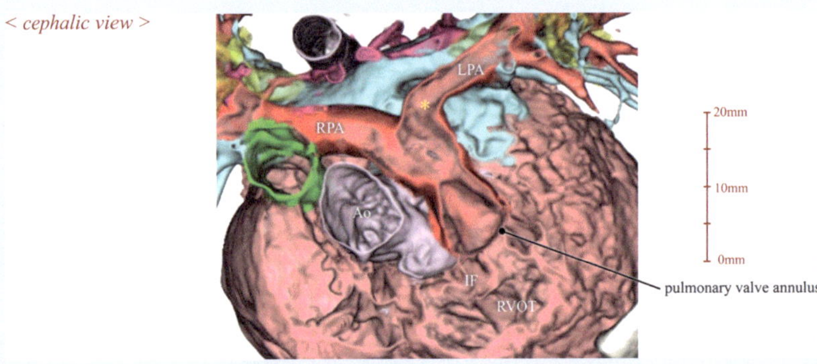

- An anteriorly deviated infundibular septum (IF) is present in the right ventricular outflow tract (RVOT).
- Left pulmonary artery (LPA) bifurcated at an acute angle with stenosis at the bifurcation (*).
- Caliber difference between the right pulmonary artery (RPA) and LPA (Case 6.1, Scene 1).

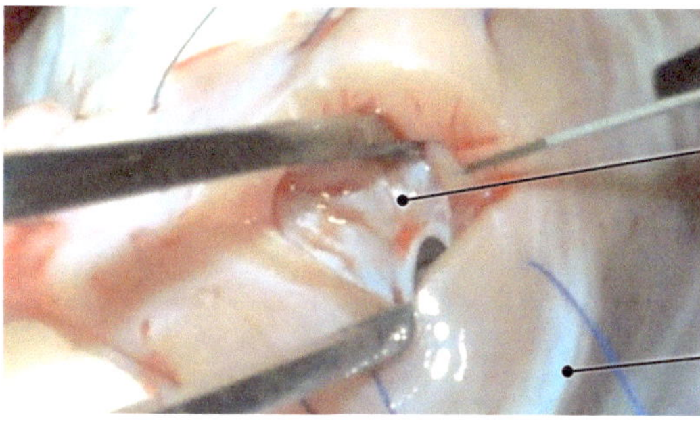

Case 6.1, Scene 1 Incise the right ventricular outflow tract (Video 00 min 32 s)

1. The right ventricular outflow tract incision line is the line passing through the midpoint of the anterior descending branch of the left coronary artery and the right ventricular branch of the right coronary artery, parallel to the anterior descending branch.
2. Supporting sutures (5-0 monofilament) are placed on either side of the incision line, and a longitudinal incision is made through the right ventricular outflow tract (Case 6.1, Scene 2).

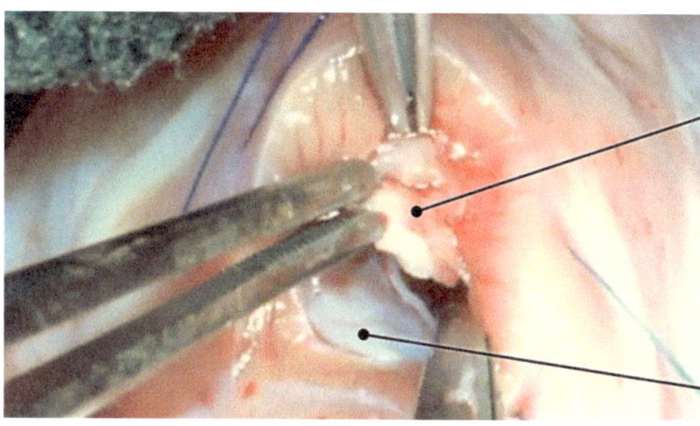

Case 6.1, Scene 2 Resection of RVOT hypertrophied muscle bundle 1 (Video 00 min 44 s)

1. Resect the hypertrophied muscle bundle that connects the anterior wall of the right ventricular outflow tract to the ventricular septum (Case 6.1, Scene 3).

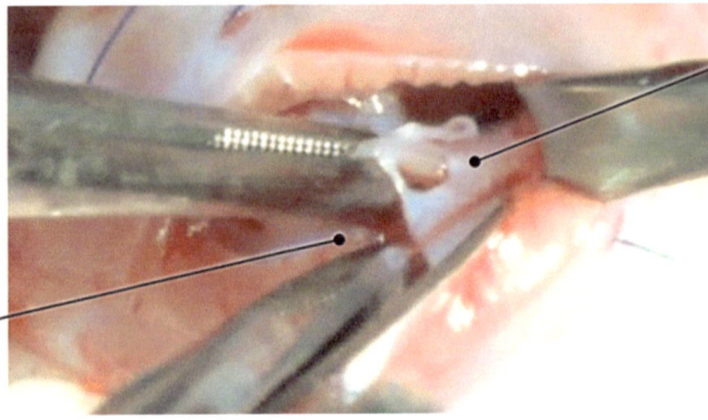

Case 6.1, Scene 3 Resection of RVOT hypertrophied muscle bundle 2 (Video 01 min 18 s)

1. Resection of hypertrophied muscle bundles connecting the right ventricular anterior wall and the ventricular infundibular fold (VIF) to the infundibular septum (IF) (Case 6.1, Scene 4).

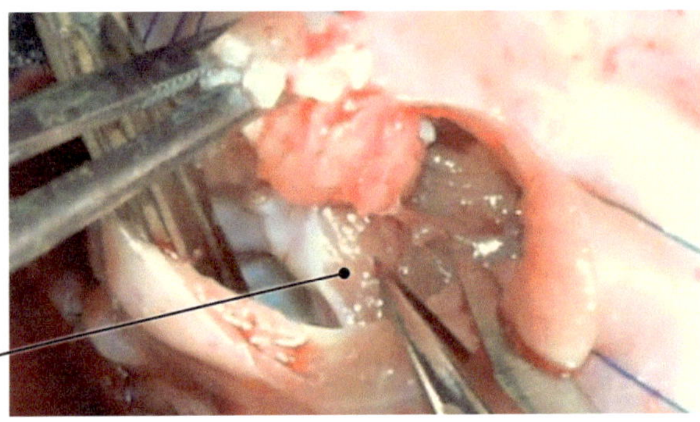

Case 6.1, Scene 4 Resection of RVOT hypertrophied muscle bundle 3 (Video 01 min 56 s)

1. Resect the anteriorly deviated infundibular septum (Case 6.1, Scene 5).

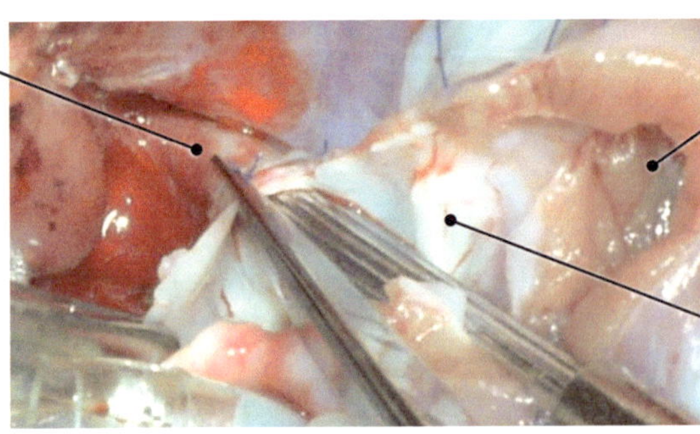

Case 6.1, Scene 5 Incision of the left pulmonary artery (Video 02 min 53 s)

1. Using the pre-sutured marker as a guide, incise the left pulmonary artery to just before the upper lobe branch (Case 6.1, Scene 6).

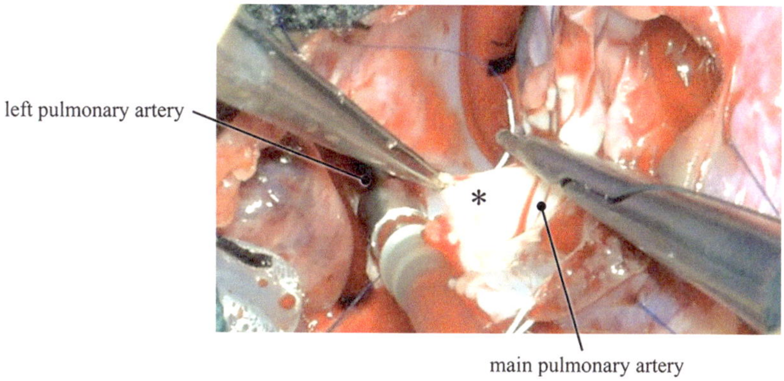

Case 6.1, Scene 6 Augmentation of the left pulmonary artery bifurcation (Video 03 min 38 s)

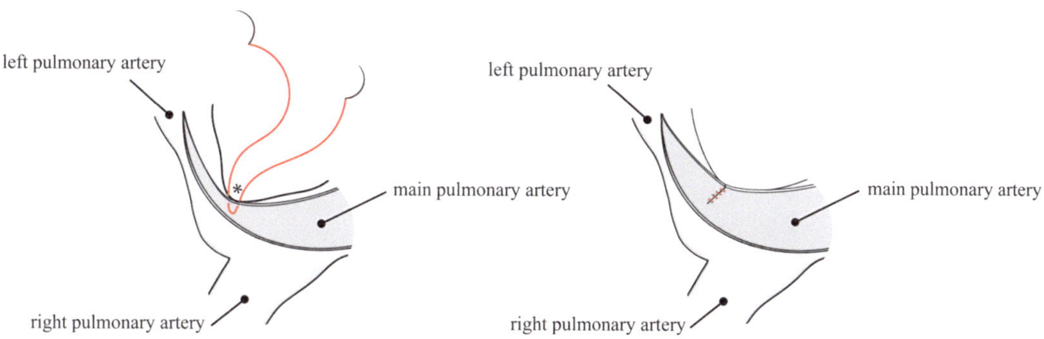

1. Lateral anastomosis of the incised surface of the left pulmonary artery bifurcation (*) to moderate the bifurcation angle (Case 6.1, Scene 7).

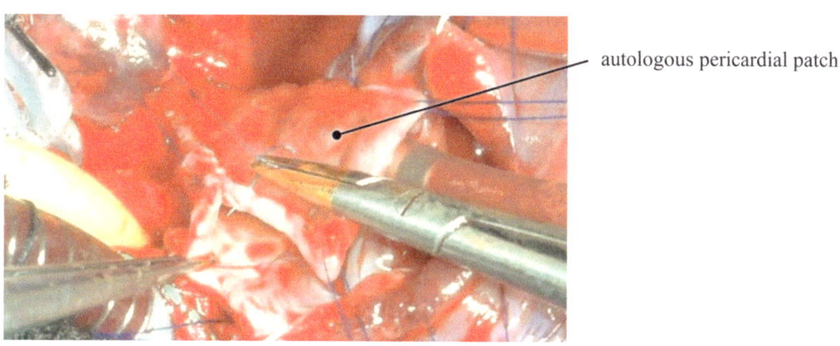

Case 6.1, Scene 7 Augmentation of the left and main pulmonary artery using autologous pericardial patch (Video 05 min 20 s)

1. Anastomose the autologous pericardial patch from the left pulmonary artery to the main pulmonary artery with a continuous 7-0 monofilament suture (Case 6.1, Scene 8).

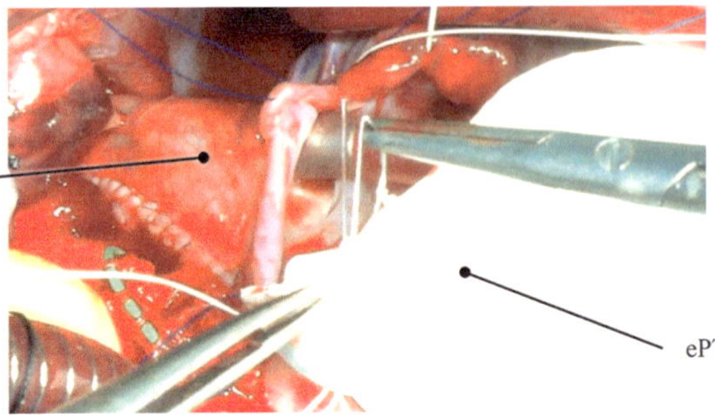

Case 6.1, Scene 8 RVOT augmentation using monocuspid ePTFE patch 1 (Video 14 min 49 s)

1. Anastomose the ePTFE monocuspid patch with bulging sinus to the main pulmonary artery with continuous ePTFE CV-6 suture.
2. Position the ePTFE valve commissure of the ePTFE monocuspid patch slightly cranial to the autologous valve commissure (Case 6.1, Scene 9).

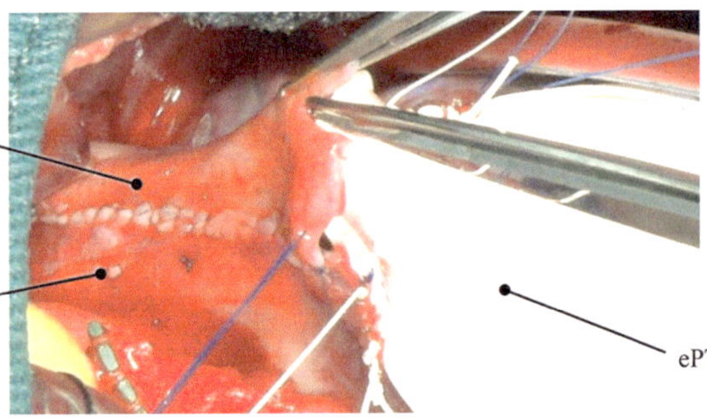

Case 6.1, Scene 9 RVOT augmentation using monocuspid ePTFE patch 2 (Video 17 min 12 s)

1. Assuming the ePTFE monocuspid patch is dilated, identify the location where the distal edge of the patch coincides with the edge of the autologous pericardial patch.
2. Make a longitudinal incision through the autologous pericardial patch to the point of coincidence and trim the cut edge (Case 6.1, Scene 10).

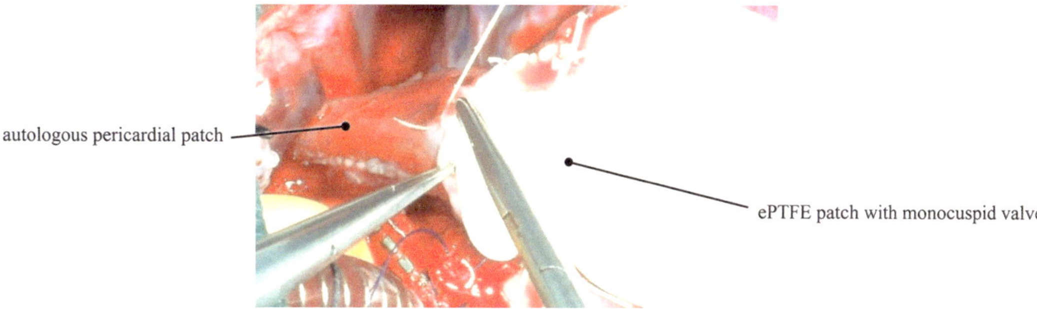

Case 6.1, Scene 10 RVOT augmentation using monocuspid ePTFE patch 3 (Video 17 min 42 s)

1. Anastomose the distal end of the ePTFE monocuspid valve patch to the autologous pericardial patch with continuous ePTFE CV-6 suture (Case 6.1, Scene 11).

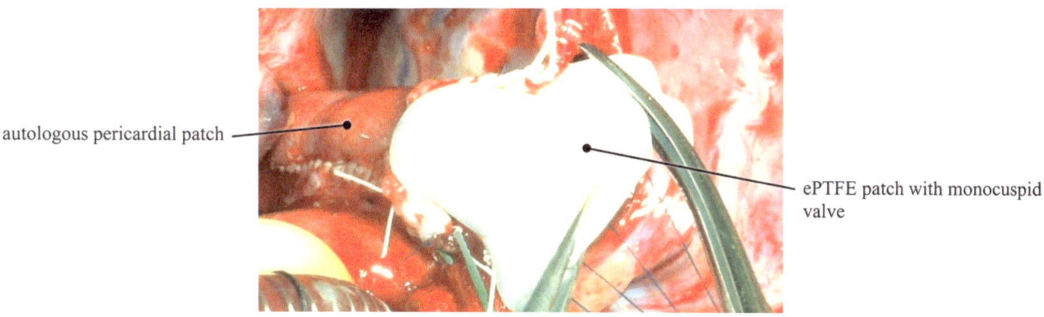

Case 6.1, Scene 11 RVOT augmentation using monocuspid ePTFE patch 4 (Video 20 min 30 s)

1. Trim the lower edge of the ePTFE monocuspid valve patch to match the shape of the right ventricular outflow tract opening (Case 6.1, Scene 12).

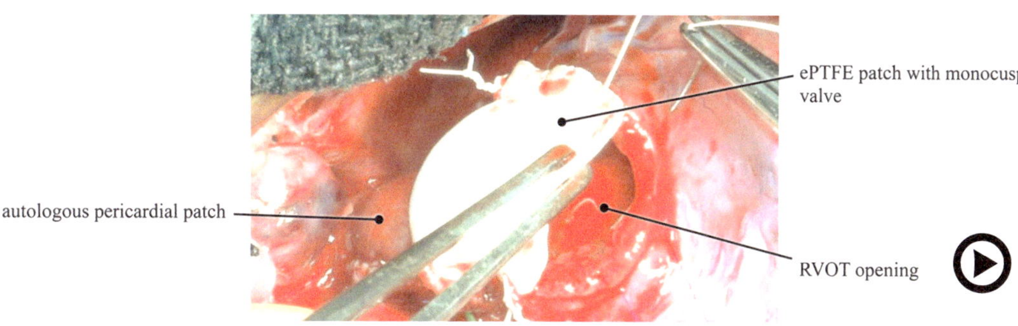

Case 6.1, Scene 12 RVOT augmentation using monocuspid ePTFE patch 5 (Video 20 min 56 s) (▶ https://doi.org/10.1007/000-hkd)

1. Anastomose ePTFE monocuspid valve patch to right ventricular outflow tract incision with continuous ePTFE suture CV-5 suture.

Case 6.1 Pre and Postoperative CT Images

< Horizontal cross-section >

< Preop >

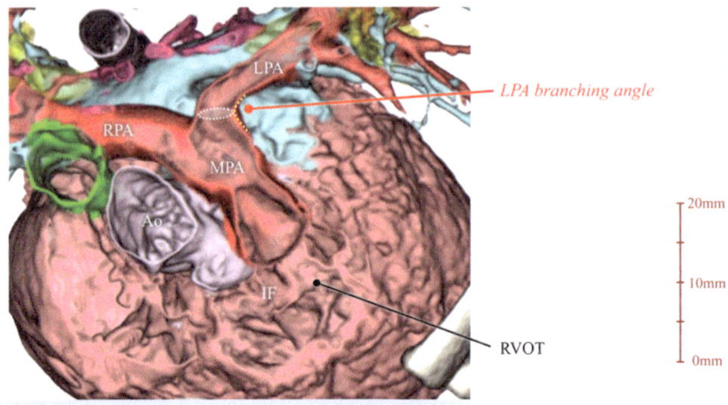

< Postop >

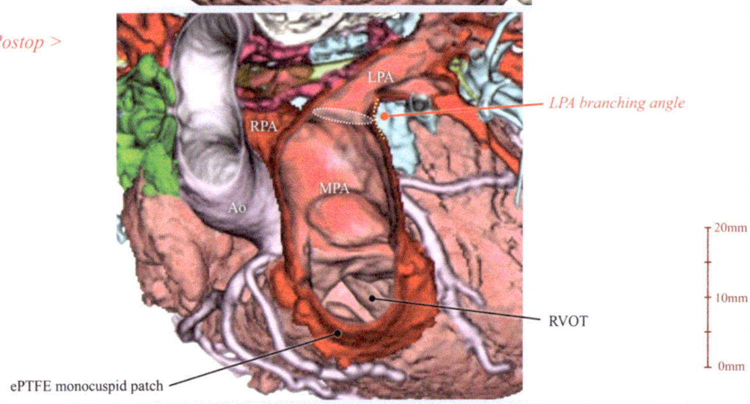

- The left pulmonary artery (LPA) bifurcation angle (*yellow dashed line*) is more gentle postoperatively than preoperatively due to the LPA bifurcation plication.
- The LPA orifice is also widened (oval with white dashed line).
- The thickened myocardial bundle of the right ventricular outflow tract (RVOT) has been resected, allowing a wider blood flow pathway.
- The pulmonary artery valve annulus is also widened by the ePTFE monocuspid patch.

< Postop >

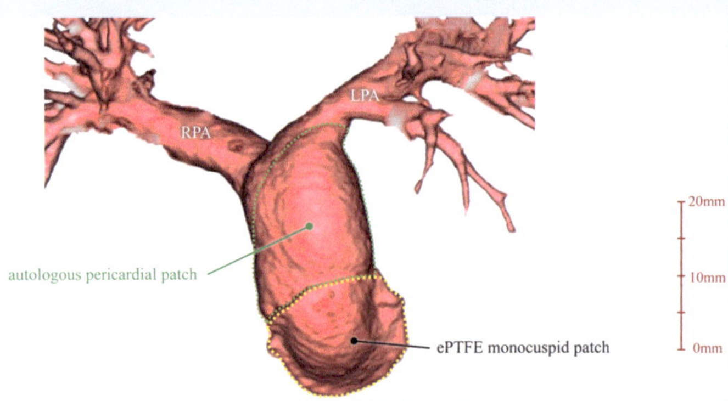

- Autologous pericardial patch (*green dashed line*) and ePTFE monocuspid patch (*yellow dashed line*) are shown.
- The autologous pericardial patch enlarges the main pulmonary artery (MPA) from the proximal LPA.
- The ePTFE patch is short and limited to the RVOT.

4 Right Ventricular Outflow Reconstruction (Surgical Video)

Case 6.2

- Tetralogy of Fallot, severe pulmonary valve stenosis, subvalvular stenosis, right aortic arch
- 10-year-old girl, body weight 9300 g, body surface area 0.43 m^2
- Prior operation (2 months old): division of patent ductus arteriosus (PDA), ligation of main pulmonary artery, Blalock-Taussig (BT) shunt (4 mm ePTFE tube)
- RPA diameter = 11.7 mm, LPA diameter = 6.9 mm
- Pulmonary artery index = 362 mm^2/m^2
- Right ventricular end-diastolic volume = 115% of normal value
- Left ventricular end-diastolic volume = 141% of normal value

In this case, the patient had severe hypoplasia of the pulmonary valve, so the pulmonary artery was not expected to develop, and the patient had muscular stenosis of the right ventricular outflow tract, which could cause instability of the antegrade pulmonary blood flow. In order to maintain stable pulmonary blood flow, we decided to ligate the main pulmonary artery (interruption of progressive pulmonary blood flow) along with PDA dissection.

At 2 months of age (5.9 kg), the patient underwent a BT shunt (left brachiocephalic artery—main pulmonary artery) with a 4-mm ePTFE graft, PDA division, and main pulmonary artery ligation.

After waiting for weight gain, the patient was scheduled for definitive Rastelli operation at 1 year of age (weight 9.4 kg, preoperative arterial oxygen saturation 85%, nasal oxygen 5 L).

■ Pre Blalock-Taussig shunt (1 month-old)

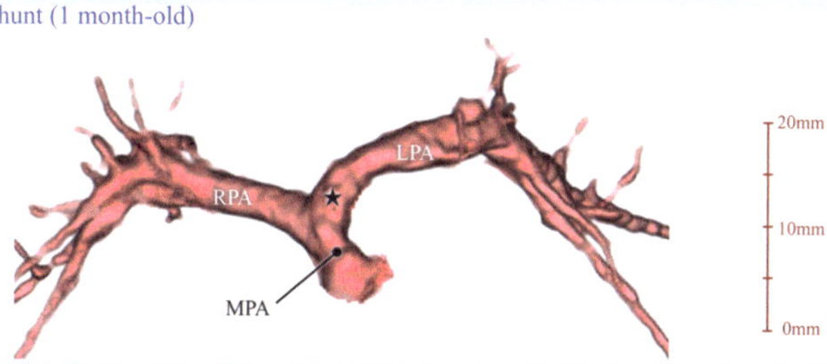

- Pulmonary valve annulus and main pulmonary artery (MPA) are hypoplastic.
- There is no stenosis at the pulmonary artery bifurcation or ductus arteriosus (★).
- There is no local stenosis in the left and right pulmonary arteries (LPA, RPA), but overall hypoplasia is present.

■ Post Blalock-Taussig shint, pre Rastelli operation (1 year-old)

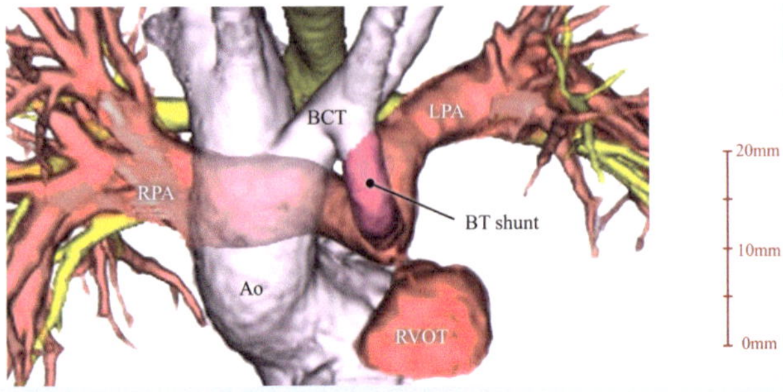

- BT shunt between left brachiocephalic artery (BCT) and MPA.
- No stenotic lesion is seen in the BT shunt.
- The MPA is ligated, and the right ventricular outflow tract (RVOT) is seen at the proximal end.
- The right and left pulmonary arteries are well grown and there is no stenotic lesion, but the right ventricular to pulmonary artery conduit (18 mm conduit planned) is too narrow to be anastomosed.
- Therefore, we decided to enlarge the anastomosis site of the conduit (pulmonary artery bifurcation) with autologous pericardium.

■ Post Blalock-Taussig shint, pre Rastelli operation (1 year-old)

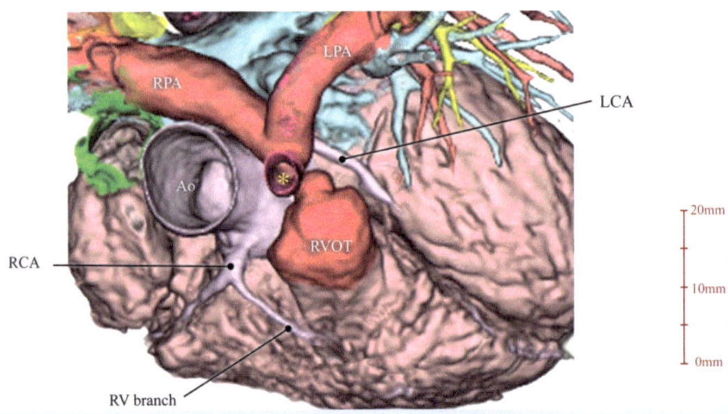

- The left coronary artery (LCA) runs posterior to the RVOT, and care must be taken not to damage it during the RVOT incision and conduit anastomosis.
- In this case, the LCA is somewhat distant from the dorsal RVOT (conduit anastomosis).
- In this case, the origin of the right coronary artery (RCA) is far from the RVOT. Care should be taken in cases where the RCA originates from the left side of the right coronary sinus, as it may come in contact with the conduit.
- The right ventricular branch (RV branch) runs below the RVOT and may be amputated when the RVOT is opened. However, the RV branch passing through in this area perfuses the RVOT thickened myocardium, and because the thickened myocardium is also resected, right ventricular function is not compromised even if the RV branch is amputated.

Asterisk (*) shows a cross-section of the BT shunt anastomosis (Case 6.2, Scene 1).

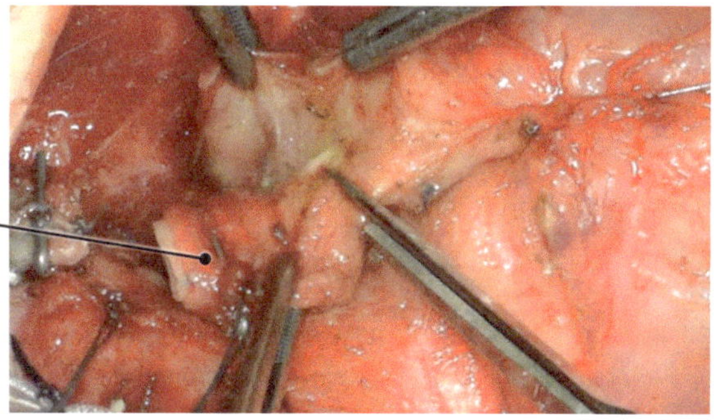

Case 6.2, Scene 1 Transect BT shunt (Video 00 min 12 s)

1. Start extracorporeal circulation and transect the Blalock-Taussig shunt (ePTFE graft).
2. Remove the ePTFE graft from the pulmonary artery anastomosis (Case 6.2, Scene 2).

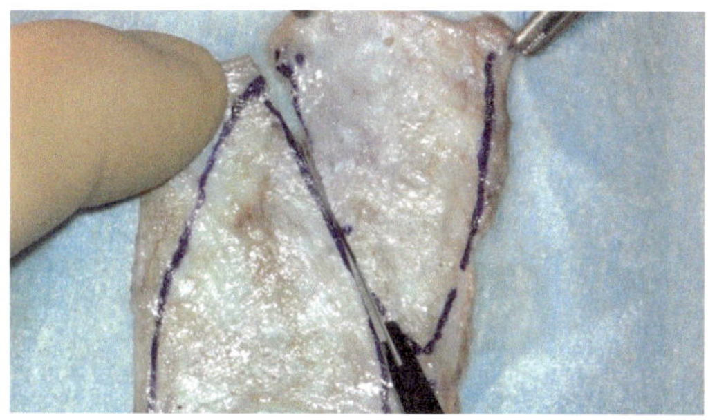

Case 6.2, Scene 2 Trim the autologous pericardium (Video 00 min 37 s)

1. Trim ethanol-treated autologous pericardium into a spindle shape (for each of the left and right pulmonary arteries) (Case 6.2, Scene 3).

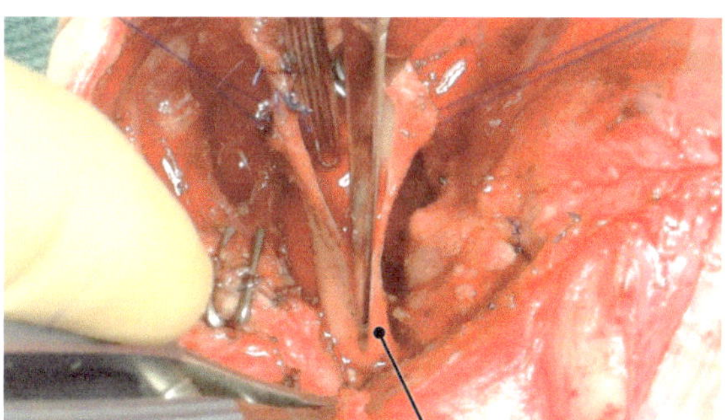

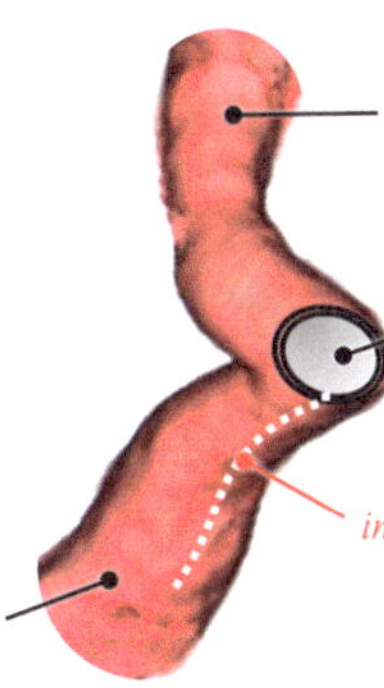

Case 6.2, Scene 3 Incise the right pulmonary artery (Video 01 min 09 s)

1. Incise the right pulmonary artery from the anastomotic opening of the ePTFE graft to just before the upper lobe bifurcation (Case 6.2, Scene 4).

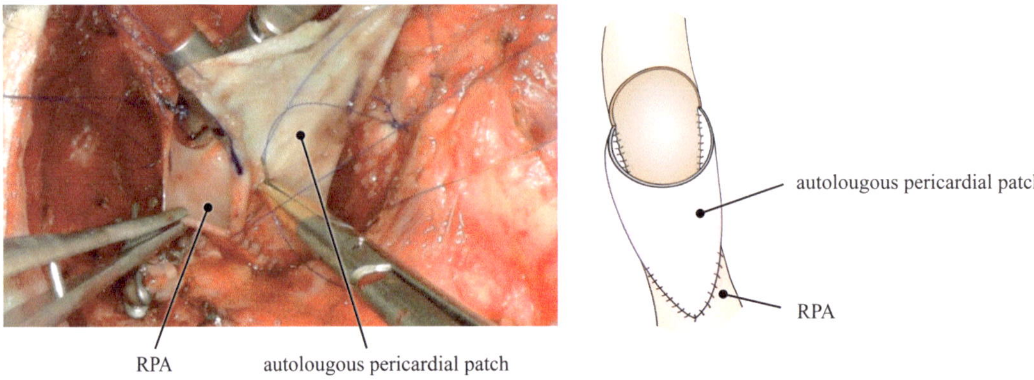

Case 6.2, Scene 4 RPA augmentation using autologous pericardial patch (Video 01 min 14 s)

1. Anastomose an autologous pericardial patch to the right pulmonary artery incision with a continuous 6-0 monofilament suture (Case 6.2, Scene 5).

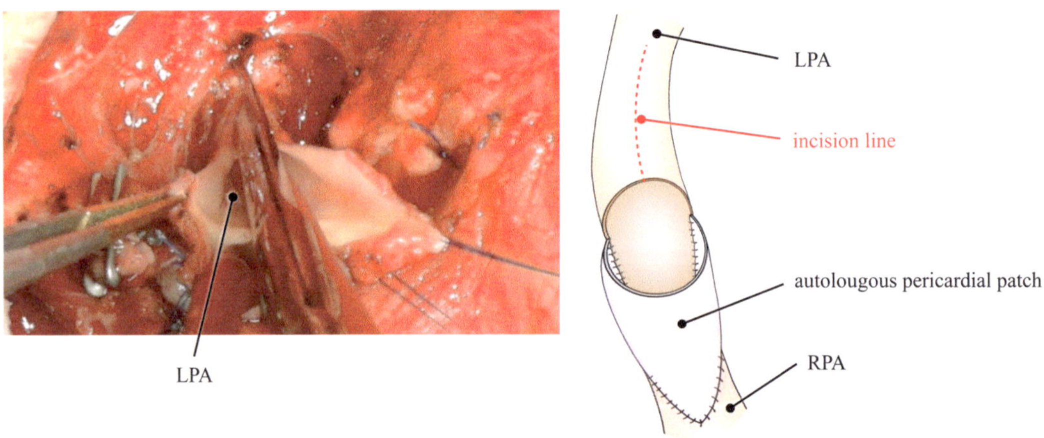

Case 6.2, Scene 5 Incise the left pulmonary artery (Video 04 min 08 s)

1. Incise the left pulmonary artery to just before the upper lobe bifurcation (Case 6.2, Scene 6).

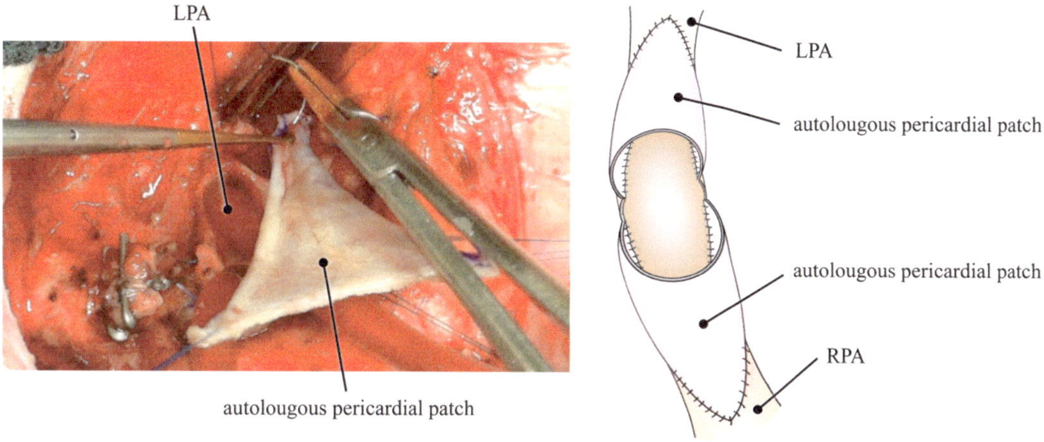

Case 6.2, Scene 6 LPA augmentation using autologous pericardial patch (Video 04 min 23 s)

1. Anastomose an autologous pericardial patch to the left pulmonary artery incision with a continuous 6-0 monofilament suture (Case 6.2, Scene 7).

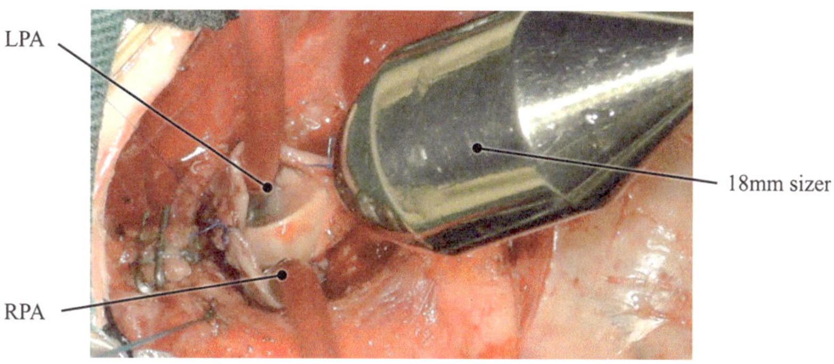

Case 6.2, Scene 7 Sizing of the pulmonary artery opening (Video 05 min 48 s)

1. Sizing of the newly formed pulmonary artery bifurcation opening.

- In this case, an 18-mm ePTFE conduit (ePTFE tricuspid valve) was selected.
- An oversized conduit may cause stenosis of the pulmonary artery bifurcation.

ESSENTIALS **Trimming of the Distal End of an ePTFE Conduit with ePTFE Tricuspid Valve**

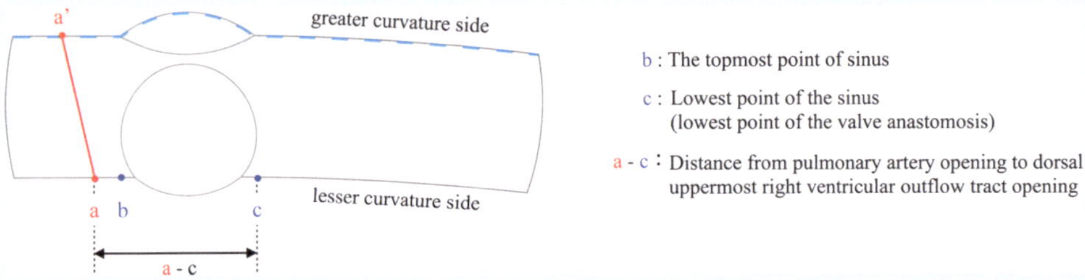

Adjust the conduit so that a valve is always placed on the greater curvature side (where the blood flow velocity is higher).

Cut the distal end of the conduit in a straight line from a point approximately 2 mm from the top of the sinus (point (b) on the lesser curvature side) (point (a)) to point (a') on the greater curvature side, slightly obliquely.

The cutting angle should not be too oblique.

Point (a) is anastomosed with the lower end of the pulmonary artery opening.

Point (c) is the dorsal uppermost point of the right ventricular outflow tract incision.

In some cases, the length between the lower end of the pulmonary artery opening and the uppermost end of the right ventricular outflow tract opening may be short (in such cases, move point a closer to point (b)) (Case 6.2, Scene 8).

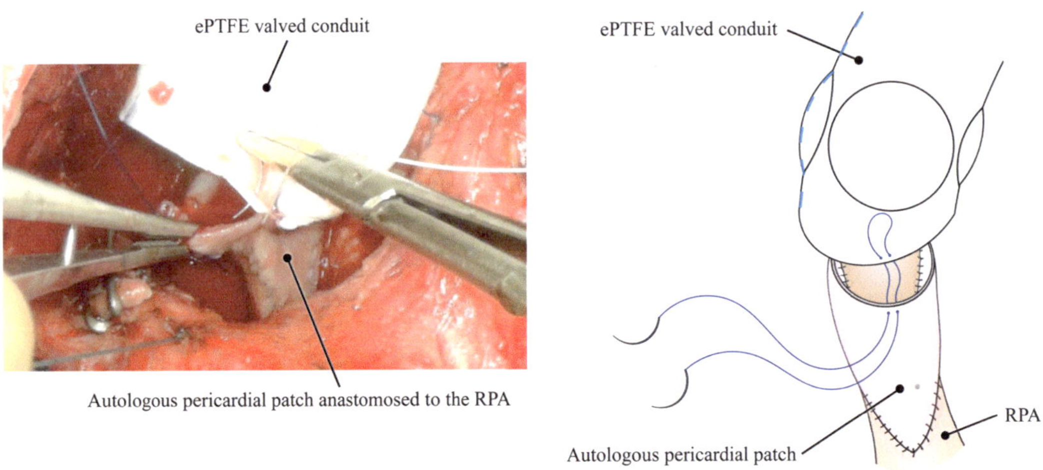

Case 6.2, Scene 8 Anastomosis of the distal end of the ePTFE valved conduit 1 (Video 06 min 31 s)

1. Anastomose the distal end of the valved ePTFE conduit to the opening of the pulmonary artery bifurcation with a continuous ePTFE CV-6 suture.

- Anastomosis is started from the right end of the opening (aortic side).
- Adjust the anastomosis at the left end of the opening (it is difficult to adjust the anastomosis at the right end of the opening due to the presence of the ascending aorta).
- The autologous pulmonary artery wall and autologous pericardium are stretched sufficiently to anastomose with the valved ePTFE graft (anastomose the stretched autologous tissue and the vascular prosthesis so that the width of the steps is approximately the same) (Case 6.2, Scene 9).

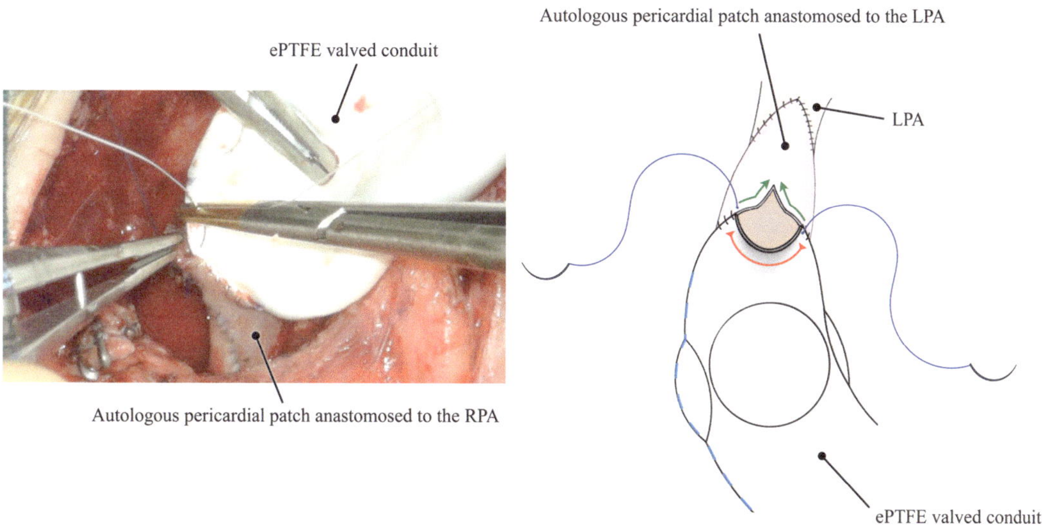

Case 6.2, Scene 9 Anastomosis of the distal end of the ePTFE valved conduit 2 (Video 08 min 52 s)

1. Anastomose the cephalic side of the pulmonary artery bifurcation.
2. Anastomose the caudal side of the pulmonary artery opening and adjust the caliber of the ePTFE valved conduit at the left end of the opening (left pulmonary artery side).
3. Check the remaining diameter of the ePTFE valved conduit (*solid red line*) against the margins of the remaining pulmonary artery opening.
4. If the autologous tissue opening is narrow, incise the autologous pericardium on the left pulmonary artery side to enlarge the opening (*green arrow*) (Case 6.2, Scene 10).

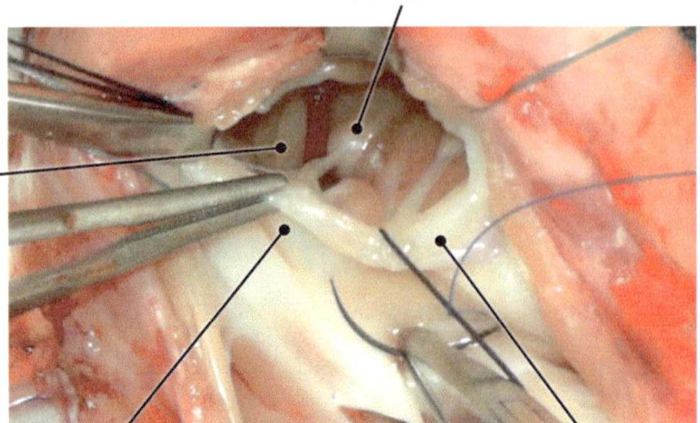

Case 6.2, Scene 10 Closure of the VSD 1 (Video 12 min 25 s)

1. Induce cardiac arrest and begin the VSD closure procedure via a trans-tricuspid approach.
2. 5-0 monofilament sutures with pledget are applied to the anterior leaflet of the tricuspid annulus.

- The closure technique is similar to standard VSD closure (Case 6.2, Scene 11).

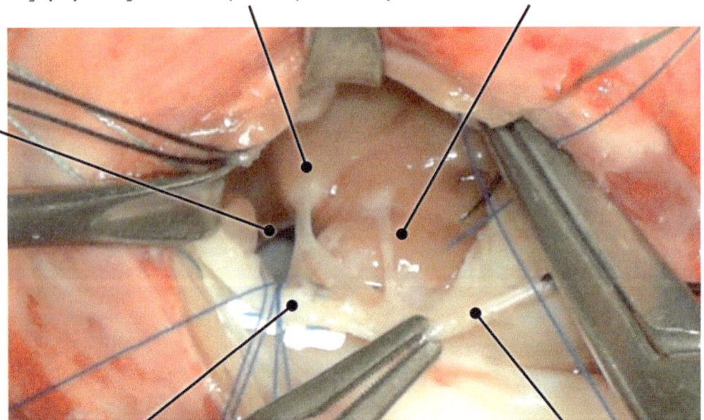

Case 6.2, Scene 11 Closure of the VSD 2 (Video 13 min 05 s)

1. 5-0 monofilament sutures with pledget are applied to the posterior edge of the VSD (posterior limb of the TSM) (Case 6.2, Scene 12).

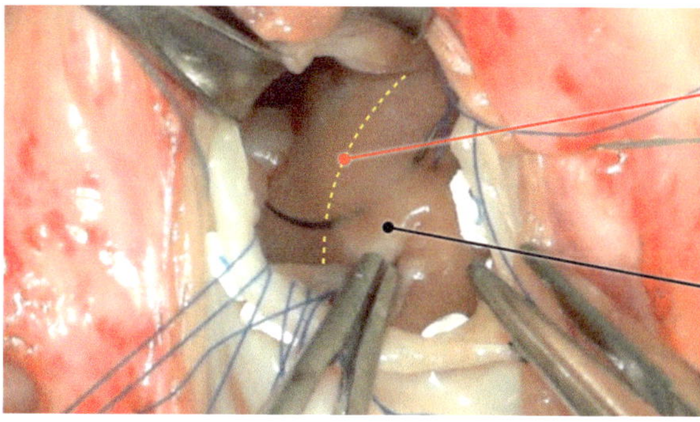

Case 6.2, Scene 12 Closure of the VSD 3 (Video 14 min 05 s)

1. Place the sutures across the right bundle branch.

- Insert the suture needle into the base of the medially papillary muscle, protrude into the subendocardium slightly short of the assumed line of the right bundle branch (yellow dashed line), and then protrude approximately 1 mm short of the assumed line of the right bundle branch after sliding under the endocardium (Case 6.2, Scene 13).

- The attachment of the infundibular septal muscle bundle to the TSM is cut (*green dashed line*) or wedge resected.
- The suture needle is inserted into the stump of the muscle bundle from the outflow tract side and then pierced just anterior to the aortic valve annulus.
- This muscle bundle may be cut through the right ventricular outflow tract incision (Case 6.2, Scene 14).

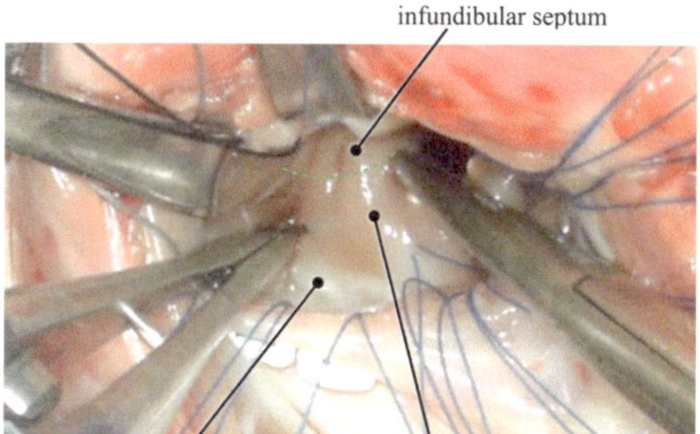

Case 6.2, Scene 13 Closure of the VSD 4 (Video 16 min 16 s)

1. Anastomosis of the anterior edge of the VSD.

- In this area, a thickened muscle bundle of the infundibular septum is attached to the anterior limb of the trabecular septomarginalis (TSM).

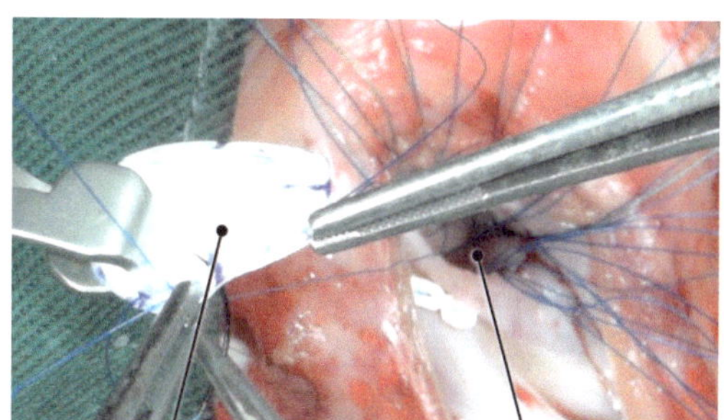

Case 6.2, Scene 14 Closure of the VSD 5 (Video 18 min 05 s)

1. Anastomose a 0.4-mm thick ePTFE patch (Case 6.2, Scene 15).

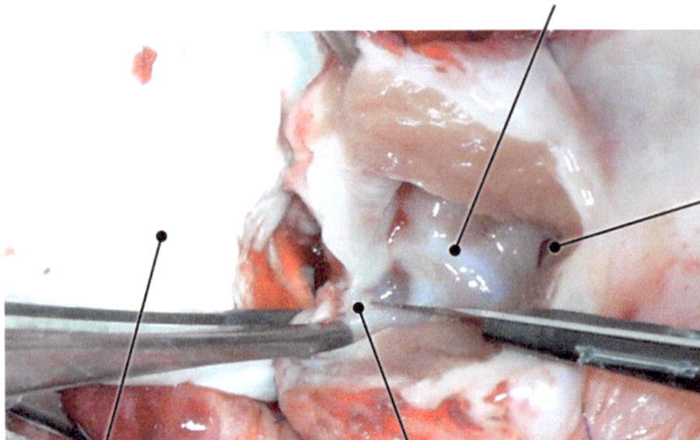

Case 6.2, Scene 15 Incise the right ventricular outflow tract (Video 18 min 56 s)

1. Make a longitudinal incision through the right ventricular outflow tract.
2. The superior edge of the incision should extend to the pulmonary valve annulus (which may be a blind edge).

- Because the left coronary artery runs dorsal to the pulmonary valve annulus, do not incise too far to avoid damaging the left coronary artery (be sure to leave a suture allowance) (Case 6.2, Scene 16).

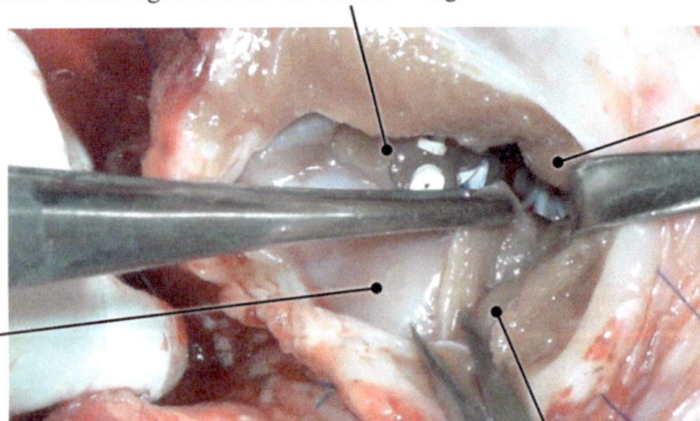

Case 6.2, Scene 16 Resection of the RVOT hypertrophied muscle bundle (Video 19 min 52 s)

1. Resect the hypertrophied muscle bundles through the RVOT opening.

ESSENTIALS Muscle Bundle Resection Areas as Seen Through the Right Ventricular Outflow Tract Incision

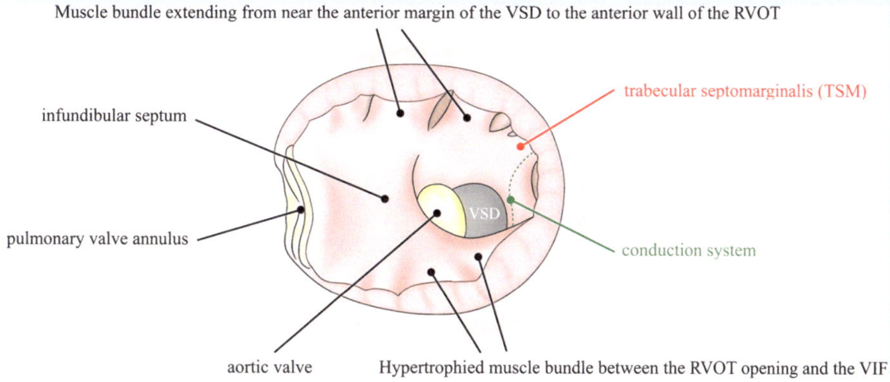

< Muscle bundle resection areas >

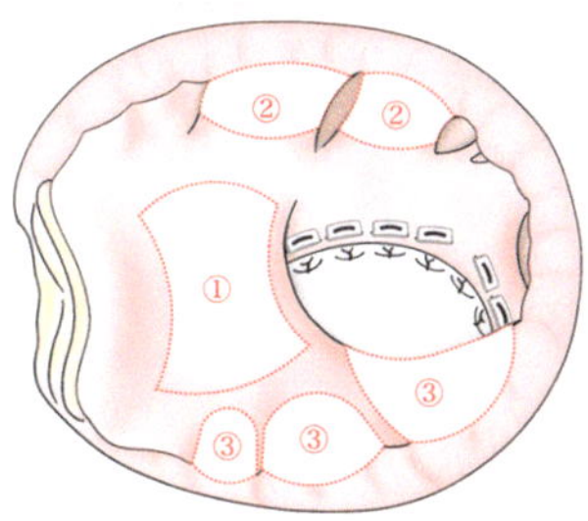

1. *Anteriorly deviated infundibular septum*
   - If the infundibular septum is thickened, shave off any protrusion into the right ventricular outflow tract lumen.
   - Be careful not to cut the VSD closure suture.
   - Be careful not to cut too deeply to avoid damaging the aortic valve.
2. *Muscle bundle extending from near the anterior margin of the VSD to the anterior wall of the RVOT*
   - The myocardial bundle in this area must be resected because it can cause postoperative residual stenosis.
   - Be careful not to incise the TSM where the right bundle branch is located (also check through the tricuspid valve).
3. *Hypertrophied muscle bundle between the RVOT opening and the VIF*
   - Since this area is the inflection point of the blood flow from the inflow to the outflow tract, the remaining muscle bundle in this area causes turbulence.
   - Therefore, the muscle bundle in this area (especially on the inflow side) should be resected in a wedge shape as much as possible (Case 6.2, Scene 17).

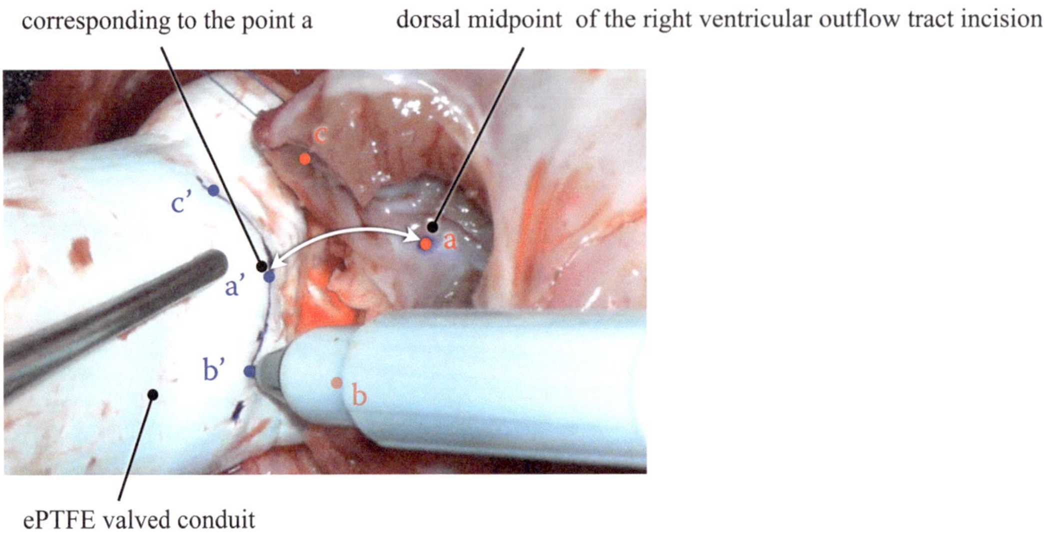

Case 6.2, Scene 17 Trimming of the RV-PA conduit 1 (Video 20 min 46 s)

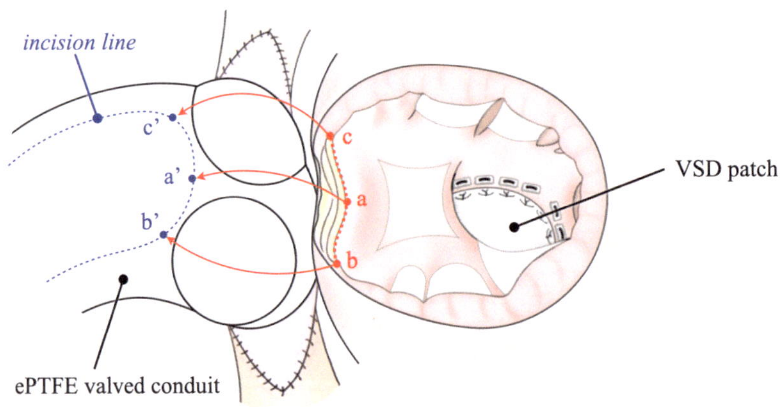

1. The dorsal midpoint of the right ventricular outflow tract incision is point (a), and the left and right sides of the incision are points (b) and (c).
2. Correspond to the right ventricular outflow tract with a natural shape so that the ePTFE valved conduit does not twist.
3. Mark point (a') on the ePTFE valved conduit corresponding to the center (point (a)) of the dorsal opening of the right ventricular outflow tract opening.
4. Next, mark points (b') and (c') corresponding to the right (point (b)) and left (point (c)) sides of the dorsal opening.
5. Determine the incision line so that c'-a'-b' becomes a smooth curve (*blue dashed line* in the figure below) (Case 6.2, Scene 18).

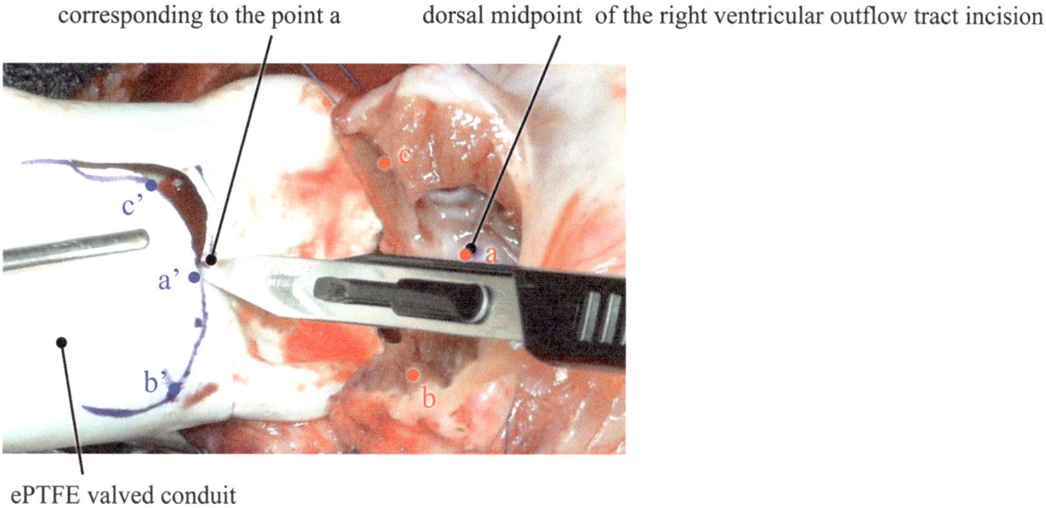

Case 6.2, Scene 18 Trimming of the RV-PA conduit 2 (Video 21 min 17 s)

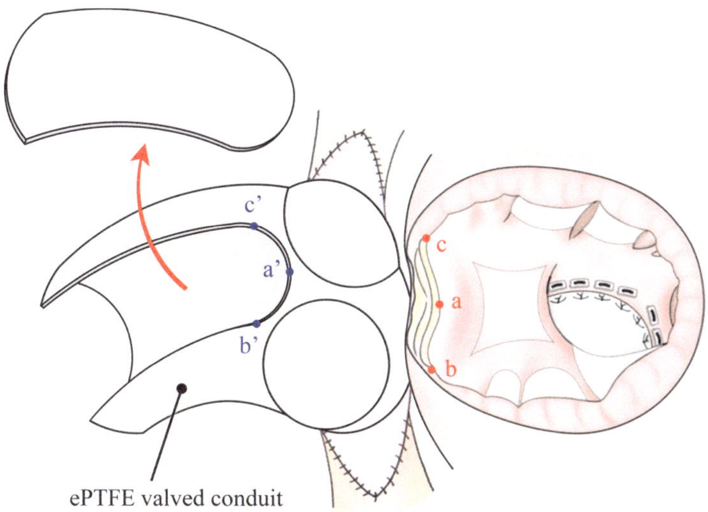

1. Incise the dorsal (lesser curvature) side of the ePTFE valved conduit with a scalpel.

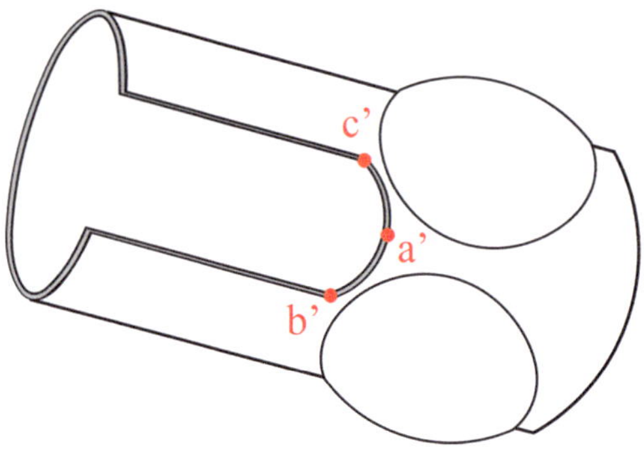

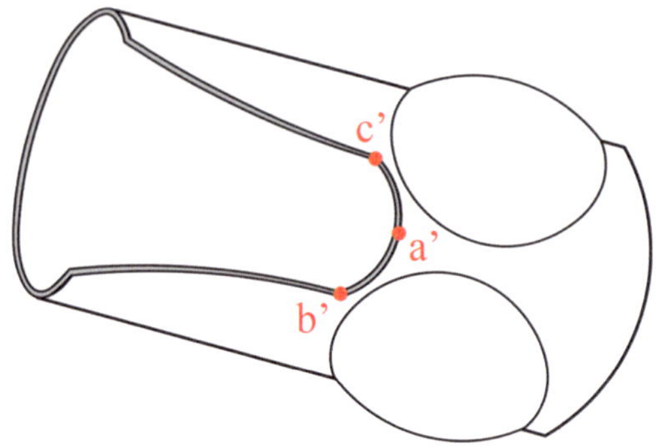

- Make a U-shaped incision on the dorsal (less curved) side of the ePTFE valved conduit.
- Instead of incising as shown in Figure A, it is better to incise the dorsal end as shown in Figure B.
- In Figure A, the end of the ePTFE valved conduit does not expand, making it difficult to suture (Case 6.2, Scene 19).

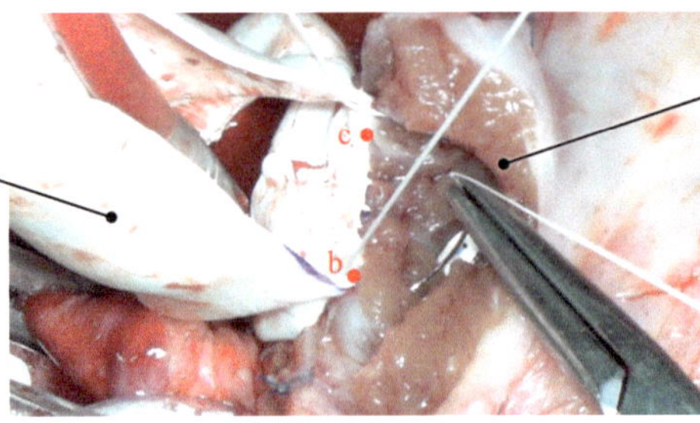

Case 6.2, Scene 19 Anastomosis of RV-PA conduit 1 (Video 21 min 48 s)

1. Anastomose the proximal end of the conduit opening to the right ventricular outflow tract opening (b-c) with a continuous ePTFE CV-5 suture.

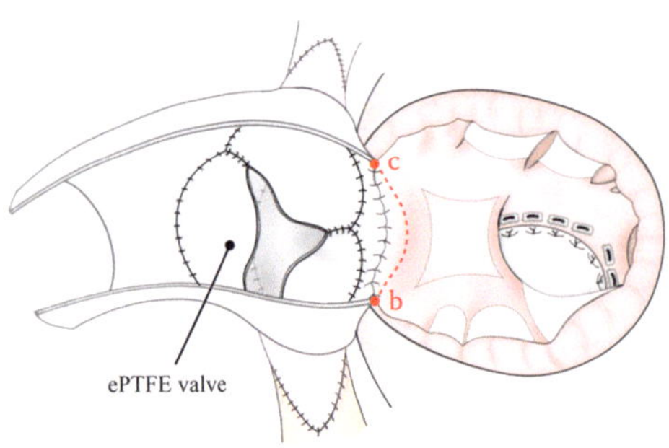

- In cases where the pulmonary artery bifurcation is close to the superior end of the right ventricular outflow tract incision, the lesser curvature side of the ePTFE valved conduit must be shortened and the cut end of the conduit may be over the suture line of the ePTFE valve.
- In such cases, the cut end of the conduit can be anastomosed closer to the right ventricular cavity (*red dashed line* b-c) (Case 6.2, Scene 20).

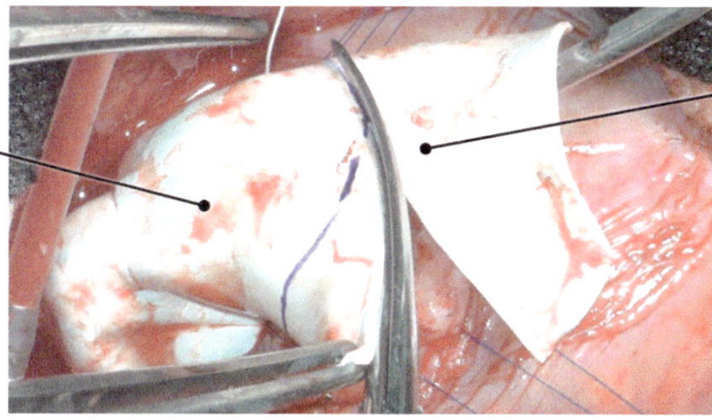

Case 6.2, Scene 20 Anastomosis of RV-PA conduit 2 (Video 24 min 00 s)

1. Draw incision lines on the ePTFE valved conduit to match the shape of the right ventricular outflow tract incision and resect the excess conduit wall.

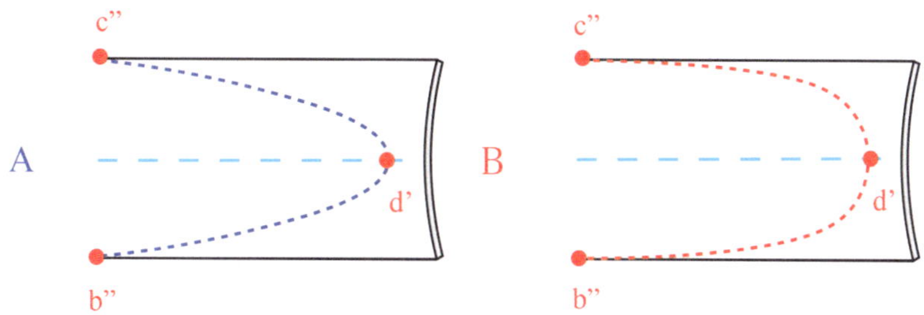

- Cut the ePTFE valved conduit wall along the curve (*red dashed line*) connecting b″-d'-c″.
- In this case, the cut line should not look like Figure A, but should bulge out as shown in Figure B.
- If cut as in Figure A, the proximal end (apical side) of the conduit will be flattened.
- Trimming in this manner allows the proximal end of the conduit to have a natural bulge.

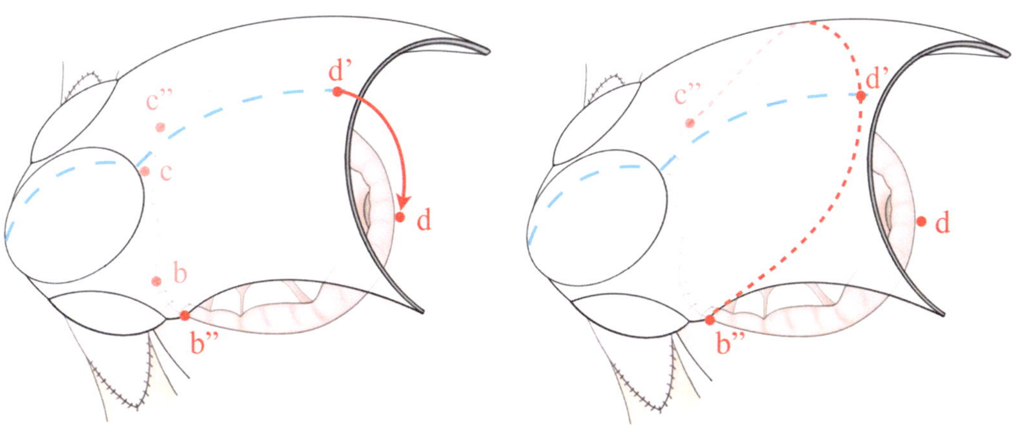

- Advance the anastomosis approximately 5–8 mm from the upper left edge of the right ventricular outflow tract incision (point (c)) to point (c″).
- Do not suture point (c-c") too long (as this will cause excessive redundancy in the conduit wall).
- In the same way, anastomose 5–8 mm from the upper right edge (point (b)) to point (b").
- Similarly, do not suture too long at point (b-b") (because the conduit wall will be too redundant).
- Determine point (d') corresponding to the lower end of the right ventricular outflow tract incision (point (d)) (Case 6.2, Scene 21).

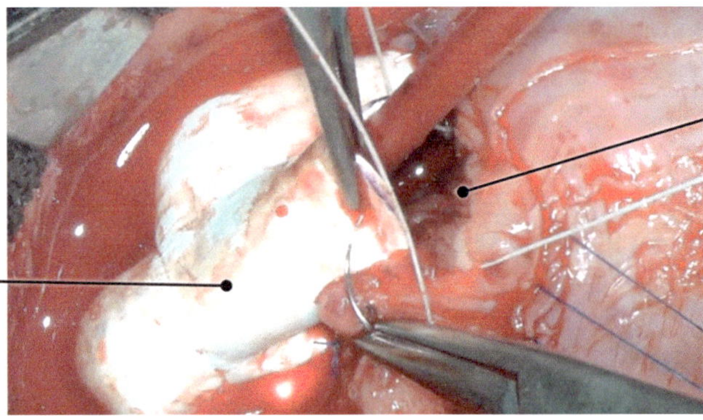

Case 6.2, Scene 21 Anastomosis of RV-PA conduit 3 (Video 24 min 56 s)

1. Anastomose so that the suture step width on the conduit side is longer than the step width of the right ventricular opening.
2. The suture at the right ventricular opening should be inserted firmly into the right ventricular opening from a point away from the edge to avoid rupture of the myocardium, and be careful not to protrude from a point away from the edge.

- The endocardial side is particularly prone to myocardial rupture.
- If the myocardium is thick, it can be inserted into one sectional area after protruding once and then inserted into the adjacent sectional area (Case 6.2, Scene 22).

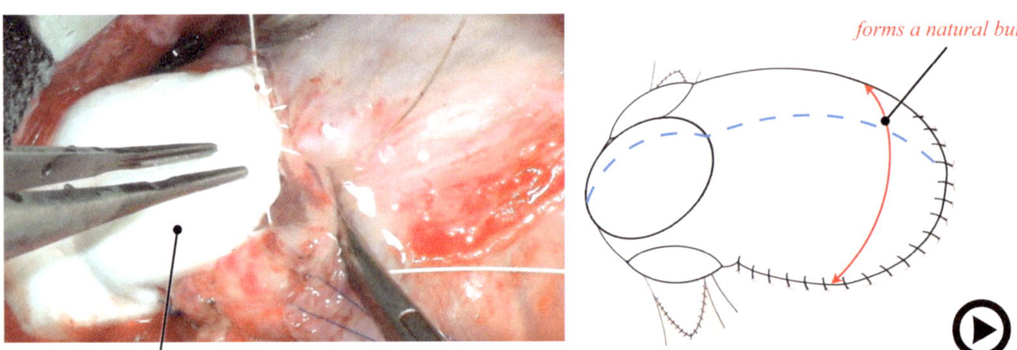

Case 6.2, Scene 22 Anastomosis of RV-PA conduit 4 (Video 28 min 38 s) (▶ https://doi.org/10.1007/000-hkc)

1. The proximal side of the conduit forms a natural bulge by making the suture width on the conduit side slightly larger than the suture width on the right ventricular opening side.

ESSENTIALS CT Images After the RVOT Reconstruction Using ePTFE Valved Conduit

The dorsal aspect of the right ventricular outflow tract opening (point (a)) coincides with the upper edge of the ventricular septum. The opening of the pulmonary artery bifurcation (point (b)) approximately coincides with the dorsal aspect of the ascending aorta. The distance between point (a) and the caudal point of the bifurcation opening (point (b)) determines the length of the lesser curvature (dorsal) side of the conduit. A preoperative CT lateral view should be taken to confirm that this distance is sufficient. The left anterior descending branch of the coronary artery is located just dorsal to point (a). The location of the left coronary artery should be kept in mind, especially for reoperations.

< Case 1 >

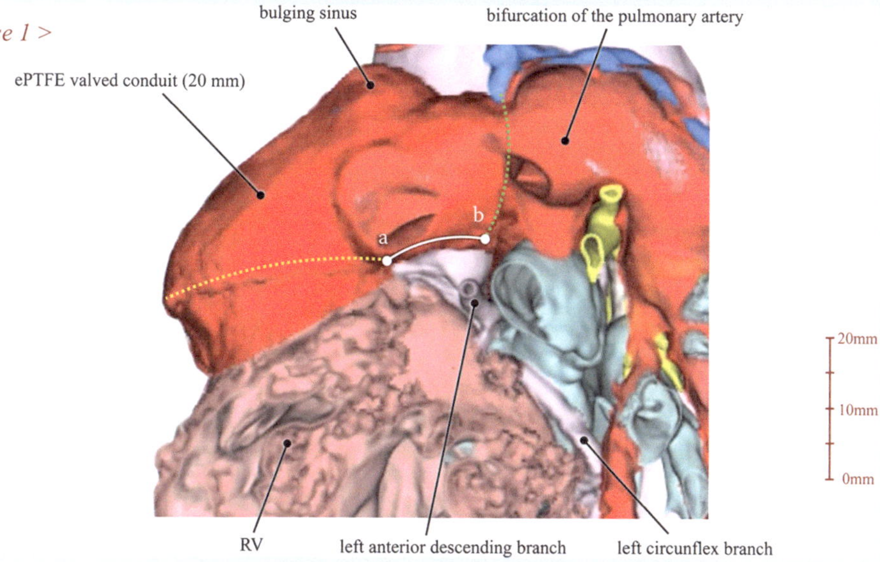

- The distance between the pulmonary artery bifurcation opening (*green dashed line*) and the right ventricular outflow tract opening (*yellow dashed line*) is short.
- Therefore, the length of the dorsal side of the conduit (white solid line) should be shortened.
- The left anterior descending branch of the coronary artery is present on the dorsal side of the conduit.

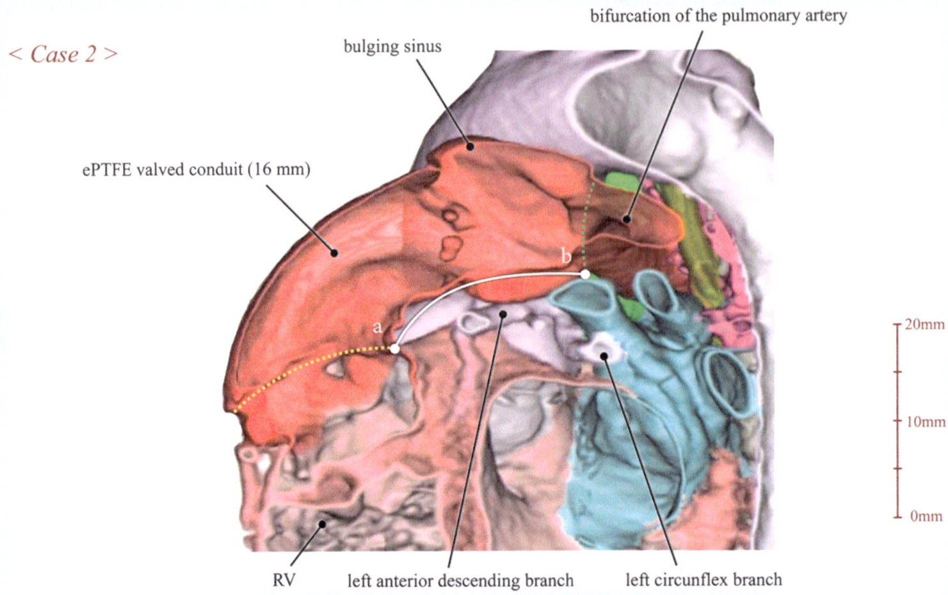

- In this case, the distance between the pulmonary artery bifurcation opening (*green dashed line*) and the right ventricular outflow tract opening (*yellow dashed line*) is long.
- The dorsal side of the conduit (*white solid line*) can be long enough.
- The left anterior descending branch of the coronary artery is present on the dorsal side of the conduit.

ESSENTIALS Fluid Analysis After the Rastelli Procedure

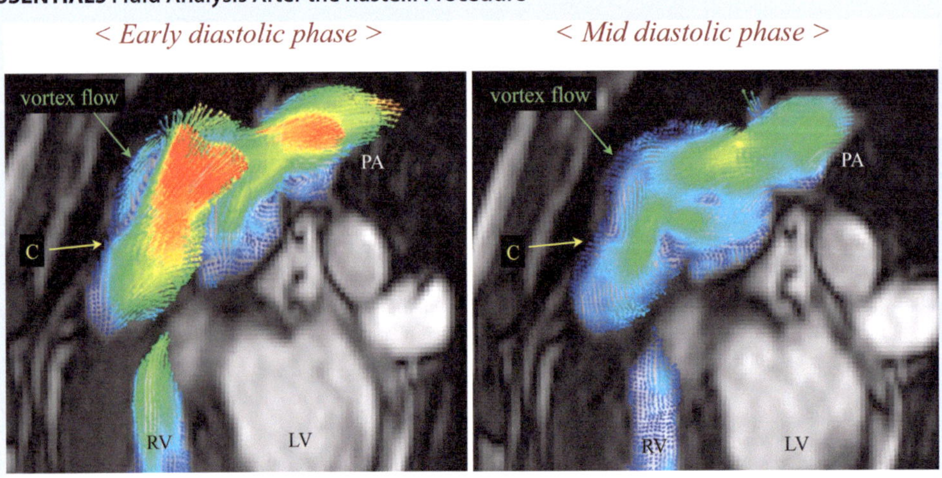

C : ePTFE valved conduit with bulging sinus

- Fluid analysis after the Rastelli procedure with fan-shaped ePTFE tricuspid valve, ePTFE conduit with bulging sinus is shown.
- Vortex flow is observed in the bulging sinus of the conduit during early and mid-diastole.
- This vortex flow may contribute to ePTFE valve motion, especially valve closure.

References

ePTFE Pulmonary Valve, ePTFE Conduit with Bulging Sinus and ePTFE Valve

Yamagishi M, Kurosawa H. Outflow reconstruction of tetralogy of Fallot using a Gore-Tex valve. Ann Thorac Surg. 1993;56:1414–7.

Yamagishi M, Kurosawa H, Nomura K, et al. Fan-shaped expanded polytetrafluoroethylene valve in the pulmonary position. J Cardiovasc Surg (Torino). 2002;43:779–86.

Yamagishi M. Right ventricular outflow reconstruction using a polytetrafluoroethylene conduit with bulging sinuses and tricuspid fan-shaped polytetrafluoroethylene valve. Oper Tech Thorac Cardiovasc Surg. 2016;21:211–29.

Pathological Considerations of the ePTFE Valve

Yamamoto Y, Yamagishi M, Maeda Y, et al. Histopathologic analysis of explanted polytetrafluoroethylene-valved pulmonary conduits. Semin Thorac Cardiovasc Surg. 2020;32:990–9.

Small Caliber ePTFE Conduit with Bulging Sinus and ePTFE Valve

Yamashita E, Yamagishi M, et al. Smaller-sized expanded polytetrafluoroethylene conduits with a fan-shaped valve and bulging sinuses for right ventricular outflow tract reconstruction. Ann Thorac Surg. 2016;102:1336–44.

Long-Term Results of the ePTFE Conduit with Bulging Sinus and ePTFE Valve

Hongu H, Yamagishi M, Maeda Y, et al. Expanded polytetrafluoroethylene conduits with bulging sinuses and a fan-shaped valve in right ventricular outflow tract reconstruction. Semin Thorac Cardiovasc Surg. 2022;34:972–80.

Fujita S, Yamagishi M, et al. Long-term results of large-calibre expanded polytetrafluoroethylene-valved conduits with bulging sinuses. Eur J Cardiothorac Surg. 2020;58:1274–80.

Engineering Investigation of the ePTFE Valve

Suzuki I, Shiraishi Y, Yamagishi M, et al. Engineering analysis of the effects of bulging sinuses in a newly designed pediatric pulmonary heart valve on hemodynamic function. J Artif Organs. 2012;15:49–56.

Tsuboko Y, Shiraishi Y, Yamagishi M, et al. Engineering based assessment for a shape design of a pediatric ePTFE pulmonary conduit valve. Annu Int Conf IEEE Eng Med Biol Soc. 2016:4313–6.

Shiraishi Y, Narracott AJ, Yamagishi M, et al. In Vitro modelling for bulging sinus effects of an expanded polytetrafluoroethylene valved conduit based on high-speed 3d leaflet evaluation. Annu Int Conf IEEE Eng Med Biol Soc. 2022:4001–4.

Major Aorto-Pulmonary Collateral Arteries (MAPCA)

7

1 Major Aorto-Pulmonary Collateral Arteries (MAPCA)

1.1 Morphological Characteristics of MAPCA

In heart disease associated with pulmonary atresia and ventricular septal defect, the blood flow pathway from the ventricle to the pulmonary artery is defective, resulting in hypoplasia of the pulmonary artery and the development of collateral blood vessels from the aorta or neck branches (brachiocephalic and subclavian arteries) to the pulmonary artery. The relatively large vessels in this pathway are called major aorto-pulmonary collateral arteries (MAPCAs). The MAPCAs originate from the aorta or cervical artery and then join the pulmonary artery. Pulmonary blood flow is often reduced, but pulmonary areas perfused by MAPCAs that do not have stenotic lesions have high pulmonary flow. The MAPCAs have the following characteristics (Fig. 7.1).

1. *Originating from the Systemic Artery*
   - Most commonly originates from the anterior or lateral aspect of the descending thoracic aorta near the tracheobronchial bifurcation (carina).
   - Very rarely from a systemic artery other than the descending thoracic aorta and the cervical branch.
   - The origin is the same, but after the origin, it may branch to the left, right, and superior side.
   - May originate even lower than near the carina (e.g., MAPCA to the left inferior lobe).

2. *Running Pattern*
   - Runs dorsal to the bronchus, dorsal to the pulmonary vein.
   - Runs anterior or dorsal to the esophagus.
   - Runs in a tortuous fashion.
   - May be stenotic near its origin, adjacent to the bronchus, or in communication with the pulmonary artery.
   - Vessels with different areas of perfusion may join (bypass) in the lung (arborization anomaly).

1. *Characteristics*
   - Unlike patent ductus arteriosus, not affected by prostaglandin E1.
   - Morphology may change with age (depending on the extent of stenotic lesions).

Supplementary Information The online version contains supplementary material available at https://doi.org/10.1007/978-981-96-6194-7_7. The videos can be accessed individually by clicking the DOI link in the accompanying figure caption or by scanning this link with the SN More Media App.

M. Yamagishi, *Surgical Treatment of Congenital Heart Disease*,
https://doi.org/10.1007/978-981-96-6194-7_7

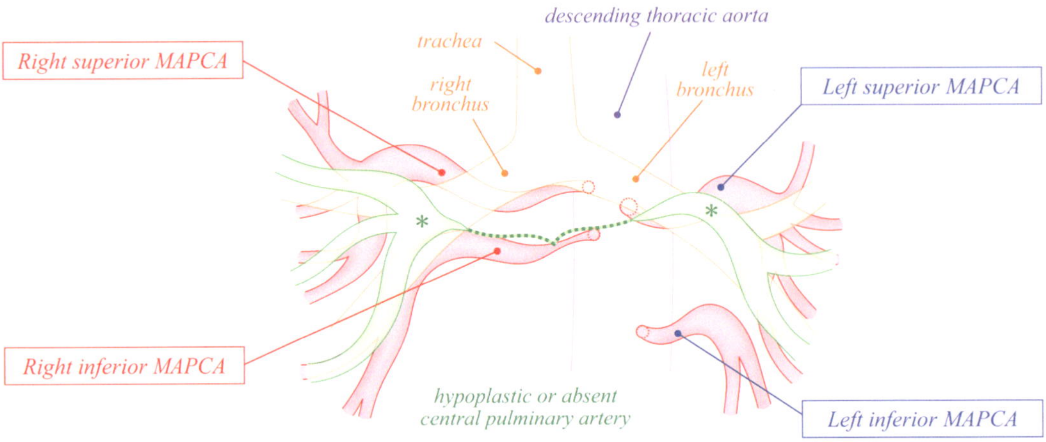

Fig. 7.1 Morphological characteristics of MAPCAs

- MAPCA wall is more fragile and less extensible than normal pulmonary arteries.

The morphology of MAPCA (number, branching, course, etc.) is highly variable, but often has the following characteristics depending on the location.

Right Superior MAPCA
- Origins from the descending thoracic aorta near the level of the carina.
- May run dorsal to the esophagus.
- Runs dorsal to the right main bronchus.
- Adjacent to the dorsal surface of the right main bronchus near the bifurcation of the superior lobe branch.
- May run anterior to the right main bronchus.

Right Inferior MAPCA
- Origins from the descending thoracic aorta near the level of the carina.
- May branch from the right superior MAPCA.
- Runs slightly inferior to the right main bronchus.
- Adjacent to the dorsal inferior right lower lobe bronchus.

Left Superior MAPCA
- Origins from the descending thoracic aorta near the level of the carina.
- Runs dorsal to the left main bronchus.
- Adjacent to the dorsal surface of the left main bronchus near the bifurcation of the superior lobe branch.

Left Inferior MAPCA
- May originate independently from the descending thoracic aorta one to two vertebrae below the carina.

**Peripheral Pulmonary Arteries Connecting from Hypoplastic Central Pulmonary Artery*
- Runs in front of the bronchi and pulmonary veins (Fig. 7.2).

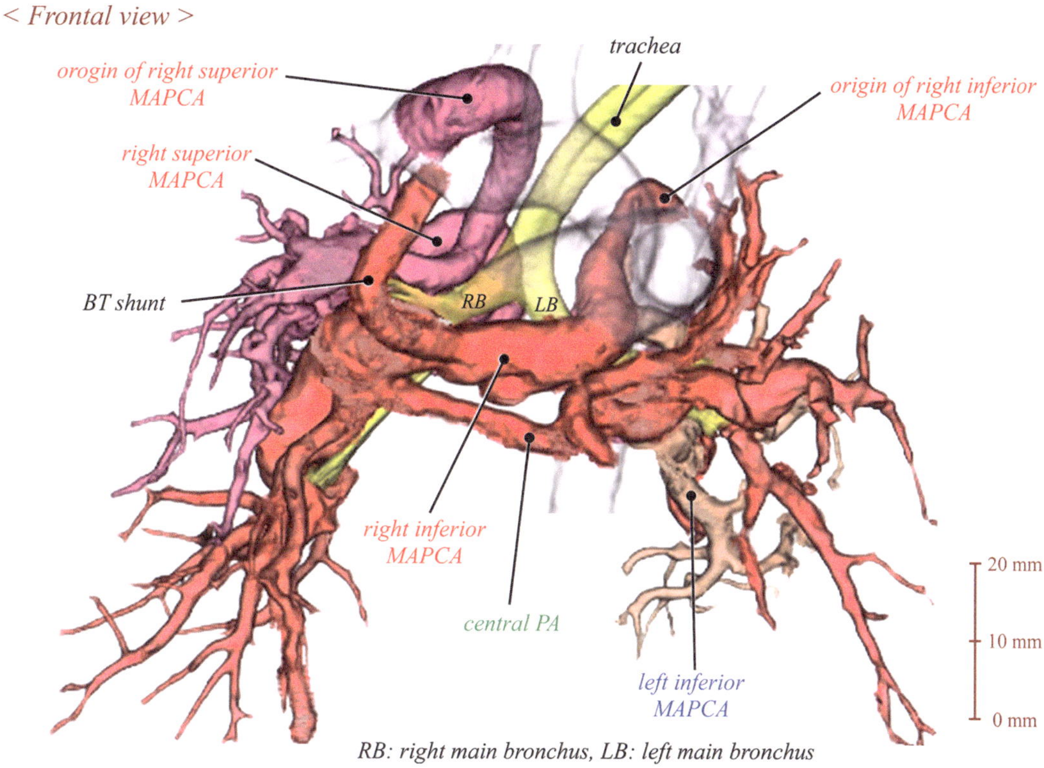

Fig. 7.2 CT images of MAPCA (case 1: hypoplastic central pulmonary artery)

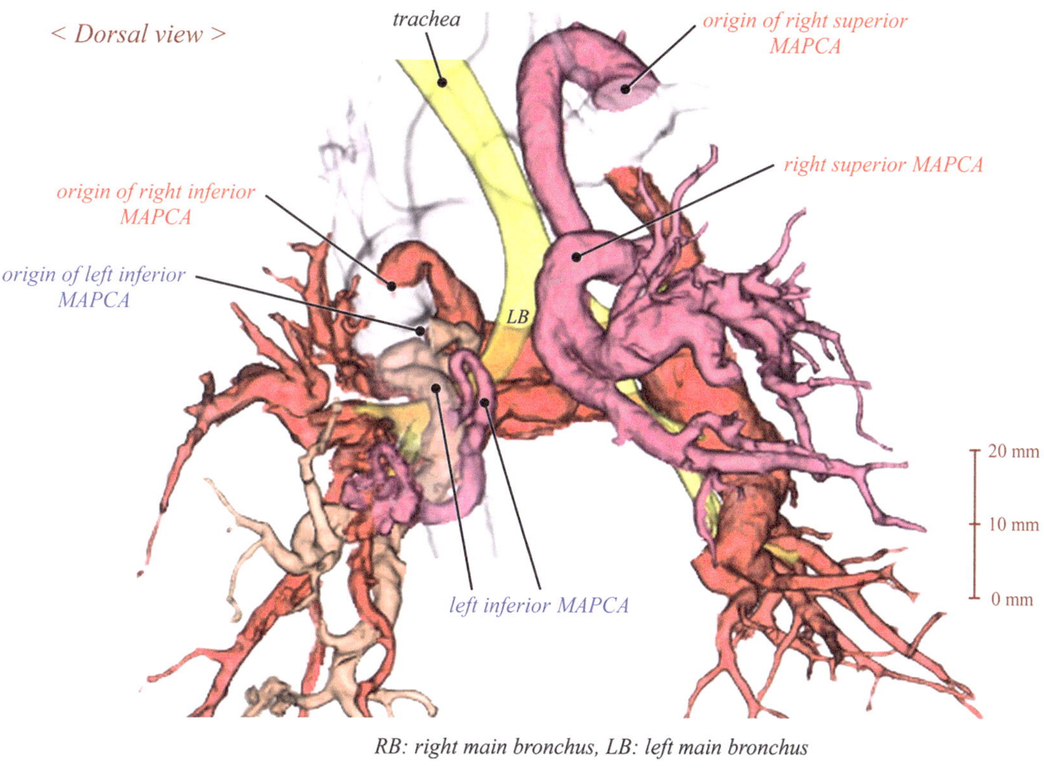

Central Pulmonary Artery The central pulmonary artery is hypoplastic. It is distributed in the lower lobe of the right lung and in the upper and middle lobes of the left lung.

Right Superior MAPCA It originates from the cervical vessels and runs just dorsal to the right main bronchus. It distributes to the upper and middle lobes of the right lung.

Right Middle and Inferior MAPCAs It originates from the cervical vessels and runs horizontally from left to right in front of both bronchi and distributes to the upper lobe of the right lung. It is anastomosed to the BT shunt. It is connected to the central pulmonary artery (arborization anomaly).

Left Inferior MAPCAs Two left inferior MAPCAs arise from the descending aorta. The MAPCA arising from the caudal side is thin (Fig. 7.3).

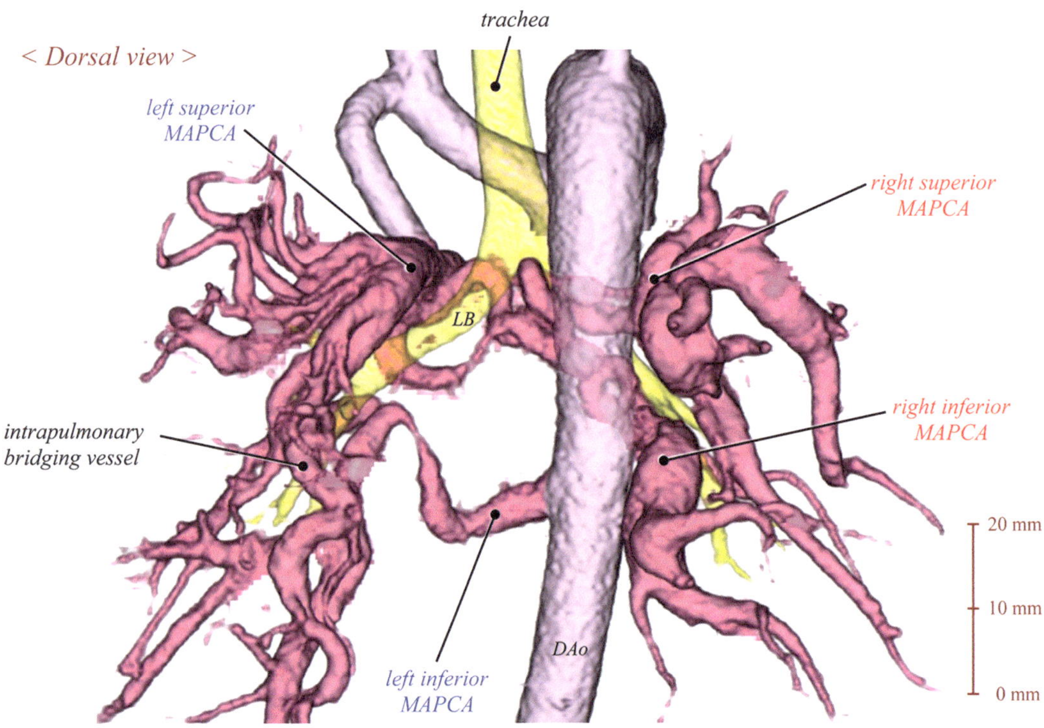

LB: left main bronchus

Right Superior MAPCA It originates from the descending thoracic aorta near the level of the carina and runs dorsal to the right main bronchus. Adjacent to the dorsal surface of the right main bronchus near the bifurcation of the superior lobe branch. Peripheral pulmonary arteries are distributed ventrally and dorsally across the left upper bronchus.

Right Inferior MAPCA It originates from the descending thoracic aorta near the level of the carina and runs slightly inferior to the right main bronchus. Adjacent to the dorsal inferior right lower lobe bronchus.

Left Superior MAPCA It originates from the descending thoracic aorta near the level of the carina and runs over the left main bronchus.

Left Inferior MAPCA It originates independently from the descending thoracic aorta one to two vertebrae below the carina and runs slightly

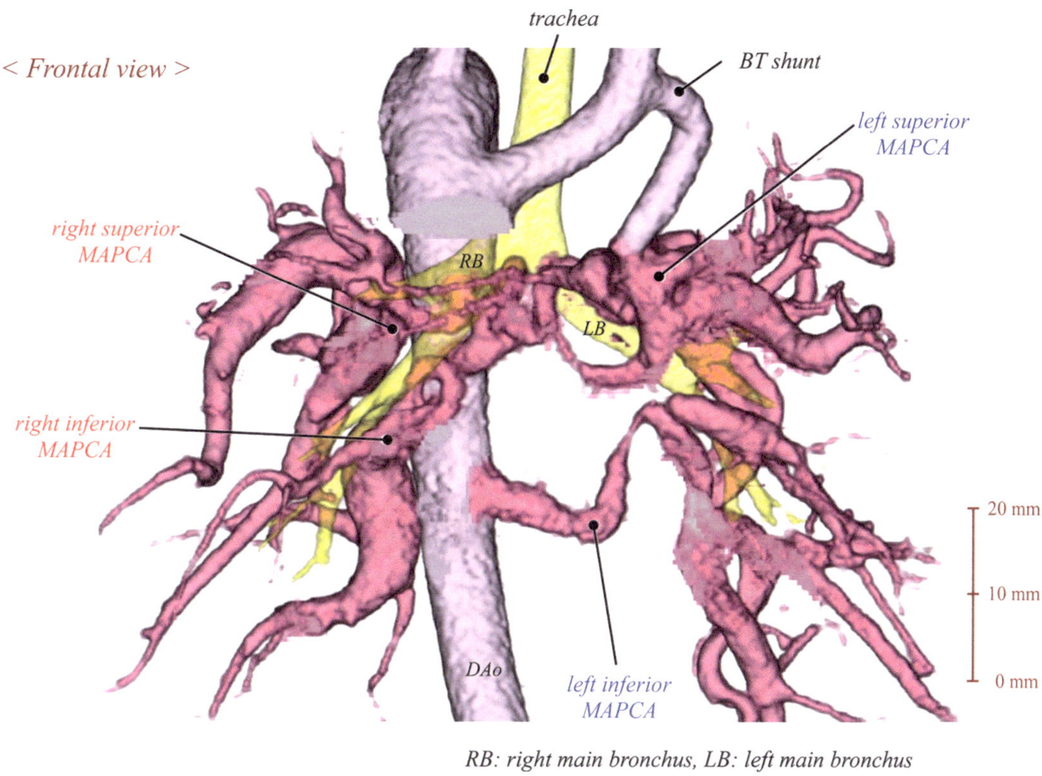

Fig. 7.3 CT images of MAPCA (case 2: absent central pulmonary artery)

inferior to the left inferior lobe branch. A bridging vessel is recognized between the superior and inferior intrapulmonary arteries.

1.2 Factors Affecting Surgical Treatment Planning for MAPCA

1. *Configuration of the MAPCAs*
   The following MAPCA configurations should be considered when planning a unifocalization procedure.
   - *Origin*: Point of origin (descending thoracic aorta, cervical vessels), often bifurcated near the origin.
   - *Number of vessels, area of perfusion.*
   - *Running pattern*: Relationship to esophagus, bronchus, and pulmonary veins is important.
   - *Presence of stenosis*: Stenosis may be present near the origin or at the crossing with the bronchus. Balloon angioplasty may be ineffective.
   - *Presence of arborization anomaly*: If there is a large intrapulmonary connection (arborization anomaly), only the origin should be amputated (unifocalization is not necessary).
2. *Configuration of the Central Pulmonary Artery*
   For hypoplastic or absent central pulmonary arteries, determine whether to enlarge the artery using the remaining central pulmonary artery or to create a central pulmonary artery using an autologous pericardial roll. Consider the perfusion zone from the central pulmonary artery and whether or not it is connected to the MAPCA.

3. *Arterial Blood Oxygen Saturation*
   Arterial blood oxygen saturation (SaO_2) is often decreased in this syndrome due to stenotic lesions of the MAPCA and hypoplasia of the peripheral pulmonary artery. If SaO_2 cannot be maintained at 75–80% even with medical therapy (oxygen inhalation, vasodilators), a prior BT shunt should be considered.
4. *Months of Age (Years of Age)*
   The optimal age range for unifocalization is from late infancy (around 8 months of age) to before 2 years of age. In the neonatal period and early infancy, the MAPCA caliber is narrow, and there is a risk of anastomotic stenosis even if unifocalization is performed. On the other hand, after 2 years of age, there are many cases in which pulmonary vascular growth and pulmonary vascular resistance do not decrease after unifocalization.

1.3 Treatment Strategies for MAPCA Based on Growth Rate of the Central Pulmonary Artery

The surgical treatment plan is highly dependent on the presence or absence and the degree of growth of the central pulmonary artery. In cases of mild hypoplasia, definitive surgery can be performed in a single stage, but in cases of moderate or severe central pulmonary artery dysplasia, multi-stage surgery consisting of unifocalization and palliative right ventricular outflow tract reconstruction is required.

- Treatment Strategy for Cases of Mild Hypoplasia of the Central Pulmonary Artery

In cases of mild hypoplasia of the central pulmonary artery (PA index > 160), the area of blood perfusion from the central pulmonary artery is relatively wide, and there are often only one or two MAPCAs. In such cases, definitive surgery (Rastelli operation) with unifocalization can be performed in early infancy (1–3 years of age).

In cases where arterial oxygen saturation (> 75–80%) cannot be maintained, BT shunt should precede unifocalization. BT shunt through a lateral thoracotomy approach is preferable, but a median sternotomy approach can be used in cases where pulmonary artery augmentation is not considered necessary (Fig. 7.4).

- Treatment Strategy for Cases of Moderate or Severe Hypoplasia of the Central Pulmonary Artery

The treatment strategy is similar for cases of moderate hypoplasia of the central pulmonary artery (PA index less than 160) and for cases of severe hypoplasia or defects. The only difference is the method of creation of the central pulmonary artery.

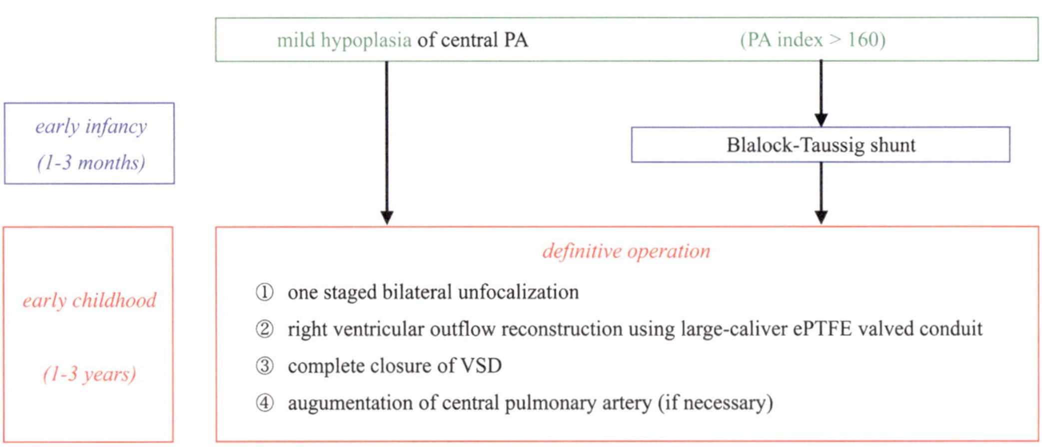

Fig. 7.4 Treatment strategy for MAPCA with mild hypoplasia of the central PA

In cases of severe cyanosis, a B-T shunt is preceded by a lateral open chest in early infancy. If there is a MAPCA that is difficult to approach through a median sternotomy, unifocalization of the MAPCA should be performed at the same time, if possible. From late infancy (8 months) to early childhood (2 years), a median sternotomy approach and extracorporeal circulation should be used for (1) one staged bilateral unifocalization and (2) palliative right ventricular outflow tract reconstruction (small-caliber conduit).

In cases of moderate hypoplasia of the central pulmonary artery, an augmentation using an autologous pericardial patch is performed, and in cases of severe hypoplasia or deficit, a central pulmonary artery creation using a Y-shaped autologous pericardial roll is performed (Fig. 7.5).

2 Basic Surgical Treatment Strategies for MAPCA

The surgical treatment of patients with MAPCA is based on a two-stage surgical approach consisting of a first-stage bilateral unifocalization and palliative right ventricular outflow tract creation followed by a second-stage Rastelli operation. This two-stage procedure allows for growth of the pulmonary arteries and complete closure of the ventricular septal defect. Both phases are approached through a median sternotomy.

Unilateral unifocalization, in which one lung is treated separately through a lateral open chest approach, results in unequal pulmonary blood flow to the right and left lungs, necessitating the use of artificial materials such as heterogeneous pericardium or homograft patch, and inevitably leads to future stenotic lesions.

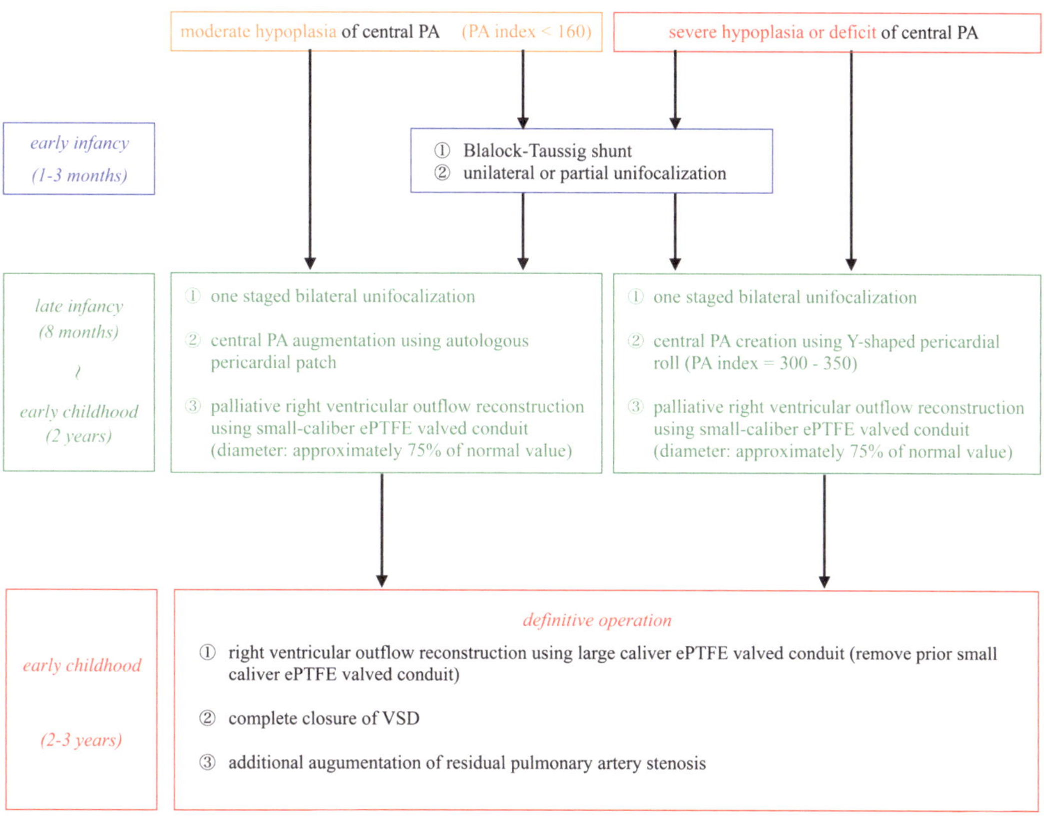

Fig. 7.5 Treatment strategy for MAPCA with moderate or severe hypoplasia of the central PA

2.1 Stage 1: Unifocalization of the MAPCAs and Palliative Right Ventricular Outflow Reconstruction

1. One-Stage Unifocalization Through a Median Sternotomy

Unifocalization of both right and left MAPCAs through a median sternotomy approach should be performed to ensure equal distribution of pulmonary blood flow. In bilateral one-stage unifocalization, the origins of the MAPCAs from the descending thoracic aorta or other cervical vessels are cut under extracorporeal circulation, and the MAPCA orifices are basically unifocalized at both pulmonary hilums. The following is an example of a one-stage unifocalization through a median sternotomy (Fig. 7.6).

Right MAPCAs

- The right MAPCA originates from the descending aorta at the dorsal side of the right main bronchus, and then the superior lobe artery (R1) branches off at the dorsal side of the bronchus.
- After R#1 branches, another superior lobe artery (R2) branches off from the bifurcation of the right upper and right lower bronchi
- R1 and R2 join together (arborization anomaly) in front of the right upper bronchus (*).
- The right lower lobe artery (R3) passes over the right lower bronchus and distributes to the lower lobe.
- Another thin lower lobe artery (R4) originates independently from the descending aorta and runs below the right lower bronchus.

Left MAPCAs

- The MAPCA, which supplies blood flow to the upper and middle lobes of the left lung, originates from the descending aorta and immediately branches into L1 and L2.
- L1 runs along the dorsal side of the left main bronchus after branching.
- L2 runs along the front of the left lower bronchus after branching.
- Another MAPCA (L3) originates independently from the descending aorta and distributes to the dorsal middle and lower lobes. It also runs from the bifurcation of the left upper and lower lobes to the anterior aspect of the bronchus and joins L2 (#) (arborization anomaly) (Figs. 7.7, 7.8, 7.9, and 7.10).

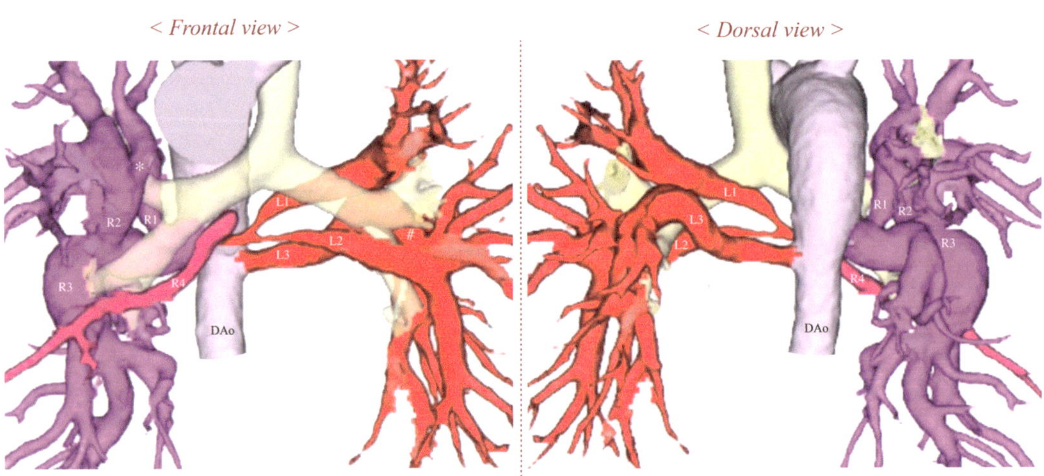

Fig. 7.6 CT images of MAPCA with deficit of the central PA

Fig. 7.7 Treatment strategy of MAPCA with deficit of the central PA (1)

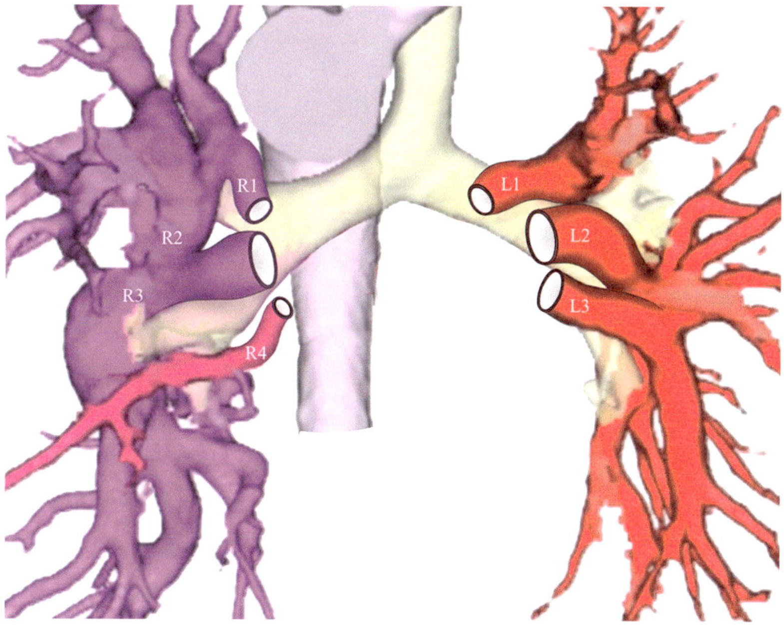

Fig. 7.8 Treatment strategy of MAPCA with deficit of the central PA (2)

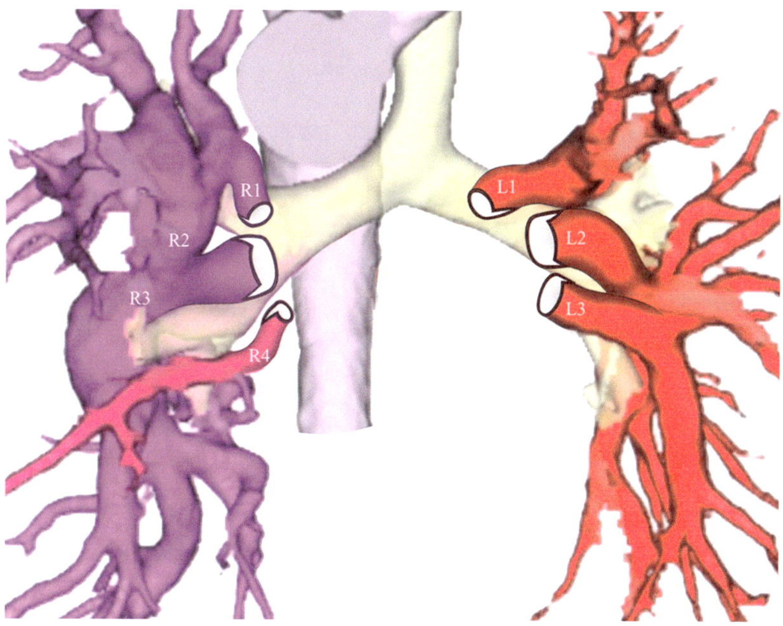

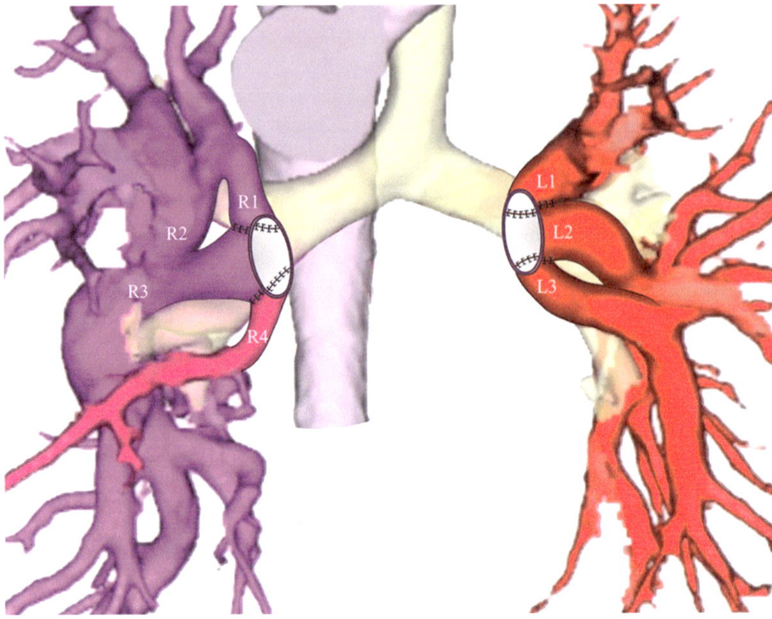

Fig. 7.9 Treatment strategy of MAPCA with deficit of the central PA (3)

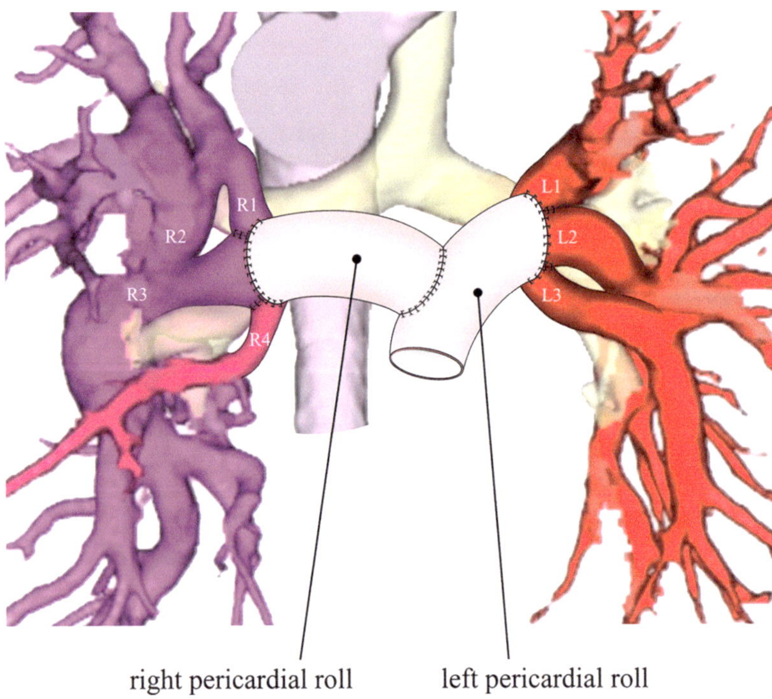

Fig. 7.10 Treatment strategy of MAPCA with deficit of the central PA (4)

Right MAPCAs

- Cut the right MAPCA at the origin. Cut it at the bifurcation of the superior lobe artery (R1). Extract the R1 stump from the dorsal side of the right upper bronchus and displace it anteriorly.
- Cut the proximal portions of another superior lobe artery (R2) and the right lower lobe artery (R3). Extract the stump from between the upper and lower bronchi and displace it anteriorly.
- Cut the another lower lobe artery (R4) at the origin. Dissect the R4 stump and displace it anteriorly.

Left MAPCAs

- Cut the left MAPCA at the origin. Cut L1 before the bifurcation. Extract the L1 stump from the dorsal side of the left upper bronchus and displace it anteriorly.
- Cut L2 at the bifurcation. Extract the L2 stump from between the upper and lower bronchi and displace it anteriorly.
- Cut L3 at the origin.

ESSENTIALS Strategy for MAPCA Running Posterior to the Bronchus

1. If all intrapulmonary pulmonary arteries are distributed on the posterior side of the bronchus on the peripheral side, perform unifocalization on the anterior side of the bronchus by transposing the origin to the anterior side of the bronchus after cutting the origin.
2. If the intrapulmonary arteries are distributed on the ventral and dorsal sides of the bronchi on the peripheral side, it is difficult to perform unifocalization on the anterior side of the bronchi, so unifocalization must be performed on the dorsal side of the bronchi.
3. If unifocalization is not possible through the median sternotomy approach, unifocalization and Blalock-Tsussig shunt should be performed through the lateral thoracotomy as a prior operation.

Right MAPCAs

- Make a longitudinal incision on the lower wall of R1, the upper and lower walls of R2+R3, and the upper wall of R4 toward the peripheral side.

Left MAPCAs

- Make a longitudinal incision on the lower wall of L1, the upper and lower walls of L2, and the upper wall of L3 toward the peripheral side.
- Create a single orifice of the right pulmonary artery at the right hilum by side-to-side anastomosis of R1, R2+R3, and R4.
- Create a single orifice of the left pulmonary artery at the left hilum by side-to-side anastomosis of L1, L2, and L3.

2. Reconstruction of the Central Pulmonary Artery and Anastomosis of MAPCAs

In cases of hypoplastic central pulmonary artery, the hypoplastic central pulmonary artery is augmented with a pericardial patch. The MAPCAs are anastomosed to the augmented central pulmonary artery. In cases of central pulmonary artery deficit, the central pulmonary artery is created with a pericardial roll. The right and left pericardial rolls are formed in a Y-shape.

The unifocalized MAPCA orifice is anastomosed end-to-end to the pericardial roll. The MAPCAs that cannot be unifocalized at the pulmonary hilum are anastomosed end-to-side to the pericardial roll.

- Determine the caliber of the pericardial roll with a PA index of 300–350 mm/m.
- Set the caliber slightly larger to avoid stenosis later.
- Determine the length of the pericardial roll with reference to the CT.
- End-to-end anastomosis of the pericardial roll to the unifocalized MAPCA orifice at the pulmonary hilum. The right and left autologous pericardial rolls are end-to-side anastomosed in the middle in a Y-shape so that the blood

flow from the ventricles becomes as laminar as possible.

- MAPCAs that cannot be unifocalized to the pericardial roll at the hilum are end-to-side or side-to-side anastomosed to the pericardial roll. MAPCAs that cannot reach the pericardial roll are anastomosed to the intrapulmonary artery.

3. Reconstruction of the Central Pulmonary Artery and Anastomosis of MAPCAs

An extracardiac conduit (valved ePTFE graft) is created between the right ventricle and the created central pulmonary artery. In patients with MAPCAs, the intrapulmonary pulmonary artery is often hypoplastic, and concomitant closure of the ventricular septal defect with unifocalization may cause an increase in right ventricular pressure. Therefore, the ventricular septal defect is not closed at the same time as unifocalization, and a small right ventricular-pulmonary artery conduit is used to provide adequate pulmonary blood flow (palliative right ventricular outflow tract reconstruction: palliative RVOTR). The conduit should be small in diameter (70–75% of the normal pulmonary artery annulus diameter) to avoid pulmonary hypertension due to excessive blood flow. The target ratio of pulmonary blood flow to systemic blood flow (Q_p/Q_s) is 1.0.

After unifocalization and palliative RVOTR, a slightly higher pulmonary blood flow may be allowed to promote pulmonary vascular growth. Postoperatively, pulmonary hypertension medications should be administered along with oxygen inhalation. In patients for whom Fontan surgery is indicated, a Blalock-Taussig (BT) shunt should be selected as the source of pulmonary blood flow. A slightly larger diameter graft should be selected to promote pulmonary vascular growth (Figs. 7.11 and 7.12).

2.2 Stage 2: Rastelli Operation with Complete Closure of VSD

After unifocalization and palliative RVOTR, the patient waits for pulmonary blood pressure and pulmonary vascular resistance to stabilize under

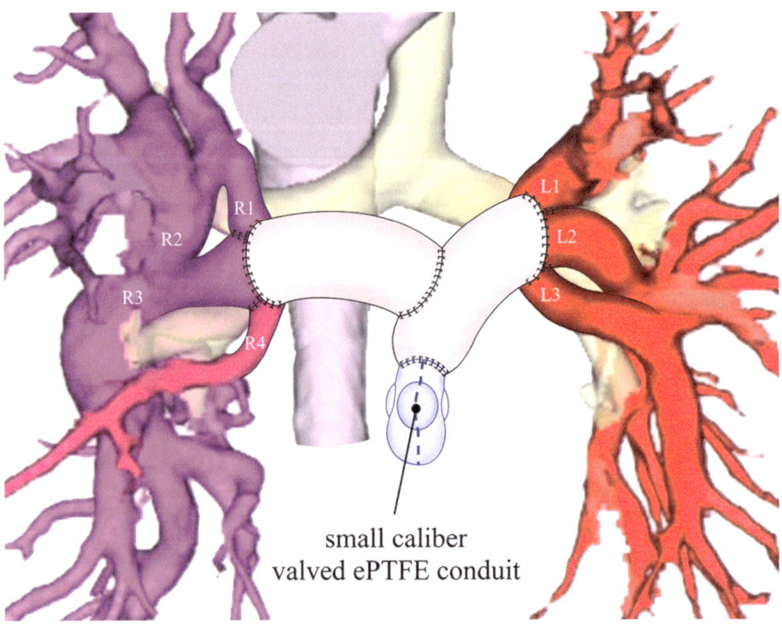

Fig. 7.11 Treatment strategy of MAPCA with deficit of the central PA (5)

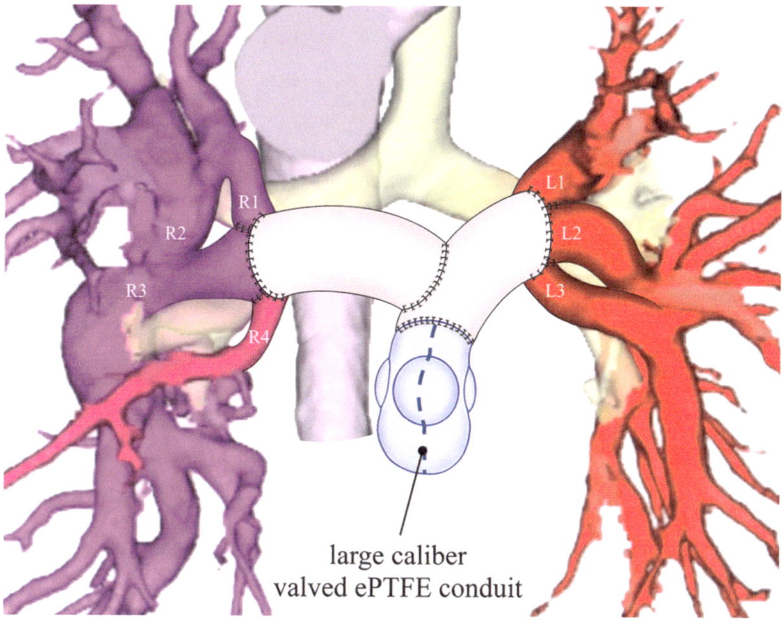

Fig. 7.12 Treatment strategy of MAPCA with deficit of the central PA (6)

the effect of medical therapy (oxygen inhalation, vasodilators).

After approximately 1 year, the second stage of surgery includes closure of the ventricular septal defect and replacement of the small conduit with a large right ventricular-pulmonary artery conduit of at least 18 mm in diameter (Rastelli procedure).

By dividing the surgical treatment of MAPCA complications into two stages (first stage unifocalization with palliative RVOTR and second stage Rastelli operation), it is possible to confirm a decrease in right ventricular pressure and sufficient growth of the pulmonary artery. As a result, complete closure of the ventricular septal defect can be achieved. If anastomotic stenosis of the pulmonary artery occurs, additional augmentation can be performed during the second stage of the Rastelli procedure.

3 Unifocalization and Palliative Right Ventricular Outflow Reconstruction (Case Presentation)

3.1 Configuration of MAPCAs and Surgical Strategy (Figs. 7.13 and 7.14)

Case 1

- 1-year-old boy, body weight: 6.4 kg, body length: 70 cm
- Diagnosis: ventricular septal defect, pulmonary atresia, central pulmonary artery deficit, MAPCAs

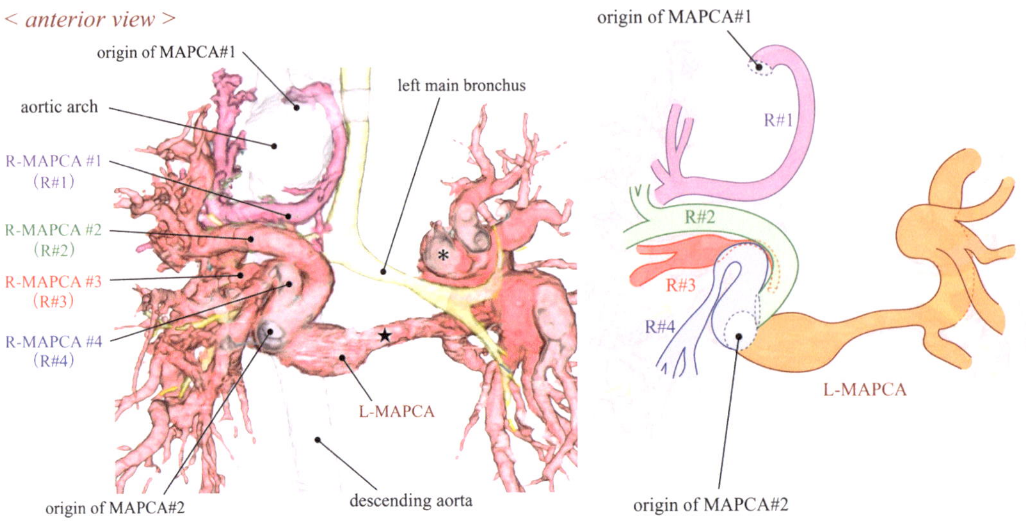

Fig. 7.13 CT findings of MAPCAs

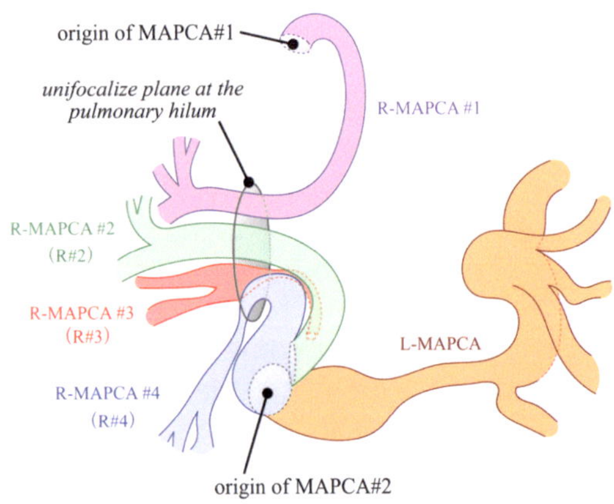

Fig. 7.14 Operation plan: unifocalization and palliative right ventricular outflow reconstruction

Right MAPCAs

- There are two orifices of the MAPCA (R-MAPCA) to the right lung.
- Orifice #1: Originates from the aortic arch (R#1).
- Orifice #2: Originates caudal to the descending thoracic aorta (approximately 1 vertebra caudal to the tracheal bifurcation) (R#2, R#3, R#4), runs anterior to the right main bronchus (R#2, R#4).

Left MAPCA

- MAPCA (L-MAPCA) toward the left lung has one origin (common with R-MAPCA).
- L-MAPCA has a stenotic lesion after its origin (*).
- L-MAPCA passes through the dorsal surface of the left main bronchus and joins the intrapulmonary artery.
- A large pulmonary artery is present on the dorsal superior surface of the left main bronchus (★).

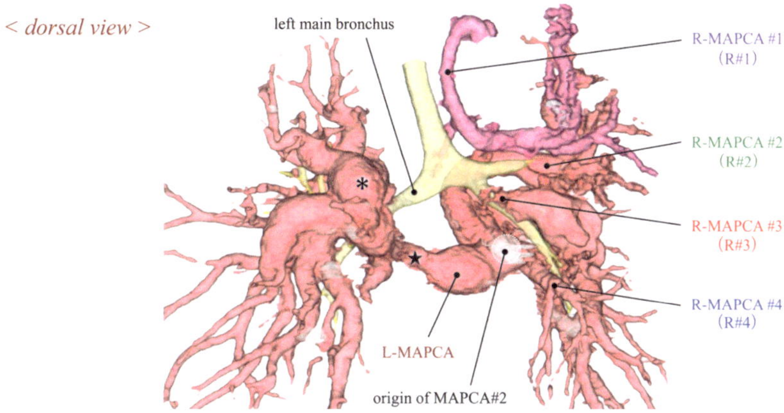

Left MAPCA

- L-MAPCA passes through the dorsal aspect of the left main bronchus and connects all intrapulmonary pulmonary arteries.
- Stenosis is present in L-MAPCA (★).
- A large pulmonary artery is present on the dorsal superior surface of the left main bronchus (*).

Right MAPCAs

- R#3 branches off from R#2 and runs dorsal to the right inferior lobe bronchus.
- R#2 and R#4 run anterior to the right main bronchus.
- R#1 is not connected to any other intrapulmonary artery.

In this case, the central pulmonary artery is deficient but the intrapulmonary pulmonary artery is growing well, so we decided to perform unifocalization and palliative right ventricular outflow tract reconstruction in a single stage.

1. The right pulmonary artery was unifocalized at the pulmonary hilar region (creation of a single orifice).
2. The left pulmonary artery was cut at its origin and anastomosed to the left pericardial roll at a site close to the pulmonary hilar region, as all left pulmonary arteries are connected within the left lung.
3. The central pulmonary artery is reconstructed with a Y-shaped pericardial roll.
4. The right ventricular outflow tract is reconstructed with a small diameter valved ePTFE conduit.

1. *Unifocalization of Right MAPCAs at the Pulmonary Hilum*

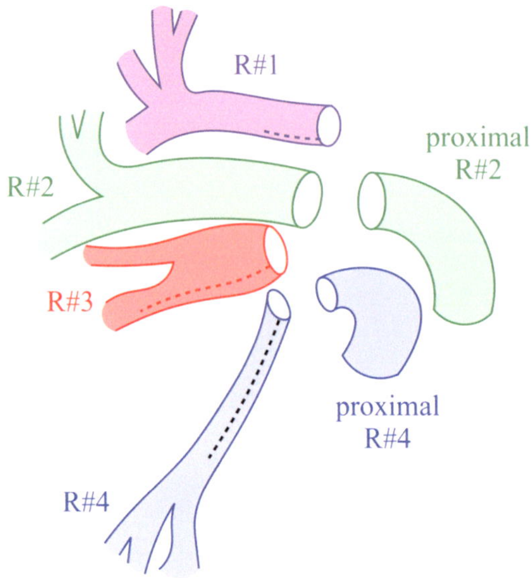

- MAPCA #2, #3, and #4 are cut at the origin.
- All MAPCAs are cut at the pulmonary hilum.

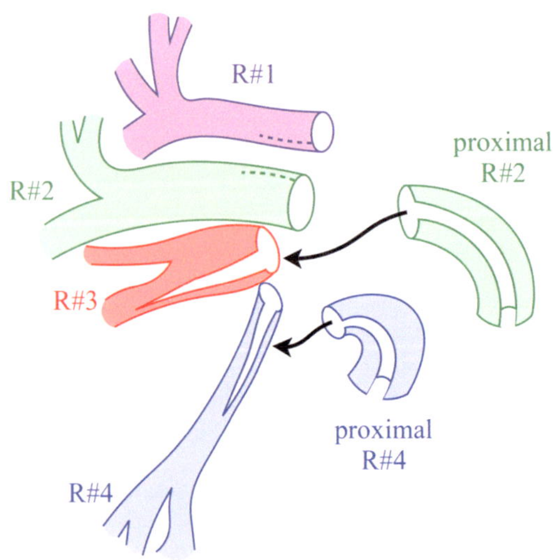

- Make a longitudinal incision in MAPCA #3 to the periphery.
- Anastomose this incision with an incised patch proximal to MAPCA #2.

- Make a longitudinal incision through MAPCA #4 to the periphery.
- Anastomose this incision with an incised patch proximal to MAPCA #4.

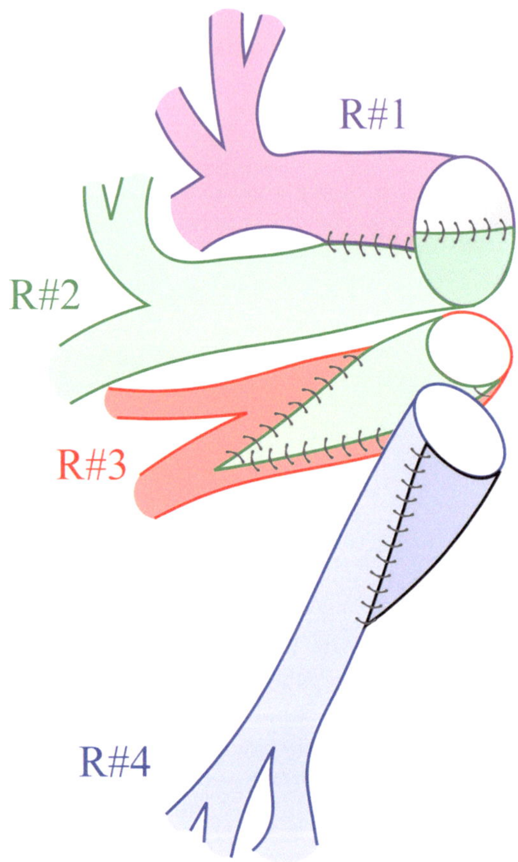

- Side-to-side anastomosis of MAPCA #1 and MAPCA #2.

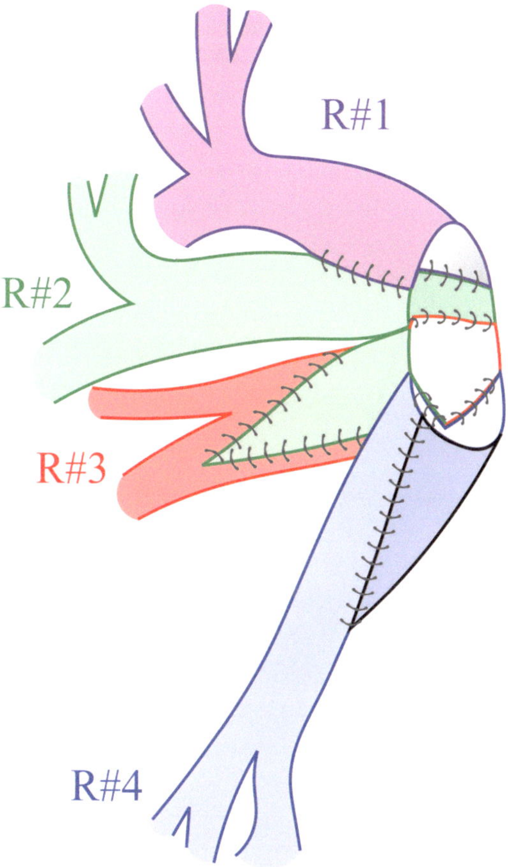

- Make a single orifice by anastomosing #1 + #2, and #3, #3 and #4 side-to-side, respectively.

2. *Augmentation of Left MAPCA Orifice*

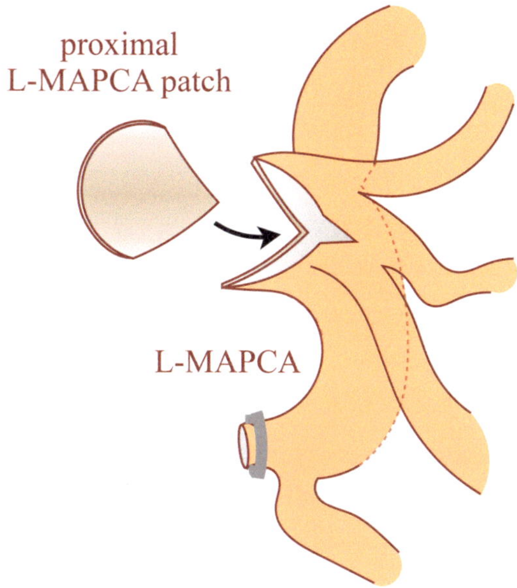

- The left pulmonary artery is divided at its origin.
- The left pulmonary artery is opened at a site cephalad to the left bronchus and the incision is enlarged with a proximal MAPCA patch.

3. *Creation of Central Pulmonary Artery*

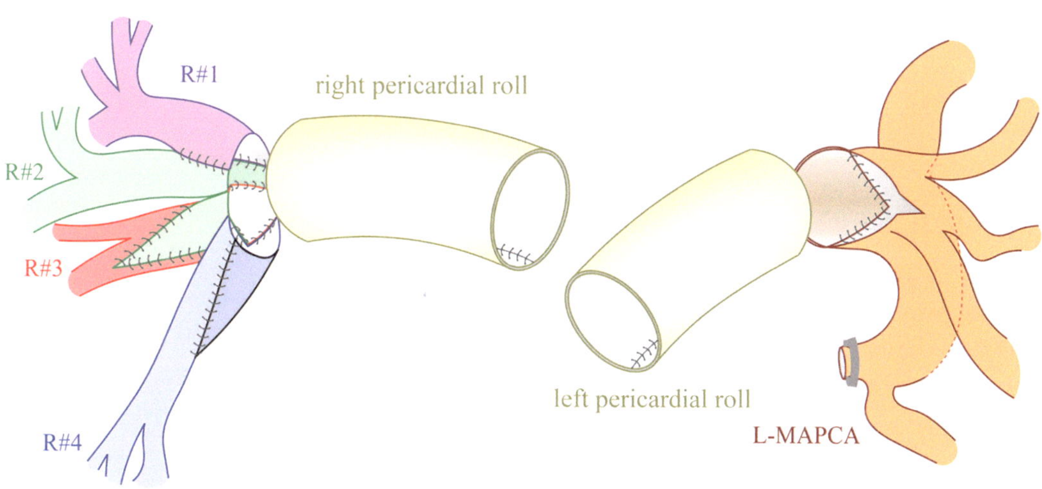

- Construct two pericardial rolls for central pulmonary artery creation (for right and left pulmonary arteries, same diameter).
- Determine the diameter of the rolls so that the PA index is 300–350 mm2/mm2 BSA (10 mm in diameter in this case).
- Determine the length of the pericardial rolls by referring to CT image.
- Anastomose the pericardial rolls at the right and left MAPCA orifices.

4. *Palliative RVOTR Using Small ePTFE Conduit*

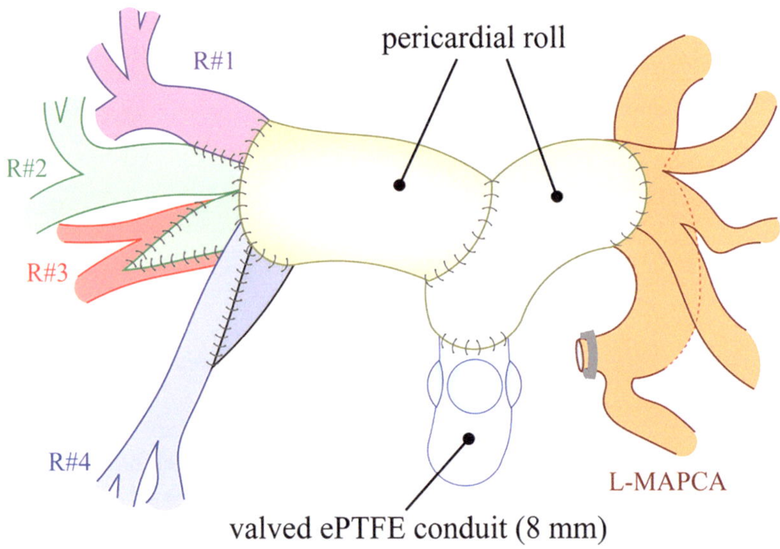

- End-to-side anastomosis of the right pericardial roll to the lateral wall of the left pericardial roll (creation of a Y-shaped central pulmonary artery).
- Reconstruction of the right ventricular-pulmonary artery blood flow pathway with a small caliber conduit (75% of the normal pulmonary valve annular diameter: 8 mm in this case).

4 Unifocalization and Palliative Right Ventricular Outflow Reconstruction (Surgical Video) (Scene 7.1)

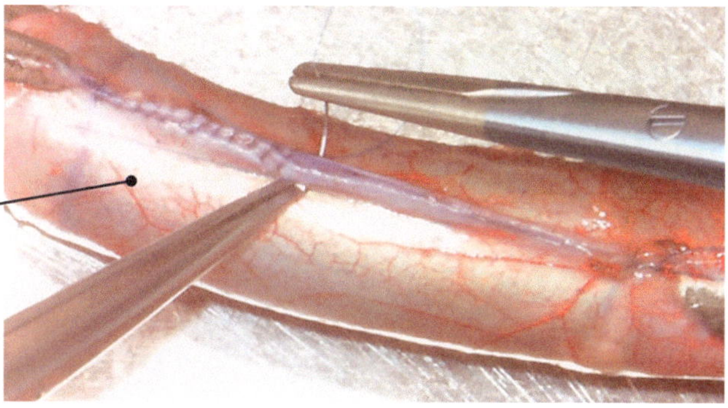

Scene 7.1 Preparing pericardial rolls (Video 00 min 06 s)

1. Harvest as large a piece of pericardium as possible.
2. Wrap the pericardium around a sizer to create a roll of pericardium for use in the central pulmonary artery with a continuous 6-0 monofilament anastomosis.
   - Determine the diameter of the pericardial roll so that the PA index is 300–350 mm^2/mm^2 BSA (10 mm diameter in this case).
   - Assume the length of the right and left pericardial rolls by referring to the distance from the left side of the ascending aorta (cephalic side of the right ventricular outflow tract) to the pulmonary hilar region on CT.
   - Ligate the sutures at −10 mm, −5 mm, and +5 mm of the assumed length of the pericardial roll to allow for cutting at the optimal length (Scene 7.2).

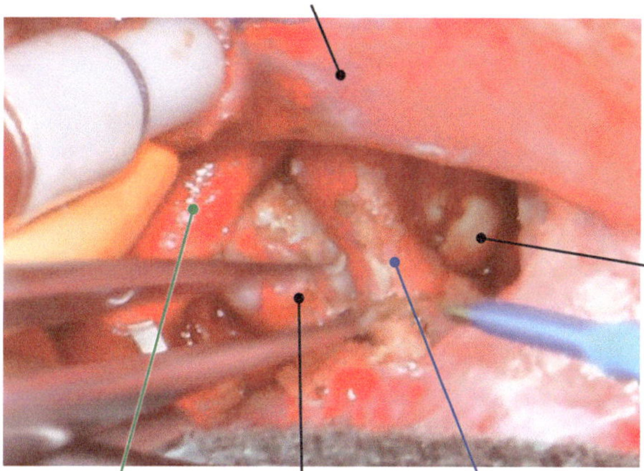

Scene 7.2 Dissection of R-MAPCA #2 and #4 (Video 00 min 43 s)

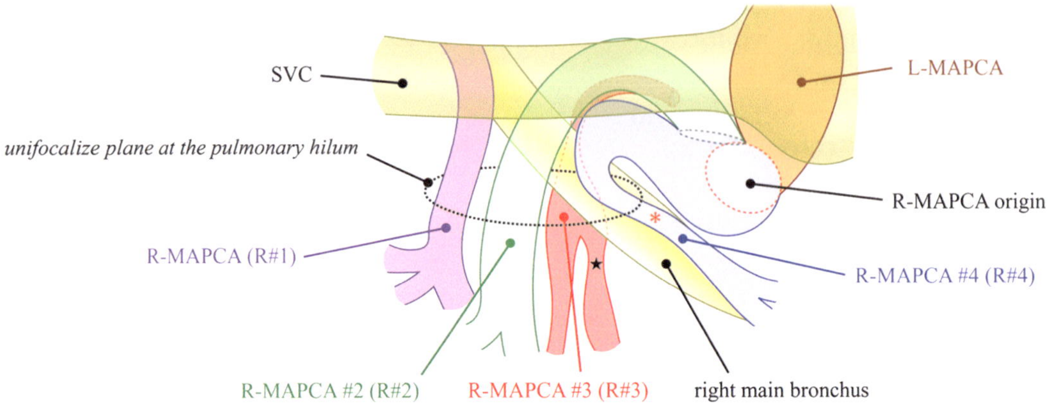

1. Using the right main bronchus as a guide, dissect R-MAPCA #2 and #4.
   - If arterial blood oxygen saturation can be maintained, dissect MAPCA as much as possible before starting extracorporeal circulation.
   - MAPCA located on the dorsal side of the heart should be dissected after extracorporeal circulation is initiated (under beating heart).
   - During dissection, carefully hemostat small blood vessels around the right main bronchus (Scene 7.3).

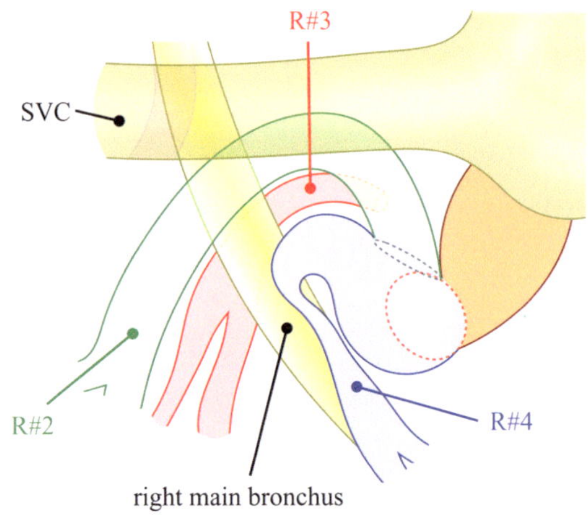

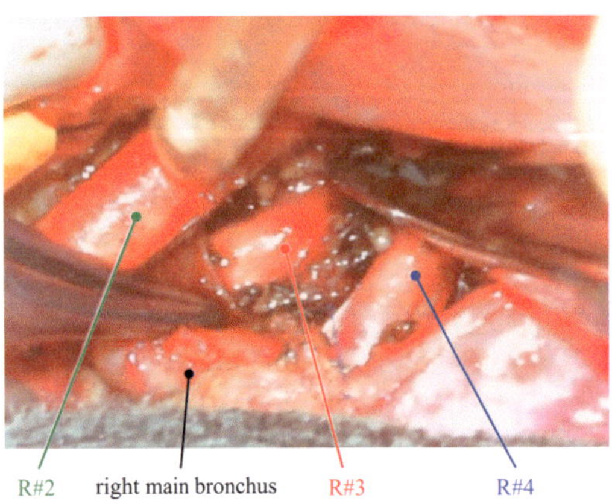

Scene 7.3 Dissection of R-MAPCA #3, Translocation of R-MAPCA #3 anterior to the right main bronchus (Video 01 min 03 s)

1. Approach from the left side of the right main bronchus and dissect R-MAPCA #3, which is located dorsally.
2. Cut R-MAPCA #3 at its origin and extract it anteriorly from the dorsal side of the right main bronchus (Scene 7.4).

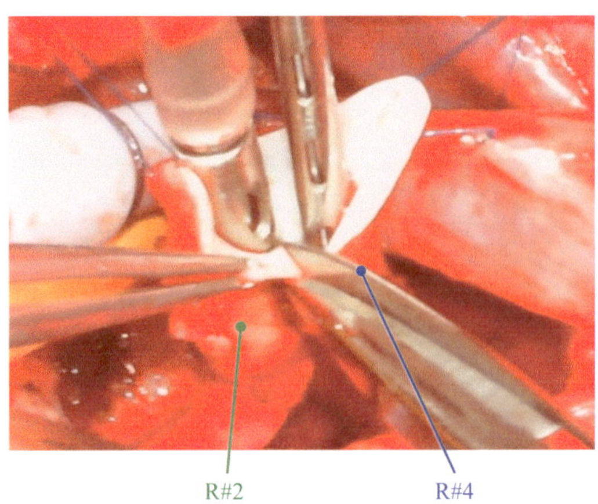

Scene 7.4 Division of R-MAPCA #4 (Video 02 min 09 s)

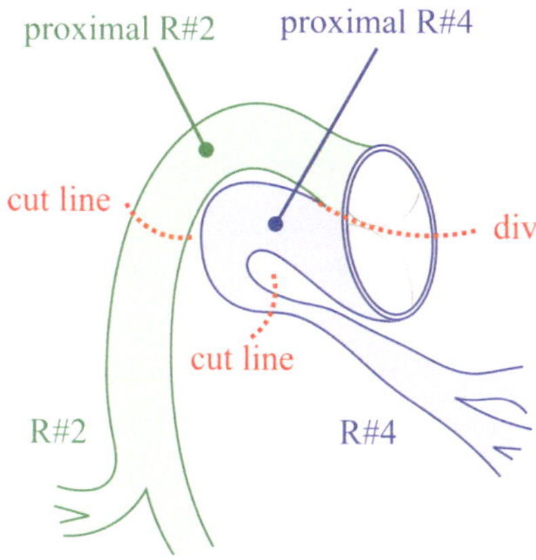

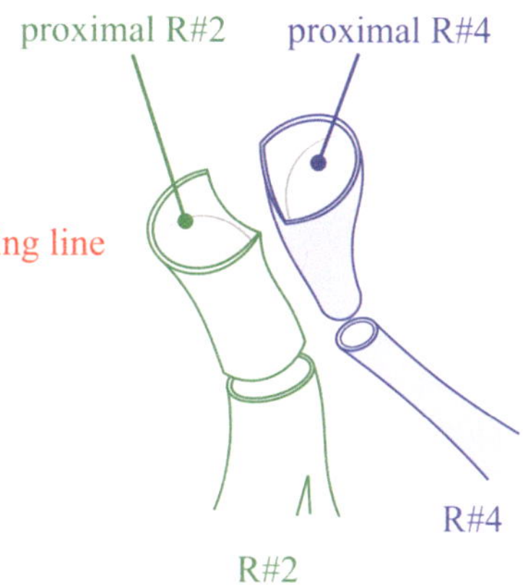

1. Cut R#2 and R#4 at the origin. R#2 is separated from R#4 at its origin. R#4 is transected at the hilar region due to a long stenosis at the distal portion of R#4. R#2 is also transected at the hilar region (Scene 7.5).

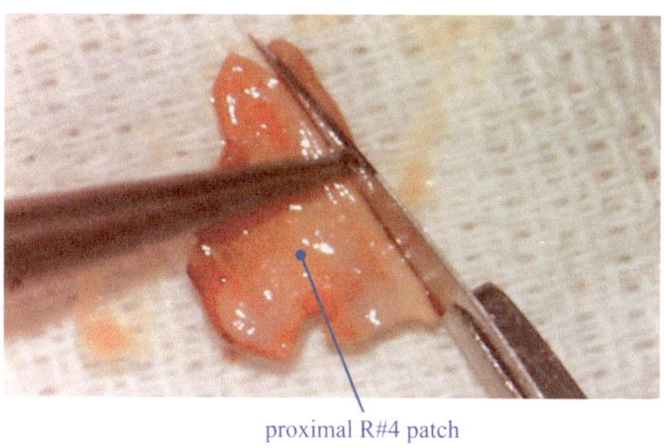

Scene 7.5 Preparing a patch by surplus R-MAPCA #4 (Video 03 min 18 s)

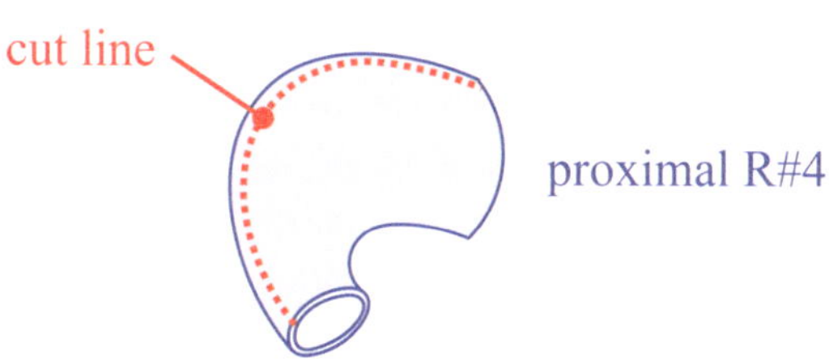

1. Cut the proximal side of the resected R#4 and use it as a patch to augment the distal portion of R#4 (Scene 7.6).

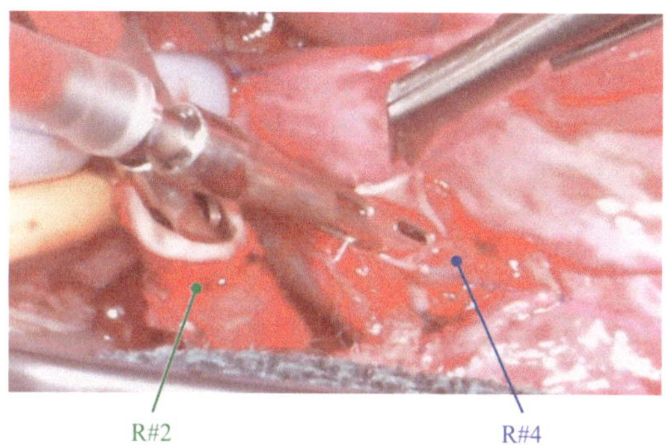

Scene 7.6 Incise of peripheral R-MAPCA #4 (Video 03 min 34 s)

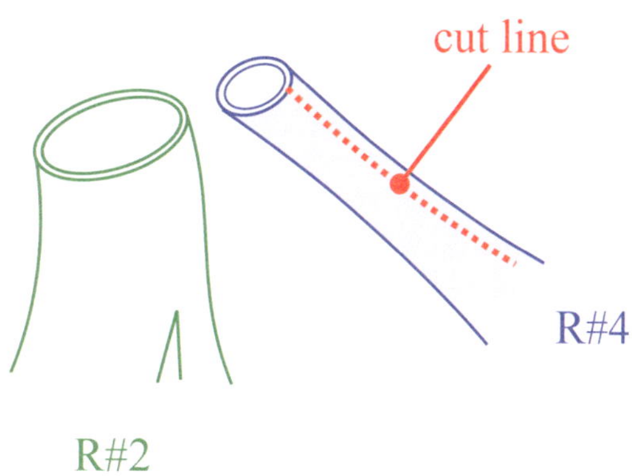

1. Incise R#4 longitudinally beyond the distal stenosis (Scene 7.7).

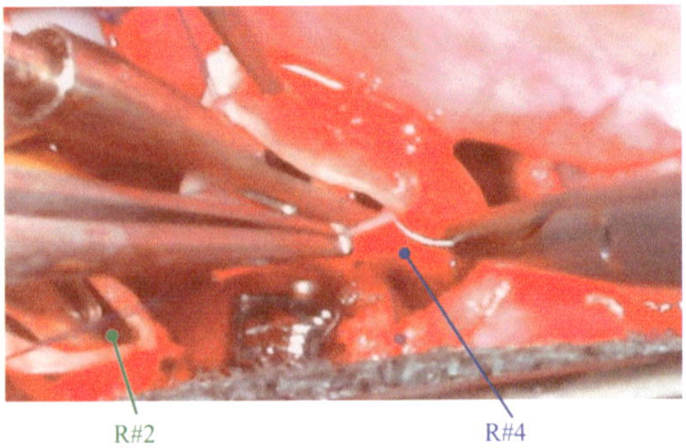

Scene 7.7 Patch augmentation of R-MAPCA #4 (Video 04 min 09 s)

1. Augment the peripheral stenotic site of R#4 by suturing the cut open R#4 proximal patch with a continuous 7-0 monofilament suture (Scene 7.8).

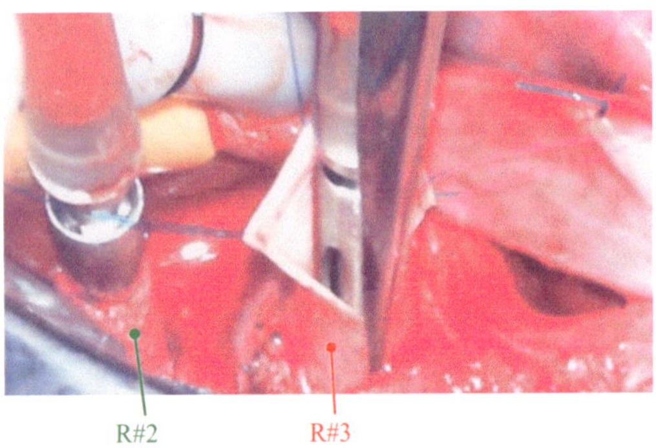

Scene 7.8 Incise of R-MAPCA #3 (Video 07 min 59 s)

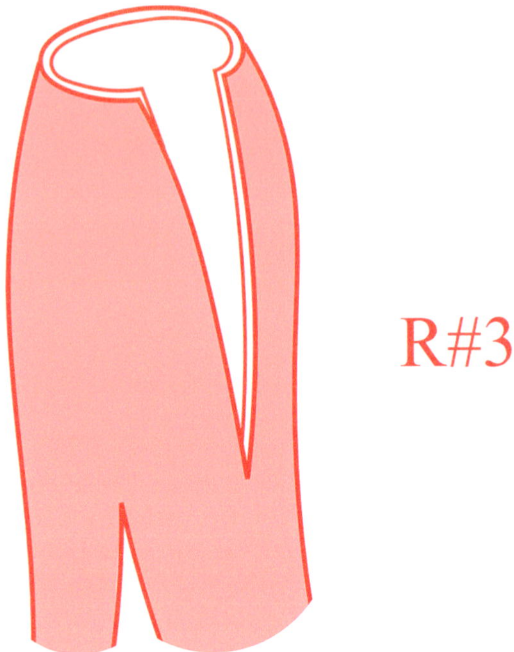

1. Incise R#3 to the distal side (Scene 7.9).

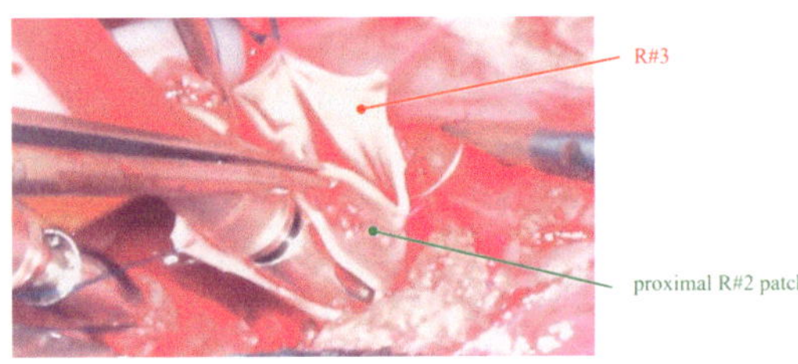

Scene 7.9 Patch augmentation of R-MAPCA #3 (Video 08 min 08 s)

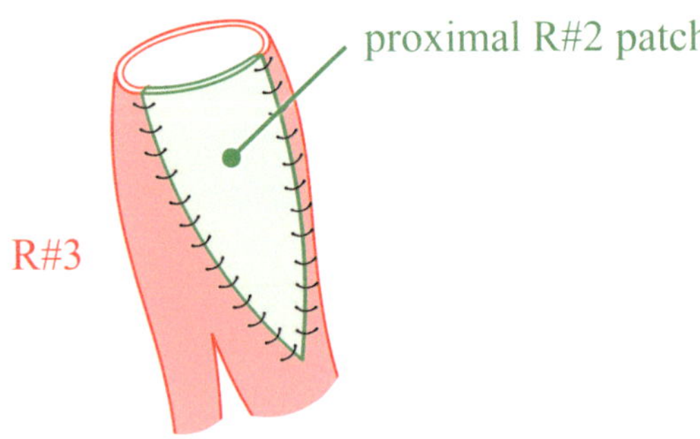

1. Augment the peripheral site of R#3 by suturing the cut open R#2 proximal patch with a continuous 7-0 monofilament suture (Scene 7.10).

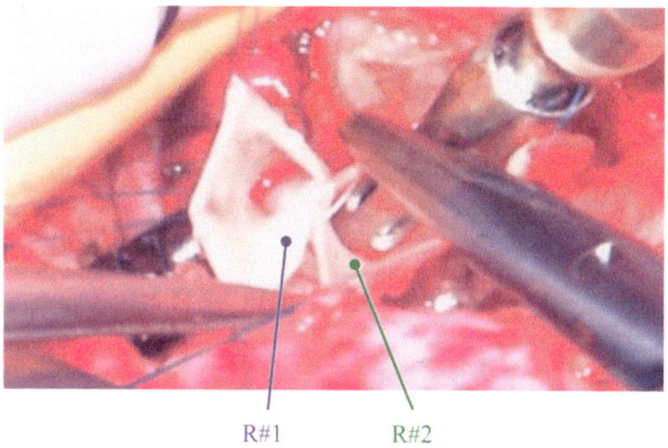

Scene 7.10 Side-to-side anastomosis of R-MAPCA #1 and #2 (Video 11 min 41 s)

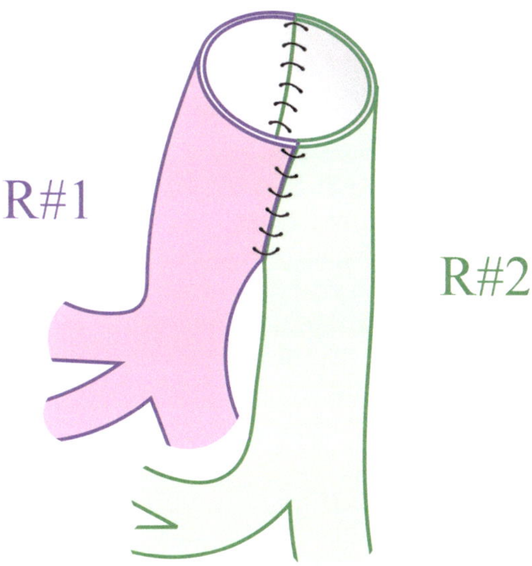

1. Cut R#1 at the proximal portion and make a longitudinal incision in the caudal wall.
2. Make a longitudinal incision in the cephalolateral wall of R#2.
3. Anastomose each incision with a continuous 7-0 monofilament suture (Scene 7.11).

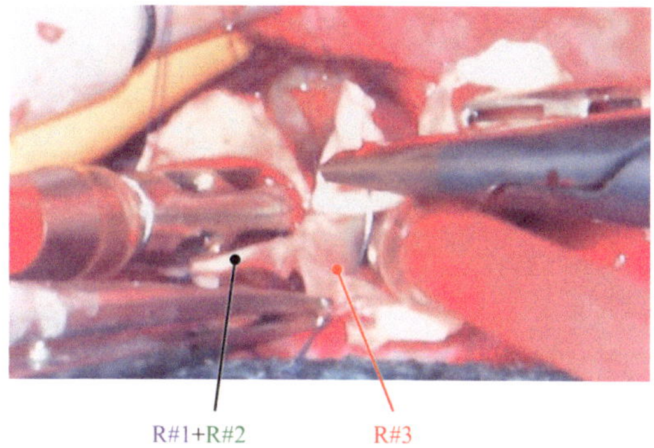

Scene 7.11 Side-to-side anastomosis of R-MAPCA #1+#2 and #3 (Video 15 min 08 s)

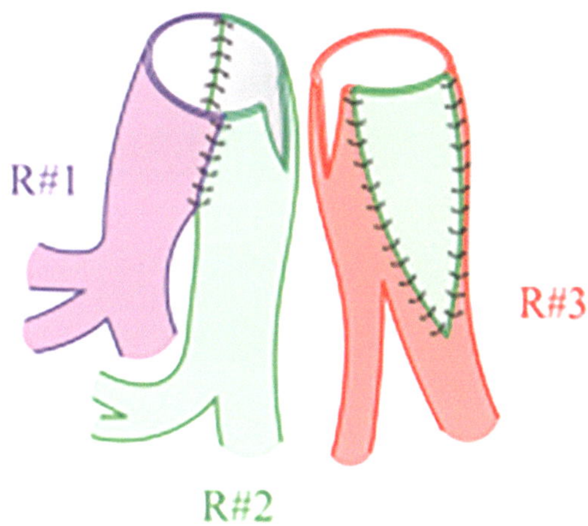

1. Make a longitudinal incision in the caudal wall of R#2.
2. Make a longitudinal incision in the cephalic wall of R#3.
3. Anastomose each incision surface with a continuous 7-0 monofilament suture (Scene 7.12).

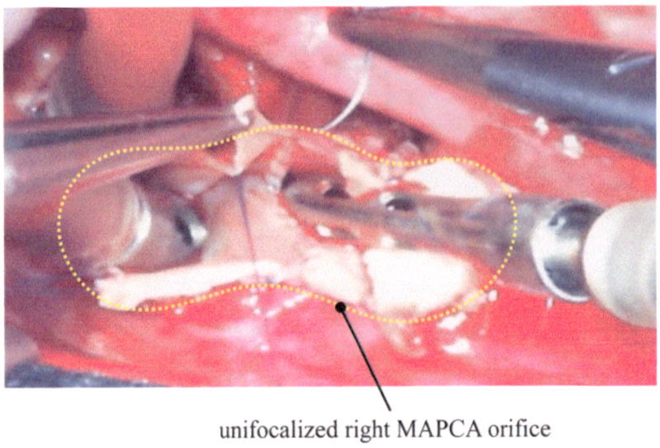

Scene 7.12 Side-to-side anastomosis of R-MAPCA #1+#2+#3 and #4 (Video 17 min 31 s)

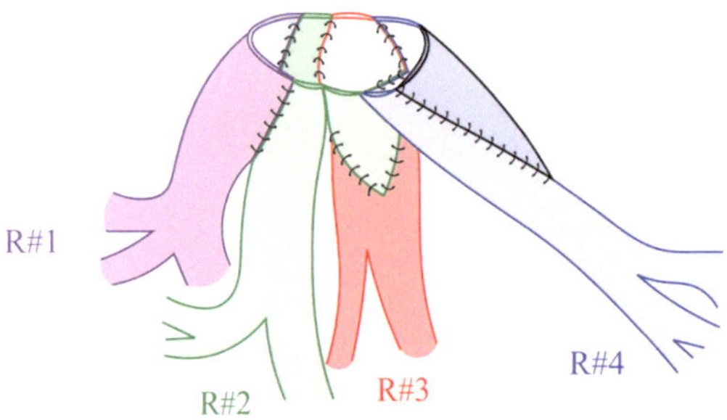

1. Incise the caudal wall of unifocalized R#1, R#2, and R#3.
2. Also incise the cephalic wall of R#4.
3. Lateral anastomose each side with a continuous 7-0 monofilament suture (Scene 7.13).

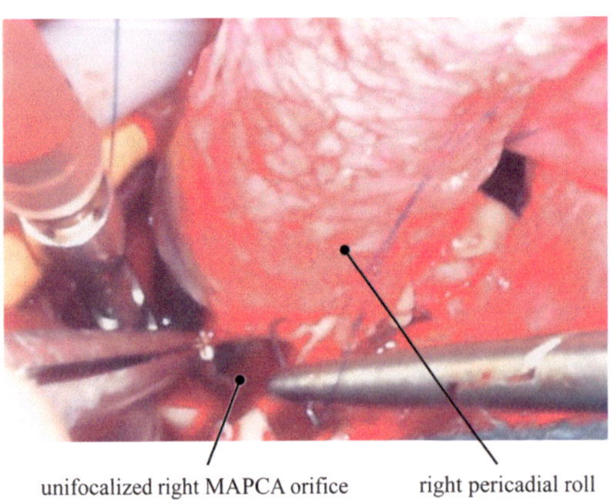

Scene 7.13 End-to-end anastomosis between unifical-ized R-MAPCA orifice and right autologous pericardial roll (Video 20 min 09 s)

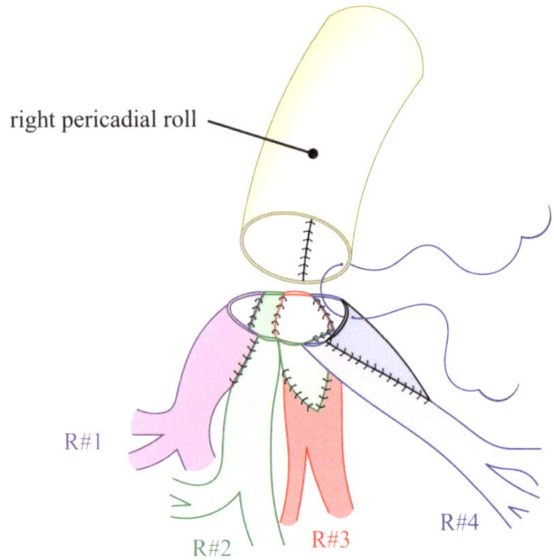

1. The autologous pericardial roll is trimmed and anastomosed end-to-end to the unifocalized right MAPCA orifice with a continuous 6-0 monofilament suture.
   - The autologous pericardial roll has a gentle curve with a convex anterior surface, so the suture line should be positioned on the dorsal side, which is the lesser curvature side (Scene 7.14).

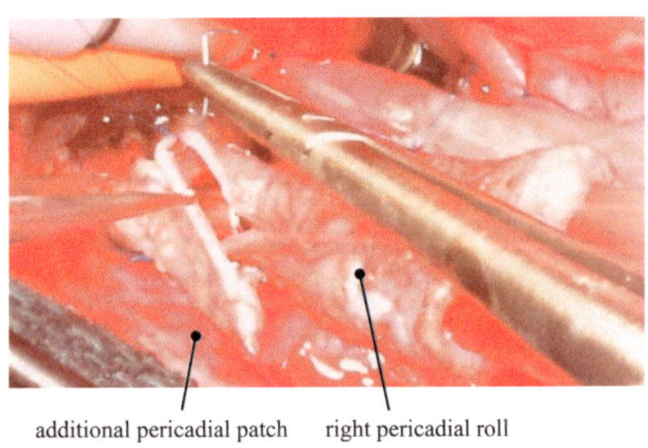

Scene 7.14 Calibration of the anastomosis (Video 24 min 02 s)

1. Because the diameter of the unifocalized MAPCA orifice is larger, a longitudinal incision is made in the autocardial roll to compensate for the excess autocardium and increase the diameter of the autocardial roll.
   - If the diameter of the MAPCA orifice is smaller, the diameter of the MAPCA orifice is increased by patch augmentation (Scene 7.15).

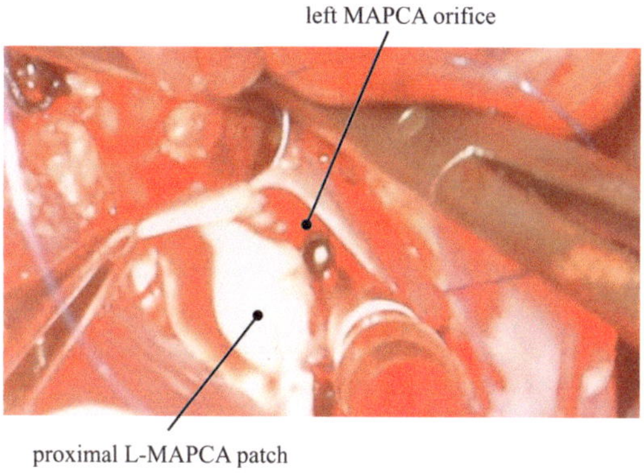

Scene 7.15 Augmentation of the L-MAPCA opening (Video 28 min 30 s)

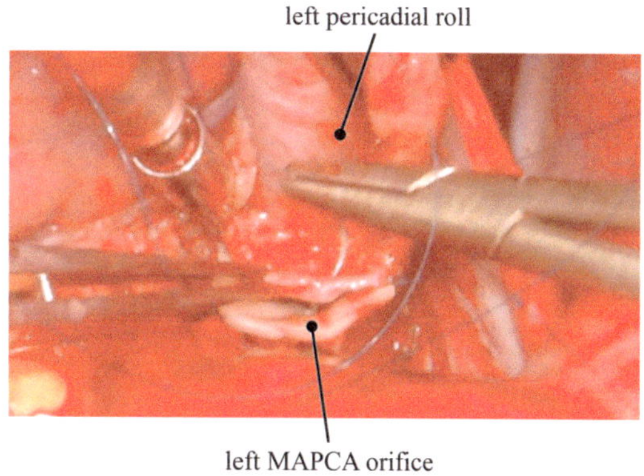

Scene 7.16 Anastomosis left autologous pericardial roll to the L-MAPCA orifice (Video 30 min 44 s)

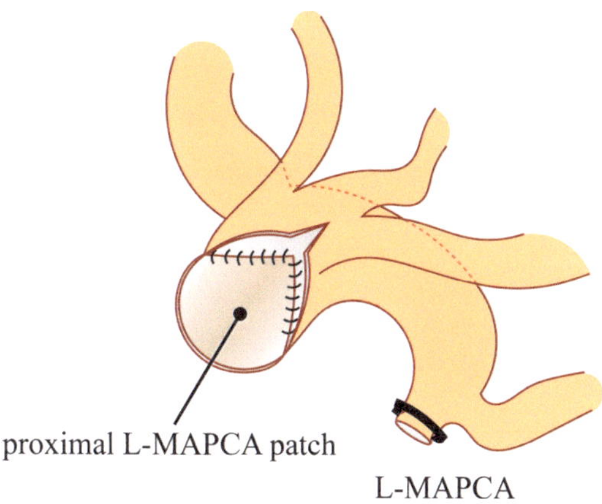

1. Incise the L-MAPCA located on the superior surface of the left main bronchus.
2. The L-MAPCA patch taken from the L-MAPCA origin is sutured to the incision to form an enlarged opening.
3. An additional incision is made caudally on the anterior surface of the L-MAPCA orifice (Scene 7.16).

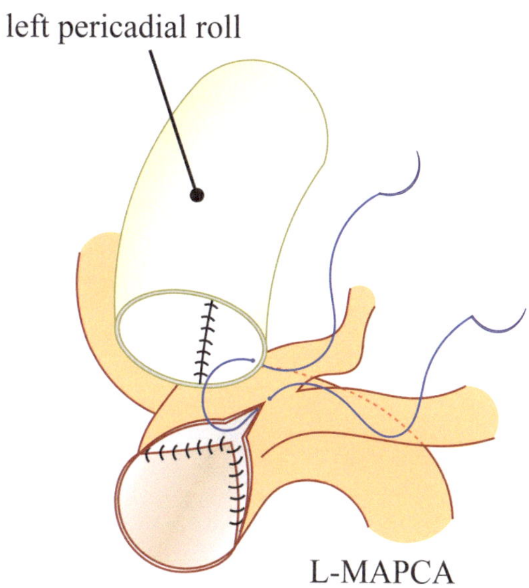

1. The left autologous pericardial roll is trimmed and anastomosed end-to-end at the L-MAPCA orifice with a continuous 6-0 monofilament suture (Scene 7.17).

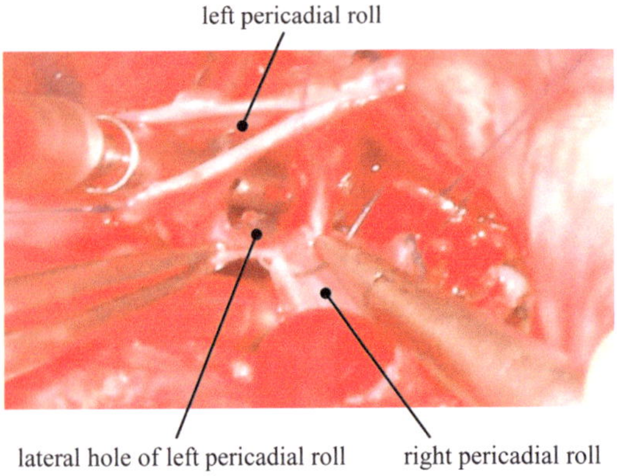

Scene 7.17 End-to-side anastomosis the right pericardial roll to the left pericardial roll (Video 33 min 17 s)

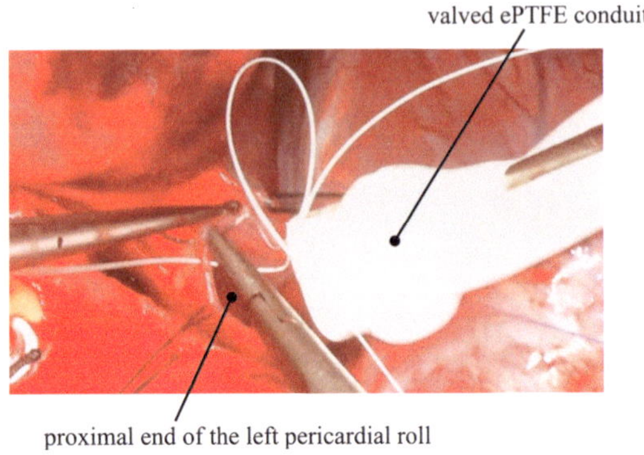

Scene 7.18 End-to-end anastomosis between the left pericardial roll and distal end of 8-mm ePTFE valved conduit (Video 35 min 15 s)

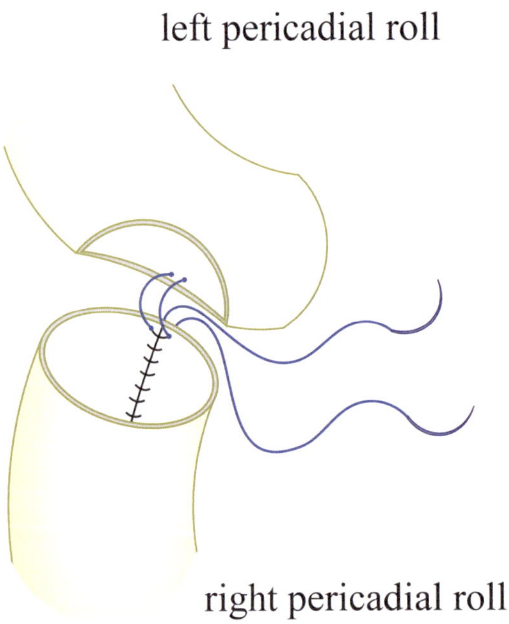

1. Open the lateral hole at the right lateral aspect of the left pericardial roll and anastomose the proximal end of the right pericardial roll end-to-side to the lateral hole with a continuous suture of 6-0 monofilament.

   - The lateral hole of the left pericardial roll is opened large enough so that it is not too small (Scene 7.18).

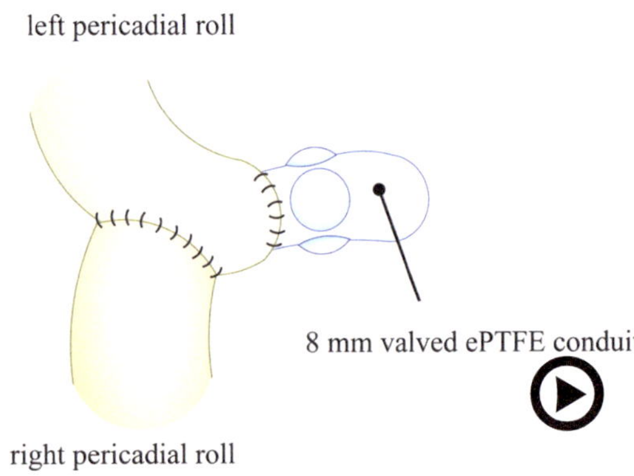

(▶ https://doi.org/10.1007/000-hke)

1. The valved ePTFE conduit (8 mm diameter) is anastomosed end-to-end to the proximal end of the left pericardial roll with a continuous ePTFE CV-6 suture (Scene 7.19).

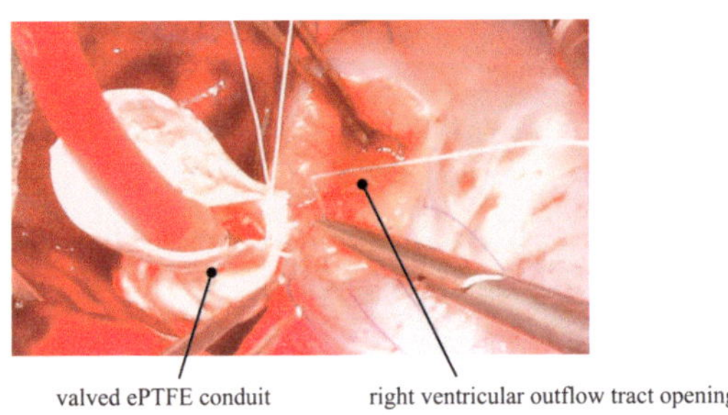

Scene 7.19 Anastomosis the ePTFE valved conduit to right ventricular outflow opening (Video 37 min 13 s)

1. After cardiac arrest, incise the right ventricular outflow tract.
2. Resect the thickened myocardial bundle of the outflow tract and create an opening of sufficient size.
3. Anastomose the proximal end of the valved ePTFE conduit to the right ventricular outflow tract opening with a continuous ePTFE CV-5 suture.

ESSENTIALS Fluid Analysis After Unifocalization and Palliative RVOT Reconstruction

- Central pulmonary artery creation by Y-shaped pericardial roll and unifocalization were performed in case of absent central pulmonary artery.
- Blood flow analysis was performed after unifocalization and central pulmonary artery creation.
- Blood flow in the central pulmonary artery showed laminar flow, and wall shear stress, a factor in stenotic lesions, was low.

- *Preoperative CT Image of MAPCA*

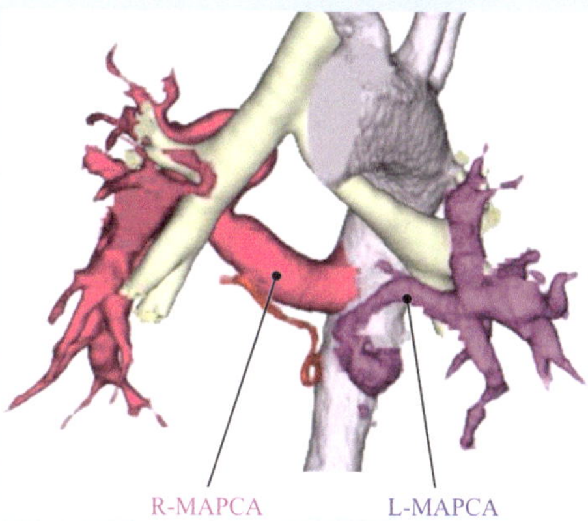

- The central pulmonary artery is absent.
- One MAPCA is present on each side.

- *Post Unifocalization, Central PA Creation, and Palliative RVOT Reconstruction*

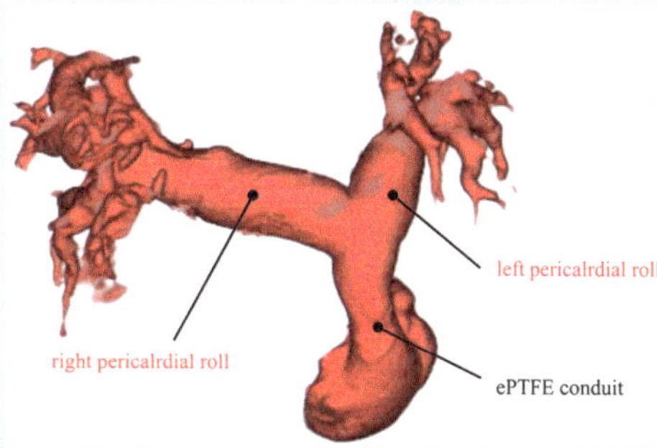

- Right MAPCA transposed anteriorly from posterior bronchus.
- Central pulmonary artery is created with a Y-shaped pericardial roll.
- Right ventricular outflow tract is reconstructed with a small-diameter ePTFE valved conduit.

(continued)

- *Fluid Analysis After Creation of Y-Shaped Central Pulmonary Artery*

< Streamline >

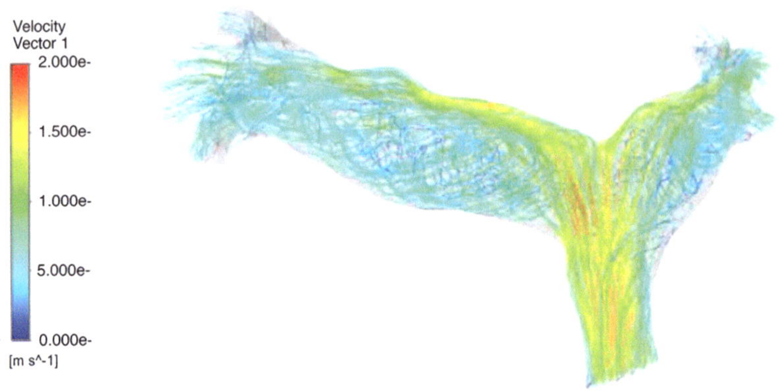

- Systolic streamline shows a gentle spiral flow in the central pulmonary artery, almost laminar flow.
- No acceleration or turbulence is observed.

< Wall shear stress >

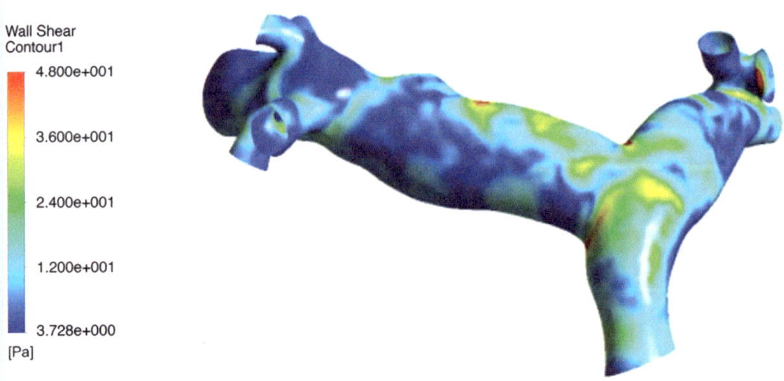

- Overall low wall shear stress in the Y-shaped pericardial roll.
- *Post Definitive Rastelli Operation with Complete Closure of the VSD*

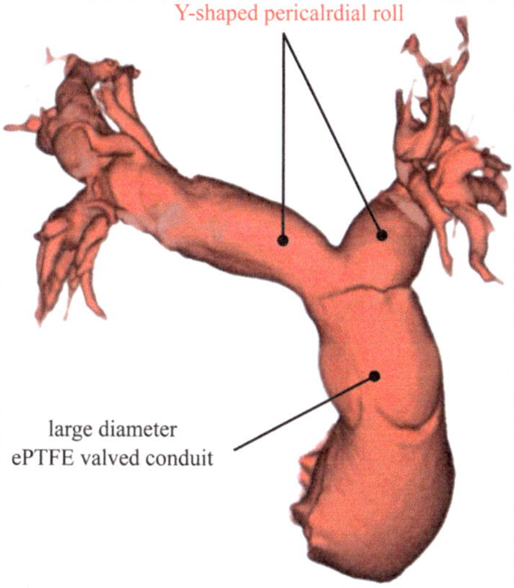

- Central pulmonary artery (pericardial roll) aneurysm or stenosis and anastomotic stenosis with MAPCA are not detected.
- The right ventricular outflow tract is reconstructed with a large diameter ePTFE valved conduit.

Reference

Fluid Analysis After Unifocalization and Y-Shaped Reconstruction of the Central Pulmonary Artery

Kato N, Yamagishi M, Itatani K, et al. Effects of blood dynamics on autologous pericardial degeneration in reconstructed pulmonary arteries. Interact Cardiovasc Thorac Surg. 2018;26:293–300.

Normal Great Artery Type Double Outlet Right Ventricle (NGA Type DORV)

8

1 Morphology of Double Outlet Right Ventricle

1.1 Definition of Double Outlet Right Ventricle

Double outlet right ventricle (DORV) is defined as a disease that fulfills two conditions: (1) in addition to one great vessel, at least 50% of the other great vessel originates from the right ventricle, and (2) the fibrous continuity between the semilunar and atrioventricular valves has disappeared and a muscular tissue ventricular infundibular fold (VIF) exists between both valves (Figs. 8.1 and 8.2).

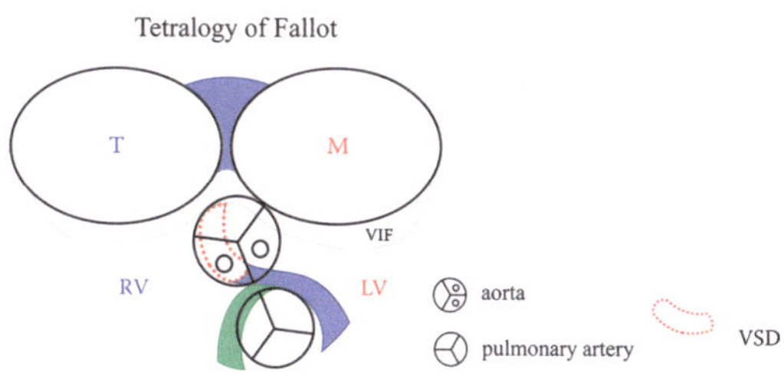

Fig. 8.1 Definition of normal great artery (NGA) type DORV

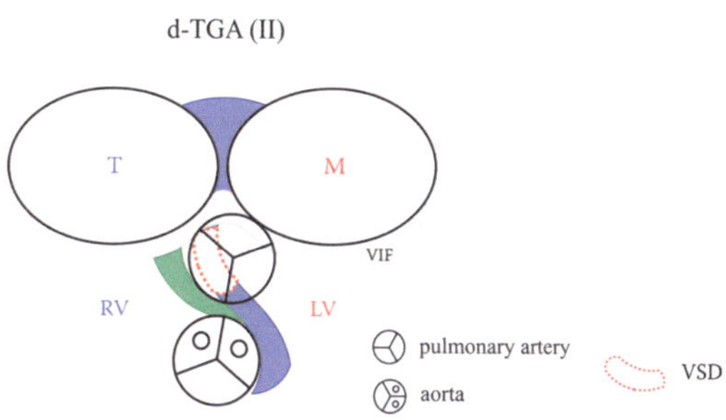

Fig. 8.2 Definition of transposition (TGA) type DORV

- In the normal great arteries (NGA) and the transposition of the great arteries (TGA) types, the basic types of disease are the presence of fibrous continuity with the mitral valve (tetralogy of Fallot in the NGA type and d-TGA II in the TGA type).
- When the posterior great vessels are deviated to the right from this basic type, the fibrous continuity with the mitral valve is disappeared and a muscular ventriculo-infundibular fold (VIF) is interposed between the mitral valve and the semilunar valve. When the posterior great artery overrides more than 50% into the ventricular septum, the definition of DORV is fulfilled.
- The location of the VSD is unrelated to the definition and classification of the disease.
- The basic form of NGA type DORV is tetralogy of Fallot.
- Posterior great artery (aorta) is slightly deviated to the right and overrides on the ventricu-

Supplementary Information The online version contains supplementary material available at https://doi.org/10.1007/978-981-96-6194-7_8. The videos can be accessed individually by clicking the DOI link in the accompanying figure caption or by scanning this link with the SN More Media App.

M. Yamagishi, *Surgical Treatment of Congenital Heart Disease*,
https://doi.org/10.1007/978-981-96-6194-7_8

lar septum, but the degree of overriding is less than 50%.

- Fibrous tissue is interposed between the aortic annulus and mitral annulus (aortic-mitral fibrous continuity)
- These are morphologic features of tetralogy of Fallot.

rightward deviation of posterior grear artery (aorta)

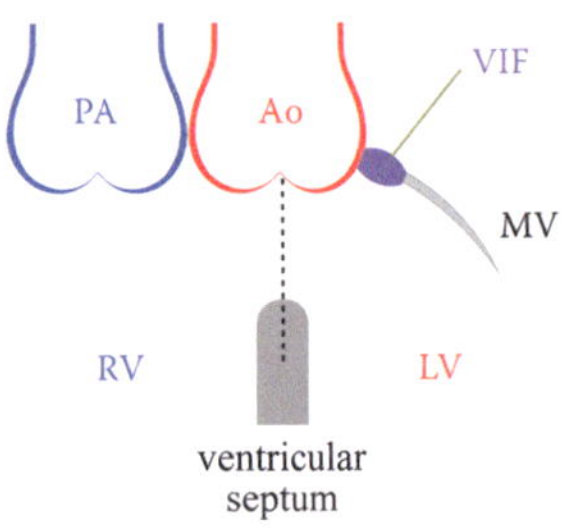

- The aorta overrides more than 50% to the ventricular septum, and muscular tissue (ventriculo-infundibular fold: VIF) appears between the aortic and mitral valves. (fulfilling the definition of DORV)

NGA type DORV

{SDN}DORV

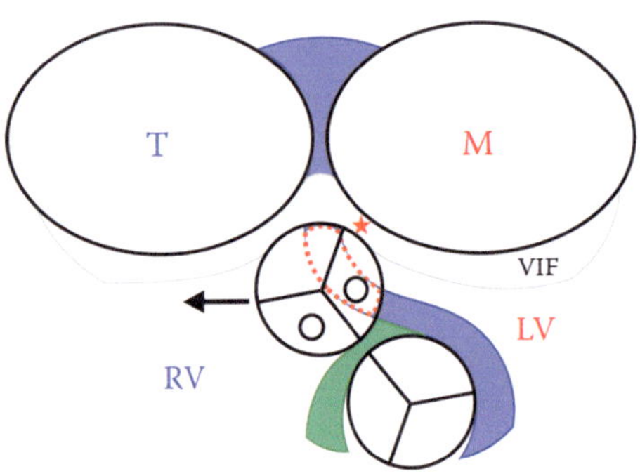

- Rightward deviation of the posterior great artery (aorta) from the basic type of tetralogy of Fallot results in the disappearance of the aortic-mitral valve fibrous continuity and the interposition of muscular tissue (VIF) between the two valves (★).
- More than 50% of the posterior great arteries (aorta) overrides the ventricular septum.
- These are morphologic features of NGA type DORV.
- Fibrous continuity remains between the posterior great artery (pulmonary) and mitral valve.
- This is a morphologic feature of d-TGA (II).

rightward deviation of posterior grear artery (pulmonary artery)

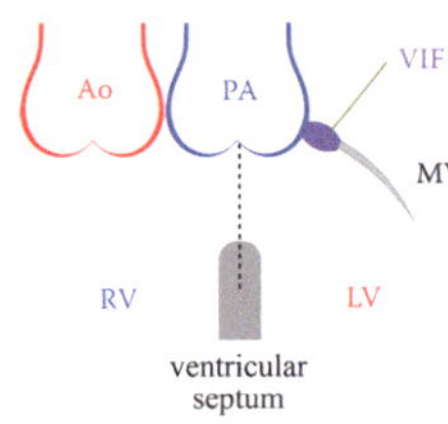

- The pulmonary artery overrides more than 50% to the ventricular septum, and muscular tissue (ventriculo-infundibular fold: VIF) appears between the pulmonary and mitral valves. (fulfilling the definition of DORV)

TGA type DORV

false Taussig-Bing

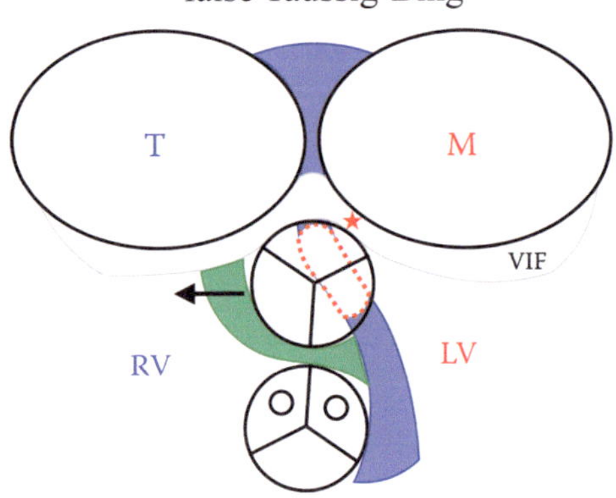

- Rightward deviation of the posterior great artery (pulmonary artery) from the basic type of d-TGA (II) results in the disappearance of the pulmonary-mitral valve fibrous continuity and the interposition of muscular tissue (VIF) between the two valves (★).
- More than 50% of the posterior great arteries (pulmonary artery) overrides the ventricular septum.
- These are morphologic feature of false Taussig-Bing.

2 Embryology of Double Outlet Right Ventricle

2.1 Malseptation Theory (Van Mierop)

There are many types of DORV, causing confusion in determining the diagnosis and surgical indications. In order to understand the types of DORV, it is useful to look back at the cardiogenic process of the great arteries and the cardiac base during the development of the heart. Visceral-atrial situs and atrioventricular situs are the primary factors. In this chapter, we discuss visceral-atrial situs solitus and atrioventricular concordance.

Although there are various theories regarding the pathogenesis of this disease, the malseptation theory proposed by Van Mierop is useful for understanding the type of the disease and selecting a surgical technique. The important factors that determine the intracardiac morphology in malseptation theory are the septation of the great arteries (truncal septation) and migration of great arteries (conotruncal rotation due to medial shift of the conus cordis). With migration of the great arteries, the overriding of the great arteries, the change in position of the VSD, and the rotation of the infundibular septum result in a variety of disease types. In addition, an anterior or posterior deviation of the infundibular septum may also occur (Figs. 8.3 and 8.4).

2.2 Malseptation Theory: Septation of Arterial Trunk

Depending on the type of septation of the great arteries during heart development, there are two types: normal great arteries (NGA) type and transposition of the great arteries (TGA) type.

In the normal pattern, the aorta and pulmonary artery are divided into spiral septation by the spiral joining of the opposite arterial trunk walls. As a result, the morphology of both great arteries becomes spiral, with the anterior great artery being the pulmonary artery (PA) and the posterior great artery being the aorta (Ao) (normal great artery type: NGA). The Ao of the posterior great artery is adjacent to the mitral valve.

On the other hand, when the truncal walls, which differ by 90°, join each other, the aorta and pulmonary artery are divided parallel (parallel septation). Parallel septation results in a parallel morphology of both great arteries, with the anterior great artery becoming the aorta (Ao) and the posterior artery becoming the pulmonary artery (PA) (transposition of the great arteries: TGA). The posterior great artery, the PA, is adjacent to the mitral valve.

2.3 Malseptation Theory: Medial Shift of Conus Cordis

In addition to the septation of the great arteries, the degree of rightward migration of the posterior great arteries and leftward migration of the anterior vessels results in a variety of disease types. This great artery migration is caused by the degree of medial shift of the conus cordis during the cardiogenic phase (Van Mierop) (Fig. 8.5).

- In the NGA type, a rightward deviation of the posterior pulmonary artery (PA) and a leftward deviation of the anterior aorta (Ao) occur.

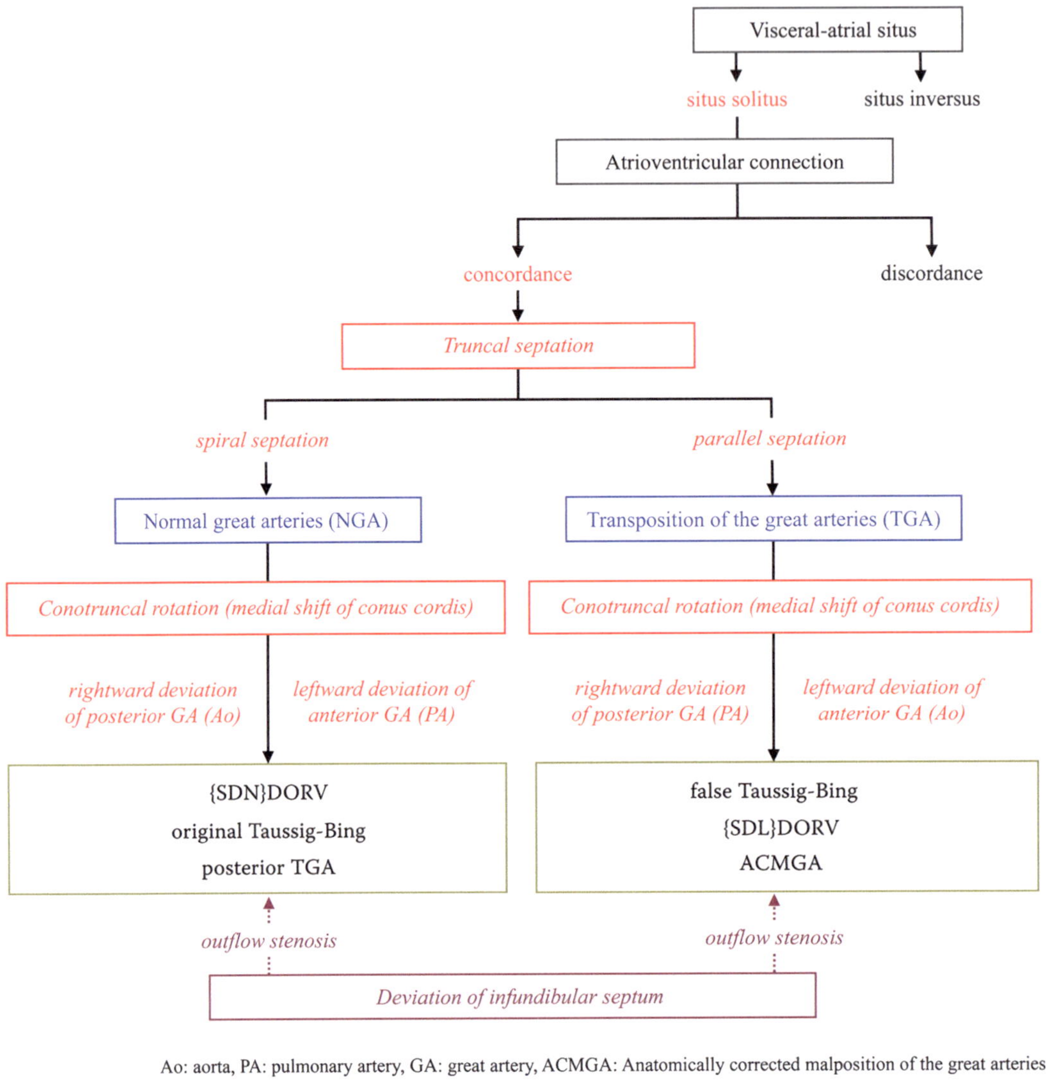

Fig. 8.3 Embryology of DORV. (Malseptation theory by Van Mierop) *Ao* aorta, *PA* pulmonary artery, *GA* great artery, *ACMGA* anatomically corrected malposition of the great arteries

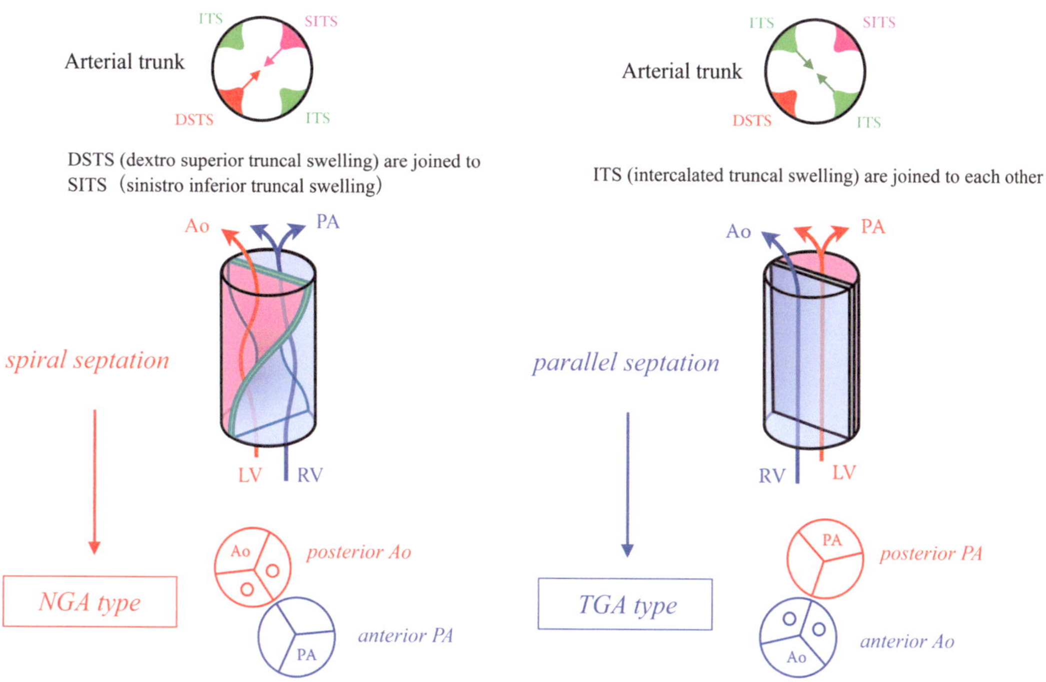

Fig. 8.4 Septation of arterial trunk (normal great artery and transposition)

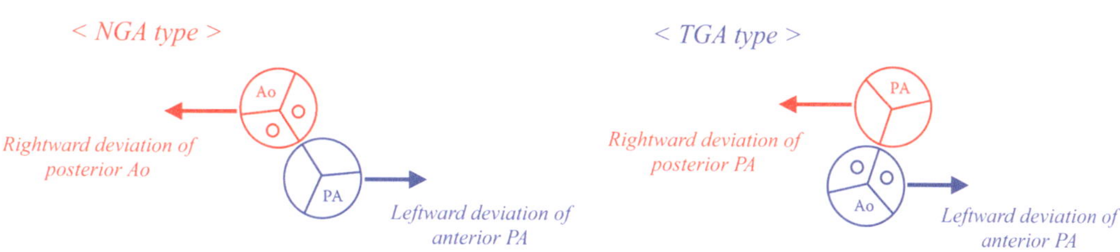

Fig. 8.5 Rightward deviation of posterior great artery and leftward deviation of anterior great artery

- In the TGA type, rightward deviation of the posterior PA and leftward deviation of the anterior Ao occur.

2.4 Malseptation Theory: Spectrum of NGA Type DORV

Depending on the degree of rightward migration of the posterior great artery (Ao) and leftward migration of the anterior great artery (PA), the spectrum of disease types is {SDN}DORV, original Taussig-Bing, and posterior TGA type DORV for the normal great artery type. Various transitional types are recognized in each type.

The great arteries become right oblique to parallel, and the infundibular septum, which was orthogonal to the ventricular septum, rotates counterclockwise to become parallel to the ventricular septum. The VSD also extends anteriorly. The site of attachment (direction) of the posterior border of the infundibular septum is important (Fig. 8.6).

Fig. 8.6 Spectrum and morphological characteristics of NGA type DORV

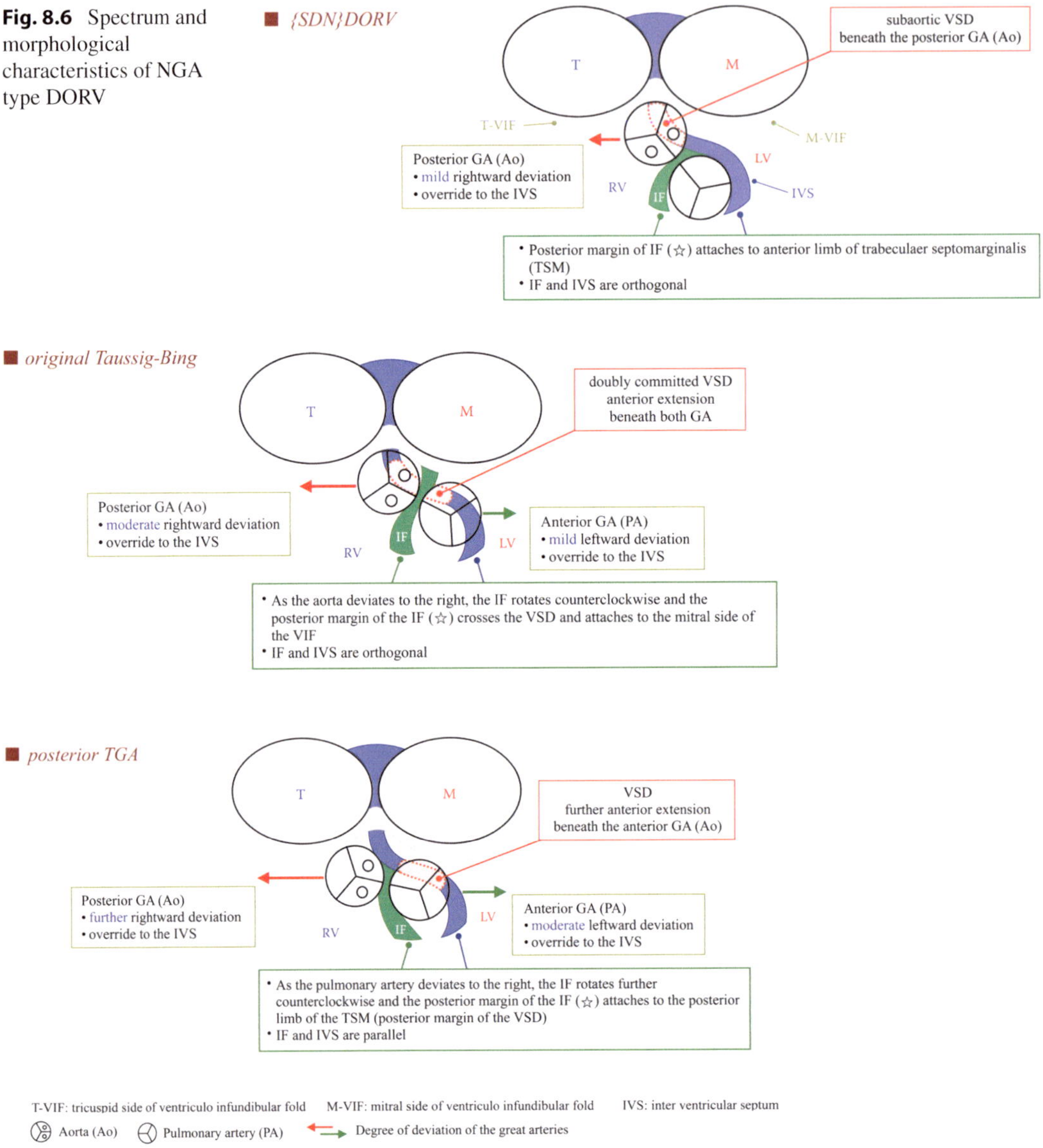

2.5 Malseptation Theory: Spectrum of TGA Type DORV

Depending on the degree of rightward migration of the posterior great artery (PA) and leftward migration of the anterior great artery (Ao), the spectrum of disease types is false Taussig-Bing, {SDL}DORV, and anatomically corrected malposition of the great arteries (ACMGA) for the transposition great artery (TGA) type. Transitional type between false Taussig-Bing and {SDL} DORV is recognized.

The relationship of the great arteries is antero-posterior in false Taussig-Bing and is parallel in [SDL}DORV and ACMGA. The infundibular septum is parallel in in false Taussig-Bing and ACMGA, and is orthogonal in {SDL}DORV. The VSD extends anteriorly in [SDL}DORV and ACMGA (Fig. 8.7).

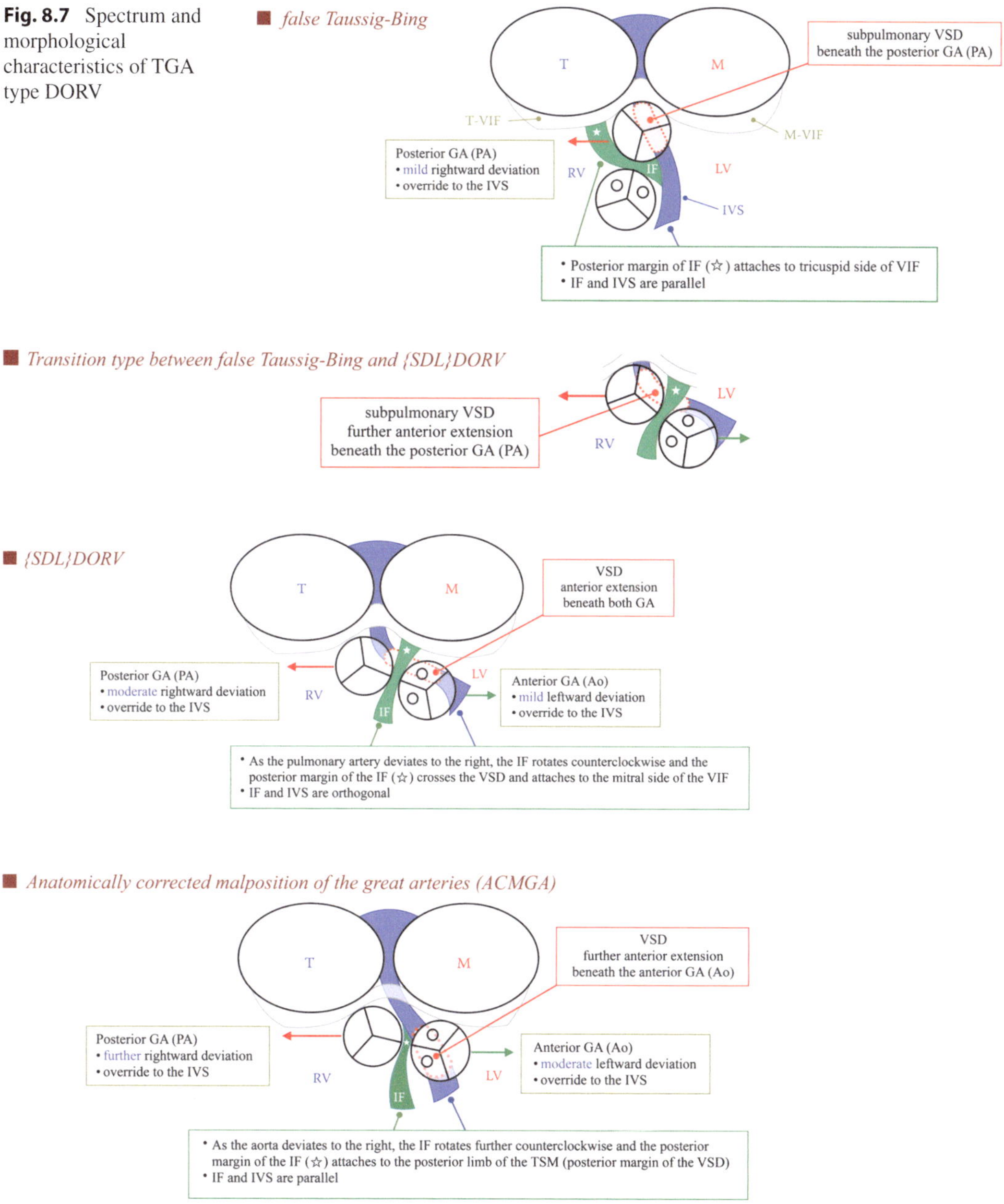

Fig. 8.7 Spectrum and morphological characteristics of TGA type DORV

2.6 Malseptation Theory: Anterior or Posterior Deviation of the Infundibular Septum

In addition to left-to-right deviation of the great arteries, anterior or posterior deviation of the infundibular septum, which lies beneath the great arteries, is associated with outflow tract stenosis on the side of the deviation (Fig. 8.8).

< *Posterior Deviation of the Infundibular Septum* >
Posterior deviation of the infundibular septum is complicated by posterior outflow tract stenosis of the great arteries (aortic stenosis in NGA type and pulmonary stenosis in TGA type).

< *Anterior Deviation of the Infundibular Septum* >
Anterior deviation of the infundibular septum is associated with anterior outflow tract stenosis of the great arteries (pulmonary stenosis in NGA type and aortic stenosis in TGA type).

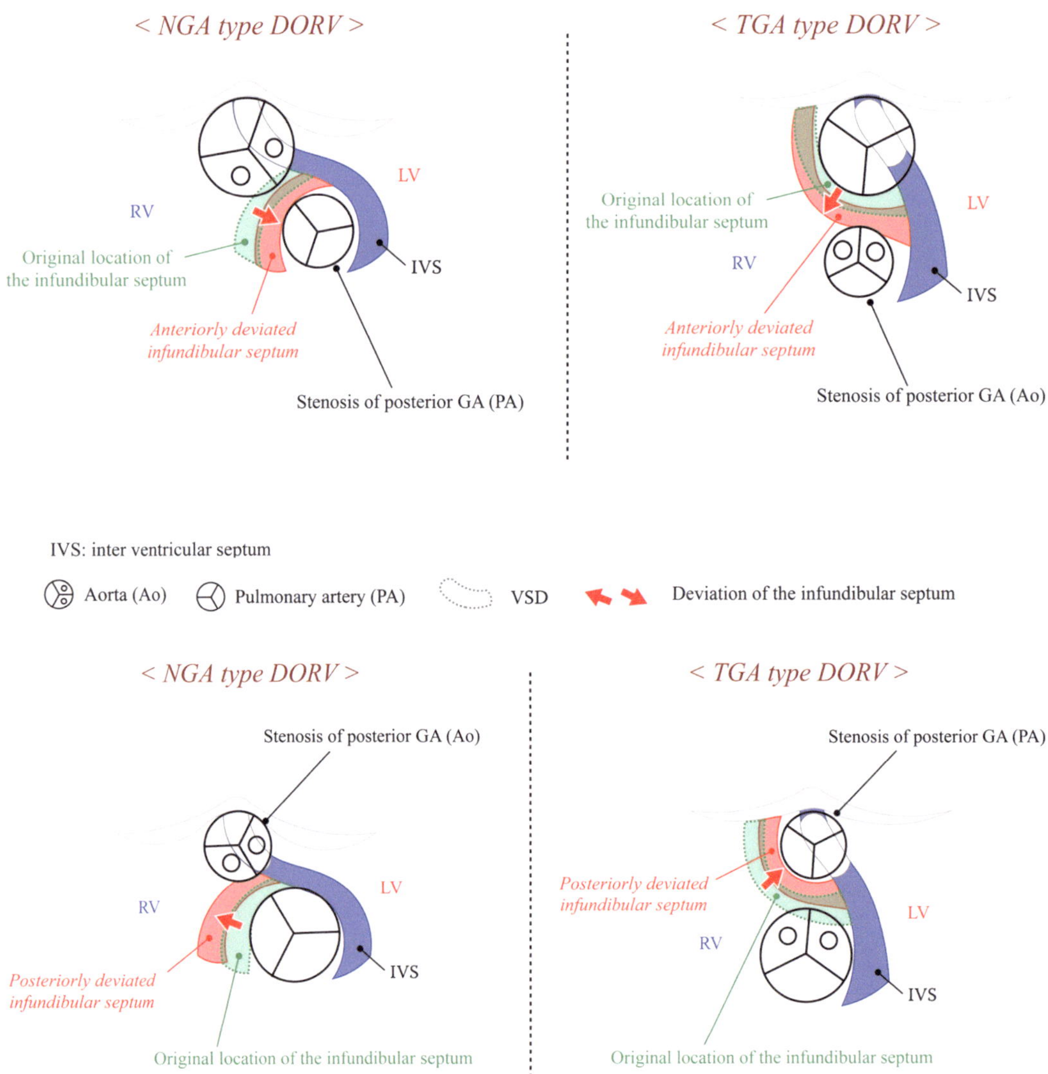

Fig. 8.8 Posterior or anterior deviation of the infundibular septum

3 Intraventricular Rerouting for DORV

3.1 Types of DORV for Intraventricular Rerouting Is Indicated

{SDN}DORV and original Taussig-Bing in NGA type group and {SDL}DORV and anatomically corrected malposition of the great artery in TGA type group have subaortic VSD or doubly committed VSD that have a large subaortic component, allowing intraventricular rerouting can direct blood flow from the left ventricle to the aortic valve through the VSD (Fig. 8.9).

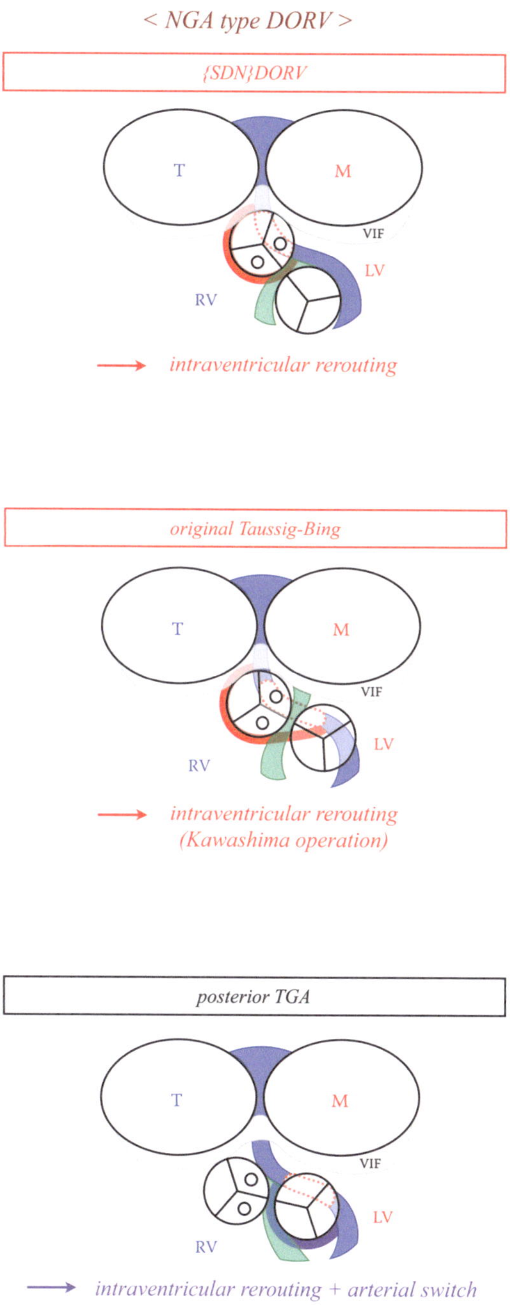

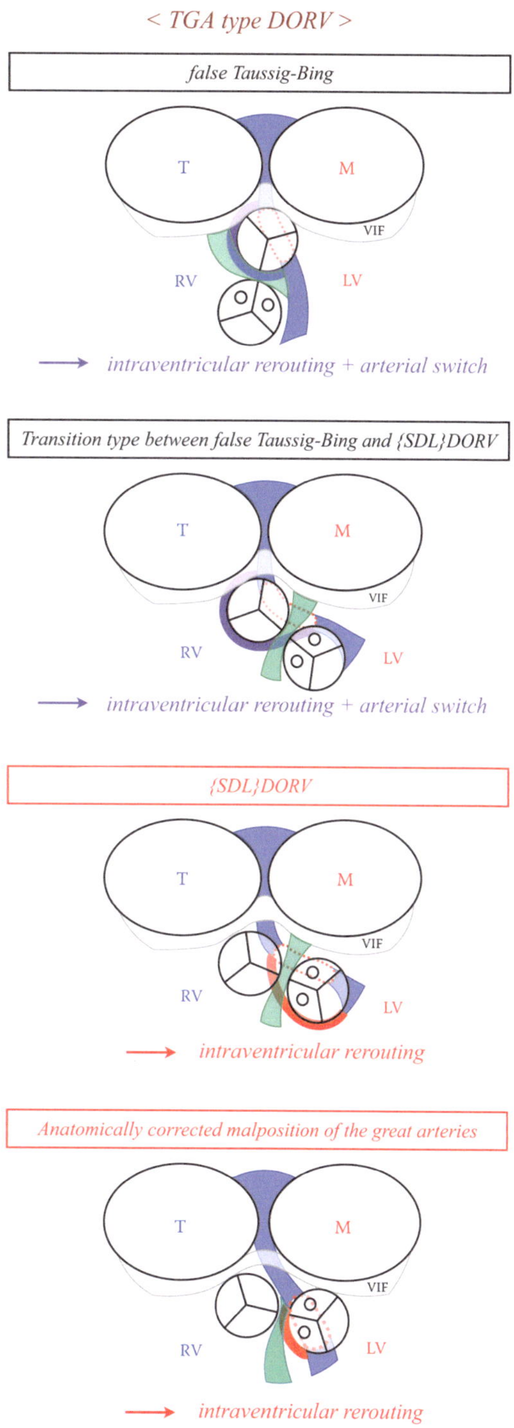

Fig. 8.9 Variation of DORV and operative procedure

3.2 {SDN} DORV: Morphology and Intraventricular Rerouting

- Relationship of the great arteries is left anterior to pulmonary artery (PA) and right posterior to aorta (Ao).
- The intracardiac morphology of {SDN} DORV is similar to that of tetralogy of Fallot.
- The differences are that the aorta originates more than 50% from the right ventricle and there is muscular tissue (VIF) between the aortic and mitral valves (Figs. 8.10, 8.11, and 8.12).
- Muscular tissue (ventriculo-infundibular fold: VIF) is interposed between the mitral and pulmonary valves.
- The posterior margin of the infundibular septum (☆) connects to the anterior limb of the trabecular septomarginalis (TSM).
- The anterior margin of the infundibular septum connects to the right ventricular anterior wall.
- The infundibular septum (IF) and ventricular septum (IVS) are orthogonal (malalign).
- Subaortic VSD.
- More than 50% of aortic valves are attached to the ventricular septum.
- The posterior inferior margin of the VSD may be present in the membranous portion. In such cases, a membranous flap is present at the posterior inferior margin.
- Blood flow from the left ventricle is directed to the aorta.
- Intraventricular rerouting from VSD to the aorta is easily possible.
- Black dotted line: patch suture line (as in tetralogy of Fallot).
- The anterior aortic margin (⟼) is difficult to visualize trans-tricuspidally (also difficult to

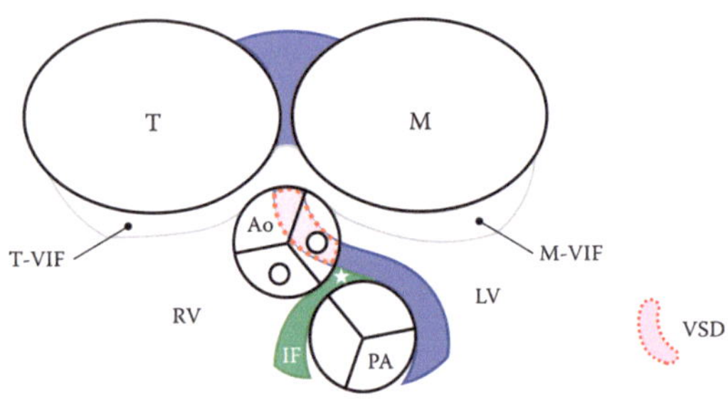

Fig. 8.10 {SDN} DORV: intracardiac morphology

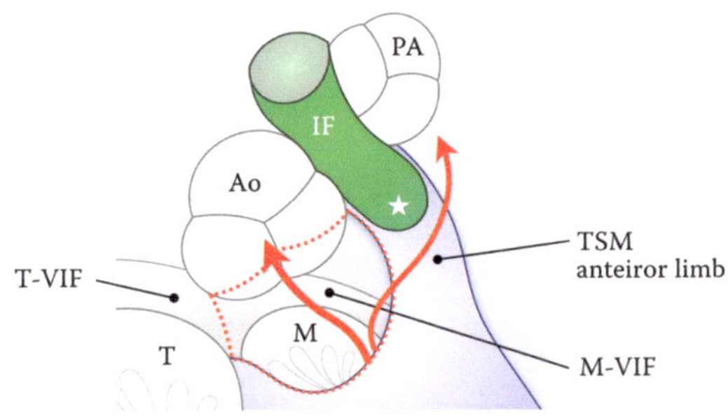

Fig. 8.11 {SDN} DORV: blood flow

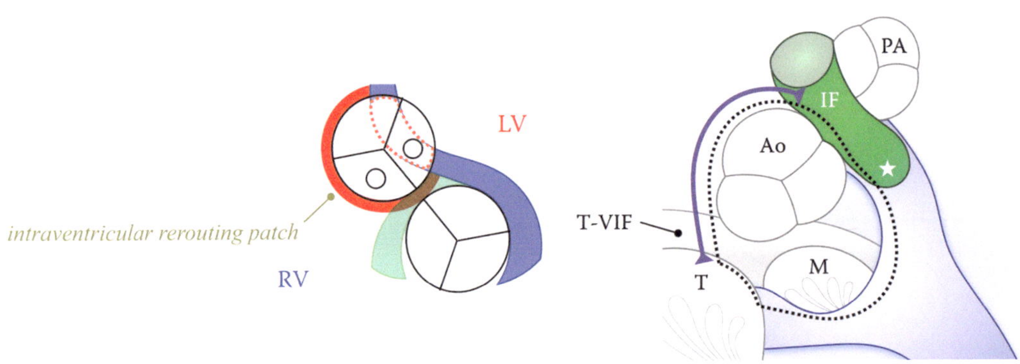

Fig. 8.12 {SDN} DORV: intraventricular rerouting

see through the right ventricular outflow tract) because the aorta is deviated to the right ventricle.

- Intraventricular rerouting patch should be slightly larger with room to spare.

3.3 False Taussig-Bing Anomaly: Morphological Variation and Intraventricular Rerouting

- The configuration of the connection between the infundibular septum and the VIF results in variations in intracardiac morphology (route from the VSD to the great arteries).
- Whether the posterior margin of the infundibular septum (☆) is connected to the mitral or tricuspid VIF is related to the success or failure of the intraventricular rerouting (Figs. 8.13, 8.14, 8.15, 8.16, 8.17, and 8.18).

< *False Taussig-Bing with Doubly-Committed VSD* >

- The rightward deviation of the posterior great artery results in a parallel great artery relationship.
- The VSDs are extended anteriorly and are also present below the pulmonary valve, fulfilling the diagnostic criteria for a false Taussig-Bing anomaly.
- Relationship of the great arteries is side by side.
- Muscular tissue (ventriculo-infundibular fold: VIF) is interposed between the mitral and pulmonary valves.
- The posterior margin of the infundibular septum (IF: ☆) connects to the mitral side ventricular infundibular fold (M-VIF).
- The anterior margin of the infundibular septum connects to the right ventricular anterior wall.
- Doubly committed VSD, major portion of the VSD is below the aortic valve.
- The posterior inferior margin of the VSD may be present in the membranous portion. In such cases, a membranous flap is present at the posterior inferior margin.
- Blood flow from the left ventricle is directed to both great arteries.

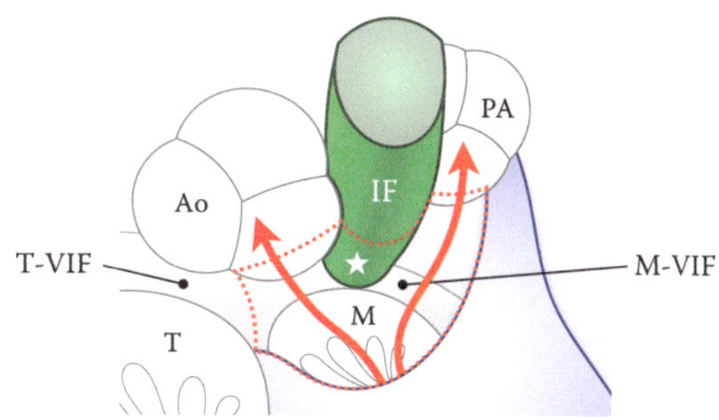

Fig. 8.14 False Taussig-Bing with doubly committed VSD: blood flow

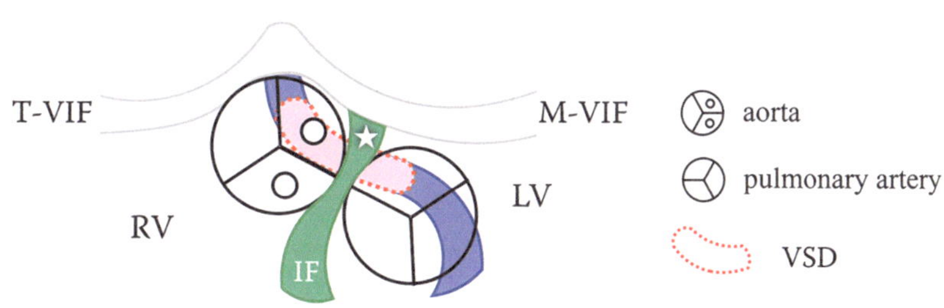

Fig. 8.13 False Taussig-Bing with doubly committed VSD: intracardiac morphology

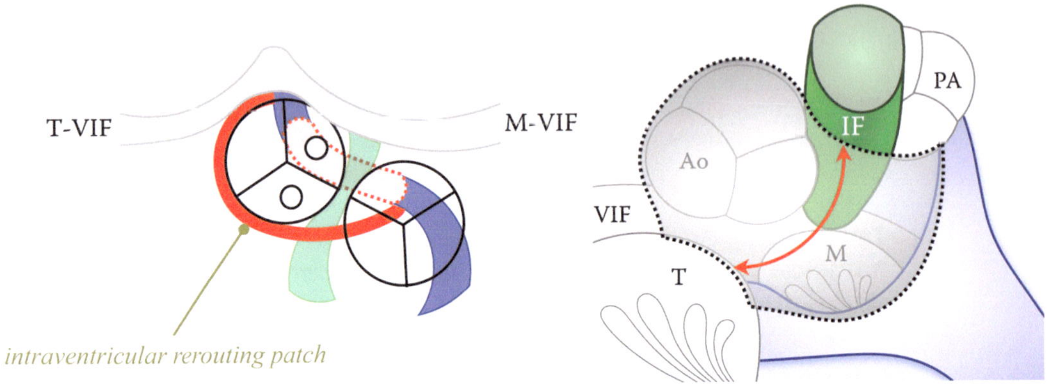

Fig. 8.15 False Taussig-Bing with doubly committed VSD: intraventricular rerouting

Fig. 8.16 False Taussig-Bing with subpulmonary VSD

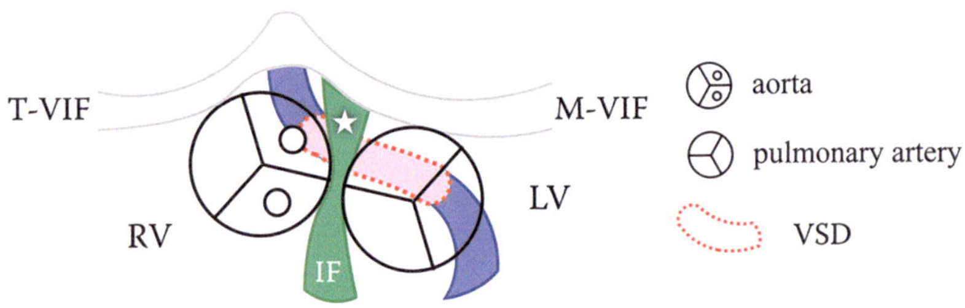

Fig. 8.17 False Taussig-Bing with subpulmonary VSD: blood flow

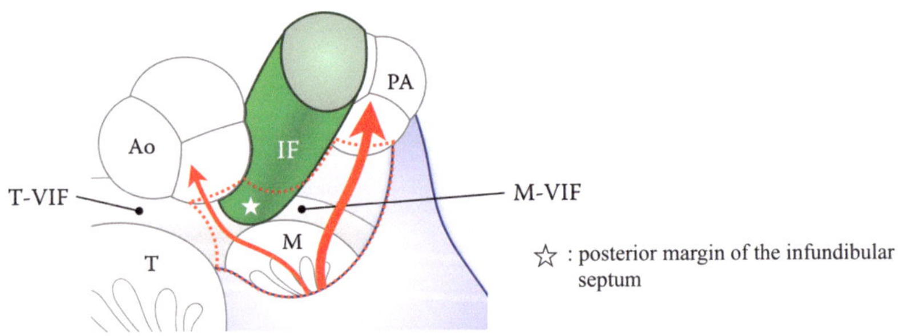

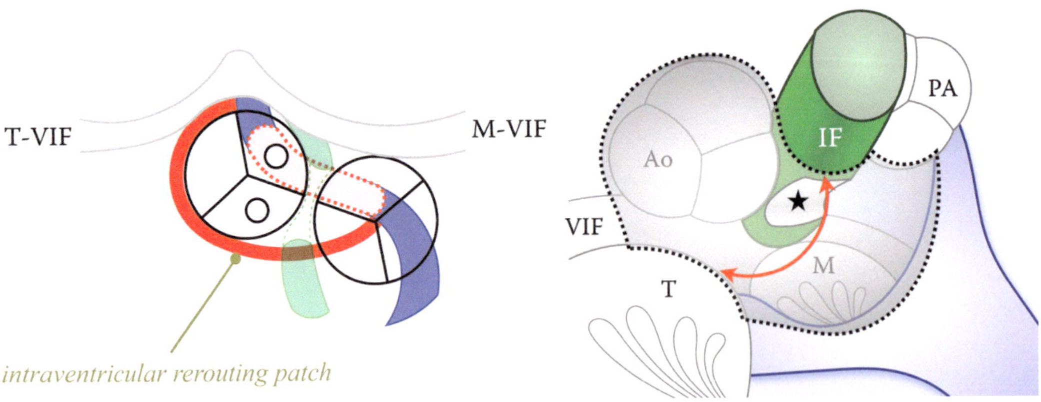

Fig. 8.18 False Taussig-Bing with subpulmonary VSD: intraventricular rerouting

- Intraventricular rerouting from VSD to the aorta is possible because the blood flow pathways to both great arteries are kept wide.
- Intraventricular rerouting (Kawashima operation) is feasible.
- Black dotted line: patch suture line.
- The anterior margin of the VSD is often difficult to visualize trans-tricuspidally.
- Intraventricular rerouting patch should be slightly larger with room to spare. To avoid left ventricular outflow tract stenosis, the patch width should be wide enough, especially in the area indicated by the red arrow.

< *False Taussig-Bing with Subpulmonary VSD* >.

- The posterior aorta is further deviated to the right.
- The VSD is further extended anteriorly and located below the pulmonary artery valve.

- Relationship of the great arteries is side by side.
- Muscular tissue (ventriculo-infundibular fold: VIF) is interposed between the mitral and pulmonary valves.
- The rightward deviation of the posterior Ao and the leftward deviation of the anterior PA cause the posterior border of the infundibular septum (IF: ☆) to connect to the VIF and come closer to the tricuspid valve, narrowing the blood flow pathway from the VSD to the Ao.
- The VSD is located below both semilunar valve.
- Anterior margin of the VSD is extended anteriorly.
- Major portion of the VSD is below the pulmonary valve (subpulmonary VSD).
- Blood flow from the left ventricle is directed mainly to the pulmonary artery.
- The red dotted line indicates the margin of the VSD.
- Right ventricular outflow tract incision is required to visualize the anterior border of the VSD.
- For intraventricular rerouting, the infundibular septum, which is orthogonal to the ventricular septum, obstructs the blood flow path from the left ventricle to the aorta.
- Black dotted line: patch suture line.
- The anterior margin of the VSD is not visible through the trans-tricuspid valve and should be approached through the right ventricular outflow tract incision.
- Part of the infundibular septum should be resected to secure the left ventricular outflow tract (★).
- Intraventricular rerouting patch should be slightly larger with room to spare. To avoid left ventricular outflow tract stenosis, the patch width should be wide enough, especially in the area indicated by the red arrow.
- If the majority of the VSD is located below the pulmonary valve, the VSD should be closed and an arterial switch operation should be performed.

SPOTLIGHT Specimen of Taussig-Bing Anomaly with Subpulmonary VSD

- The infundibular septum (IF) crosses the VSD and posterior edge of the IF (☆) attaches to the mitral side of the ventriculo-infundibular fold (M-VIF).
- IF and the interventricular septum are orthogonal.
- The VSD is located beneath both aortic and pulmonary valves (doubly committed VSD).
- Postero-inferior margin of the VSD (*) is in close proximity to the membranous area.

< Right ventricular morphology through the anterior wall incision >

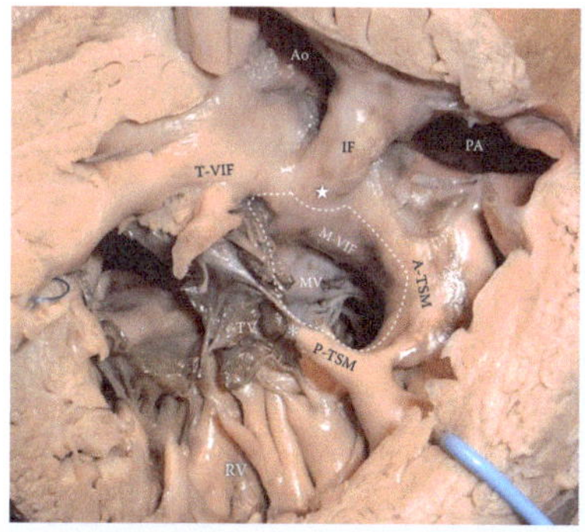

(continued)

Ao aortic valve, *PA* pulmonary valve, *MV* mitral valve, *TV* tricuspid valve, *A-TSM* anterior limb of the trabecular septomarginalis, *P-TSM* posterior limb of the trabecular septomarginalis, *M-VIF* mitral side of the ventriculo-infundibular fold, *T-VIF* tricuspid side of the ventriculo-infundibular fold, *RV* right ventricle. White dashed line: margin of the VSD.

4 Intraventricular Rerouting for DORV

Case

- Age: 5 years 2 months old.
- Body weight: 14.2 kg.
- Diagnosis: Original Taussig-Bing, doubly committed VSD.
- Coronary artery: [1LCx: 2R], Yacoub type A (Shaher type 1).
- Previous operation: Pulmonary artery banding (2 months old).
- Pulmonary valve: Tricuspid, no regurgitation.
- Pulmonary annular diameter = 13.1 mm (135% of normal value).
- Pressure gradient at pulmonary banding site = 23 mmHg (v = 5.56 m/s).
- Aortic valve: Tricuspid, no regurgitation.
- Aortic annular diameter: 14.5 mm (124% of normal value).
- Left ventricular end-diastolic volume = 186% of normal value.
- Right ventricular end-diastolic volume = 106% of normal value.

In this case, both great arteries were nearly parallel, and more than 50% of both great arteries originated from the right ventricle. The VSD extended anteriorly from below the aortic valve to below the pulmonary valve. Based on the above, the diagnosis of original Taussig-Bing was made.

Because the VSD was not confined beneath the pulmonary valve, arterial switch operation was not indicated, and intraventricular rerouting (Kawashima operation) was indicated (Fig. 8.19).

< Frontal image >

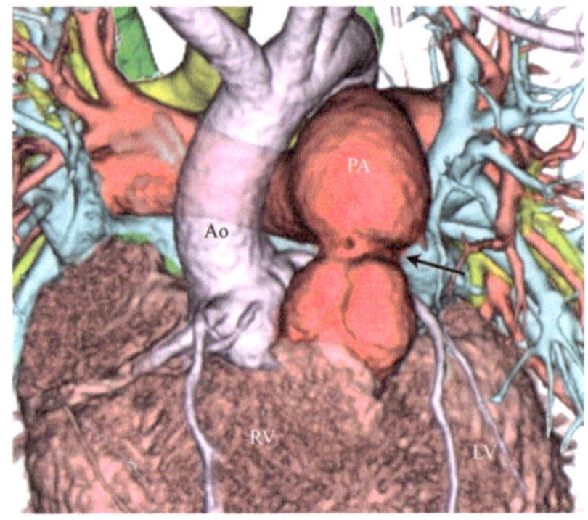

Fig. 8.19 Preoperative CT images

- Both great arteries nearly parallel.
- Pulmonary artery slightly anterior to the left, aorta slightly posterior to the right.
- Coronary artery morphology is [1LCx: 2R], Yacoub A (Shaher type 1).
- Stenosis due to previous pulmonary artery banding (black arrow) and deformation of the sinus of Valsalva.

< Horizontal cross-section image >

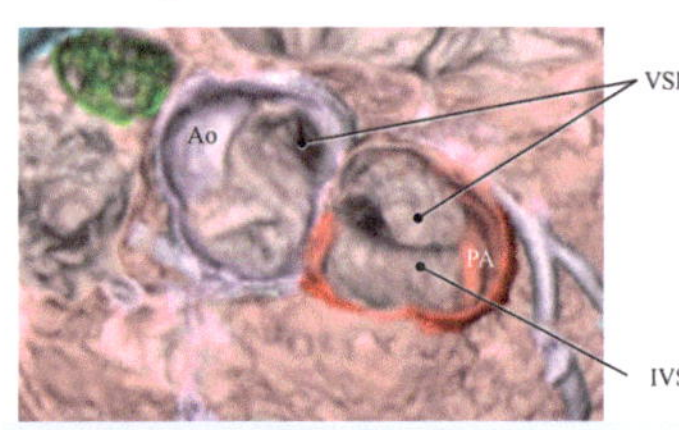

Ao aorta, *PA* pulmonary artery, *LV* left ventricle, *RV* right ventricle

- VSD is present in both great arteries.
- Both semilunar valves originate more than 50% from the right ventricle.
- If the VSD extends further anteriorly and becomes confined beneath the pulmonary valve, and the infundibular septum and ventricular septum become

(continued)

parallel, the diagnosis is posterior TGA and an arterial switch is indicated.

- In this case, the posterior margin of the VSD is located near the perimembranous area, so even if an arterial switch is performed, intraventricular rerouting to the pulmonary valve is required.
- Since it is easier to create a blood flow route from the VSD to the aortic valve and coronary artery grafting is not required, intraventricular rerouting is indicated.
- In addition, because the pulmonary valve and sinus of Valsalva were deformed due to pulmonary artery strangulation, arterial switch operation was not indicated.

< Frontal cross-section image >

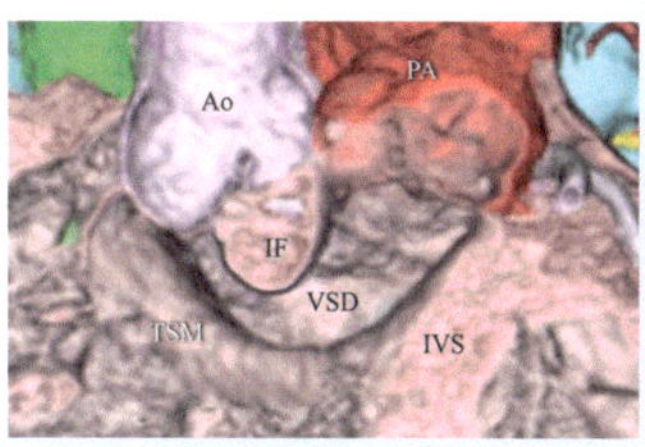

IVS interventricular septum, *TSM* trabecular septomarginalis, *IF* infundibular septum

- The infundibular septum is orthogonal to the interventricular septum.
- The infundibular septum is extended apex ward, requiring resection of the infundibular septum for intraventricular rerouting.
- The intraventricular rerouting patch protrudes into the right ventricular cavity, requiring enlargement of the right ventricular outflow tract.
- The anterior cephalic side of the intraventricular rerouting patch must be sutured to the pulmonary valve annulus (a longitudinal incision is made through the anterior commissure of the pulmonary valve for visualization and the valve annulus is reconstructed after suturing the patch) (Scene 8.1).

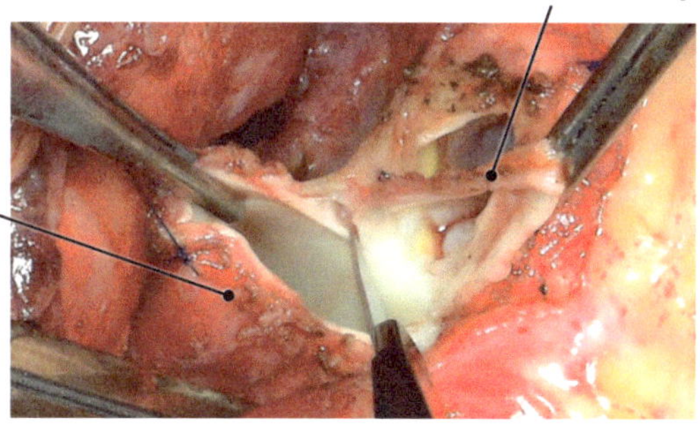

Scene 8.1 Resection of pulmonary wall at the banding site (Video 00 min 09 s)

1. Remove the pulmonary artery tape of the previous operation.
2. Resect the pulmonary artery wall in the strangulated area in the shape of a tube (Scene 8.2).

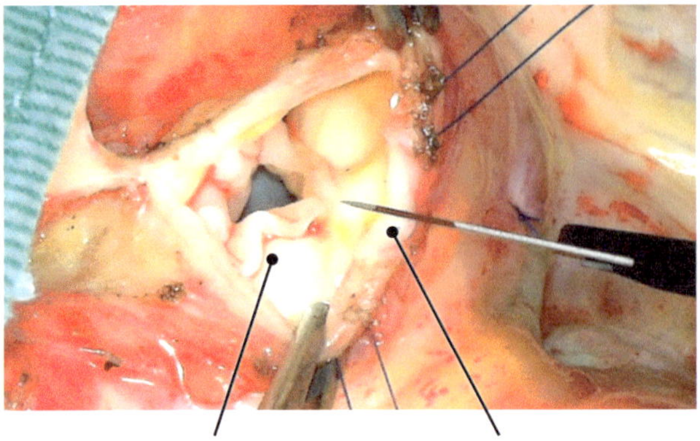

Scene 8.2 Longitudinal incision of the anterior pulmonary wall (Video 00 min 31 s)

1. Longitudinal incision of the pulmonary artery wall and valve annulus at the anterior commissure of the pulmonary artery to secure a view under the pulmonary valve.
   - Although the pulmonary valve was thickened due to pulmonary artery banding, the annular diameter was 135% of normal (Z score 1.60), so we decided to preserve the annulus by suturing the longitudinal incision after closure of the VSD (Scene 8.3).

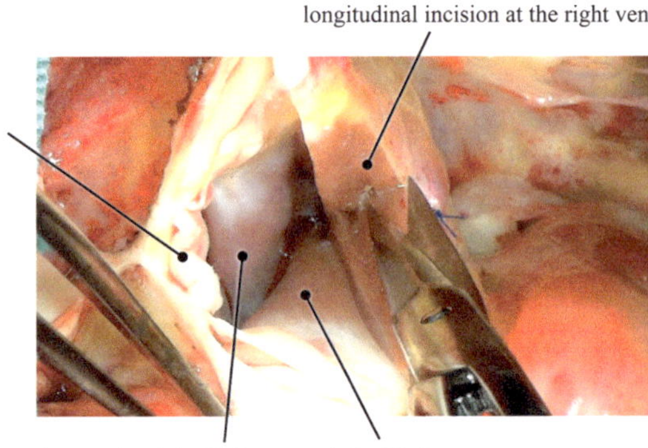

Scene 8.3 Longitudinal incision of the right ventricular outflow tract (Video 01 min 01 s)

1. The right ventricular outflow tract is incised longitudinally.
   - A long infundibular septum extending toward the apex is seen.
   - The anterior border of the VSD is seen below the pulmonary valve.
   - The right ventricular outflow tract is enlarged in the subvalvular patch, so the incision may be longer (Scene 8.4).

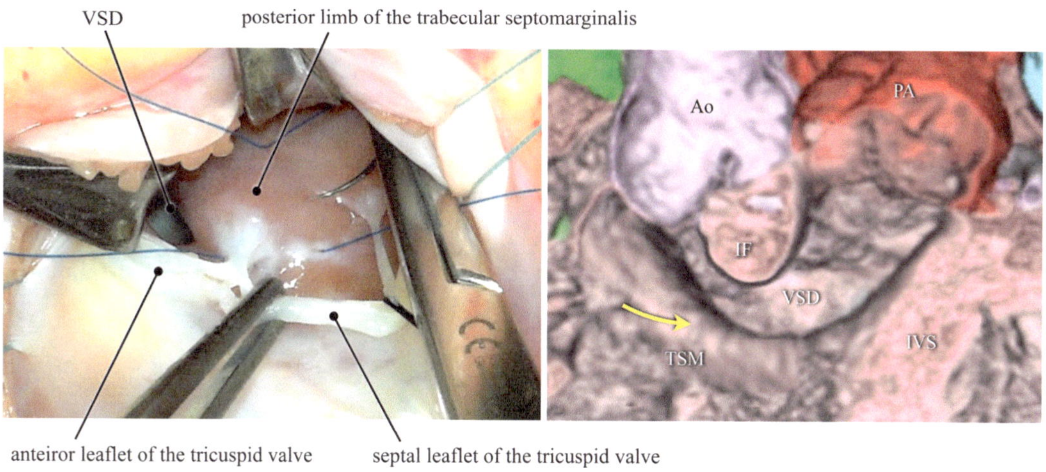

Scene 8.4 VSD closure 1 posterior limb of trabecular septomarginalis (Video 01 min 43 s)

1 Through the tricuspid valve, 5-0 monofilament sutures with pledgets are sewn to the inferior margin of the VSD (posterior limb of the trabecular septomarginalis) (right figure, yellow arrowed area) (Scene 8.5).

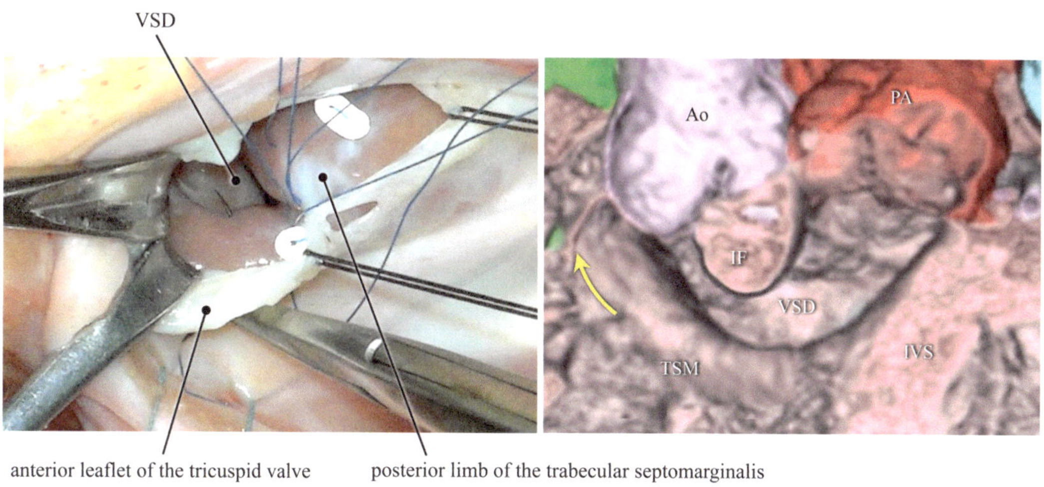

Scene 8.5 VSD closure 2 tricuspid annulus (Video 02 min 10 s)

1. 5-0 monofilament sutures with pledgets are sewn to the tricuspid annulus of the anterior leaflet (right figure, yellow arrowed area) (Scene 8.6).

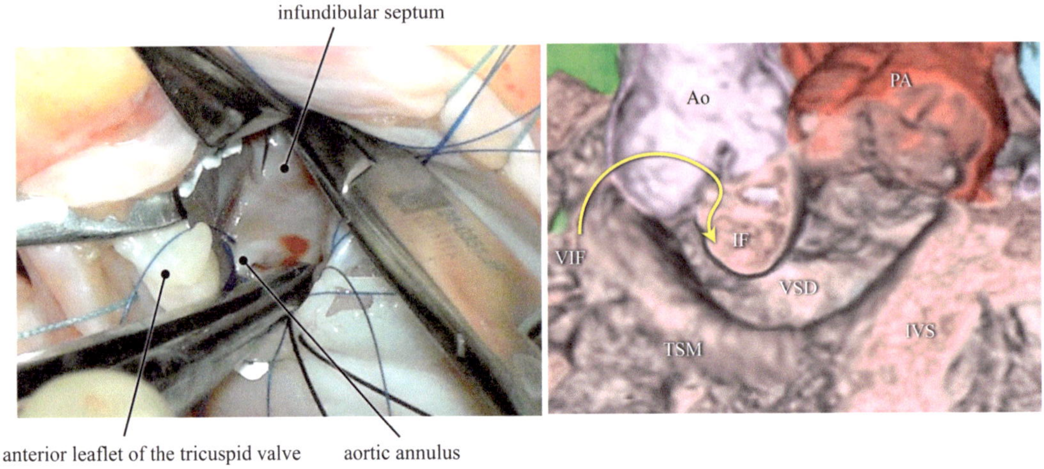

Scene 8.6 VSD closure 3 infundibular septum through the tricuspid valve (Video 02 min 37 s)

1. Through the tricuspid valve, 5-0 monofilament sutures with pledgets are sewn to the right ventricular wall anterior to the aortic annulus (*right figure, yellow arrowed area*) (Scene 8.7).

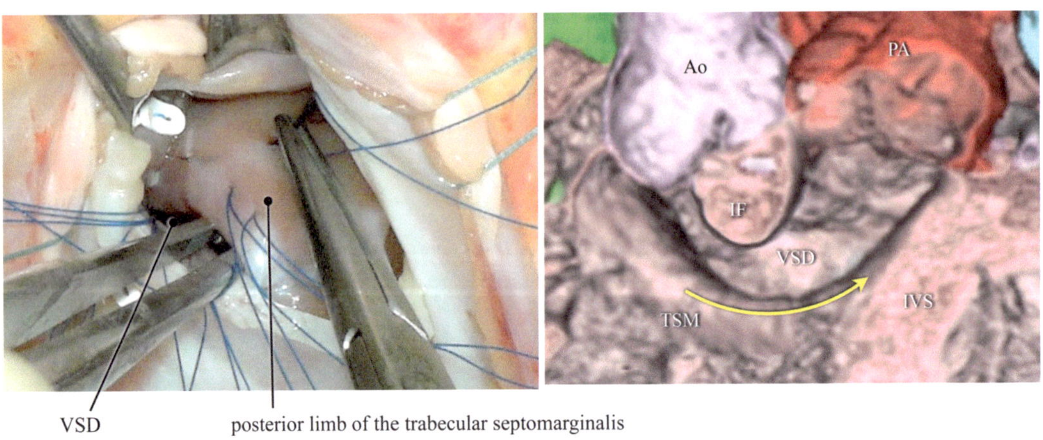

Scene 8.7 VSD closure 4 posterior limb of trabecular septomarginalis (Video 05 min 12 s)

1. Through the tricuspid valve, 5-0 monofilament sutures with pledgets are sewn to the inferior margin of the VSD (posterior limb of the trabecular septomarginalis) (*right figure, yellow arrowed area*) (Scene 8.8).

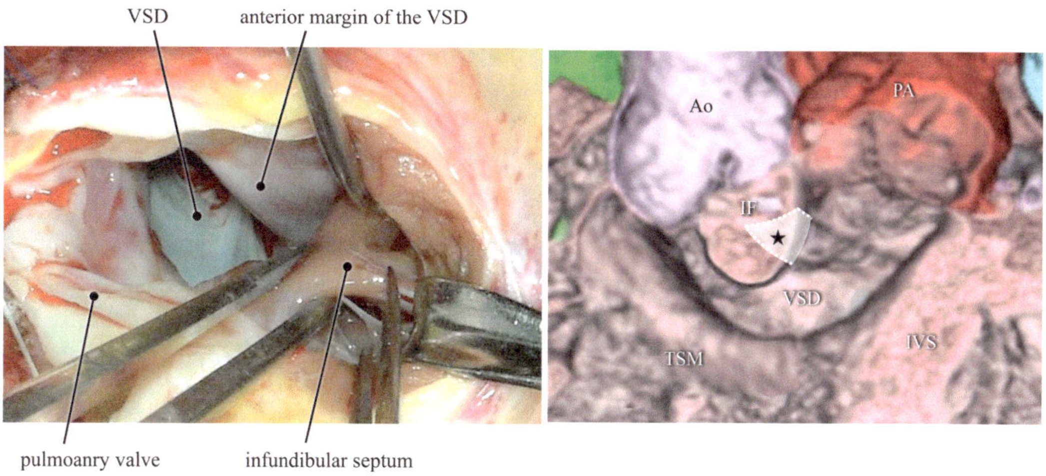

Scene 8.8 Resection of the infundibular septum 1 (Video 05 min 39 s)

1. Incise the anterior margin of the infundibular septum through the right ventricular outflow tract incision (★) (Scene 8.9).

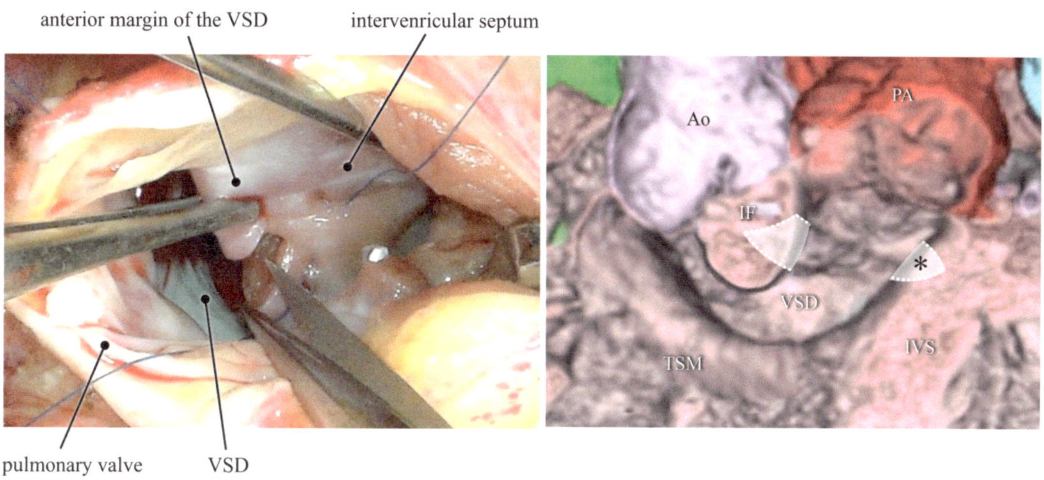

Scene 8.9 Enlargement of anterior edge of the VSD (Video 05 min 59 s)

1. Enlarge the VSD by incising the anterior margin of the VSD through the right ventricular outflow tract incision (*) (Scene 8.10).

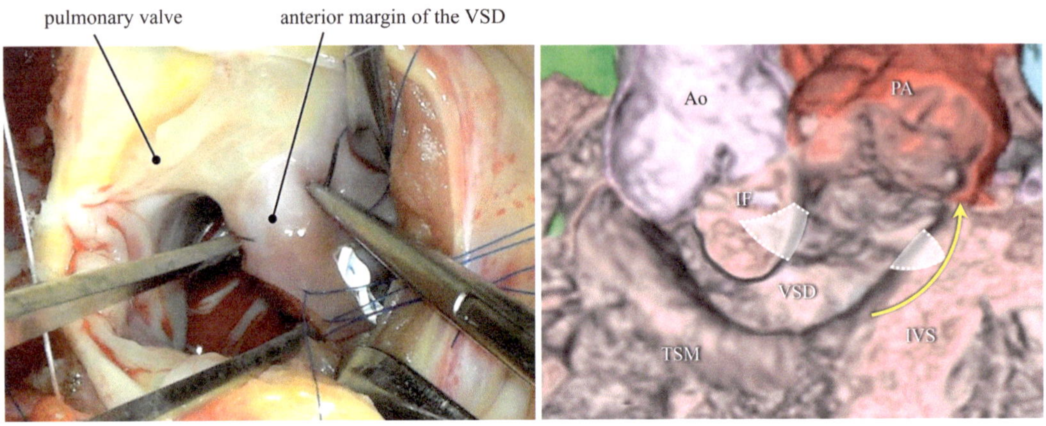

Scene 8.10 VSD closure 5 through the right ventricular outflow incision (Video 06 min 12)

1. Through the right ventricular outflow incision, 5-0 monofilament sutures with pledgets are sewn to the anterior margin of the VSD (*right figure, yellow arrowed area*) (Scene 8.11).

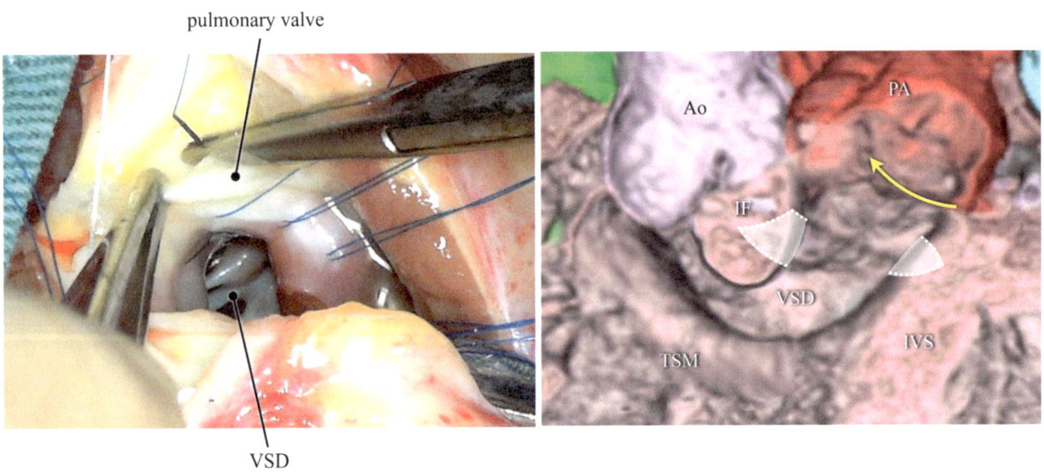

Scene 8.11 VSD closure 6 pulmonary valve annulus (Video 07 min 01 s)

1. 5-0 monofilament sutures with pledgets are sewn to the pulmonary annulus of the left posterior leaflet (*right figure, yellow arrowed area*) (Scene 8.12).

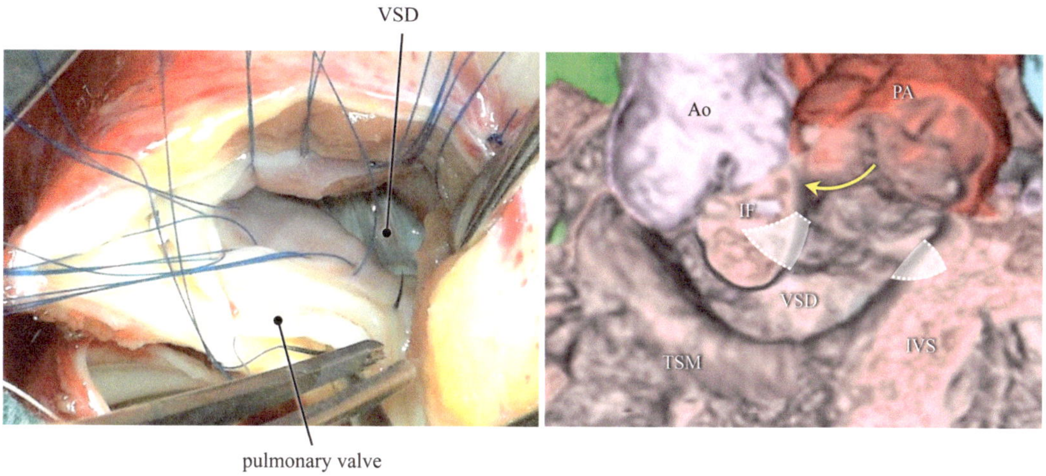

Scene 8.12 VSD closure 7 pulmonary valve annulus (Video 07 min 31 s)

1. 5-0 monofilament sutures with pledgets are sewn to the pulmonary annulus of the right posterior leaflet (*right figure, yellow arrowed area*) (Scene 8.13).

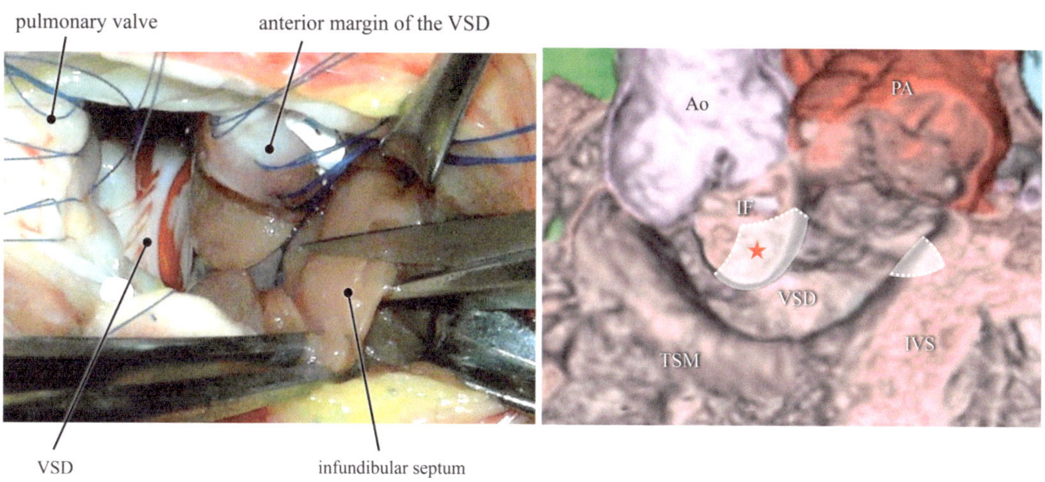

Scene 8.13 Resection of the infundibular septum 2 (Video 08 min 46 s)

1. The anterior margin of the infundibular septum is incised through the right ventricular outflow incision (Scene 8.14).

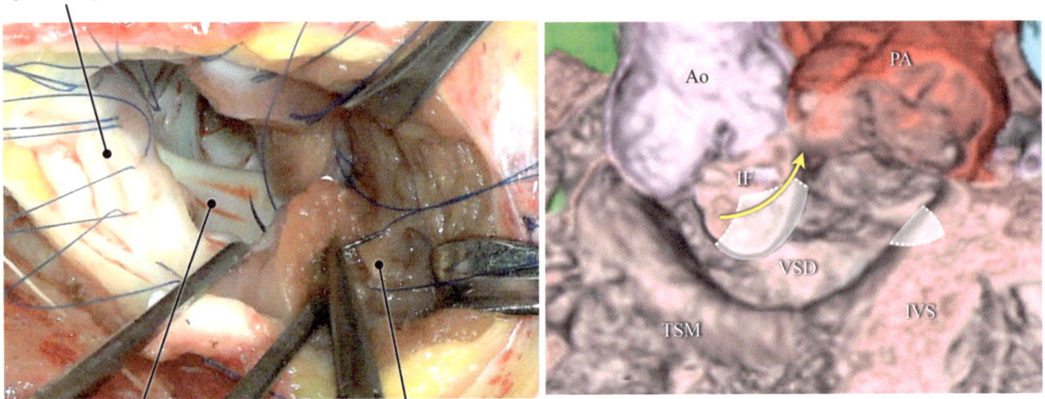

Scene 8.14 VSD closure 8 infundibular septum through right ventricular outflow (Video 09 min 20 s)

1. Through the right ventricular outflow incision, 5-0 monofilament sutures with pledgets are sewn to the anterior margin of the infundibular septum (*right figure, yellow arrowed area*) (Scene 8.15).

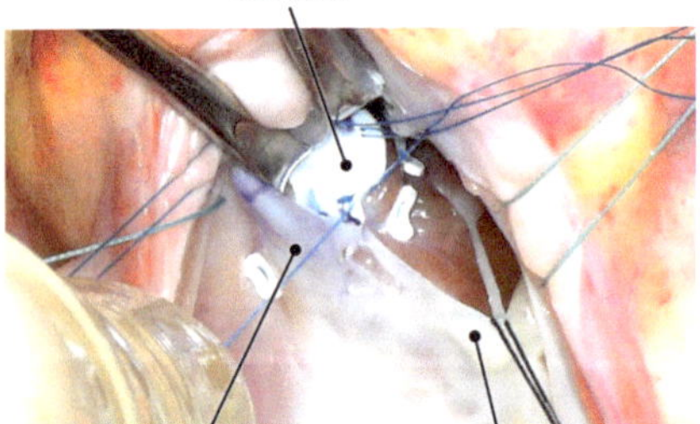

Scene 8.15 VSD patch anastomosis 1 through tricuspid annulus (Video 10 min 28 s)

1. Ligate the VSD patch sutures through the tricuspid valve (Scene 8.16).

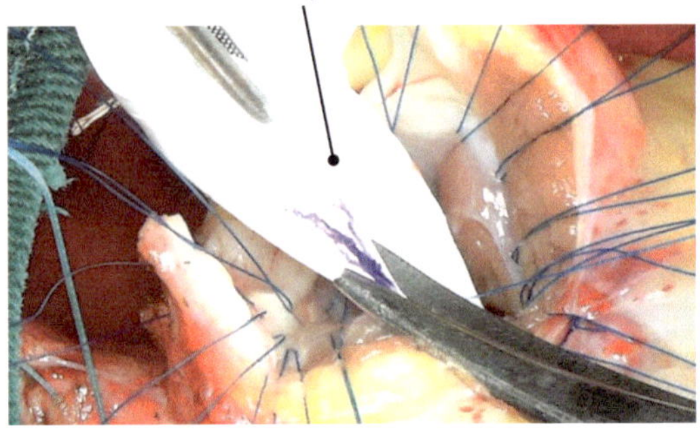

Scene 8.16 Trimming of the VSD patch 1 (Video 11 min 17 s)

1. Pull the VSD patch through the right ventricular outflow tract incision.
2. Trim the VSD patch gradually along the curvature of the suture line (Scene 8.17).

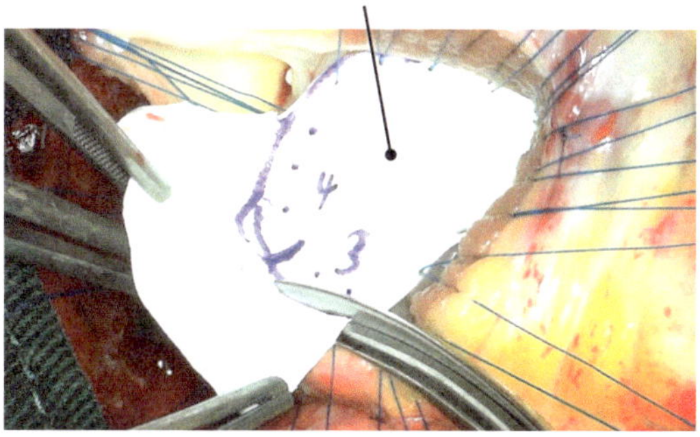

Scene 8.17 Trimming of the VSD patch 2 (Video 12 min 12 s)

1. Trim the VSD patch along the pulmonary valve annulus (Scene 8.18).

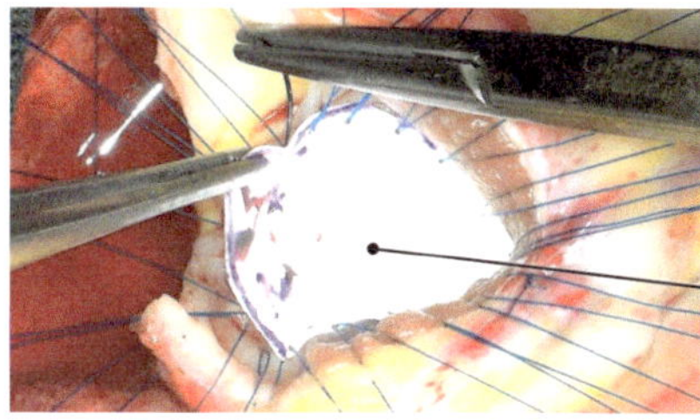

Scene 8.18 VSD patch anastomosis 2 through tricuspid annulus (Video 12 min 50 s)

1. Insert the monofilament VSD sutures into the superior edge of the ePTFE patch in sequence (Scene 8.19).

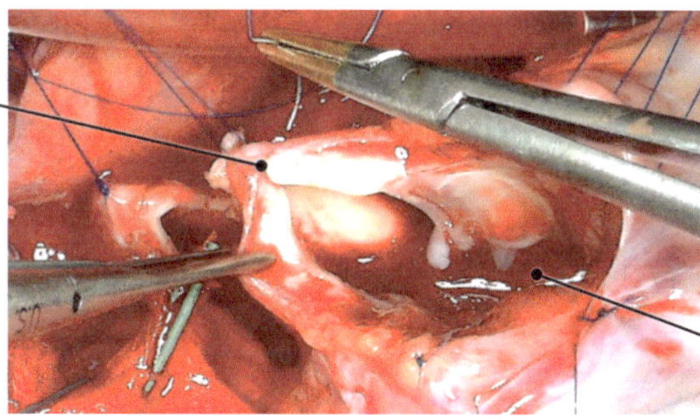

Scene 8.19 Repair of anterior wall of the pulmonary artery (Video 13 min 48 s)

1. Suture closure of the incised anterior wall of the pulmonary artery (reconstruction of the pulmonary valve annulus) (Scene 8.20).

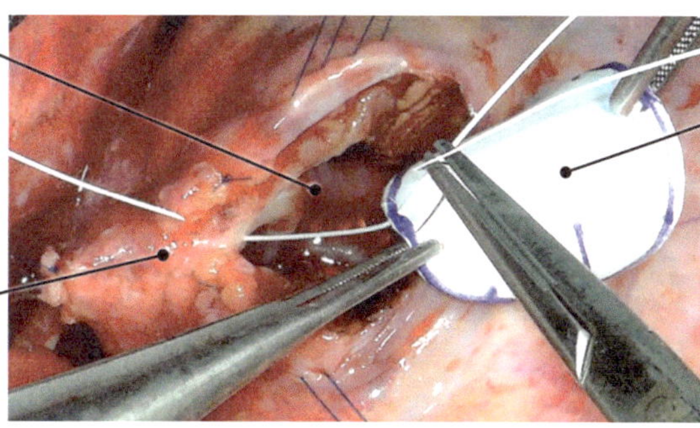

Scene 8.20 Anastomosis of right ventricular outflow patch 1 (Video 15 min 13 s)

1. The ePTFE patch is anastomosed with a CV-5 ePTFE continuous suture to augment the right ventricular outflow tract (Scene 8.21).

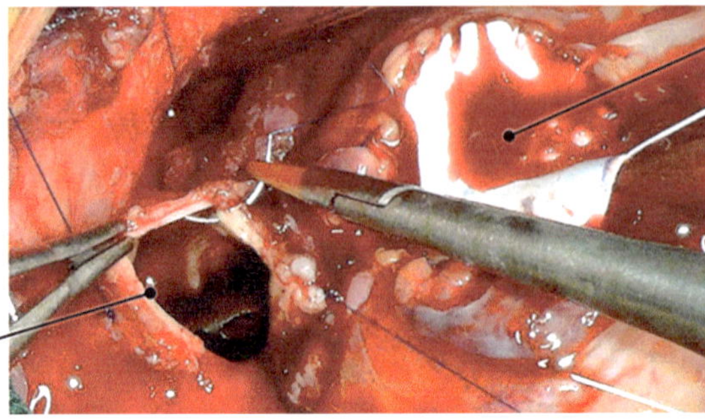

Scene 8.21 End-to-end anastomosis of the main pulmonary artery (Video 17 min 10 s)

1. The pulmonary artery with the resected banding wall is anastomosed end-to-end with a continuous 6-0 monofilament suture.

- A flexible suction is inserted into the pulmonary artery from the inferior end of the right ventricular outflow tract patch to secure the surgical field (Scene 8.22).

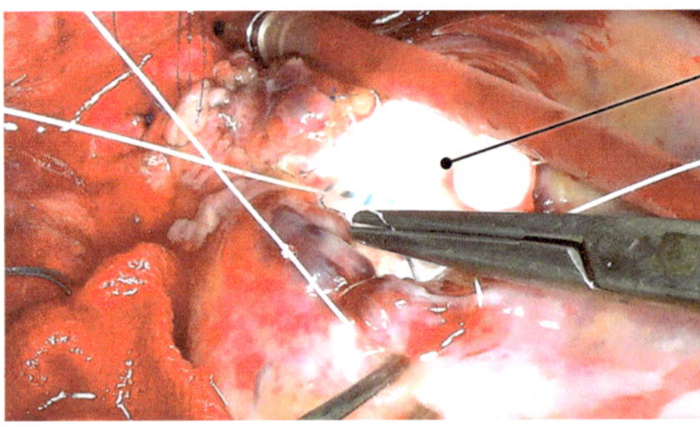

Scene 8.22 Anastomosis of right ventricular outflow patch 2 (Video 19 min 04 s) (▶ https://doi.org/10.1007/000-hkf)

1. Suture closure of the lower end of the right ventricular outflow patch and complete the procedure.

SPOTLIGHT Pre and Postoperative CT Images

< Suture lines of intraventricular rerouting >

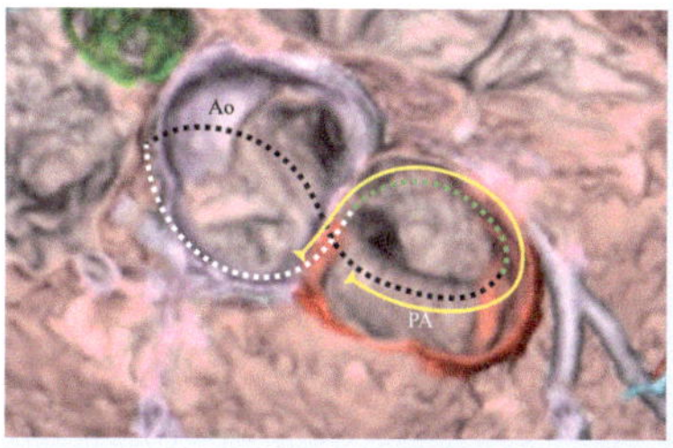

- ***The black dashed line*** indicates the suture line along the postero-inferior and anterior margins of the VSD.
- ***The white dashed line*** indicates the suture line of subaortic muscle along the aortic annulus and infundibular septum.
- ***The green dashed line*** indicates the suture line through the pulmonary annulus.
- ***The yellow line*** indicates the suture area approaching through the right ventricular outflow and pulmonary artery incisions.

< Configuration of the intraventricular rerouting patch >

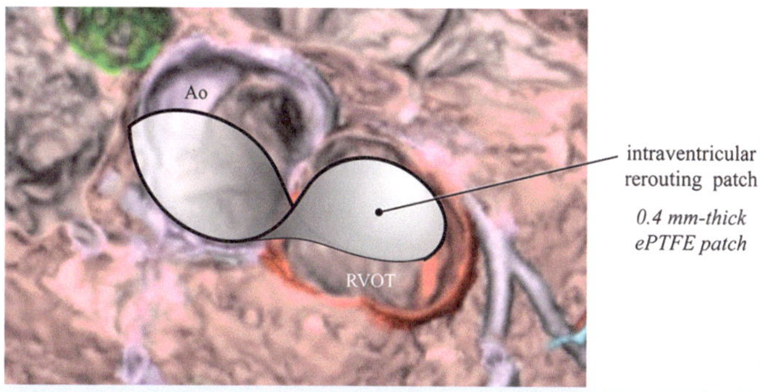

- Intraventricular rerouting patch will have a twisted shape as shown in the figure.
- Right ventricular outflow tract (RVOT) is narrowed due to intraventricular rerouting patch.

< Configuration of the intraventricular rerouting patch >

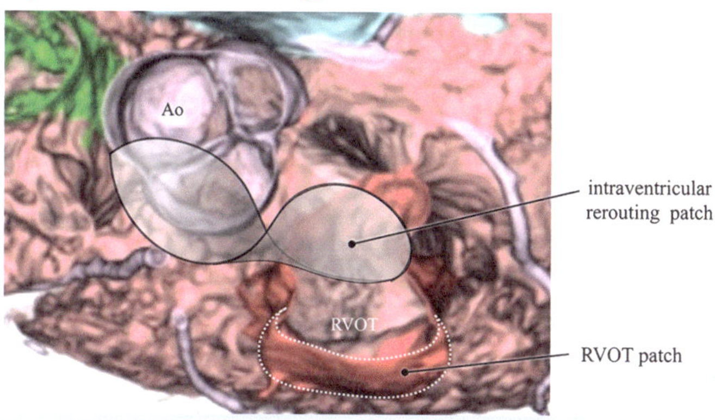

- Enlarge the right ventricular outflow tract below the pulmonary annulus by supplementing the ePTFE patch.

References

Malseptation Theory

Van Mierop LH. Transposition of the great arteries. I. Clarification or further confusion? Am J Cardiol. 1971a;28:735–8.
Van Mierop LH. Transposition of the great arteries. II. Transposition clarified. Am J Cardiol. 1971b;28:739–41.

Intraventricular Rerouting (Kawashima Operation) for Original Taussig-Bing

Kawashima Y, Fujita T, Miyamoto T, Manabe H. Intraventricular rerouting of blood for the correction of Taussig-Bing malformation. J Thorac Cardiovasc Surg. 1971;62:825–9.

9 Transposition of the Great Arteries (TGA) Transposition Type Double Outlet Right Ventricle (TGA Type DORV)

1 Morphology of Transposition of the Great Arteries

1.1 Typical Configuration of d-Transposition of the Great Arteries (d-TGA)

d-Transposition of the great arteries (d-TGA) is the basic form of TGA. Basically, relationship of the great arteries are the anterior aorta (Ao) and the posterior pulmonary artery (PA). In some cases, the PA is located slightly posterior to the left. The mitral annulus and the pulmonary annulus are connected by a fibrous continuity. The ventricular septum and the infundibular septum are parallel.

TGA type I is not associated with ventricular septal defect (VSD). In TGA type II, the posterior PA overrides on the ventricular septum.

The postero-inferior margin of the VSD is often located in the perimembranous portion. In this case, it is a perimembranous and juxtapulmonary VSD. The VSD does not extend anteriorly (Figs. 9.1 and 9.2).

- The relationship of the great arteries is anterior-posterior, with the anterior aorta and the

■ *d-TGA (I)*

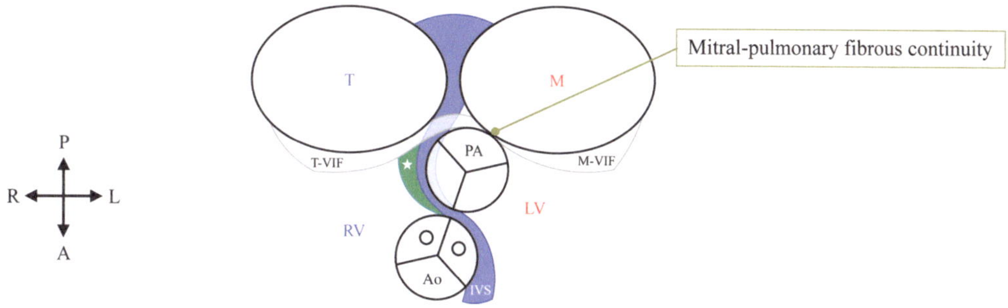

Fig. 9.1 d-TGA (I)

Supplementary Information The online version contains supplementary material available at https://doi.org/10.1007/978-981-96-6194-7_9. The videos can be accessed individually by clicking the DOI link in the accompanying figure caption or by scanning this link with the SN More Media App.

M. Yamagishi, *Surgical Treatment of Congenital Heart Disease*,
https://doi.org/10.1007/978-981-96-6194-7_9

■ *d-TGA (II)*

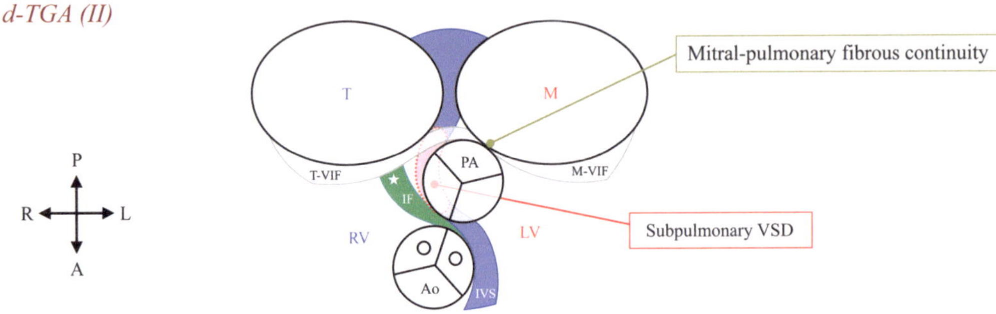

Fig. 9.2 d-TGA (II)

posterior pulmonary artery (slightly left posterior).

- Pulmonary valve annulus and mitral valve annulus are in contact (pulmonary-mitral fibrous continuity).
- Infundibular septum (IF) and interventricular septum (IVS) are parallel (*align*).
- Posterior border of the IF (☆) is connected to tricuspid side ventricular infundibular fold (*T-VIF*).
- This type is an indication of arterial switch operation.
- The relationship of the great arteries is anterior-posterior, with the anterior aorta and the posterior pulmonary artery (slightly left posterior).
- Pulmonary valve annulus and mitral valve annulus are in contact (pulmonary-mitral fibrous continuity).
- Posterior pulmonary artery deviates to the right and overrides to the IVS.
- Infundibular septum (IF) and interventricular septum (IVS) are parallel (*align*).
- Posterior border of the IF (☆) is connected to tricuspid side ventricular infundibular fold (*T-VIF*).
- The VSD is located below the pulmonary valve (*subpulmonary VSD*).
- Postero-inferior margin of the VSD is often located in the perimembranous portion.
- The VSD does not extend anteriorly.
- This type is an indication of arterial switch operation.

1.2 Morphological Spectrum of TGA Type DORV

The morphological spectrum of TGA type DORV includes false Taussig-Bing, {SDL} DORV, and anatomically malposition of the great arteries (ACMGA). There are also transitional forms of false Taussig-Bing and {SDL} DORV also exist. These morphological characteristics are shown.

The fibrous continuity between the mitral and pulmonary valve annulus is absent, and muscular tissue (ventriculo-infundibular fold: VIF) is interposed. The definition of double outlet right ventricle (DORV) is fulfilled by the 50% overriding and the disappearance of fibrous continuity between mitral and ventricular septum (VIF) (Figs. 9.3 and 9.4).

- The relationship of the great arteries is anterior-posterior, with the anterior aorta and the posterior pulmonary artery.
- Muscular tissue (ventriculo-infundibular fold: VIF) is interposed between the mitral and pulmonary valve annulus.
- Posterior pulmonary artery deviates to the right (*red arrow*) and more than 50% of the pulmonary valve overrides on the ventricular septum.
- Infundibular septum (IF) and interventricular septum (IVS) are parallel (*align*).
- Posterior border of the IF (☆) is connected to tricuspid side ventricular infundibular fold (T-VIF).

■ *false Taussig-Bing*

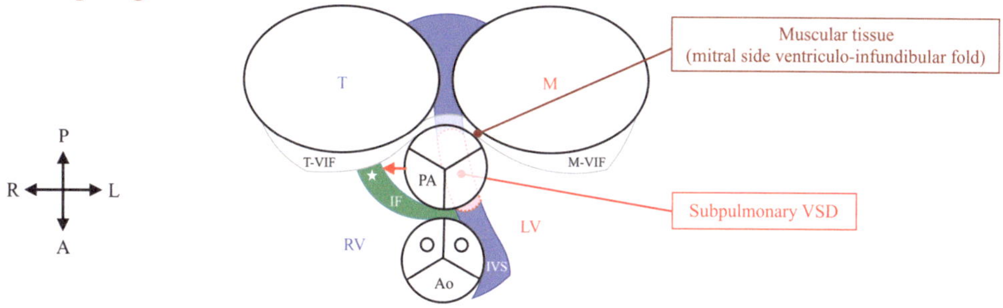

Fig. 9.3 Spectrum of TGA type DORV indicated for arterial switch operation

■ *{SDL}DORV*

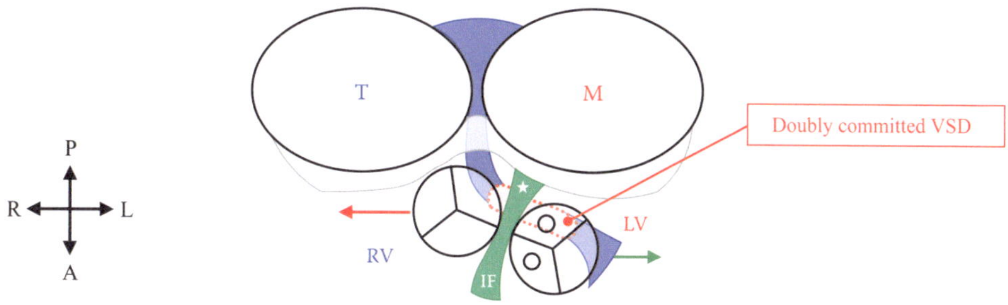

Fig. 9.4 Spectrum of TGA type DORV indicated for intraventricular rerouting

- Tricuspid chordae tendineae may be attached to the IF.
- The VSD is located below the pulmonary valve (*subpulmonary VSD*).
- Postero-inferior margin of the VSD is often located in the perimembranous portion.
- Compared to d-TGA, the VSD is slightly extended anteriorly.
- This type is an indication of arterial switch operation.

■ *Transition type between false Taussig-Bing and {SDL}DORV*

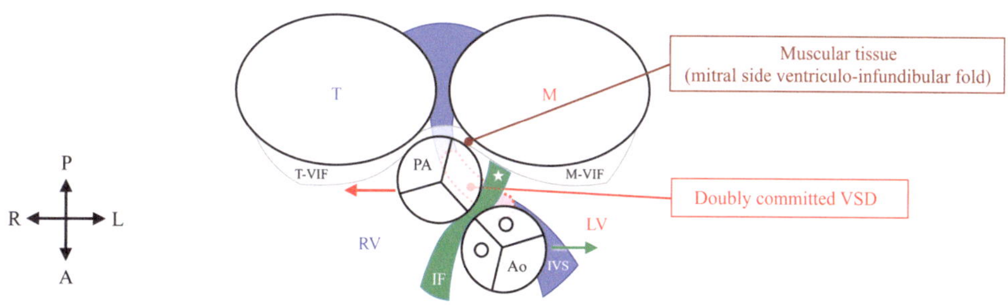

- The relationship of the great arteries is anterior-posterior, with the left anterior aorta and the right posterior pulmonary artery.
- Muscular tissue (ventriculo-infundibular fold: VIF) is interposed between the mitral and pulmonary valve annulus.
- Posterior pulmonary artery deviates to the right (*red arrow*) and more than 50% of the pulmonary valve overrides on the ventricular septum.
- The aorta slightly deviates to the left (*green arrow*).
- The infundibular septum (IF) and interventricular septum (IVS) are perpendicular (*malalign*).
- As the pulmonary artery deviates to the right, the IF rotates counterclockwise and the posterior margin of the IF (☆) crosses the VSD and attaches to the mitral side ventricular infundibular fold (*M-VIF*).
- The VSD is extended anteriorly and located under both semilunar valves, but the majority of VSD is located primarily under the PA valve (*doubly committed VSD*).
- This type is an indication of arterial switch operation.

Not all types of TGA type DORV are candidates for arterial switch operation. Types with an anterior extension of the VSD are indicated for intraventricular rerouting.

- The relationship of the great arteries is side-by-side, with the left aorta and the right pulmonary artery.
- Muscular tissue (ventriculo-infundibular fold: VIF) is interposed between the mitral and pulmonary valve annulus.
- The pulmonary artery moderately deviates to the right (*red arrow*) and overrides on the ventricular septum.
- The aorta deviates to the left (*green arrow*) and overrides on the ventricular septum more than 50% of the aortic valve.
- Posterior border of the infundibular septum (IF) (☆) is connected to mitral side ventricular infundibular fold (*M-VIF*).
- The IF and interventricular septum (IVS) are perpendicular (*malalign*).
- The VSD is further extended anteriorly and located under both semilunar valves, but the majority of VSD is located primarily under the aortic valve (*doubly committed VSD*).
- This type is an indication of intraventricular rerouting from the left ventricle to the aorta through the VSD.

■ *Anatomically corrected malposition of the great arteries (ACMGA)*

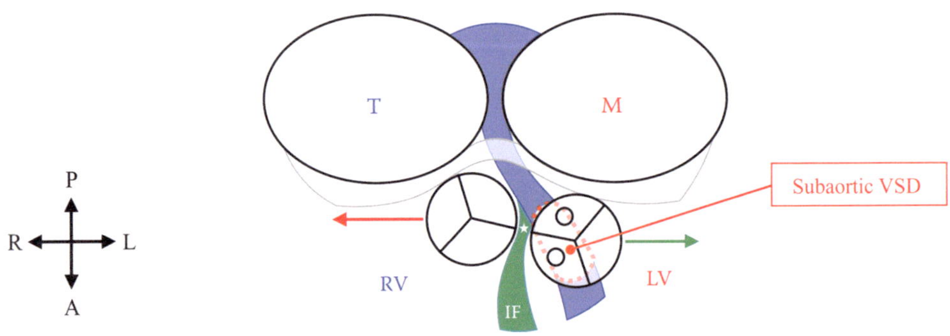

- The relationship of the great arteries is side-by-side, with the left aorta and the right pulmonary artery.
- Muscular tissue (ventriculo-infundibular fold: VIF) is interposed between the mitral and pulmonary valve annulus.
- The pulmonary artery further deviates to the right (*red arrow*) and overrides on the ventricular septum.
- The aorta moderately deviates to the left (*green arrow*) and overrides on the ventricular septum more than 50% of the aortic valve.
- As the aorta deviates to the left, the infundibular septum (IF) rotates further counterclockwise and the posterior margin of the IF (☆) attaches to the posterior limb of the TSM (posterior margin of the VSD).
- The IF and interventricular septum (IVS) are parallel (*align*).
- The VSD is further extended anteriorly and located under the aortic valve (*subaortic VSD*).
- This type is an indication of intraventricular rerouting from the left ventricle to the aorta through the VSD.

ESSENTIALS TGA Like Hemodynamics in NGA Type DORV

■ *posterior TGA (NGA typs DORV)*

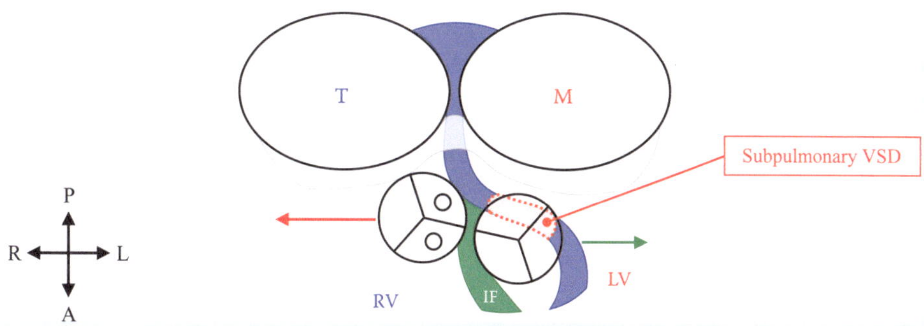

- The relationship of the great arteries is side-by-side with the right aorta and the left pulmonary artery.
- The pulmonary artery further deviates to the right (*red arrow*).
- The aorta moderately deviates to the left (*green arrow*) and overrides on the ventricular septum.
- As the pulmonary artery deviates to the left, the infundibular septum (IF) rotates further counterclockwise and the posterior margin of the IF (☆) attaches to the posterior limb of the TSM (posterior margin of the VSD).
- IF and interventricular septum (IVS) are parallel (*align*).
- The VSD is further extended anteriorly and located under the aortic valve (*subpulmonary VSD*).
- Posterior TGA is classified as NGA DORV but is indicated for arterial switch operation because of subpulmonary VSD and PA overriding the ventricular septum.

1.3 Anterior or Posterior Deviation of the Infundibular Septum (Ventricular Outflow Obstruction)

Another factor that causes variation in morphology is the deviation of the infundibular septum. An anterior or posterior deviation of the infundibular septum is associated with right ventricular outflow tract stenosis (aortic or subvalvular stenosis) or right ventricular outflow tract stenosis (pulmonary or subvalvular stenosis).

Arterial switch operation may be indicated in very mild cases or in cases of outflow tract dynamic stenosis. However, Rastelli or aortic translocation operation may be indicated in cases of moderate stenosis (Fig. 9.5).

1.4 Classification of TGA, Timing of the Operation and Operative Procedure

Patients are classified into the following types according to the presence or absence of ventricular septal defect (VSD) and pulmonary stenosis (PS). The presence of patent ductus arteriosus (PDA) or patent foramen ovale (PFO) is irrelevant for classification. Arterial switch operation (ASO) is indicated for type I, II, and mild PS. The optimal timing of definitive surgery depends on the type.

Type	*associated malformation*	*Timing of definitive operation*	*Operative procedure*
Type I	(PDA, PFO)	neonatal period (within 2 weeks after birth)	Arterial switch operation
Type II	VSD	early infantile period	Arterial switch operation
Type III	VSD, PS	early infantile period	Palliative operation (Blalock-Taussig shunt)
		early childhood	Rastelli operation Aortic translocation (Nikaidoh operation, Half-turned truncal switch operation)

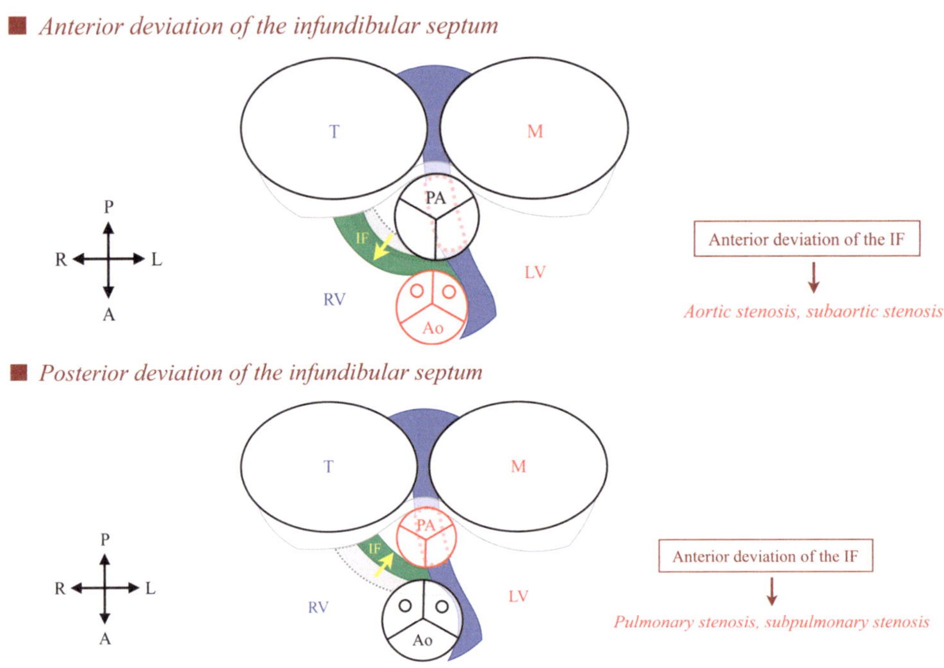

Fig. 9.5 Anterior or posterior deviation of the infundibular septum in false Taussig-Bing

1.5 Morphology of the Coronary Arteries

TGA and DORV show a variety of coronary artery morphology. The Leiden, Shaher, and Yacoub classifications of coronary artery morphology have been reported. The Leiden classification is based on the origin of the coronary arteries. The Shaher classification includes the origin, course, and branches of the coronary arteries.

The Shaher classification is useful for coronary artery transplantation because not only the origin of the coronary artery but also its course and bifurcation are important in ASO.

Shaher type 1 (Leiden; [1LCx: 2R]) is the most common type of coronary artery (approximately 60%). Shaher type 2 (Leiden [1 L: 2CxR]) is about 15%, and the other types are only a few percent of the total number of coronary arteries (Fig. 9.6).

- ***Normal Coronary Arteries.***
- LCA originates from sinus 1 (right hand sinus) and branches into the LAD and LCX.
- RCA originates from sinus 1 (right hand sinus).

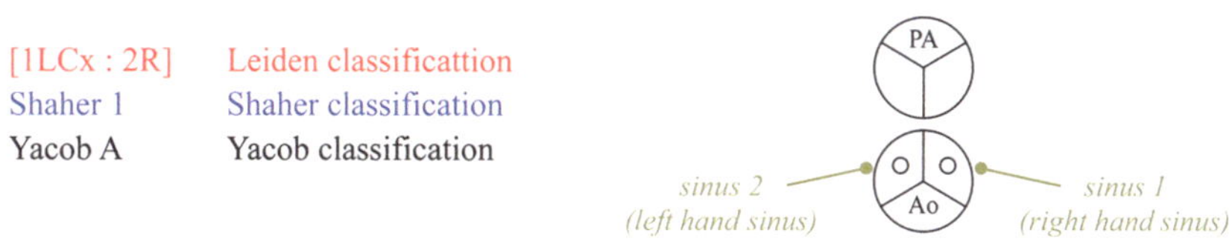

LCX : left coronary artery、LAD : left anterior descending branch 、LCX : left circumflex branch、RCA : right coronary artery

- ***LCA or LCX Running Posterior to the Pulmonary Artery.***
  The LCX or LCA may run posterior to the PA, either slightly away from or close to the PA valve annulus. When performing coronary artery reimplantation, care must be taken to avoid bending and overstretching of the coronary artery originating from sinus 2, as well as compression by the anteriorly shifted pulmonary artery bifurcation (Fig. 9.7).
- RCA and LCX originate from a single opening in sinus 2 (left hand sinus).
- LCX runs posterior to the pulmonary artery.

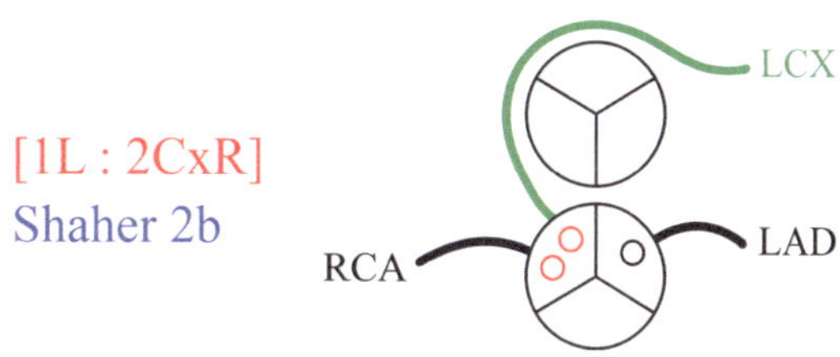

- RCA and LCX originate from separate openings in sinus 2 (left hand sinus).
- LCX runs posterior to the pulmonary artery.

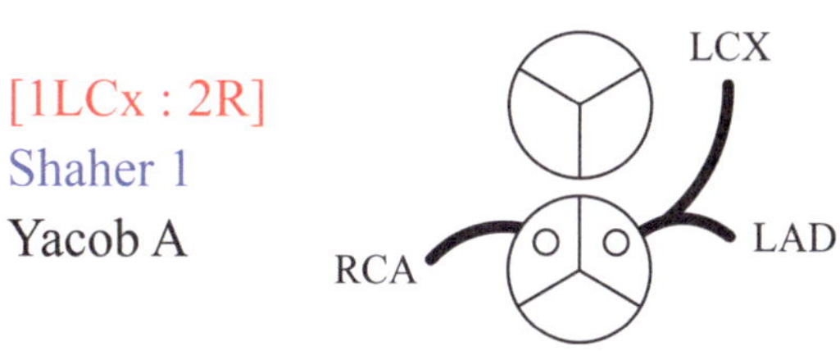

Fig. 9.6 Normal coronary pattern

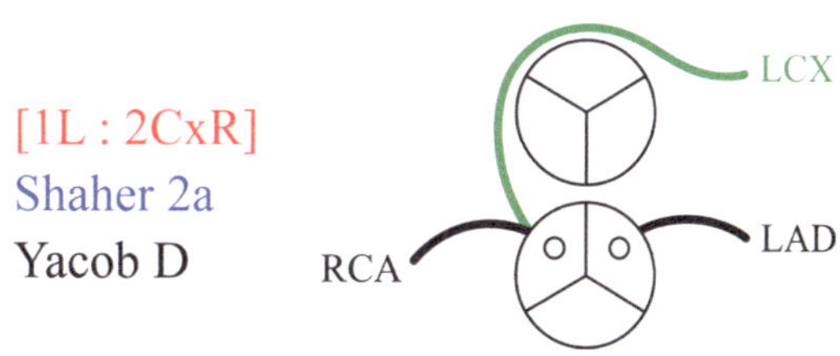

Fig. 9.7 LCA or LCX running posterior to the pulmonary artery, RCA or running anterior to the aorta

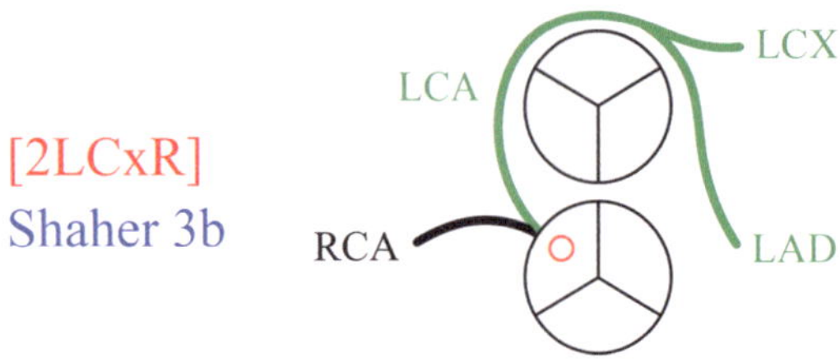

- RCA and LCA originate from a single opening in sinus 2 (left hand sinus).
- LCA runs posterior to the pulmonary artery and branches into the LAD and LCX.

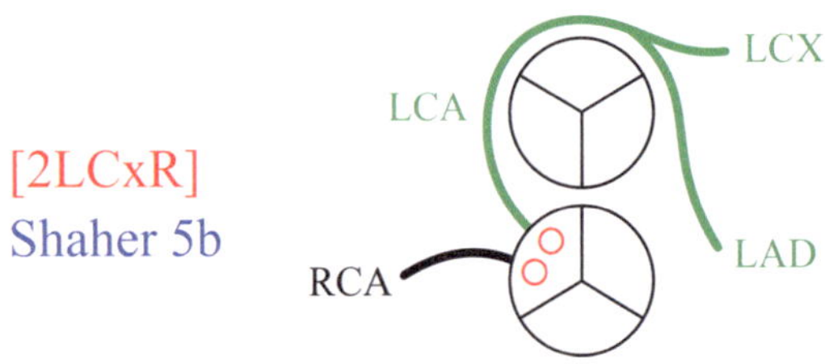

- RCA and LCA originate from separate openings in sinus 2 (left hand sinus).
- LCA runs posterior to the pulmonary artery and branches into the LAD and LCX.

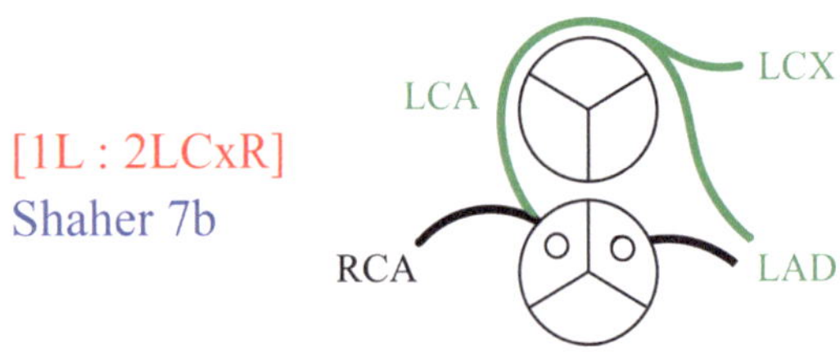

- RCA and LCA originate from a single opening in sinus 2 (left hand sinus).
- LCA runs posterior to the pulmonary artery and branches into the LAD and LCX.
- Another LAD originates from sinus 1 (right hand sinus): double LAD or accessory LAD.

< Precautions for Transplantation >

- Care should be taken to bend and overstretch each branch.
- Dissect the LCX or LCA far enough from the origin.
- The cuff including the LCA (LCX) and RCA is implanted slightly cephalad of the PA wall.

- ***LCA or LCX Running Posterior to the Pulmonary Artery, RCA or Running Anterior to the Aorta***

  The coronary artery pattern is that the LCX or LCA runs posterior to the PA and the RCA or LAD runs anterior to the Ao. Shaher types 4 and 9 are often associated with side-by-side relationships of the great arteries (Fig. 9.8).
- Common coronary pattern in DORV with side-by-side great arteries.
- RCA and LAD originate from a single opening in sinus 1 (right hand sinus).
- RCA runs anterior to the right ventricular outflow.
- LCX originates from sinus 2 (left hand sinus) and runs posterior to the pulmonary artery.

< Precautions for Transplantation >

- Care should be taken to bend and overstretch each branch.
- Dissect the LCX and RCA well above the origins.
- The LCX cuff is implanted slightly cephalad of the PA wall.
- When PA reconstruction is performed posterior to the Ao in parallel great vessel cases (original Jatene method), the compression of the LCX by the left PA should be kept in mind.

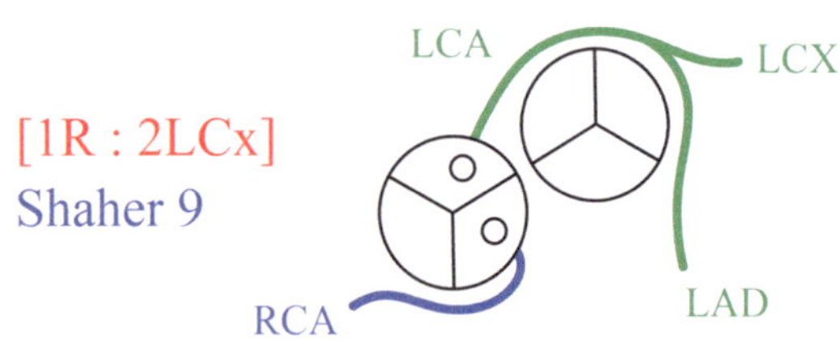

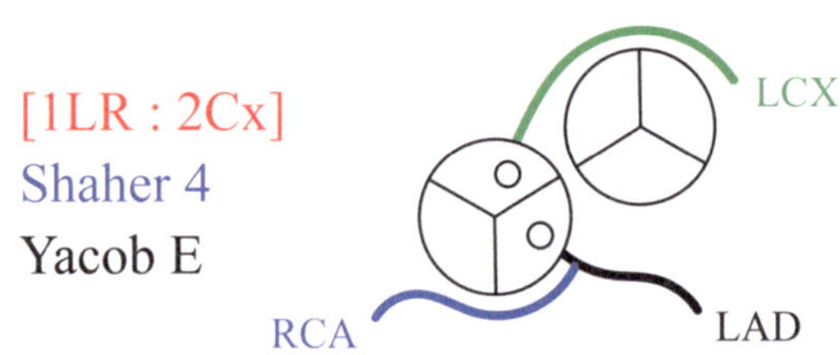

Fig. 9.8 LCA or LCX running posterior to the pulmonary artery, RCA or running anterior to the aorta

- Common coronary pattern in DORV with side-by-side great arteries.
- LCA originates from sinus 2 (left hand sinus).
- LCA runs posterior to the pulmonary artery and branches into the LAD and LCX.
- RCA originates from a single opening in sinus 1 (right hand sinus) and runs anterior to the right ventricular outflow.

< Precautions for Transplantation >

- Care should be taken to bend and over-stretch each branch.
- Dissect the LCA and RCA well above the origins.
- The LCX cuff is implanted slightly cephalad of the PA wall.
- When PA reconstruction is performed posterior to the Ao in parallel great vessel cases (original Jatene method), the compression of the LCA by the left PA should be kept in mind.

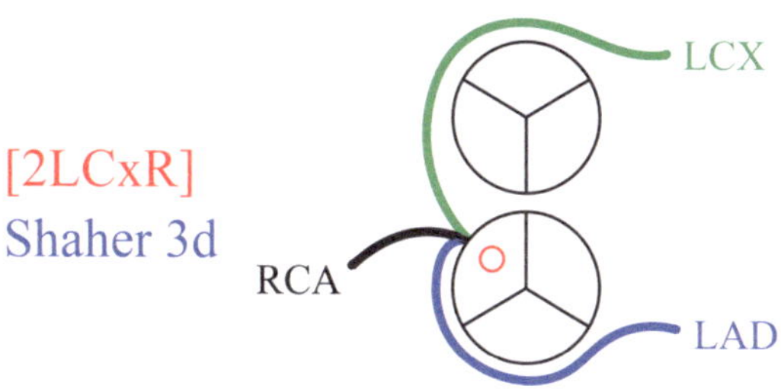

- Single coronary artery.
- All coronary arteries originate from a single opening in sinus 2 (left hand sinus).
- LCX runs posterior to the pulmonary artery.
- LAD runs anterior to the right ventricular outflow.

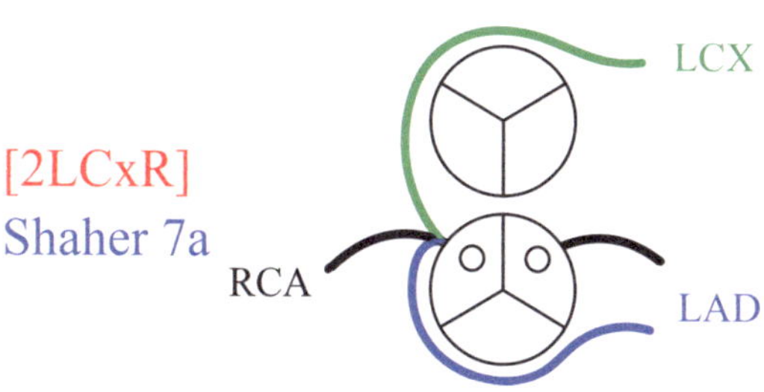

- LAD, RCA, and LCX originate from a single opening in sinus 2 (left hand sinus).
- Another LAD originates from sinus 1 (right hand sinus): double LAD or accessory LAD.
- LCX runs posterior to the pulmonary artery.
- LAD runs anterior to the right ventricular outflow.

< Precautions for Transplantation >

- Care should be taken to bend and over-stretch each branch.
- Dissect the LAD, RCA, and LCX well above the origin.
- The cuff is implanted slightly cephalad of the PA wall.

- ***RCA or LCA Running Anterior to the Aorta (Right Ventricular Outflow Tract).***
  The coronary artery pattern is that the RCA or LCA runs anterior to the right ventricular outflow. All coronary arteries originate from a single opening (Fig. 9.9).

- Single coronary artery.
- All coronary arteries originate from a single opening in sinus 1 (right hand sinus).
- RCA runs anterior to the right ventricular outflow.

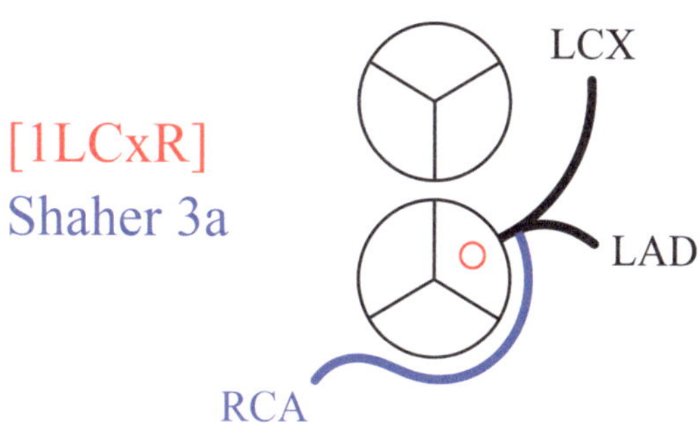

Fig. 9.9 RCA or LCA running anterior to the aorta (right ventricular outflow tract)

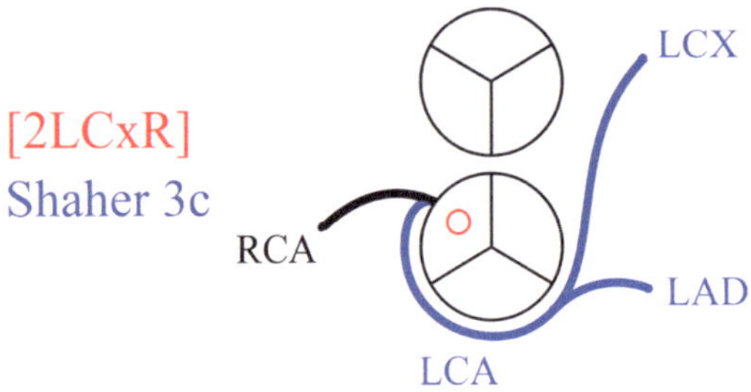

- Single coronary artery.
- All coronary arteries originate from a single opening in sinus 2 (left hand sinus).
- LCA runs anterior to the right ventricular outflow and branches into the LAD and LCX.

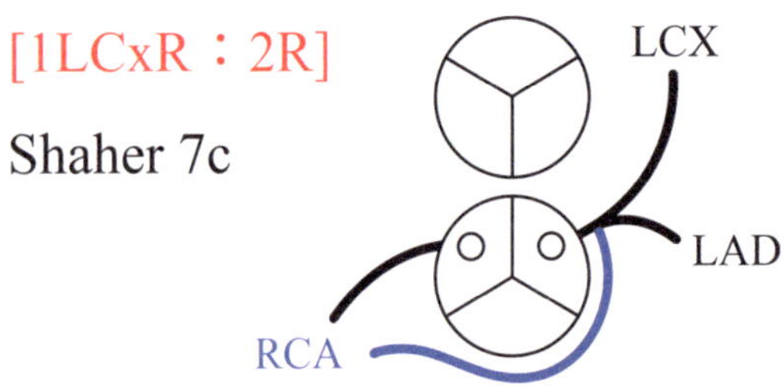

- All coronary arteries originate from a single opening in sinus 1 (right hand sinus).
- RCA runs anterior to the right ventricular outflow.
- Another RCA originates from sinus 2 (left hand sinus): double RCA or accessory RCA.

< Precautions for Transplantation >

- Care should be taken to bend and overstretch each branch.
- Dissect the RCA or LCA running anterior to the right ventricular outflow well above the origin.

- ***LCA or LAD Running Between Both Great Arteries.***
  The coronary artery pattern is that the RCA or LCA runs anterior to the right ventricular outflow. All coronary arteries originate from a single opening (Fig. 9.10).

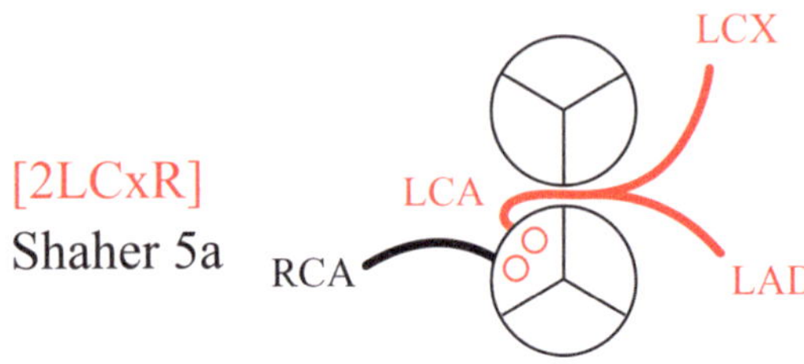

Fig. 9.10 LCA or LAD running between both great arteries

- RCA and LCA originate from separate openings in sinus 2 (left hand sinus).
- LCA runs between both great arteries and branches into the LAD and LCX.
- LCA may take an intramural course of the aorta at its origin.

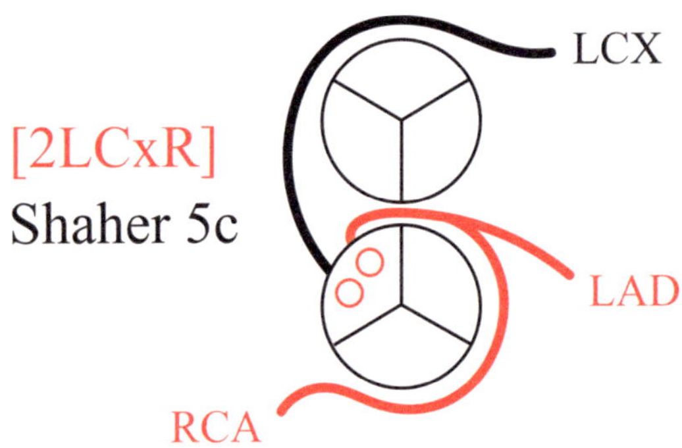

- LCX and LCA originate from separate openings in sinus 2 (left hand sinus).
- LCA runs between both great arteries and branches into the LAD and RCA.
- LCA may take an intramural course of the aorta at its origin.
- RCA runs anterior to the right ventricular outflow.

< Precautions for Transplantation >.

- Conventional grafting techniques are difficult.
- Consider a divided coronary cuff technique (Mee method) or a tunneling technique (Aubert method, Imai method, etc.).

2 Arterial Switch Operation

2.1 Horizontal Positioning of the Great Artery Origins and Coronary Artery Implantation Sites

In coronary artery transplantation, the most important point is to determine the coronary artery cuff implantation site (the center point of the coronary artery orifice) to avoid bending and overstretching of the coronary artery to be transposed to the base of the pulmonary artery. To avoid deformation of the pulmonary sinus of Valsalva, the coronary cuff should be implanted above the sinotubular junction.

In cases with an anterior-posterior relationship of the great arteries, the aortic annulus is positioned higher than the pulmonary annulus due to the presence of the subaortic conus. Therefore, it is easy to implant the valve above the sinotubular junction.

In cases where the relationship of the great arteries is parallel, the aortic and pulmonary annuli are at the same height. Therefore, the implantation site may need to be in the sinus of Valsalva, below the sinotubular junction (Fig. 9.11).

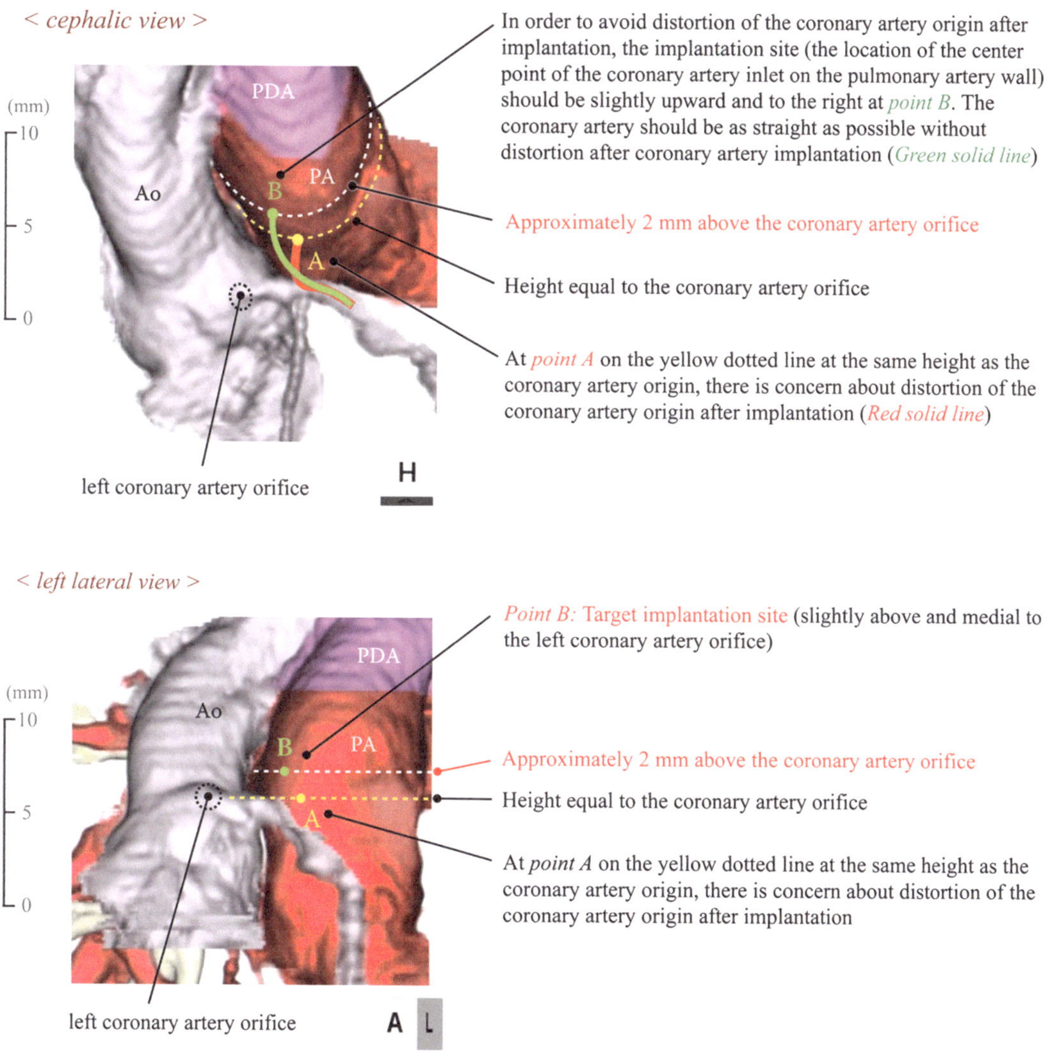

Fig. 9.11 Determination of coronary artery implantation site

2.2 Pulmonary Artery Division Site

When determining the pulmonary artery incision line, it is important to determine (1) the expected coronary artery implantation site (midpoint), (2) the beginning of the ductus arteriosus, (3) the openings of the left and right pulmonary arteries, and (4) the aortic incision line.

In the punch-out and trap-door methods, it is necessary to leave enough length at the base of the pulmonary artery for coronary artery cuff implantation. In contrast, the bay-window method requires only a few millimeters higher than the center point of the graft (lower than the punch-out and trap-door methods).

It is important to keep the residual pulmonary artery as short as possible, since leaving vulnerable pulmonary artery tissue at the base of the new aorta for a long periods of time may cause the aortic root to widen at a later stage (Fig. 9.12).

- *Case 1: d-TGA(I).*
  Antero-posterior relationship of the great arteries.
  Coronary artery pattern: [1LCx: 2R], Shaher type 1.
- In the punch-out method, the pulmonary artery is divided approximately 3 mm headword from the cuff anastomotic opening.
- In the trap-door method, the pulmonary artery is divided at a sufficient distance from the center point of the coronary artery implantation (+) (almost the same line as in the punch-out method) because the trap-door channel may narrow if the distance from the coronary artery orifice to the upper end of the cuff is not kept long enough.

< anterior view >

Pulmonary artery dividing line for punch-out and trap-door methods (yellow line)

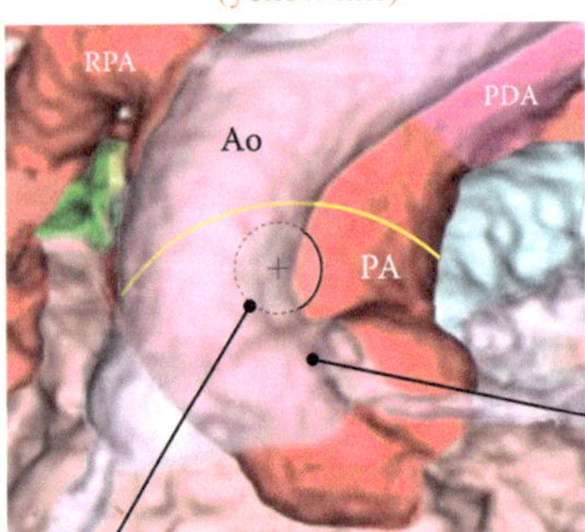

left coronary orifice

Pulmonary artery wall opening in the punch-out method

+ *the center point of the coronary artery implantation*

Pulmonary artery dividing line for bay-window method (blue line)

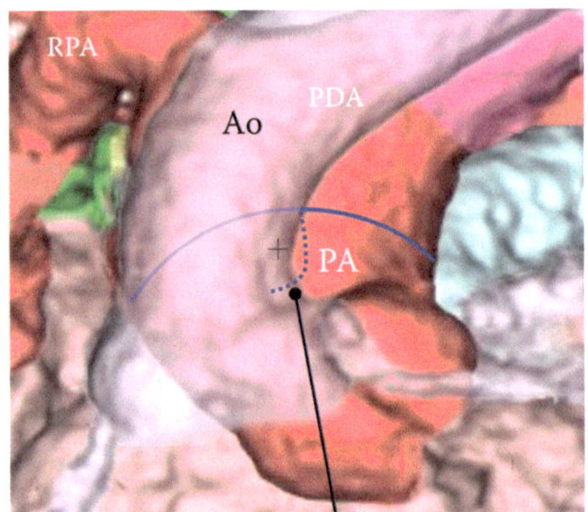

J-shaped incision line of the pulmonary artery wall

+ *the center point of the coronary artery implantation*

Fig. 9.12 Determination of pulmonary artery division site

- The dividing line should be approximately 3 mm headward from the center point of the coronary artery implantation (+).
- Lower than the punch-out method.
- Because the upper end of the cuff covers the bay-window channel, there is no risk of coronary artery orifice stenosis even if the length of the base is short.

< left lateral view >

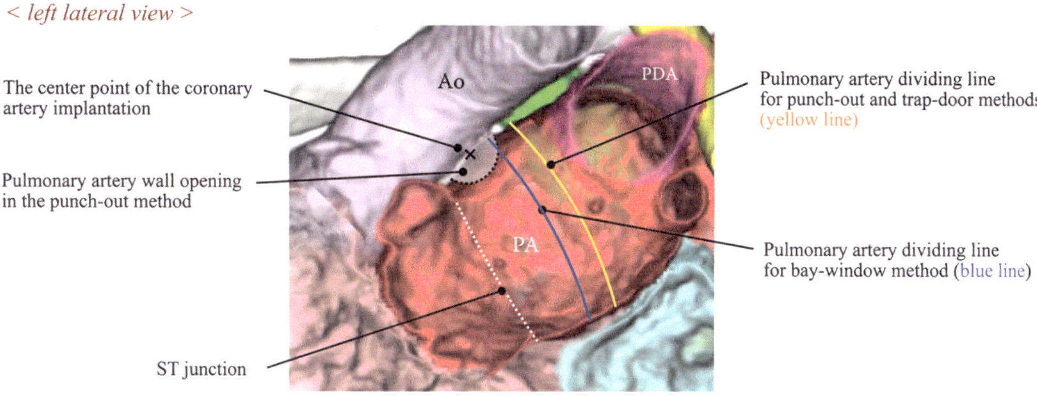

- ***Case 2: d-TGA(II).***

  Side-by-side relationship of the great arteries.

  Coronary artery pattern: [1 L: 2LCxR], Shaher type 7b.

Because both semilunar valves are at the same height in parallel great arteries, the center point of coronary artery implantation is close to the ST junction. The right pulmonary artery bifurcates just above the ST junction, so the base of the pulmonary artery cannot remain long.

In this case, the left coronary artery (LCA) runs behind the pulmonary artery in Shaher 7b, and it is necessary to place the LCA in the higher pulmonary artery wall to avoid distortion of the wall during implantation. The bay-window technique is useful in cases such as the present case where the remaining pulmonary artery wall is limited.

< anterior view >

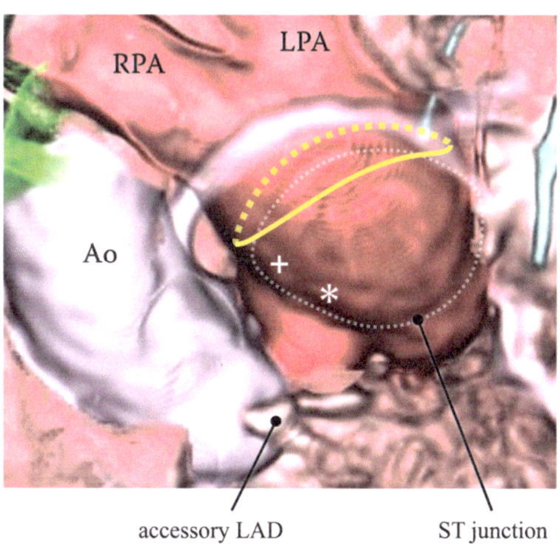

\+ *the center point of the coronary artery implantation*

< right lateral view >

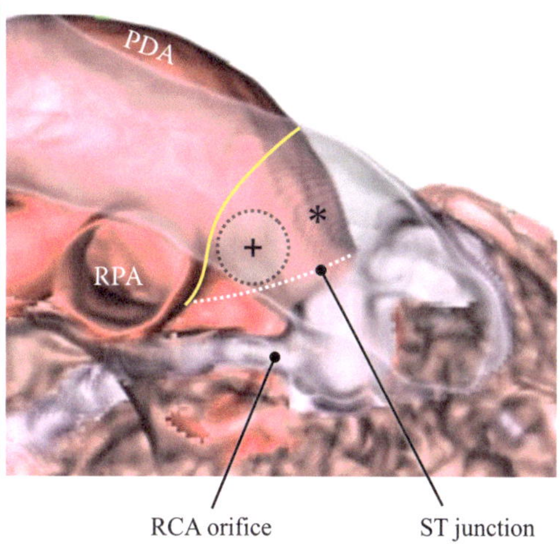

* *the center point of the accessory LAD implantation*

Pulmonary Artery Dividing Line for Punch-Out and Trap-Door Methods (Yellow Line)

- The transection line must be elevated to secure the cuff opening, but the right pulmonary artery origin is low, so the transection line is limited.
- The coronary artery implantation center (+) cannot be elevated to avoid coronary artery compression by the left pulmonary artery after reconstruction using the original Jatene method.

Pulmonary Artery Dividing Line for Bay-Window Method (Blue Line)

- The distance between the transection line and the center point of coronary artery implantation (+) should be approximately 3 mm.
- The coronary artery implantation center point (+) cannot be elevated too high to avoid coronary artery compression by the left pulmonary artery after reconstruction using the original Jatene method.

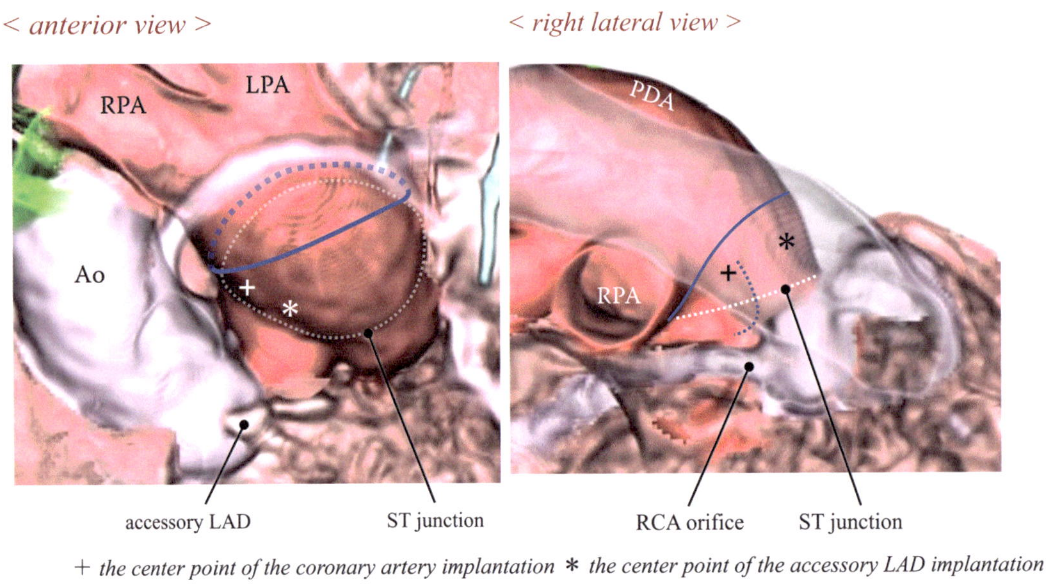

2.3 Coronary Artery Implantation Procedure (1) Punch-Out Method

It is the most common method of coronary artery implantation. It is applicable to common coronary artery morphologies such as Shaher type 1 (Fig. 9.13).

1

- The anterior wall of the pulmonary artery should be transected at a site far enough away from the target site for implantation (×).
- The implantation site should be slightly above and inside the pulmonary artery wall corresponding to the origin of the coronary artery.

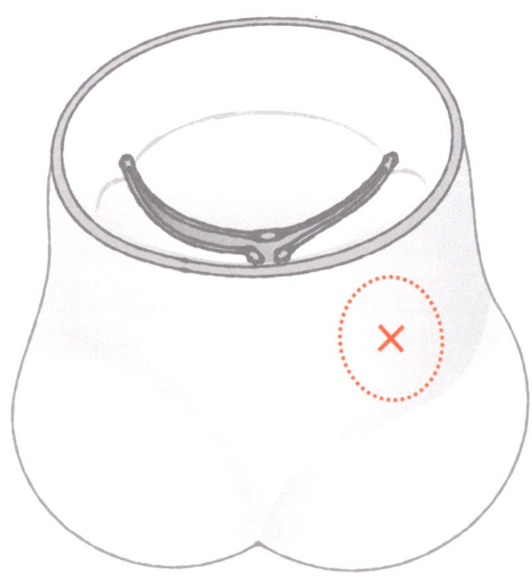

Fig. 9.13 Punch-out method

2

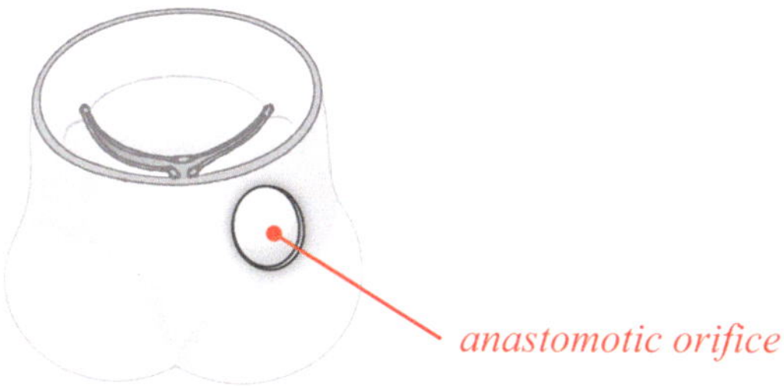

- Create an anastomotic orifice centered on the implantation target point.
- Use a coronary puncher and scissors.
- Be careful not to damage the pulmonary valve leaflets and commissures.

3

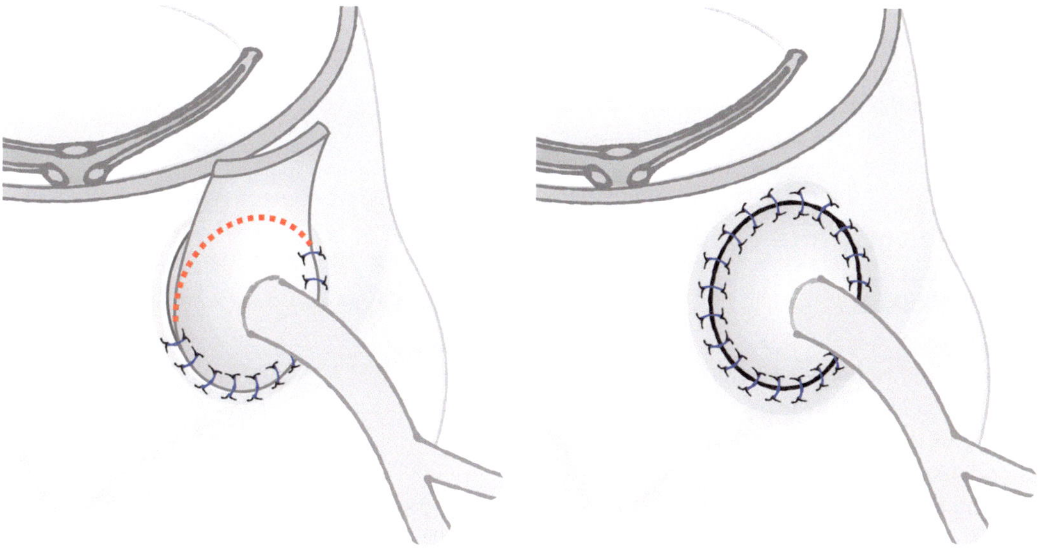

- The coronary cuff is harvested in a U-shape. The cuff is not harvested in a circular shape from the beginning.
- When the anastomosis of the lower half is completed, the upper half is trimmed to a circular shape (*red dashed line*).

4

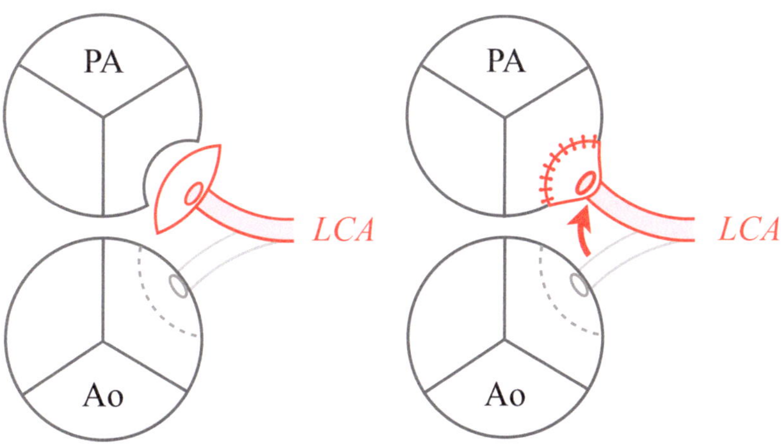

- Because the angle of the coronary cuff changes significantly with the punch-out technique, perform adequate dissection of the coronary origin.
- Open the pulmonary artery wall anastomosis opening so that it is slightly smaller than the coronary cuff. Anastomose the cuff by stretching the wall of the pulmonary artery opening sufficiently.
- Stretch the pulmonary artery wall at the opening sufficiently so that the anastomotic pitch on the cuff side (suture step width) is larger than the anastomotic pitch at the pulmonary artery orifice.
- The cuff is slightly extended funnel-shaped to allow room at the beginning of the coronary artery.

2.4 Coronary Artery Implantation Procedure (2): Trap-Door Method

The trap-door technique developed by Mee is an excellent technique that maintains the angle of the cuff of the resected coronary artery as much as possible and avoids bending the base of the coronary artery after implantation (Figs. 9.14 and 9.15).

- In conventional punch-out method, the cuff angle changes significantly after implantation (*angle a*), whereas in the trap-door method, the change in cuff angle after implantation is small (*angle b*).
- This reduces the risk of coronary artery bending after implantation.

1

- First, using the coronary artery orifice implantation center point as a guide, determine the position where the left edge of the cuff corresponds to the proximal stump of the pulmonary artery (point (a)).
- In order to get the trap-door to open well, keep in mind that point (a) should not be too far to the outside.
- From point (a), make a longitudinal incision through the wall of the pulmonary artery.

2

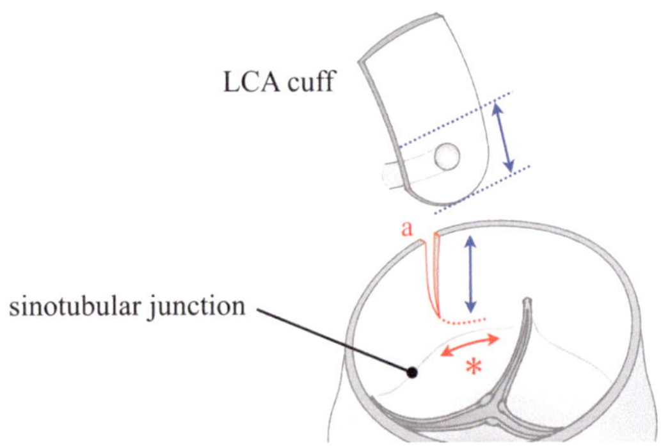

- The depth of the J-shaped incision should be approximately 2–3 mm beyond the coronary artery orifice (it is not necessary to go too deep).
- As a general rule, do not cut into the sinus of Valsalva beyond the sinotubular junction.
- Be careful that the incision should not damage the commissure.
- The length of the base of the J-shaped incision (*) should be approximately 75% of the width of the cuff (not too long).

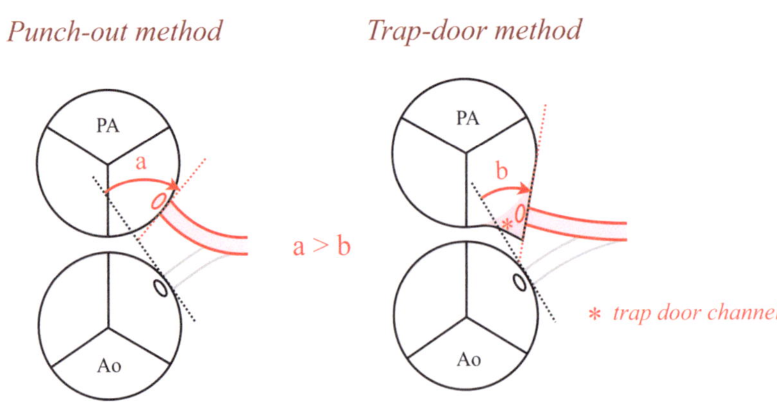

Fig. 9.14 Advantage of the trap-door method

3

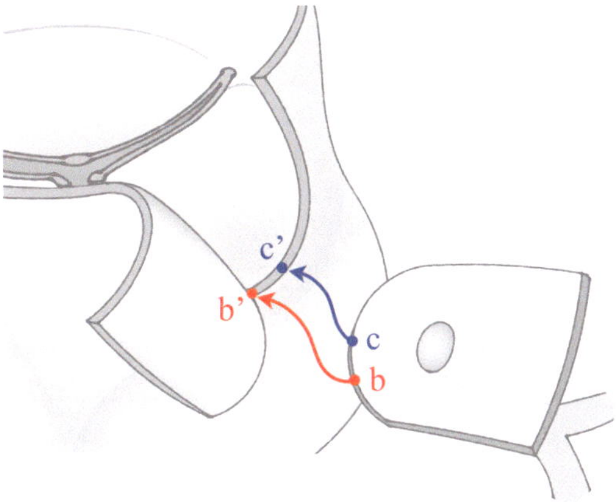

- Be careful not to twist the cuff in the short-axis direction.
- The midpoint between the center of the lower end of the cuff and the right lateral edge (point (b)) is positioned at the tip of the J-shaped incision (point (b′)).

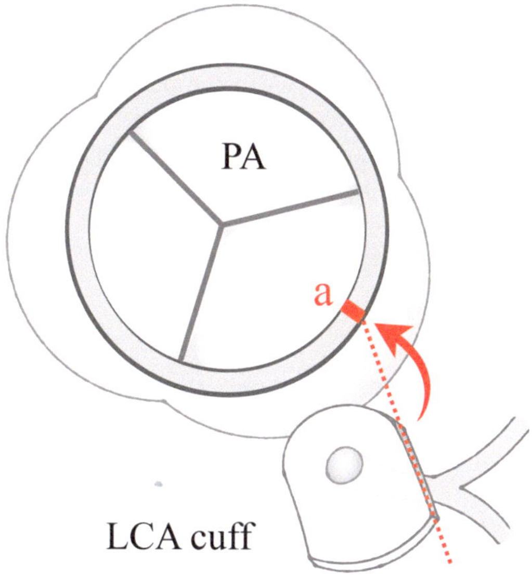

Fig. 9.15 Procedure of the trap-door method

- The center of the lower end of the cuff (point (c)) is positioned at the center of the lower end of the coronary artery orifice (point (c′)).

4

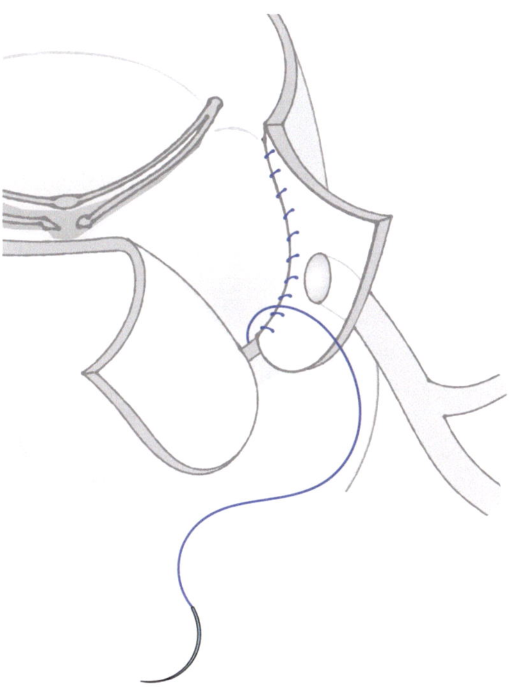

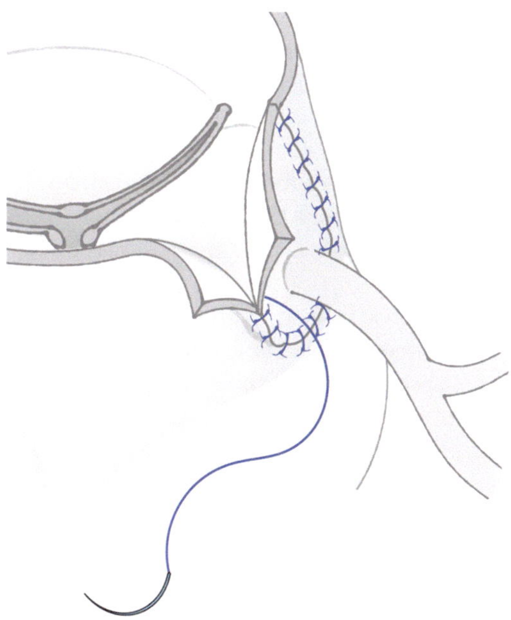

- Anastomose the cuff from the contralateral side of the trap door to the upper edge of the coronary artery opening the using a 7–0 or 8–0 monofilament suture.
- The anastomosis should not protrude into the lumen as much as possible.
- Anastomose the coronary cuff to the upper end of the trap-door.

5

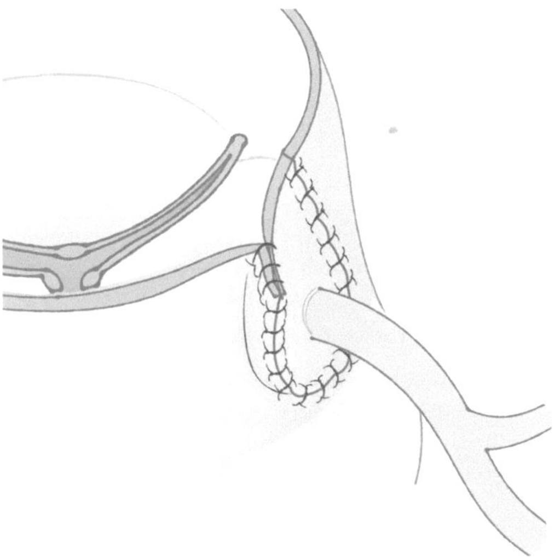

- Anastomose the top of the coronary cuff to the top of the trap-door.

2.5 Coronary Artery Implantation Procedure (3): Bay-Window Method

The trap-door method is an effective coronary implantation method, but it still has the problem of collapsing the upper end of the cuff. The purpose of the bay-window method is to secure a wider coronary channel by improving the anastomosis method of the upper end of the coronary cuff anastomosis.

The bay-window method involves a J-shaped incision in the pulmonary artery wall similar to the trap-door method, but with an improved anastomosis in the upper part of the cuff (Figs. 9.16, 9.17, and 9.18).

- The lower part of the trap-door channel is wide and functioning as it should.
- The advantage of a smaller deflection angle of the coronary cuff is lost because the upper edge of the trapdoor is directly anastomosed.
- The upper part of the trap-door channel may be narrowed and coronary blood flow may be reduced because the cuff and trap door are sewn together.
- The trap-door technique slightly widens the diameter of the base of the pulmonary artery, resulting in a larger diameter difference with the ascending aorta.
- The concept of the bay-window method is to use the upper edge of the cuff to form a ceiling over the implantation site, in addition to the advantages of the trap-door method of reducing the deflection angle of the coronary cuff.
- The cuff deflection angle can be maintained at a small angle and a wide bay-window channel is secured.
- Good coronary blood flow can be expected due to the generation of vortex flow in the wide bay-window channel.
- The difference in caliber between the pulmonary artery and the ascending aorta will not be large because the caliber at the base of the pulmonary artery will not be large.
- The aorta is transected slightly higher because the bay-window technique requires harvesting a longer upper portion of the coronary artery cuff.
- The transection line should be approximately 7 to 8 mm cephalad from the superior edge of the right coronary artery origin.
- A U-shaped suture for cardioplegia is placed on the transection line.

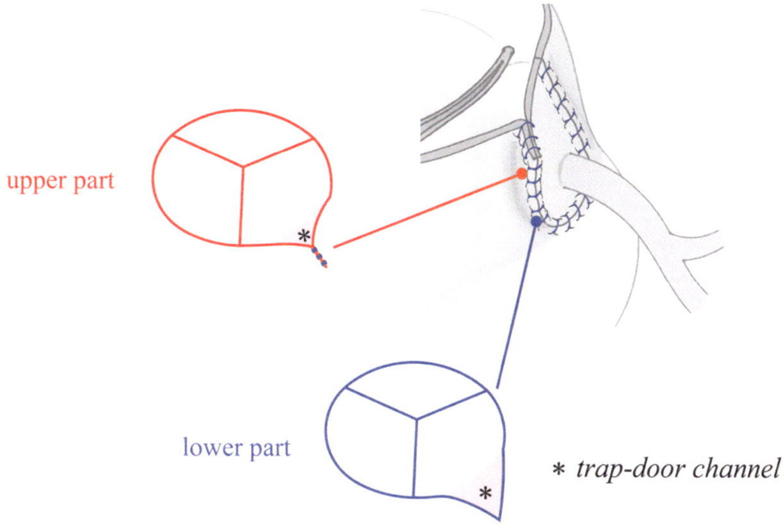

Fig. 9.16 Problem of trap-door method

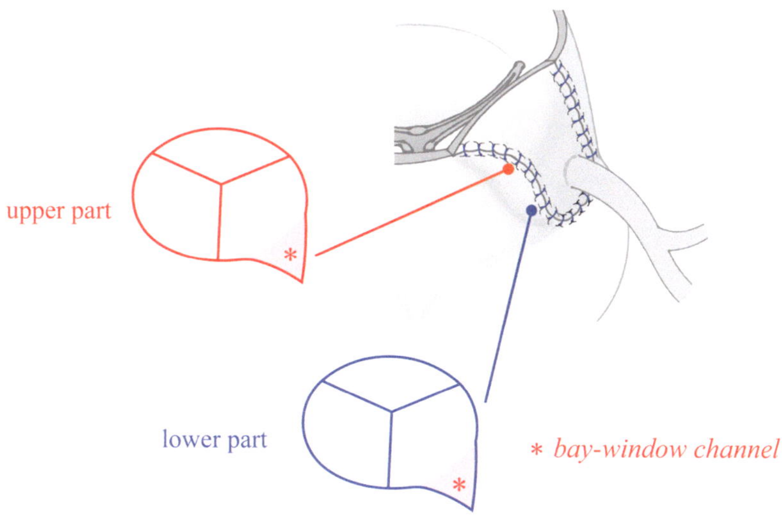

Fig. 9.17 Concept of bay-window method

1 *Transection line of the aorta*

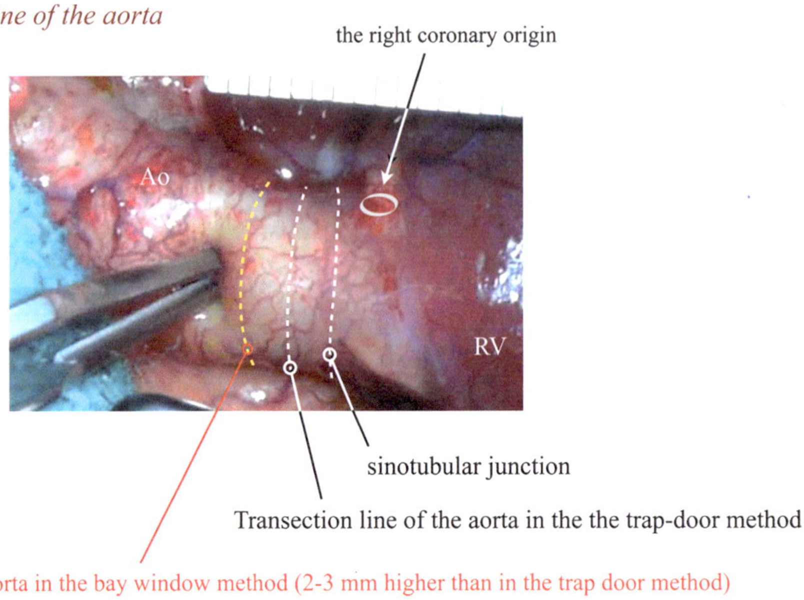

Fig. 9.18 Procedure of bay-window method

2 *Harvest of the coronary cuffs*

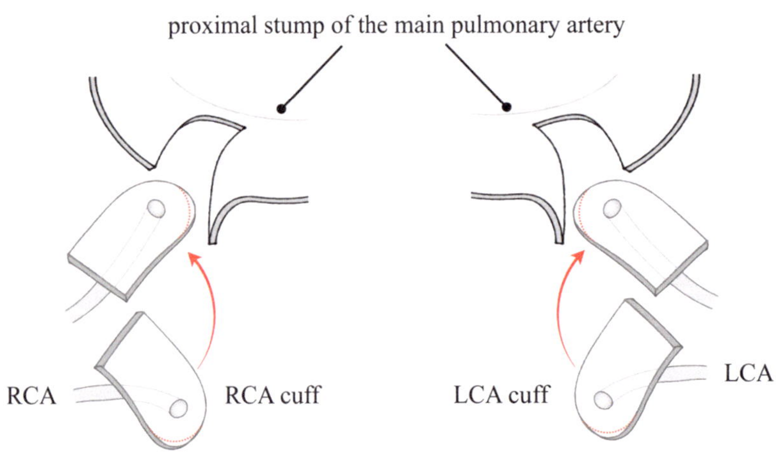

- If possible, the left and right cuffs should be cut with a slightly convex medial side (*red dashed line*) instead of a symmetrical base, since the medial side of the lower edge corresponds to the lower edge of the trap door during the coronary cuff resection.
- In practice, this cuff design may be difficult to achieve because of its proximity to the attachment site of the valve leaflet.
- The resection line of the cuff should be far enough away from the coronary artery orifice.
- If the coronary artery orifice is close to the pulmonary valve commissure, the commissure should be removed from the wall and reconstructed by suturing the commissure to the autologous pericardium that has been repaired to compensate for the coronary defect.

3 *J-shaped incision at the proximal stump of the pulmonary artery*

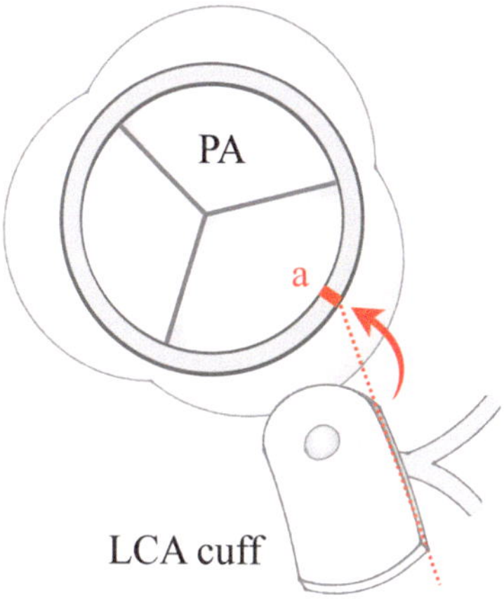

- First, using the coronary artery orifice implantation center point as a guide, determine the position where the left edge of the cuff corresponds to the proximal stump of the pulmonary artery (point (a)).
- In order to get the trap-door to open well, keep in mind that point (a) should not be too far to the outside.
- From point (a), make a longitudinal incision through the wall of the pulmonary artery.

4

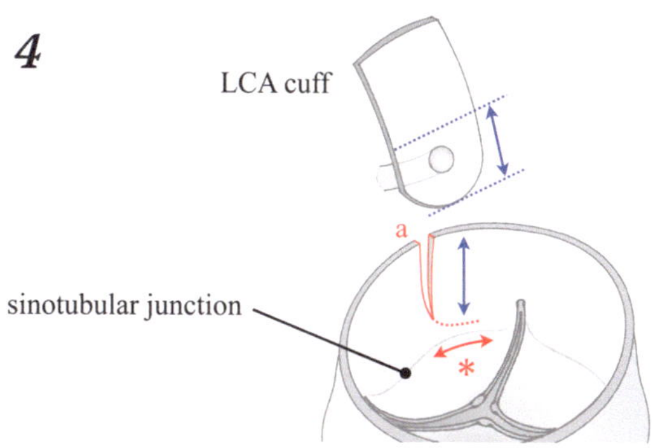

- The depth of the J-shaped incision should be approximately 2 or 3 mm beyond the coronary artery orifice (it is not necessary to go too deep).
- As a general rule, do not cut into the sinus of Valsalva beyond the sinotubular junction.
- The length of the base of the J-shaped incision (*) should be approximately 75% of the width of the cuff (not too long).

5

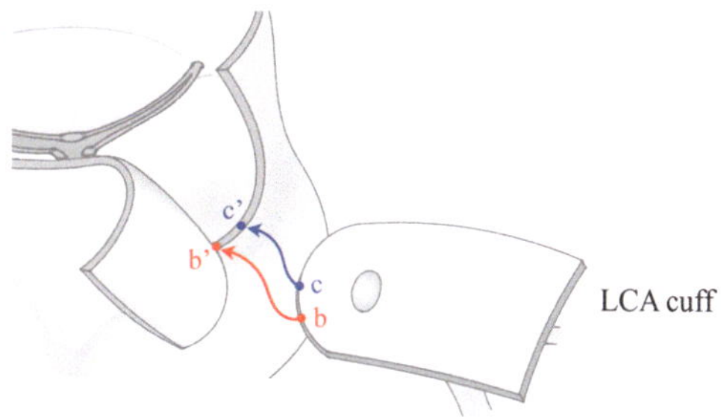

- Be careful not to twist the cuff in the short-axis direction.
- The midpoint between the center of the lower end of the cuff and the right lateral edge (point (b)) is positioned at the tip of the J-shaped incision (point (b′)).
- The center of the lower end of the cuff (point (c)) is positioned at the center of the lower end of the coronary artery orifice (point (c′)).

6

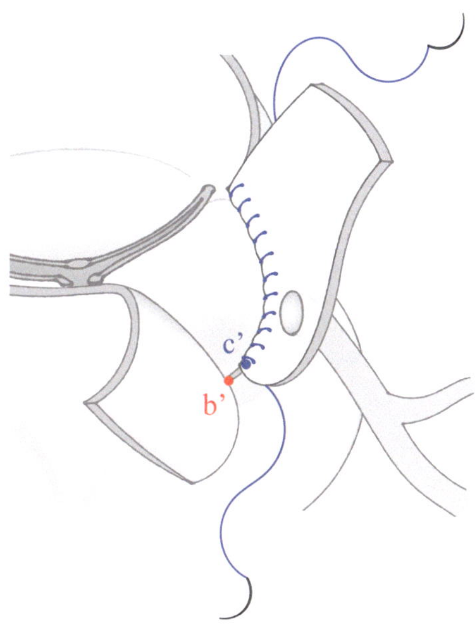

- Anastomose from the contralateral side of the trap door using a 7–0 or 8–0 monofilament suture.
- The anastomosis should not protrude into the lumen as much as possible.

7

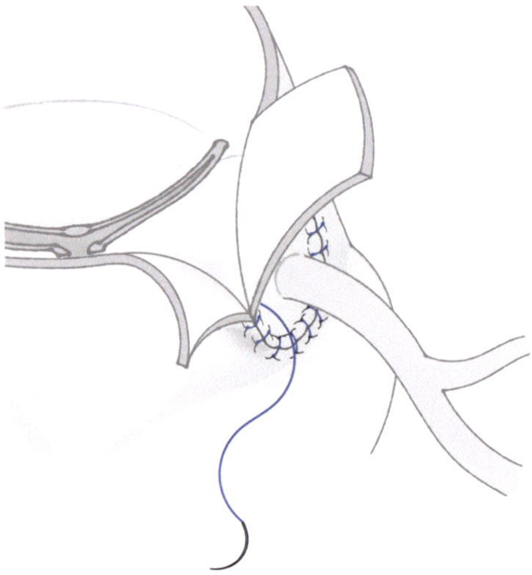

- Anastomose the trap door side of the cuff to a level just above the upper edge of the coronary artery opening.

8

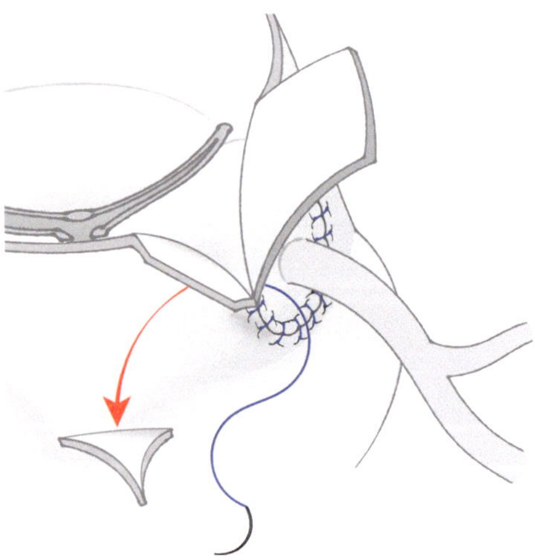

- Cut the top corner of the trap-door obliquely to smooth the shape of the bay-window channel.

9

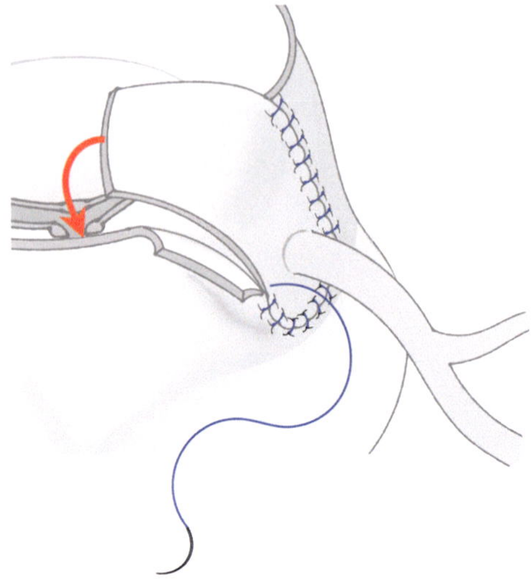

- The roof of the bay-window channel is covered with the upper part of the coronary cuff.

10

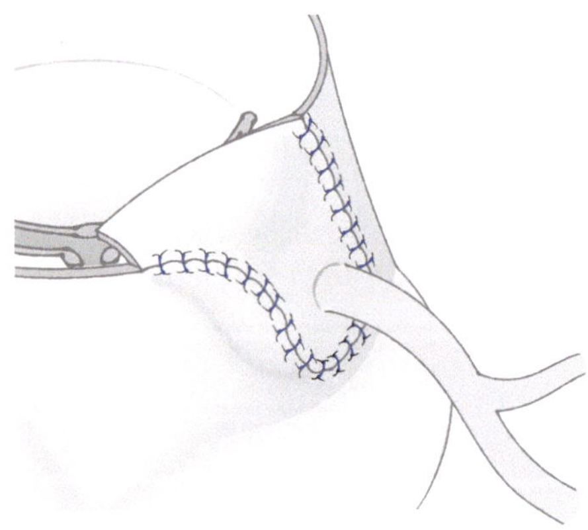

- Anastomose the upper part of the covered cuff to the trap door.

11

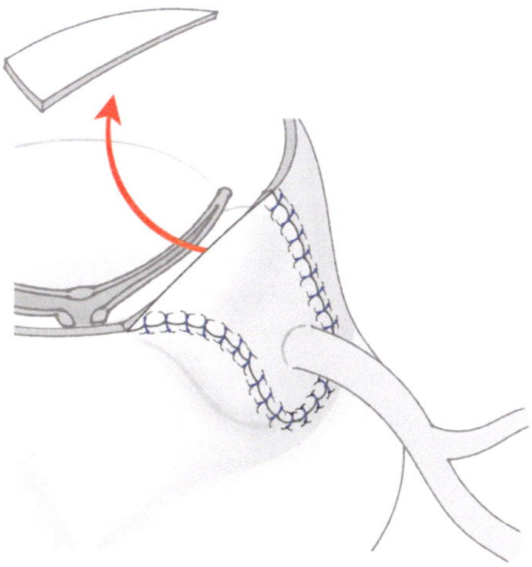

- Trim the excess of the upper cuff over the base of the pulmonary artery.

12

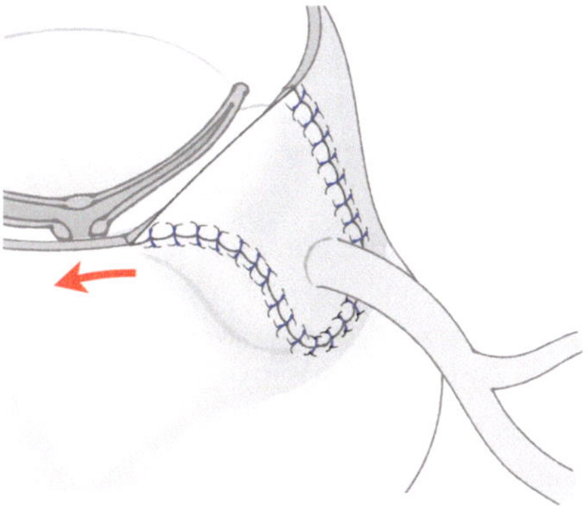

- Longer suture of the upper part of the cuff to the pulmonary artery opening can reduce the caliber of the proximal end of the pulmonary artery (new aorta).

13

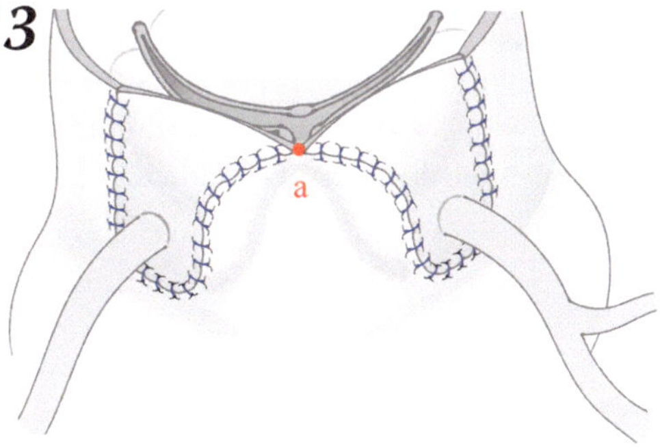

- Because the implantation centers of the left and right coronary cuffs are slightly closer to each other, the left and right bay-window channels are close together.
- In many cases, the upper edges of the left and right coronary cuffs almost touch (point (a)).

14

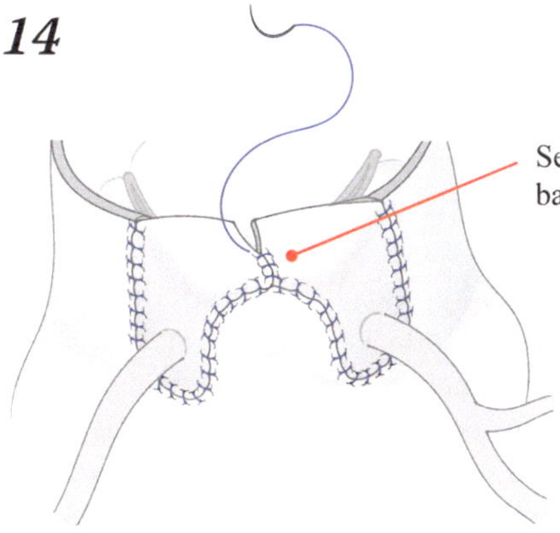

- If the two cuffs are even closer together, the top cuff will not be trimmed.
- The upper edges of the left and right coronary cuffs are sewn directly together.
- This will unite the left and right bay-window channels.
- By sewing the upper ends of the cuff together, the proximal end can be reduced in diameter to match the diameter of the ascending aorta.

15

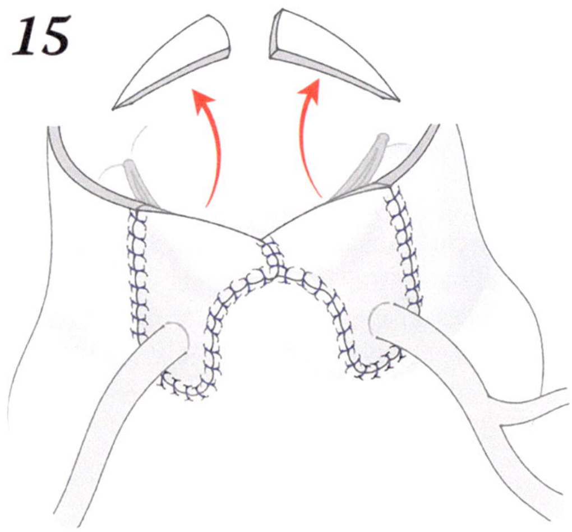

- The trimming of the upper edge of the cuff is done after the anastomosis has been completed.

ESSENTIALS The Important Point of the Coronary Implantation

- The most important point of arterial switch operation is the coronary artery implantation. Determination of the graft site (central point) is most important.
- The appropriate technique should be selected according to the morphology of the coronary artery to avoid bending, overstretching, or twisting of the coronary artery.
- To prevent turbulence at the anastomosis, it is essential to suture with fine sutures (7–0 or 8–0) so that the anastomosis is turned outward as much as possible.
- Uniform and fine anastomosis is recommended to avoid bleeding from the suture and deformation of the cuff.
- Since vortex flow in the sinus promotes coronary blood flow, it is recommended to create an appropriate bulging sinus at the origin of the coronary artery.
- However, if the difference in diameter between the sinus and the entrance of the coronary artery is too large, intimal thickening and stenosis may occur due to turbulent flow. Therefore, the creation of an excessively large sinus should be avoided.

2.6 Relationship of the Great Arteries and Pulmonary Artery Reconstruction Procedure

The great arteries are found to have various relationships from anterior-posterior to parallel in d-TGA(II) and false Taussig-Bing, depending on the case. In {SDL}DORV and posterior TGA, the angles of the great arteries are parallel, but the angles of the great arteries vary from case to case. In ASO, it is necessary to avoid overstretching or stenosis of the left and right pulmonary arteries when reconstructing the great arteries.

Considering the relationship of the great arteries, it is necessary to distinguish between (1) the original Jatene method, in which the pulmonary artery is reconstructed posterior to the neo aorta, and (2) the Lecompte's maneuver, in which the pulmonary artery branch is posteriorly translocated to the neo aorta and the pulmonary artery is reconstructed anterior to the neo aorta.

In cases of d-TGA (II) and false Taussig-Bing, where the great arteries are anterior-posterior or the pulmonary artery is slightly posterior to the left, the Lecompte's maneuver is indicated to reconstruct the pulmonary artery by posterior translocation of the pulmonary bifurcation to the anterior part of the neo aorta. In cases with anterior-posterior great arteries, there is an infundibulum under the aortic valve, and the aortic valve is positioned higher than the pulmonary valve. Therefore, the reconstructed new pulmonary artery is higher than the coronary artery implantation site, and there is little concern that the pulmonary artery bifurcation will compress the coronary artery.

In cases where the great arteries are nearly parallel, the Jatene's original method, in which the pulmonary artery is reconstructed posterior to the new great arteries, is indicated. Since both semilunar valves are of equal height in cases of parallel great arteries, it is necessary to keep in mind that the pulmonary artery reconstructed posteriorly or anteriorly may put pressure on the coronary artery implantation site (Fig. 9.19).

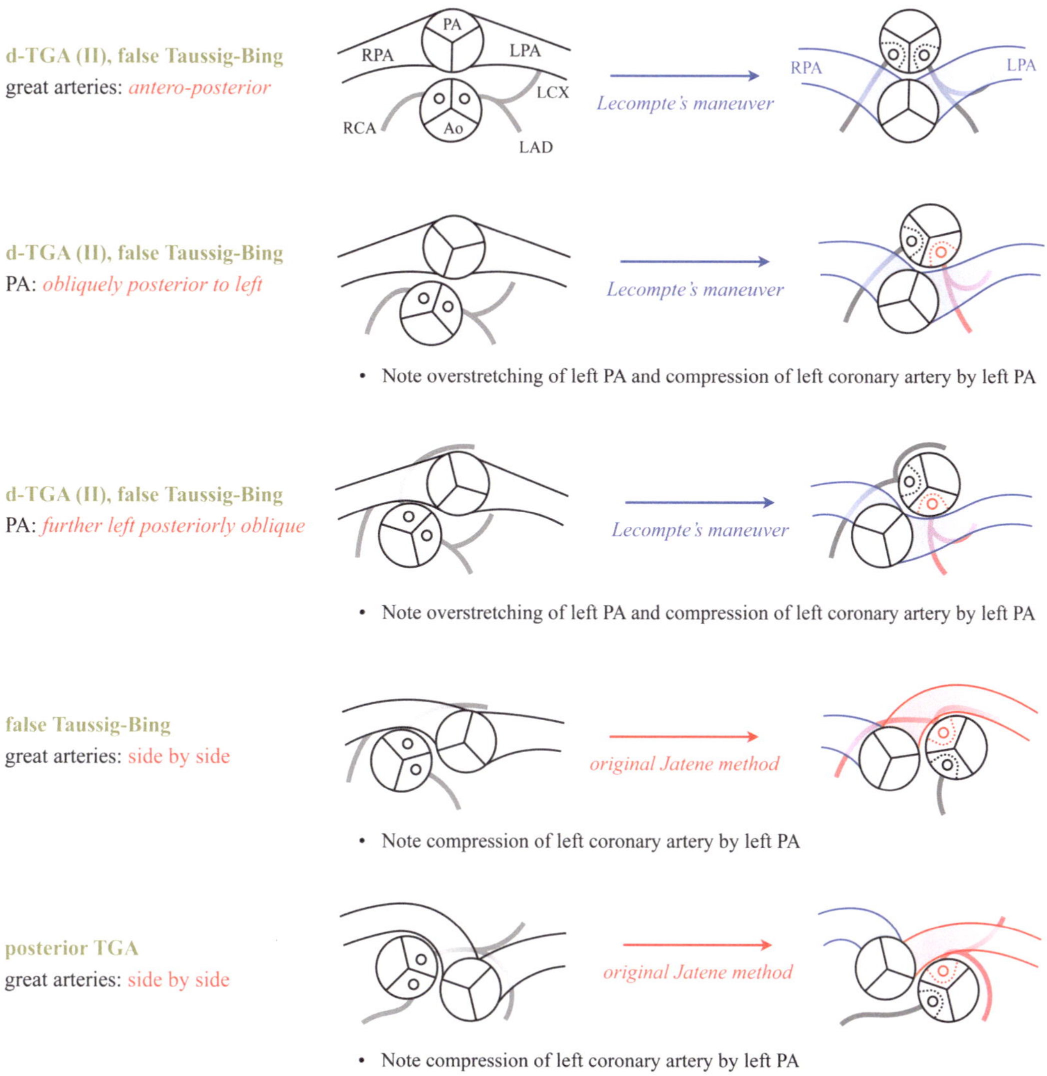

Fig. 9.19 Relationship of the great arteries and pulmonary artery reconstruction procedure

2.7 Pulmonary Artery Reconstruction Procedure: Lecompte or Original Jatene Procedure

In the arterial switch operation, the pulmonary artery is reconstructed either anterior (Lecompte maneuver) or posterior (original Jatene maneuver) to the new aorta. The choice of which method should take into consideration several factors such as the diameter of the new aorta, the location of the left pulmonary hilum, the diameter of the left and right pulmonary arteries, and the location of the coronary artery implantation, in addition to the relationship of the great arteries (relative positional relationship). It is important to avoid overstretching of the reconstructed pulmonary artery (especially the left pulmonary artery) and to avoid compression of the implanted coronary artery by the reconstructed pulmonary artery (pulmonary artery bifurcation) (Fig. 9.20).

The Lecompte maneuver is generally selected in cases of anterior-posterior great arteries. In this group of patients, the aorta is often located slightly anterior to the right, and overstretching of the left pulmonary artery should be noted after an anterior translocation of the pulmonary artery bifurcation.

In cases where the relationship of the great arteries is close to parallel, the original Jatene method is used to reconstruct the pulmonary artery posterior to the neo aorta. In cases where the coronary artery runs behind the new aorta, the left pulmonary artery should be reconstructed to avoid compression of the implanted coronary artery.

2.8 New Indicator for the Choice of Pulmonary Artery Reconstruction Method

The angle between the anterior and posterior walls of the pulmonary artery at the left pulmonary hilum and the great arteries (*pulmonary hilum-great arteries angle*) is a useful indicator for selecting the pulmonary artery reconstruction technique (Figs. 9.21 and 9.22).

- In this case, the great arteries are not in a perfect anteroposterior relationship, with the aorta anterior to the right and the pulmonary artery posterior to the left.
- The Lecompte maneuver is preferable because $\alpha > \beta$ and the angle of reconstruction is relatively gentle.
- In the original Jatene method, there is concern about compression and stenosis of the left pulmonary artery by the posterior wall of the reconstructed aorta.

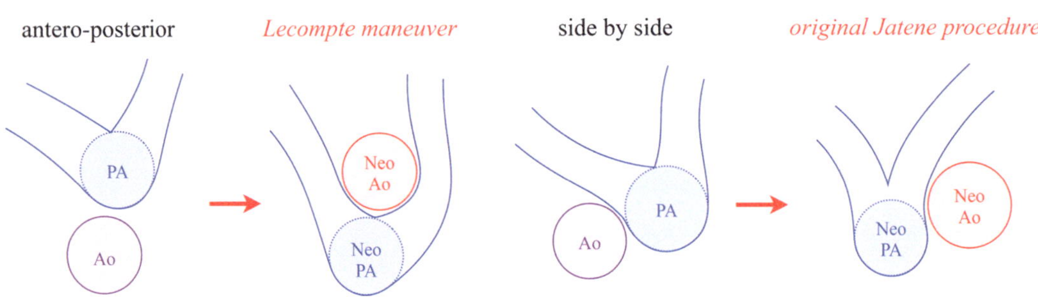

Fig. 9.20 Lecompte's maneuver or original Jatene procedure

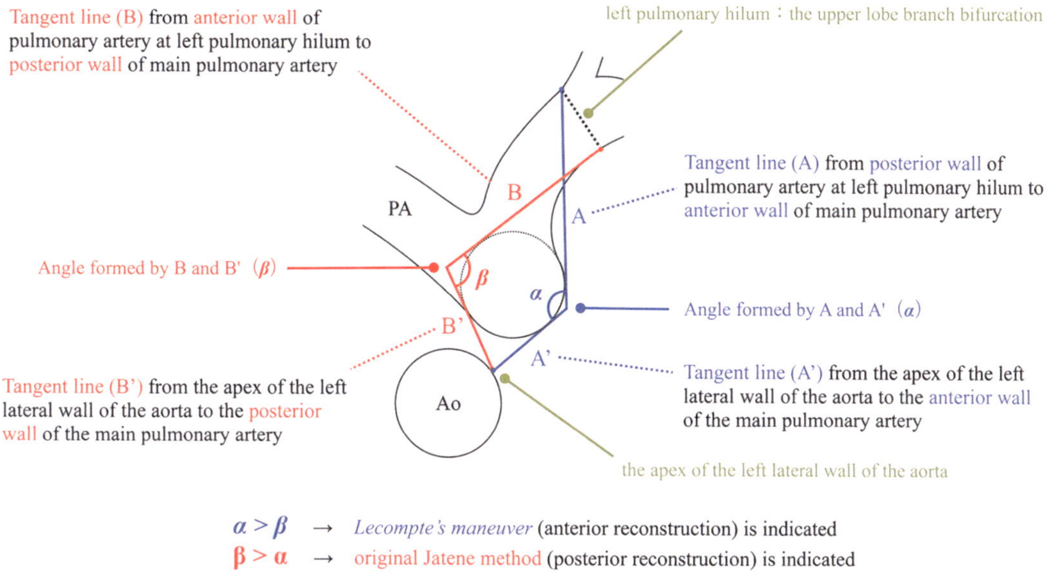

Fig. 9.21 Pulmonary hilum-great arteries angle

< Case 1: Lecompte's maneuver preferred case >

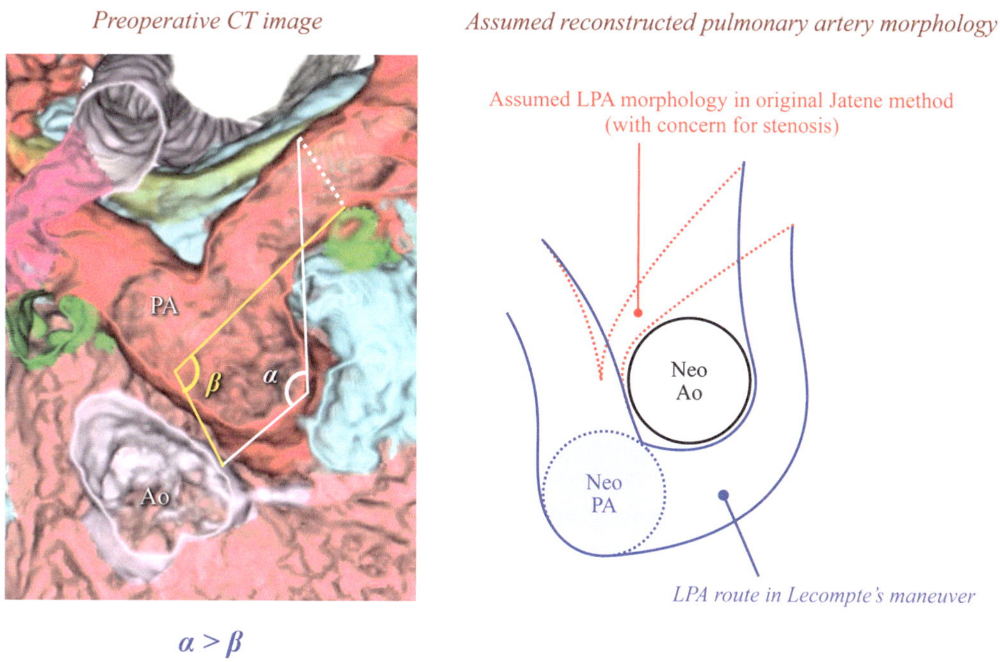

Fig. 9.22 Relationships of the great arteries indicated for the Lecompte's maneuver

< Case 2: Lecompte's maneuver preferred case >

Preoperative CT image

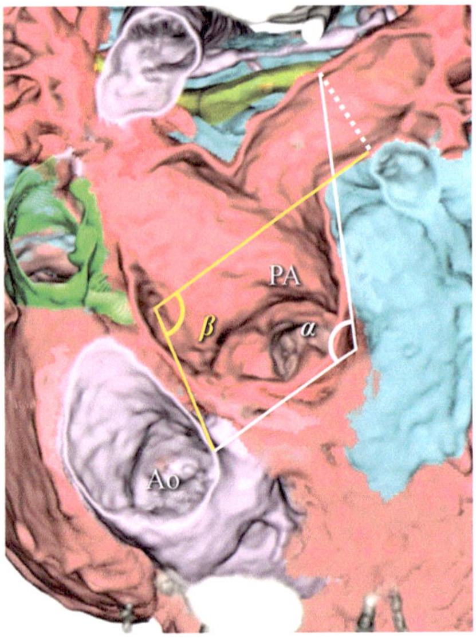

$\alpha > \beta$

Assumed reconstructed pulmonary artery morphology

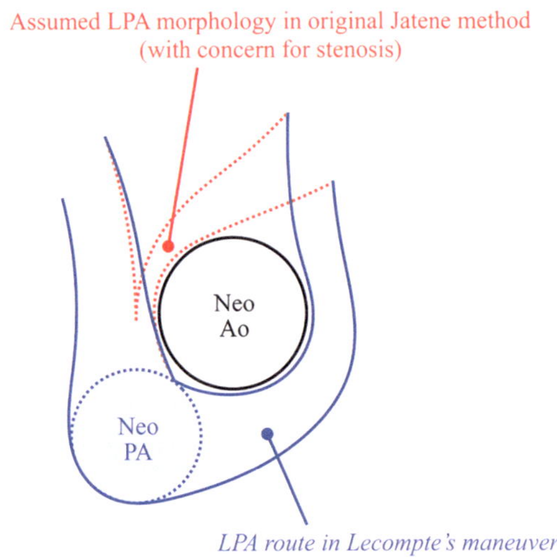

- This case is also an indication for anterior aortic pulmonary artery reconstruction (Lecompte maneuver), but the diameter of the reconstructed new aorta (old main pulmonary artery) is so large that overstretching of the left pulmonary artery is feared. Therefore, it is necessary to enlarge the pulmonary artery bifurcation (LPA origin) using autologous pericardium.
- In the original Jatene method, there is concern about compression and stenosis of the left pulmonary artery by the reconstructed posterior wall of the aorta (Fig. 9.23).
- In this case, $\beta > \alpha$, the patient is indicated for pulmonary artery reconstruction posterior to the aorta (original Jatene's method).
- The Lecompte maneuver results in overstretching and stenosis of the left pulmonary artery, and the left pulmonary artery may compress the implanted coronary artery.
- In this case, the anterior left coronary artery defect requires repair using autologous pericardium.
- The right coronary artery defect was repaired with autologous pericardium, and the pulmonary artery bifurcation was also formed by leaving a long autologous pericardium fragment.

< Case 3: original Jatene procedure preferred case >

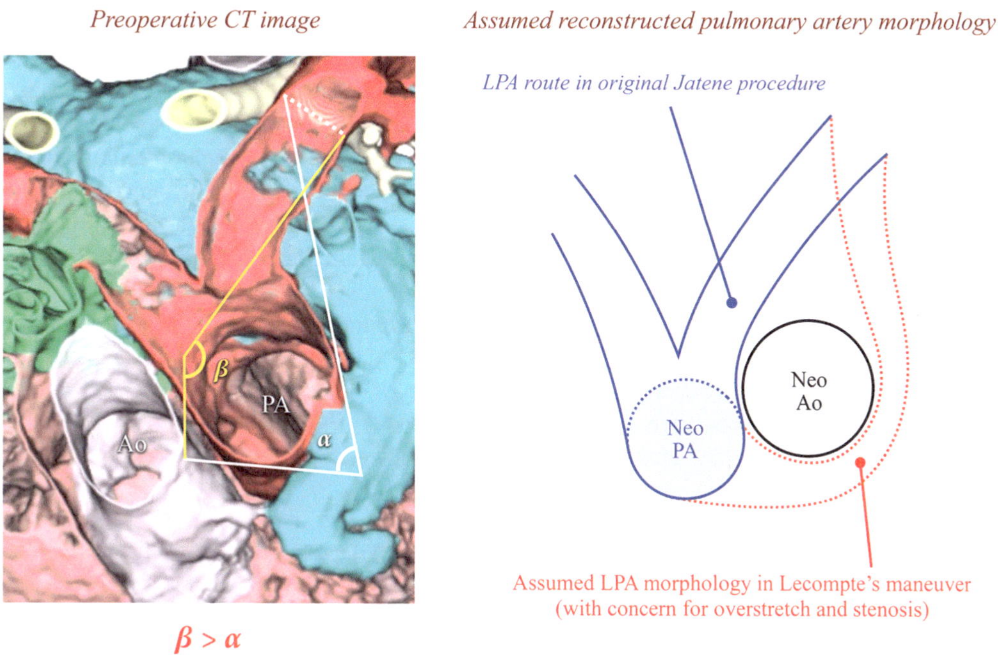

Fig. 9.23 Relationships of the great arteries indicated for original Jatene procedure

< Case 4: original Jatene procedure preferred case >

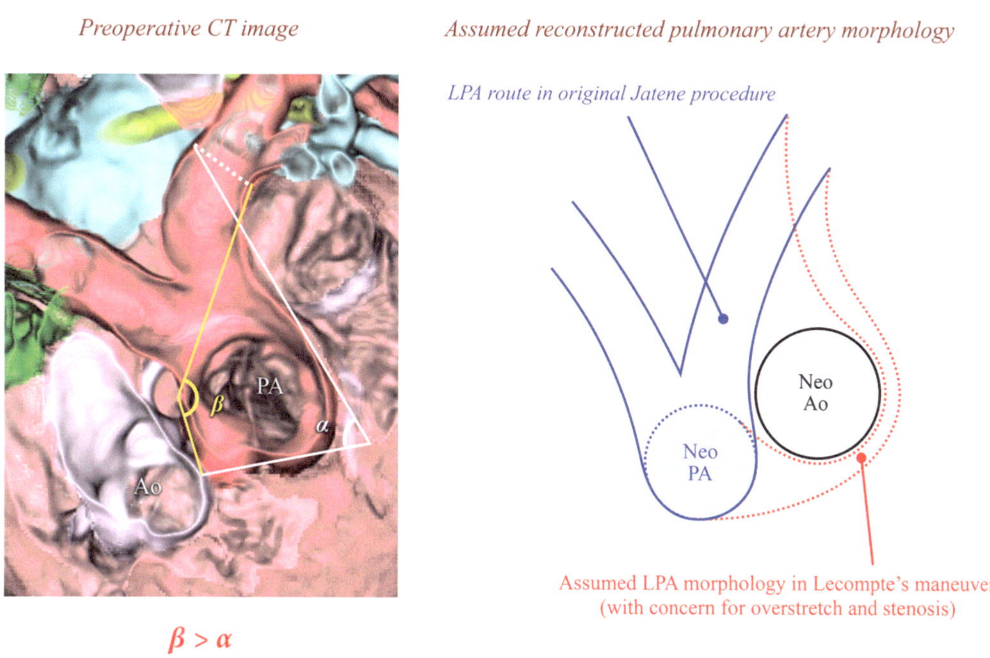

- In this case, β > α, the patient is indicated for pulmonary artery reconstruction posterior to the aorta (original Jatene's method).
- The Lecompte's maneuver results in overstretching and stenosis of the left pulmonary artery.
- The patient has Shaher 5b type coronary arteries, so care must be taken that the left pulmonary artery does not compress the implanted coronary artery.

2.9 Pulmonary Artery Reconstruction: Longitudinal Extension Procedure

Stenosis of the pulmonary artery bifurcation is a problem after arterial switch operation. Especially in the Lecompte's maneuver, which involves anterior translocation of the pulmonary artery bifurcation, the left and right pulmonary arteries are overstretched in the long axis direction due to compression from the posterior aorta, resulting in stenosis at the bifurcation. Even if the stenosis is partially enlarged with a prosthetic patch, the long-axis overstretch is not eliminated, and the possibility of restenosis cannot be denied. The overstretched pulmonary artery bifurcation may also cause stenosis of the ascending aorta.

In contrast, the concept of longitudinal extension is to avoid overstretching the pulmonary artery. The pulmonary artery bifurcation is extended longitudinally using the upper part of the autologous pericardium, which compensates for the coronary button defect (Fig. 9.24).

- Incise dorsally upward from the center of the opening (*red dashed line*) of the anteriorly displaced pulmonary artery by Lecompte's method.
- The longer the incision, the more the pulmonary artery can be extended in both directions (the incision may be made until approximately 5 mm remains: point (a)).
- The linear distance between *b-c* is the distance of the extension of the inferior (caudal) surface of the pulmonary artery.

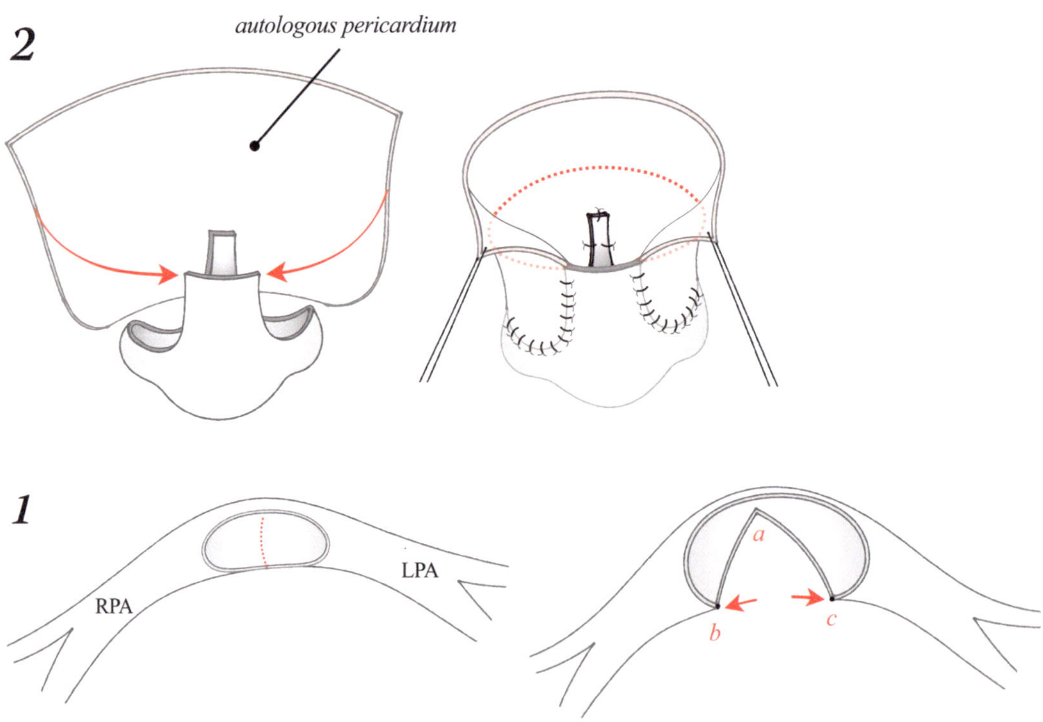

Fig. 9.24 Longitudinal extension of the pulmonary bifurcation during Lecompte procedure

- Fresh autologous pericardium (approximately 30 × 30 mm) is sutured to the coronary button defect with a continuous 7-0 monofilament suture.
- The posterior commissure is sutured to the inner wall of the autologous pericardium with interrupted sutures.
- A horizontal line is drawn on the autocardium at the level of the proximal end of the anterior pulmonary artery.

3

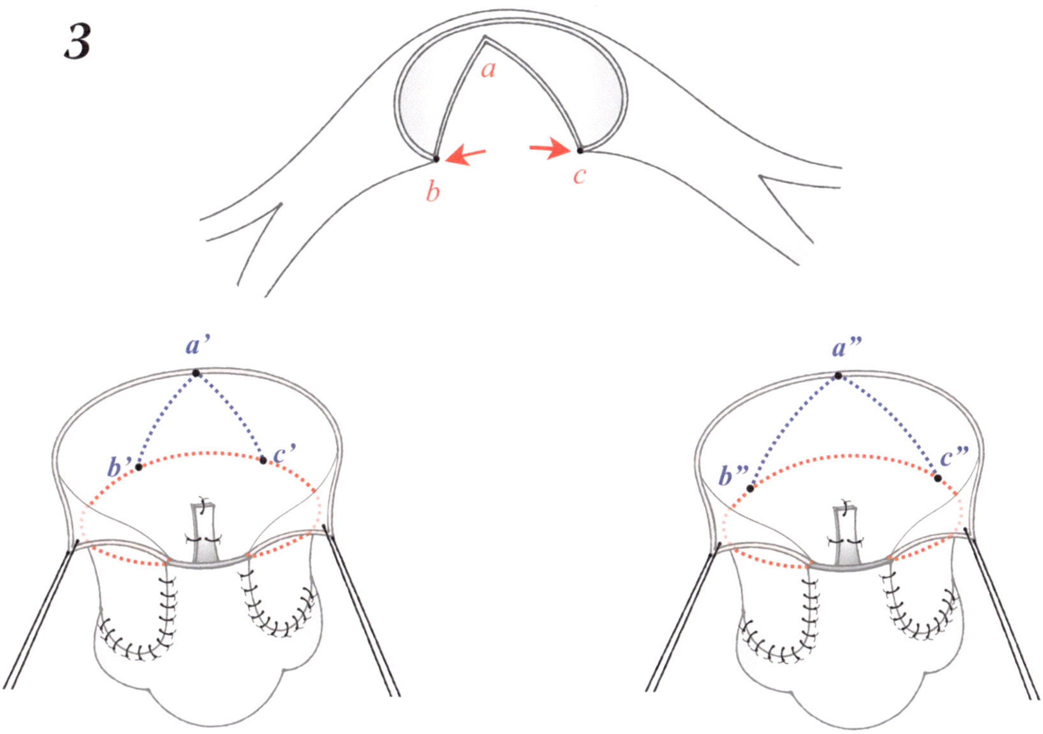

- Mark the autologous pericardium of the posterior wall portion in a triangular shape according to the length of the incision lines (*a-b*, *a-c*) at the pulmonary artery bifurcation (*a′-b′*, *a′-c′*). The distance *b′-c′* is the length of the left and right pulmonary arteries.
- If the left and right pulmonary arteries are to be lengthened, the base of the autocardium triangle is lengthened (*a″-b″*, *a″-c″*).
- The distance *b″-c″* is the length of the left and right pulmonary arteries to be extended, thus allowing for longer extension (*b″- c″* > *b′- c′*).

4

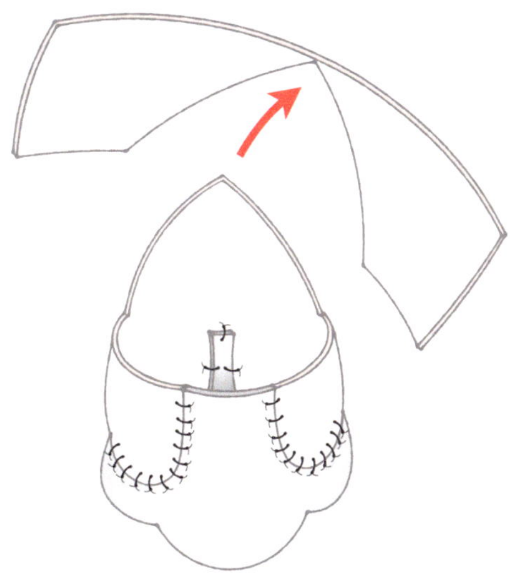

- Incise the autologous pericardium along the marked incision line.

5

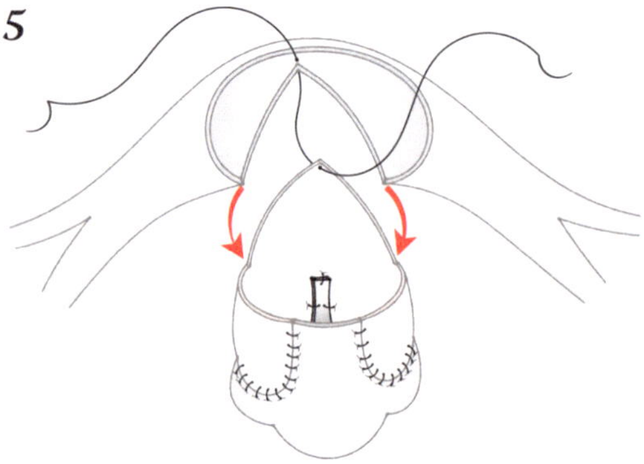

- Anastomose the pulmonary artery with the autologous pericardium using a continuous 6–0 monofilament suture, aligning the tip of the pulmonary artery incision with the triangular apex of the autologous pericardium.

6

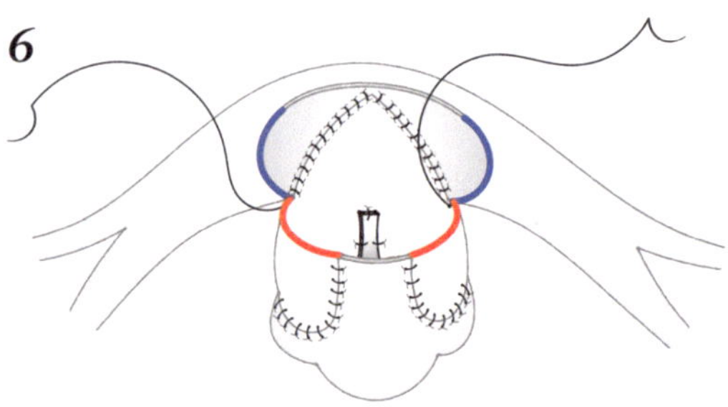

- After suturing to the triangular base of the autologous pericardium, check the length of the pulmonary artery opening and the remaining circumference of the basal part of the pulmonary artery.

- When anastomosing the upper part of the autologous pericardium (*red part*) and the orifices of the right and left pulmonary arteries (*blue part*), it is essential to suture the pulmonary artery orifices, taking care not to shrink the pulmonary artery orifices.

7

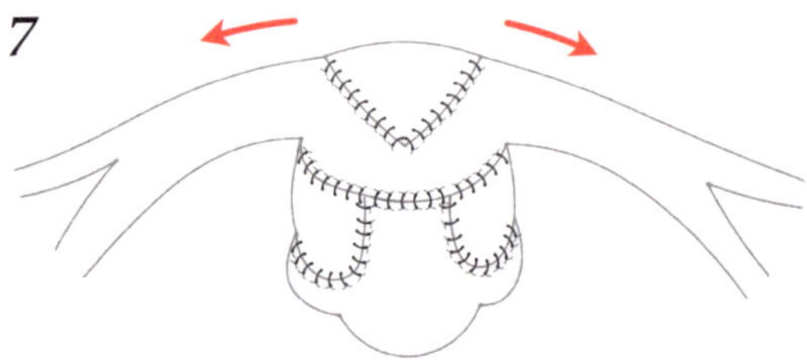

- Longitudinal extension of the pulmonary artery bifurcation is completed by the longitudinal extension method.
- Overstretching of the pulmonary artery bifurcation is eliminated in most cases.

8

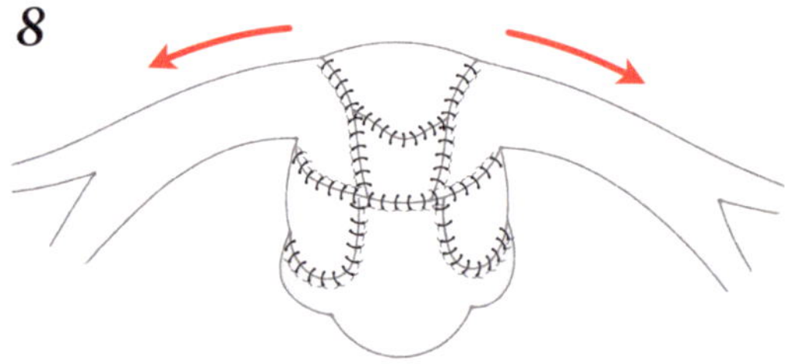

- If there is residual tension in the pulmonary artery, an autologous pericardial patch can be added to the anterior wall of the pulmonary artery to further extend the pulmonary artery bifurcation in the long axis direction.

3 Arterial Switch Operation: Bay-Window Method (Surgical Video)

Case

- Age: 2 months old.
- Body weight: 4.5 kg.
- Diagnosis: d-TGA (II), PFO, PDA.
- Coronary artery pattern: [1LCx: 2R], Shaher type 1, Yacoub type A.

< cephalic view >

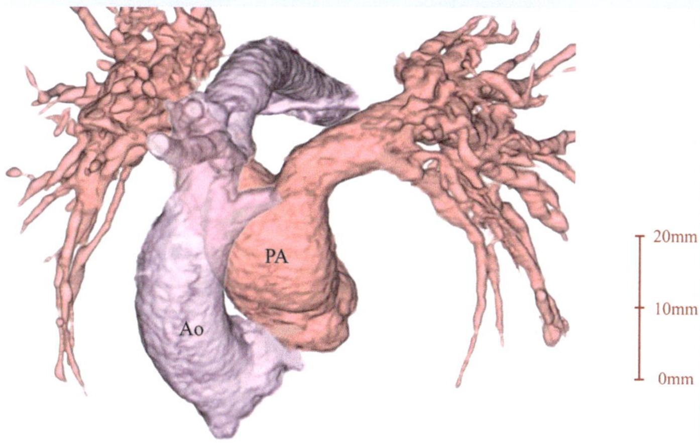

- Relationship of the great arteries: right anterior aorta, left posterior pulmonary artery (Scene 9.1).

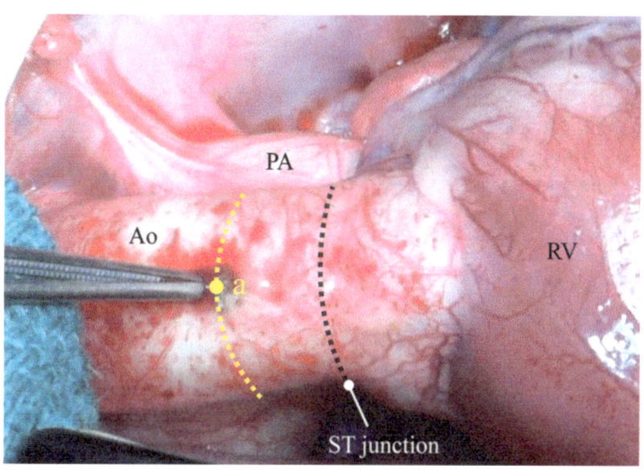

Scene 9.1 Transection site of the aorta (Video 00 min 16 s)

1 Because the bay-window method requires harvesting a longer coronary cuff, the aortic transection line (yellow dotted line) should be approximately 7–8 mm cephalad of the ST junction (approximately 3 mm cephalad of the trap door and punch-out methods).

2 A root cannula (6-0 monofilament suture, U-shaped suture) is placed over the aortic transection line to inject myocardial protection solution (point (a)).
- The aorta is sufficiently dissected near the beginning of the second branch of the cervical artery.
- The right and left pulmonary arteries are dissected to the pulmonary hilum after the start of extracorporeal circulation.
- The ductus arteriosus is dissected as far as possible before the start of extracorporeal circulation and divided after the start of extracorporeal circulation.
- If the patient is hemodynamically unstable, the ductus arteriosus should be dissected after extracorporeal circulation is started (Scene 9.2.1).

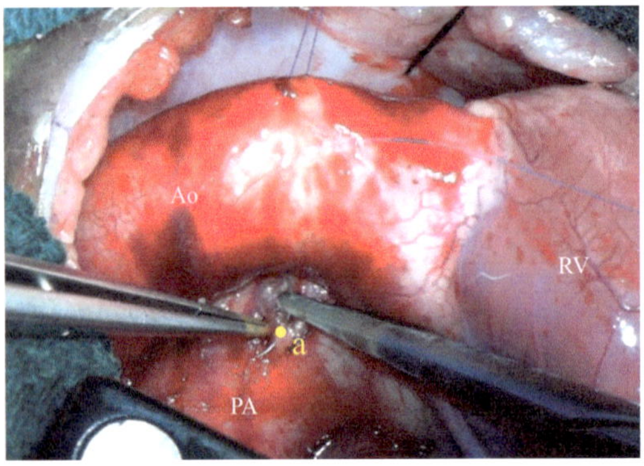

Scene 9.2.1 Marking of right coronary artery implantation site (Video 00 min 24 s)

1 With the aorta in traction to the left, mark the right coronary artery implantation site (point (a): the center point of the coronary artery orifice) on the anterior wall of the pulmonary artery with 7-0 monofilament suture.
   - The implantation site should be slightly cephalad and medial to the level of the origin of the coronary artery (Scene 9.2.2).

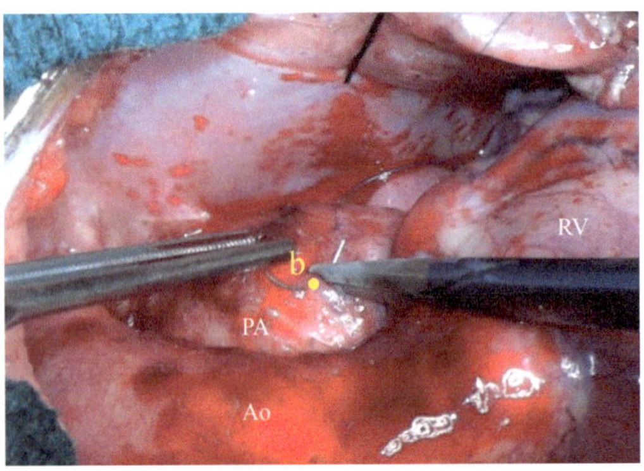

Scene 9.2.2 Marking of left coronary artery implantation site (Video 00 min 33 s)

2 Similarly, traction suture the aorta to the right and mark the left coronary artery implantation site (point (b): the center of the coronary artery orifice) on the anterior wall of the pulmonary artery with 7-0 monofilament suture.
   - The implantation site should be slightly cephalad and medial to the level of the coronary artery origin (Scene 9.3).

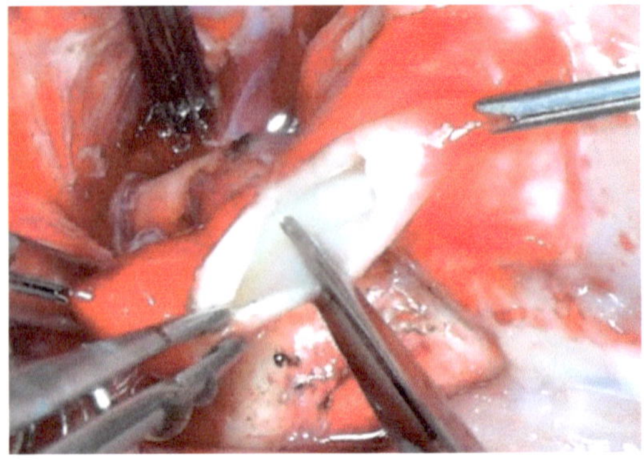

Scene 9.3 Transection of the aorta (Video 00 min 37 s)

1 Clamp the aorta and induce cardiac arrest.
2 Transect the aorta at the site of insertion of the root cannula.
   - Transect the aorta, taking care not to place the incision line too close to the coronary artery orifices.
   - Make sure that the incision line is straight and not jagged (Scene 9.4.1).

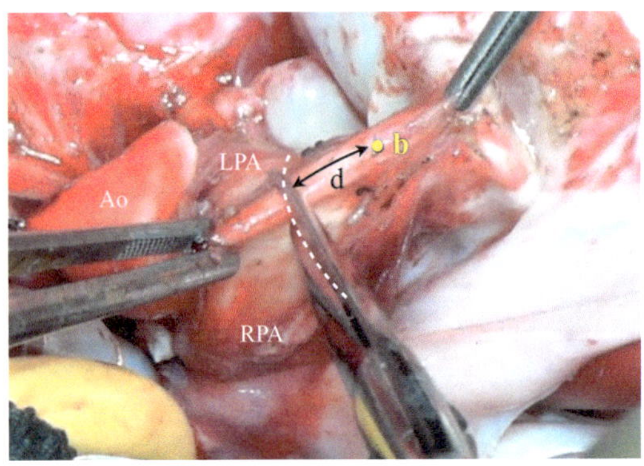

Scene 9.4.1 Transection of the pulmonary artery (Video 00 min 47 s)

1 Make a transverse incision (white dotted line) in the anterior wall of the pulmonary artery approximately 5–7 mm headword (before the bifurcation) from the marker at the coronary artery implantation site (point (b)).
   - The distance between the marker and the incision line on the anterior wall of the pulmonary artery (d) should be shorter than the distance between the incision line at the

proximal end of the aorta and the coronary artery orifice.
- The proximal end of the pulmonary artery need not be left longer than necessary.
- Care should be taken not to cut into either the left or right pulmonary artery (Scene 9.4.2).

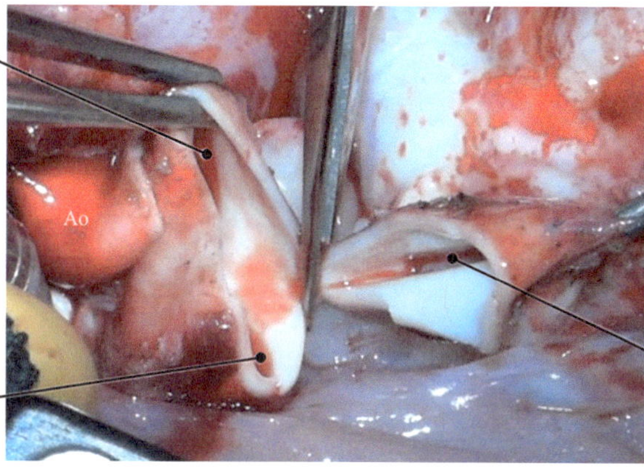

Scene 9.4.2 Transection of the pulmonary artery before the bifurcation (Video 00 min 52 sec)

2 Transect the pulmonary artery before the bifurcation, taking care not to incise the right and left pulmonary artery orifices and the pulmonary valve.
- Incise approximately midway between the apex of the dorsal commissure and the right and left pulmonary artery orifices (Scene 9.5).

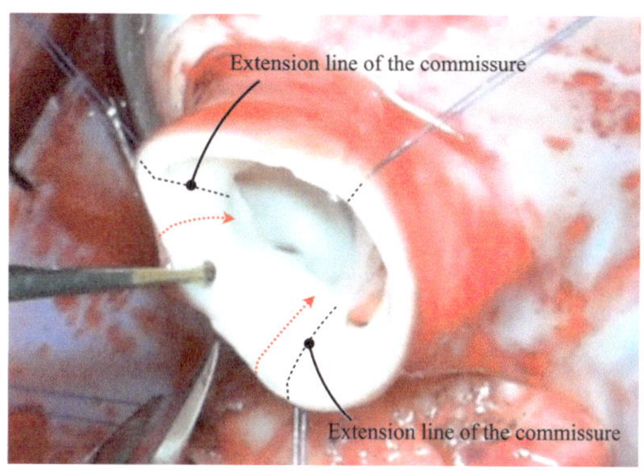

Scene 9.5 Harvest of the coronary cuff (Video 00 min 57 s)

1 Apply three 7-0 monofilament sutures on the extension of the aortic valve commissure at the proximal end of the aorta (black dotted line) and pull each of them in a 120° direction.
2 It is important to pull the traction suture in the appropriate direction with moderate tension (tension cannot be adjusted with thicker sutures).
3 Harvest the left coronary artery cuff: From the transverse side of the traction suture to the medial side of the commissure (coronary artery opening side), incise the aortic wall in a straight line using straight scissors (incision line: *red dashed line*) (Scene 9.6).

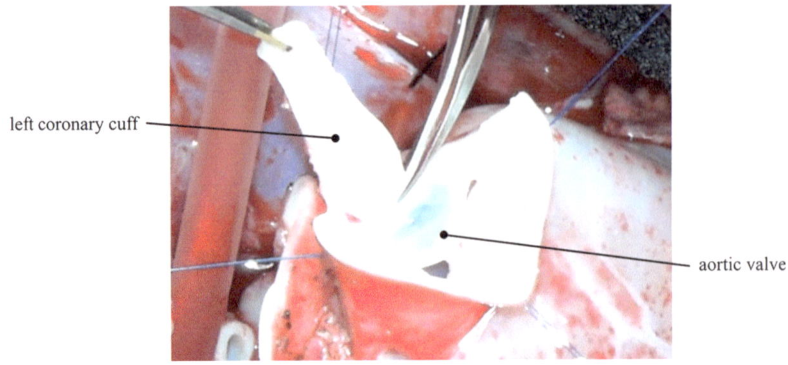

Scene 9.6 Harvest of the left coronary cuff (Video 01 min 09 s)

1 Once the incision reaches the sinus of Valsalva, continue the incision (*red dashed line* in the figure below) approximately 1 mm away from the aortic valve attachment site (*blue line* in the figure below).

- In this area, incise the intima and tunica media by inserting the curved vascular scissors below the origin of the coronary artery (*red arrows* in the figure below).
- Care should be taken not to damage the cusps and commissures of the aortic valve.
- The adventitia is incised with an electric scalpel.
- The adventitia surrounding the coronary artery is also dissected with an electric scalpel to ensure the mobility of the origin of the coronary artery (Scene 9.7).

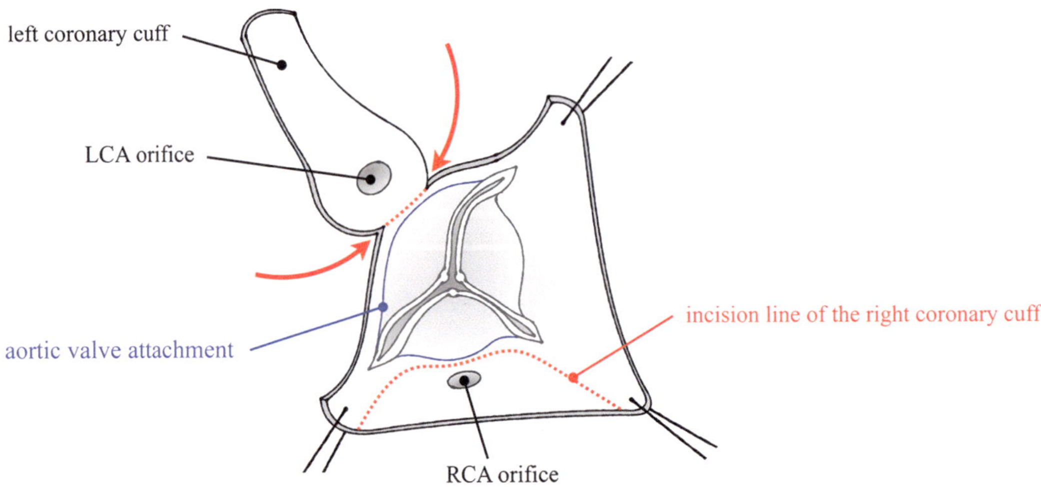

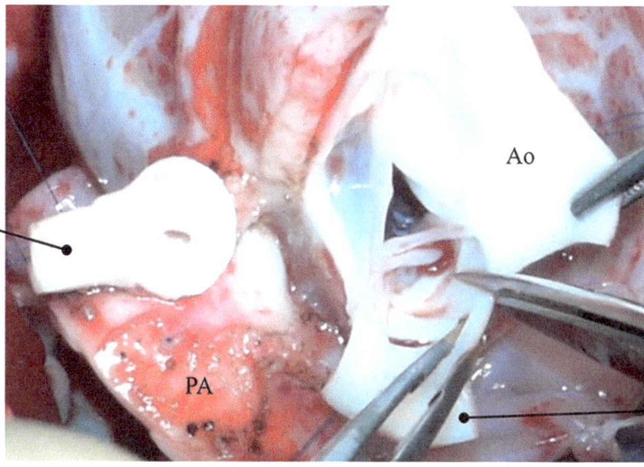

Scene 9.7 Harvest of the right coronary cuff (Video 01 min 28 s)

1 Similarly, remove the right coronary cuff.
- Dissect the adventitia at the origin with an electric scalpel.
- Since a conus branch may be present near the origin of the right coronary artery, be careful not to damage it during dissection.

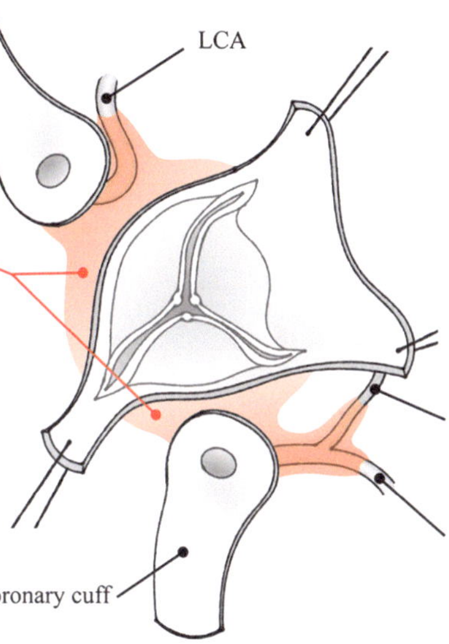

- When dissecting the right coronary artery, check for the presence of a conus branch running anterior to the aortic annulus and take care not to damage it.
- The branches should be dissected distally, as they may be overstretched after transplantation.
- Use a low-power electric scalpel to dissect the adventitia around the coronary arteries.
- The dissection should be approximately 5–7 mm from the origin of the coronary arteries.
- In cases of branching near the origin or in cases of anomalous running, the coronary arteries should be dissected distally.
- Small branches should be preserved as much as possible.
- The left circumflex branch may branch near the origin, so be careful not to damage it.

POINT Dissect the Adventitia in Case of Shaher 4

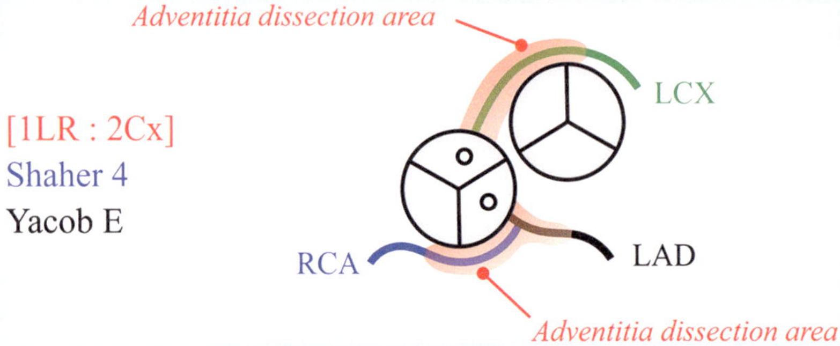

- For coronary arteries that run anterior or posterior to the great arteries, the adventitia is dissected to a point beyond the circumference of the great arteries (Scene 9.8).

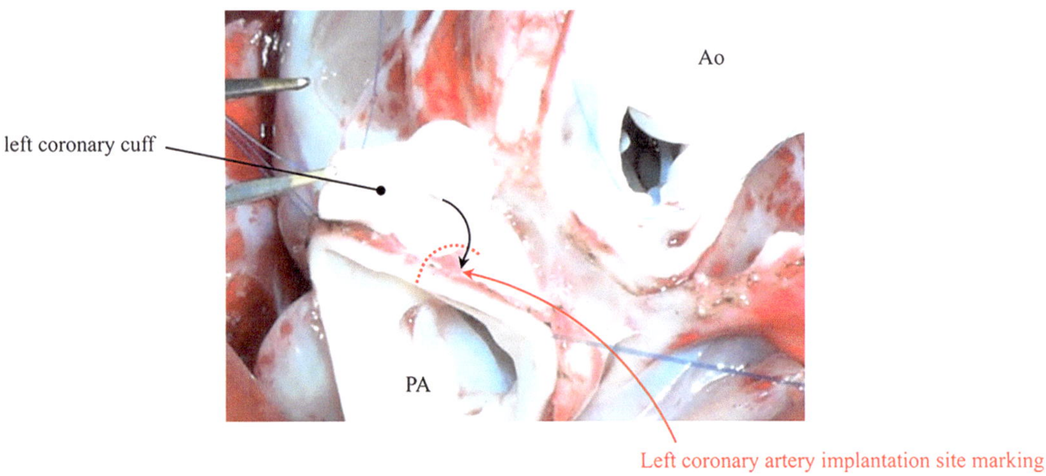

Scene 9.8 Implantation of the left coronary cuff 1 (Video 02 min 01 s)

1 Use the marking suture as a guide to determine the implantation site.
2 Make a J-shaped incision in the pulmonary artery wall so that the left coronary artery opening corresponds to the marked site (*black arrow*) (*red dashed line*).
3 Using straight vascular scissors, make a longitudinal incision in the pulmonary artery wall corresponding to the left edge of the cuff.
4 The direction of incision is changed before the ST junction, and a J-shaped transverse incision is made with a curved vascular scissors.
   - Be sure that the incise line does not enter the sinus of Valsalva.
   - The width of the lower edge of the J-shaped incision should be approximately 2/3 of the width of the cuff.

POINT Adjustment of the Implantation Site According to the Coronary Artery Morphology

< *Case 1* >

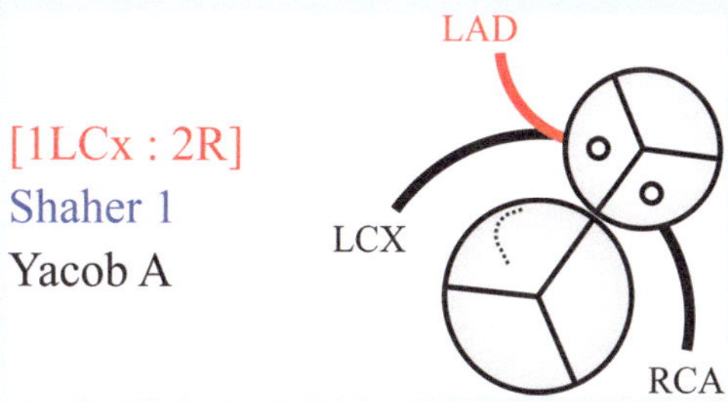

- For normal Shaher type 1, use the marker as a guide to determine the J-shaped incision site (*black dashed line*).

< *Case 2* >

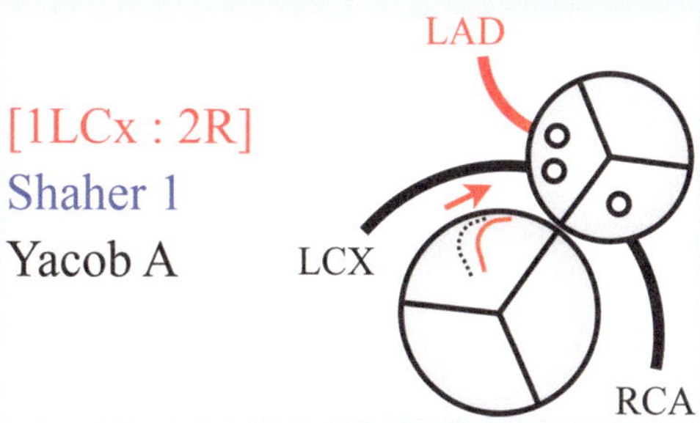

- In Shaher type 1 cases with separate LAD and LCX orifices, the J-shaped incision (vertical incision) is made slightly to the right (*red line*) to prevent bending of the implanted LCX orifice.

< *Case 3* >

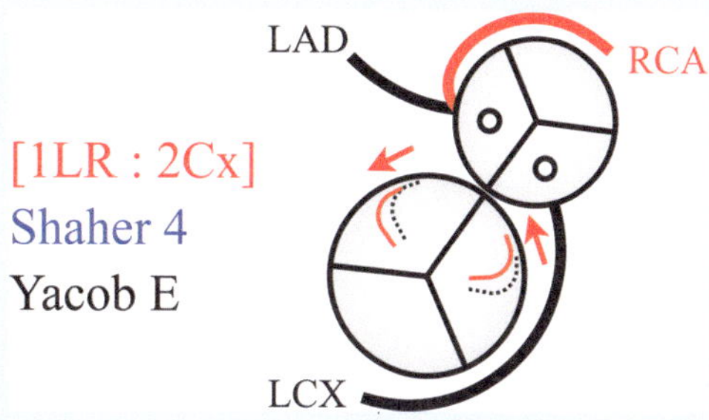

- In Shaher type 4, the J-shaped incision (longitudinal incision) is made slightly to the left (*red line*) so that the RCA running anterior to the aorta is as straight as possible without overstretching.
- The LCX is also implanted slightly medial and higher in the pulmonary artery wall to avoid bending (*red line*) (Scene 9.9).

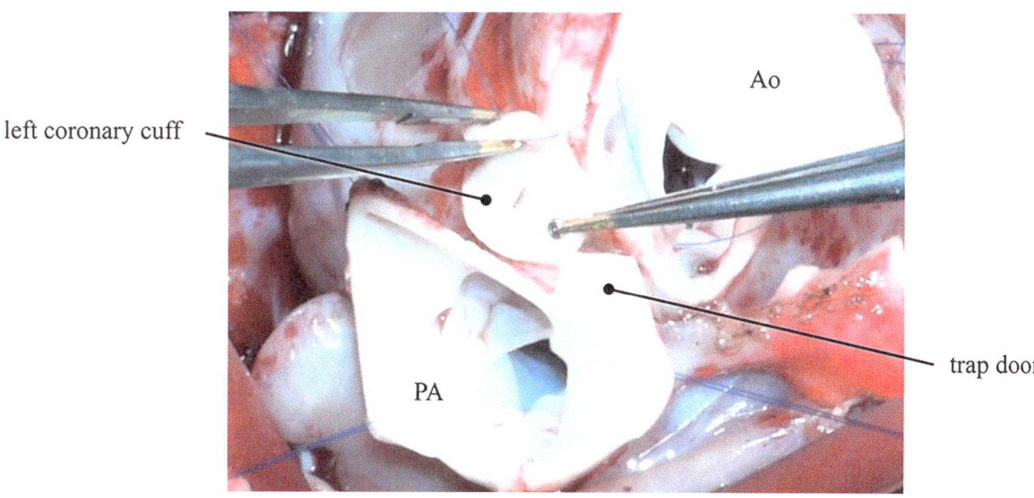

Scene 9.9 Implantation of the left coronary cuff 2 (Video 02 min 16 s)

1 Align the left coronary cuff with the pulmonary artery incision and ensure that there is no bending or overstretching of the coronary artery.

- Ensure that the coronary cuff (coronary artery origin) is not twisted (Scene 9.10).

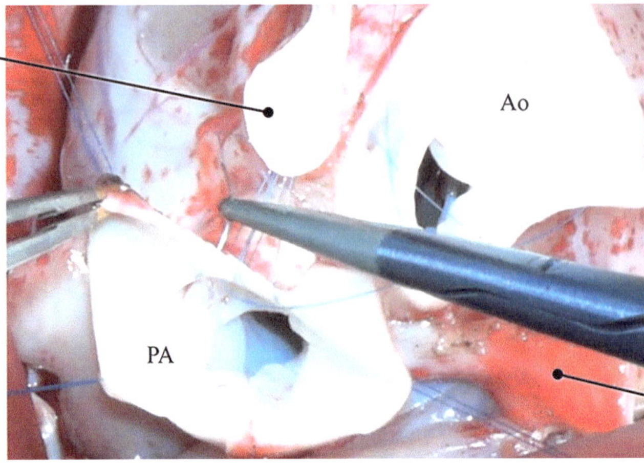

Scene 9.10 Implantation of the left coronary cuff 3 (Video 02 min 20 s)

1 Begin the anastomosis with a 7-0 (or 8-0) monofilament suture from the tip of the J-shaped incision and the lower end of the coronary cuff.
   - Insert the suture needle vertically into the vessel wall and then vertically out.

2 After anastomosis between the lower end of the cuff and the lower end of the J-shaped incision, pull the thread and drop the cuff onto the incision (parachute method).

3 The side of the cuff is sewn up from the outside of the vessel with a continuous suture.

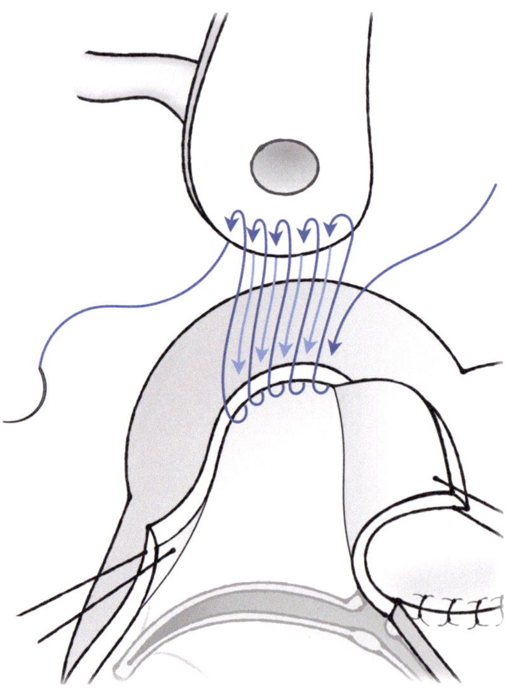

When suturing with the forehand, start suturing from the lower right edge of the J-shaped incision in the pulmonary artery wall.

In this case, the pulmonary artery is sutured from the outer surface to the inner surface, and the cuff is sutured from the inner surface to the outer surface.

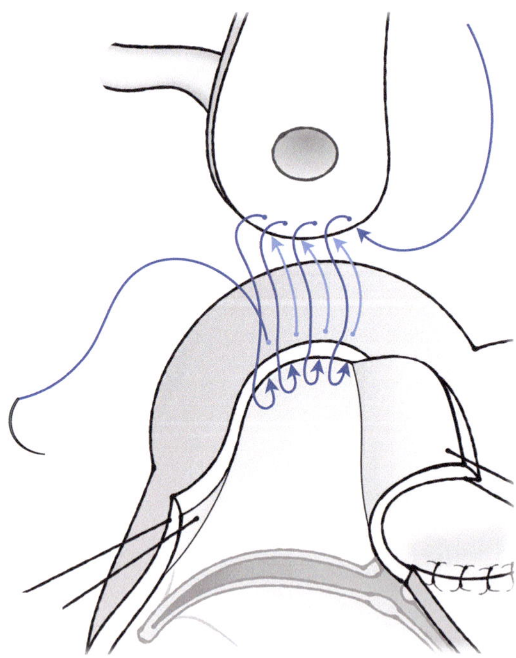

When suturing with the backhand, start suturing from the lower right edge of the cuff.

In this case, the cuff is sutured from the outer surface to the inner surface, and the pulmonary artery is sutured from the inner surface to the outer surface (Scene 9.11).

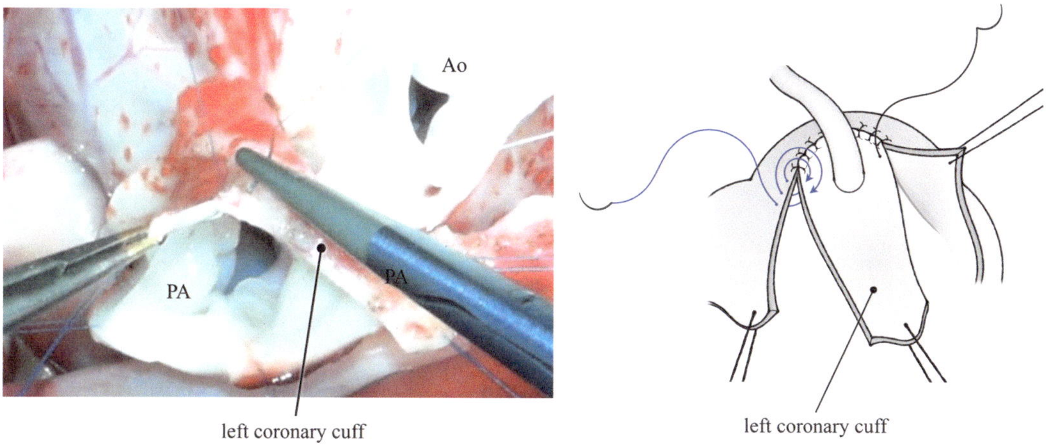

Scene 9.11 Implantation of the left coronary cuff 4 (Video 03 min 11 s)

1 Anastomose the left side of the left coronary cuff with the pulmonary artery wall incision from the outside by forehand.

- Anastomose the cuff and the pulmonary artery wall with adequate traction (Scene 9.12).

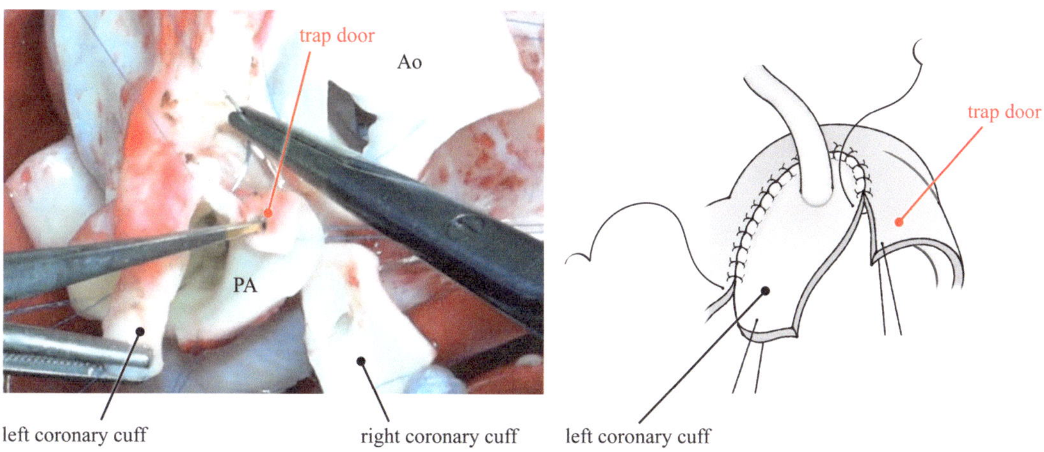

Scene 9.12 Implantation of the left coronary cuff 5 (Video 03 min 41 s)

1 The right side of the left coronary cuff is anastomosed to the pulmonary artery trap door with a continuous suture from the outside of the vessel (Scene 9.13).

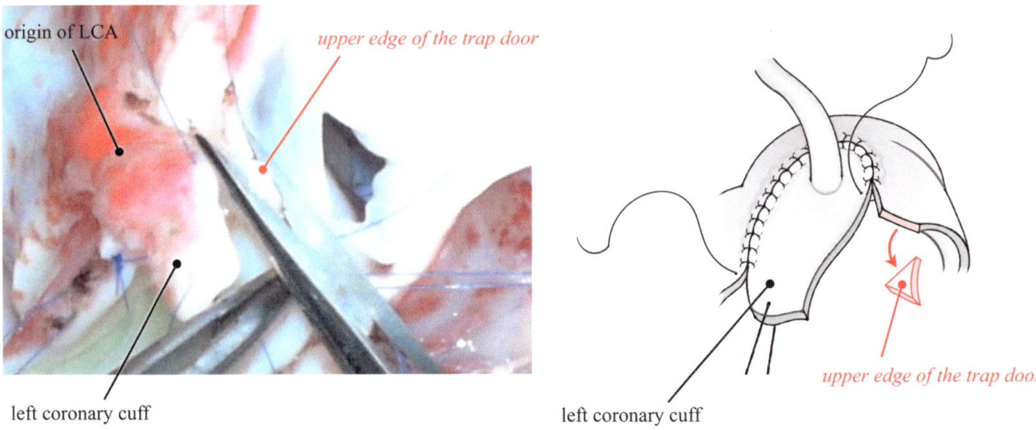

Scene 9.13 Implantation of the left coronary cuff 6 (Video 04 min 08 s)

1 Once the suture crosses the level of the coronary artery orifice, trim the tip of the pulmonary artery wall trap door obliquely to create a smooth bay-window channel (Scene 9.14).

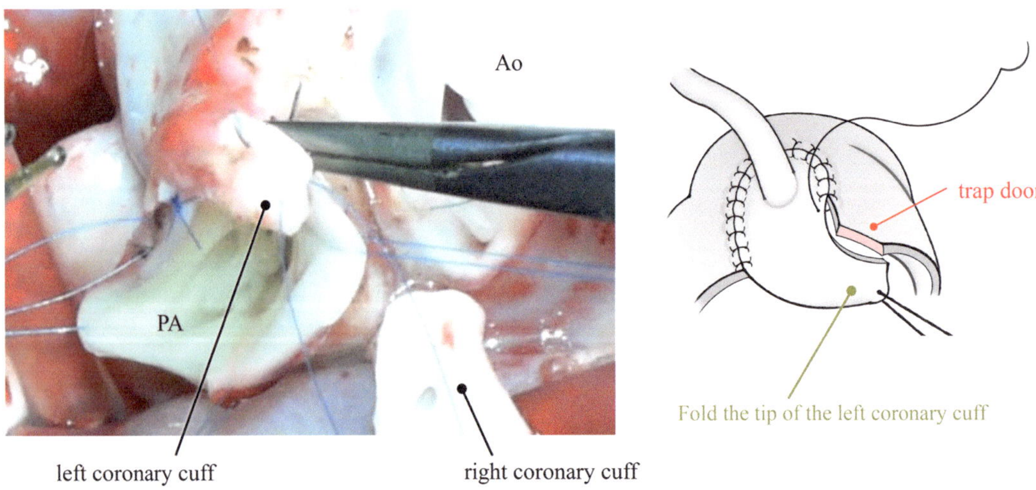

Scene 9.14 Implantation of the left coronary cuff 7 (Video 04 min 13 s)

1 Fold the tip of the left coronary cuff and anastomose it to the upper end of the pulmonary artery wall trap door (creating a bay-window channel) (Scene 9.15).

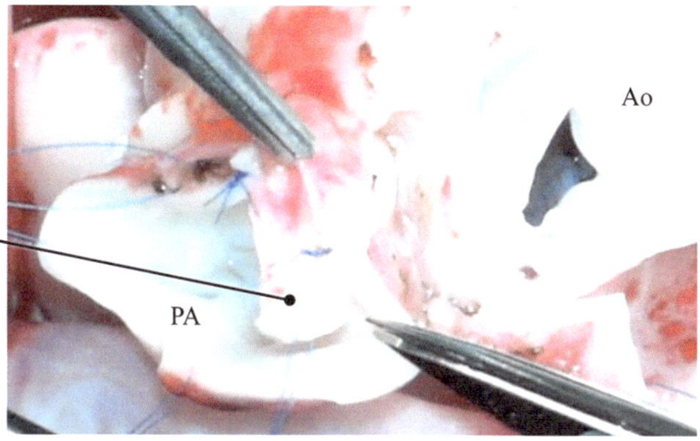

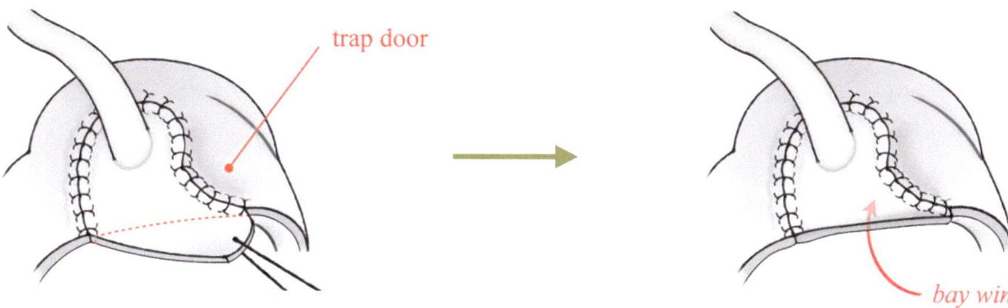

Scene 9.16 Implantation of the left coronary cuff 8 (Video 04 min 56 s)

1 Trim the upper end of the coronary cuff to prepare the cross section of the proximal end of the neo-aorta.
   - Trimming of the upper end of the cuff may be performed after the anastomosis of the right coronary cuff is also done and after checking the alignment of both bay-window channels (Scene 9.16).

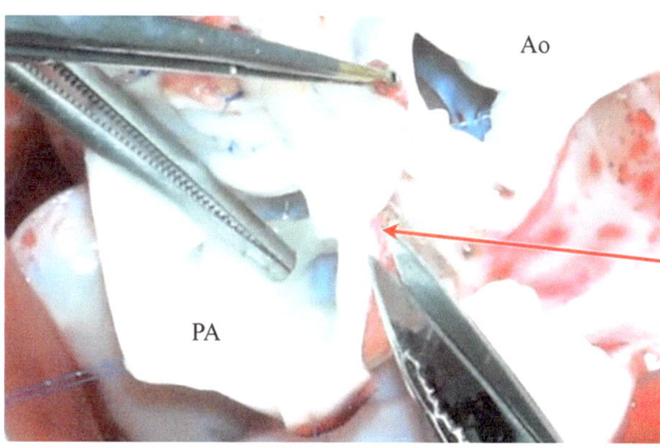

Scene 9.16 Implantation of the right coronary cuff 1 (Video 05 min 09 s)

1 Make a J-shaped incision on the wall of the pulmonary artery as well as the left coronary artery cuff.
   - Make sure that the incision does not go beyond the ST junction into the sinus of Valsalva (Scene 9.17).

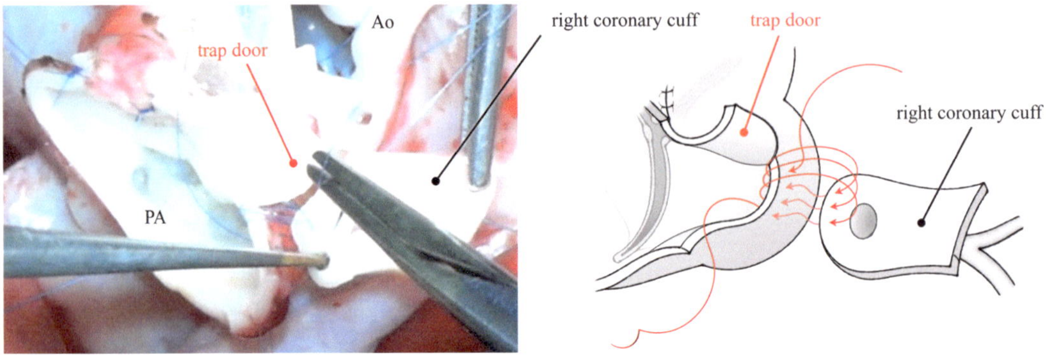

Scene 9.17 Implantation of the right coronary cuff 2 (Video 05 min 33 s)

1 Start suturing from the lower left edge of the right coronary cuff.
2 The cuff is sutured from the inner surface to the outer surface, and the pulmonary artery is sutured from the outer surface to the inner surface (Scene 9.18).

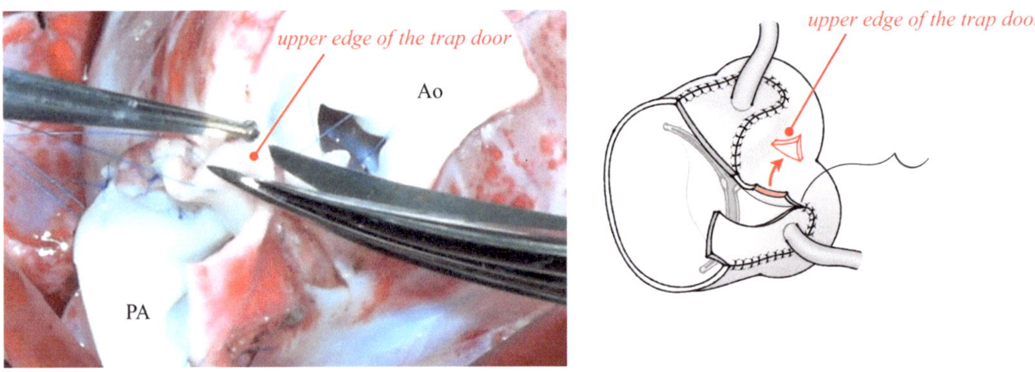

Scene 9.18 Implantation of the right coronary cuff 3 (Video 06 min 56 s)

- Trim the tip of the trap door obliquely to create a smooth bay-window channel (Scene 9.19).

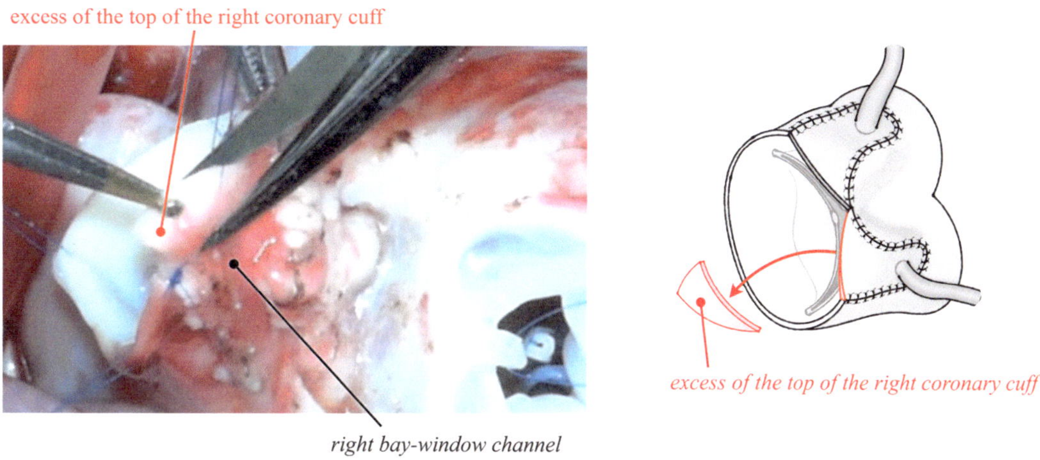

Scene 9.19 Implantation of the right coronary cuff 4 (Video 07 min 40 s)

- Trim the excess from the top of the cuff.

POINT Bay-Window Channel Top Edge Processing

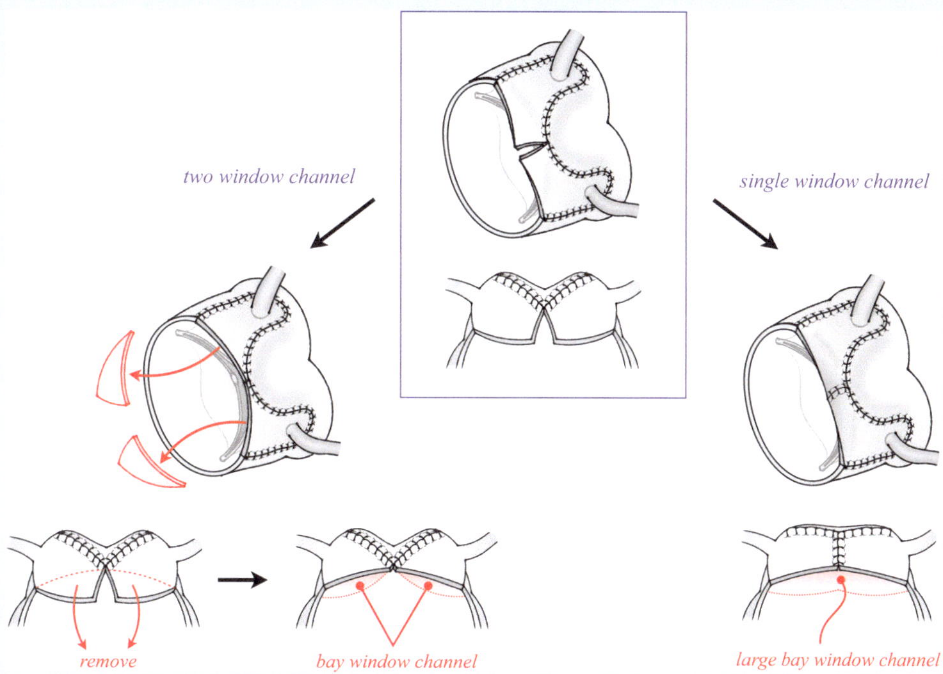

- (*Left*) Usually, the excess portion of the upper edge of the cuff on the left and right sides is removed. Two bay-window channels are created on the left and right sides.
- (*Right*) When the left and right coronary artery implantation sites are close together, the bay-window channels are also close together, so the upper ends of the left and right cuffs can be sutured together to form a single large bay-window channel.

POINT Calibration of the Distal and Proximal Aortic Stumps

In cases where there is a significant difference in caliber between the proximal pulmonary artery (base of the new aorta) and the ascending aorta, a wedge-shaped resection of the posterior wall of the base of the new aorta is performed and the caliber of the base side is sutured.

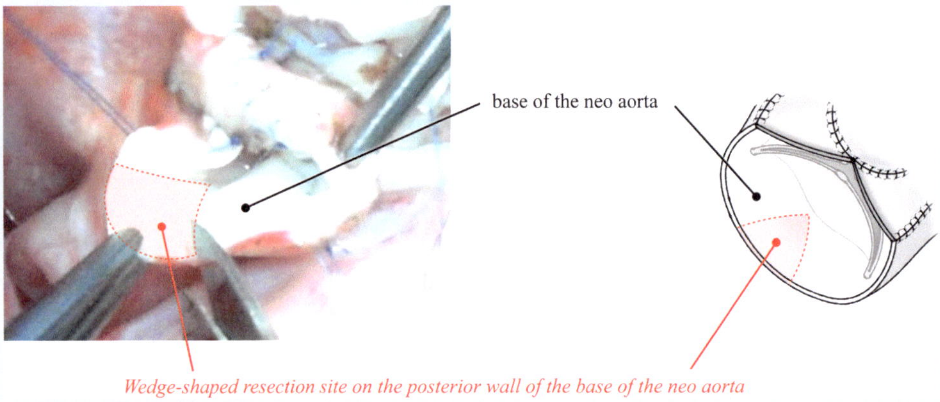

Wedge-shaped resection of the posterior neo aortic wall

1 Measure with a sizer to match the caliber of the ascending aorta, determine the width of the resection of the posterior wall of the base, and perform a wedge resection.

- Be careful not to reduce the base caliber too much.
- Be careful not to incise the ST junction.

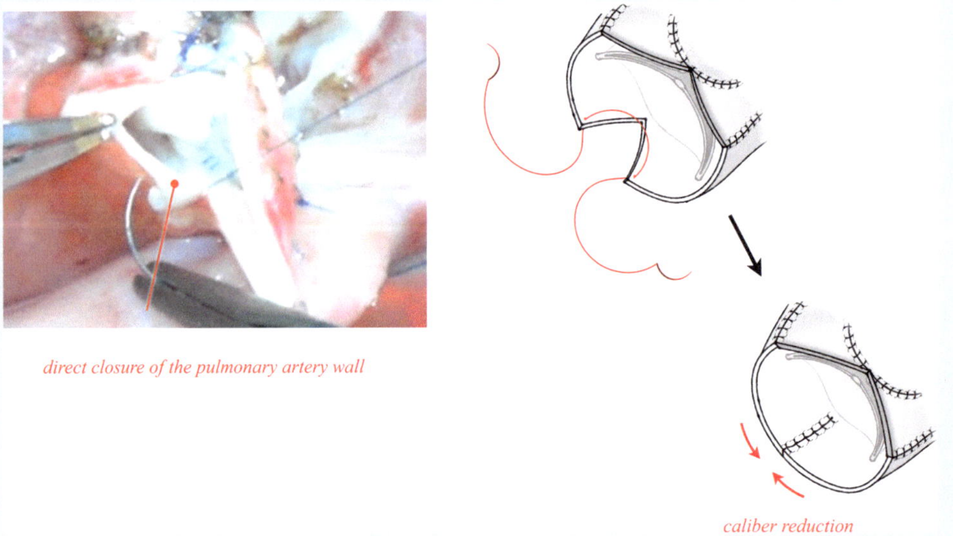

Caliber reduction by longitudinal direct anastomosis

2 Direct closure of the pulmonary artery (neo aorta) wall resected in an inverted triangular shape with continuous suture of 7-0 monofilament suture and reduction of the caliber of the proximal transected stump (Scene 9.20).

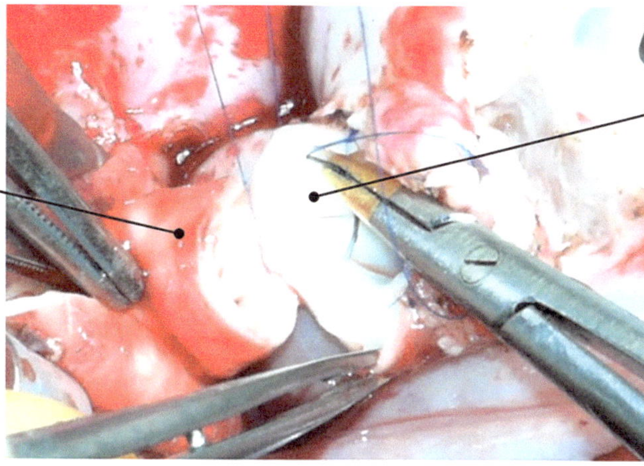

Scene 9.20 Reconstruction of the ascending aorta 1 (Video 07 min 58 s)

1 Translocate the pulmonary artery bifurcation anterior to the aorta (Lecompte maneuver).
2 Reconstruct the aorta by end-to-end anastomosis of the proximal end of the neo aorta and the ascending aorta with continuous suture of 6-0 (or 7-0) monofilament suture.

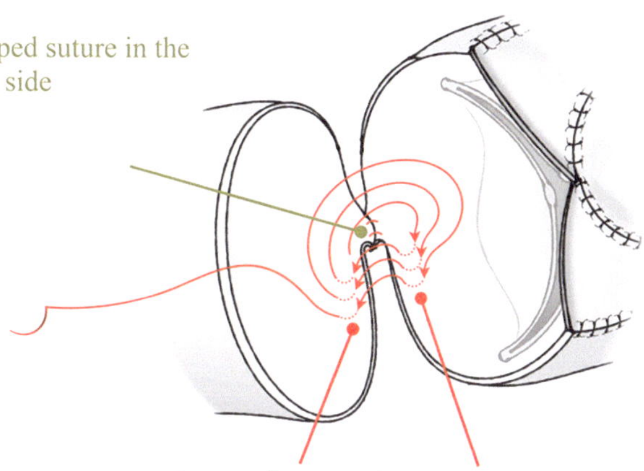

- To avoid intravascular turbulence, the dorsal aspect of the aorta is anastomosed so that the intima are connected to each other (*everting suture*).
- First, the dorsal center of the proximal and distal ends are aligned and ligated and fastened with a U-shaped suture.
- If the proximal end is undergoing caliber reduction, similarly, first ligate and fasten the center of the dorsal wall.
- (*Proximal stump*) Insert the suture needle to the proximal intima, penetrate to the tunica media, and then exit through the proximal intima.
- (*Ascending Ao*) Insert the suture needle to the distal intima, penetrate to the tunica media, and then exit through the distal intima.
- Repeat this procedure for everting suture of the dorsal wall.
- Reinforcement with U-shaped sutures is performed in several places to prevent bleeding (especially on the posterior and lateral walls) (Scene 9.21).

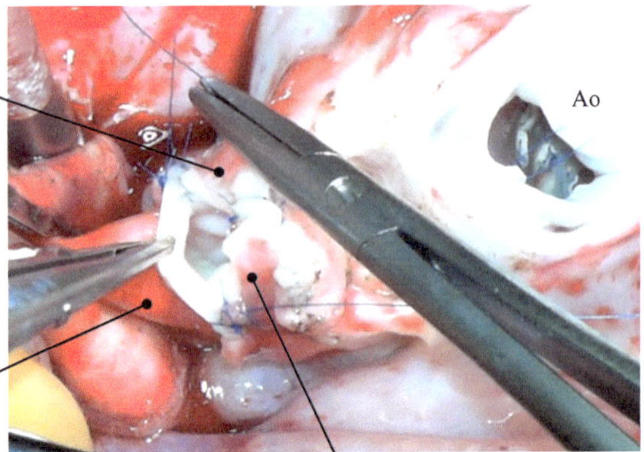

Scene 9.21 Reconstruction of the ascending aorta 2 (Video 09 min 46 s)

- When anastomosing the upper end of the bay window with the distal end of the aorta, be careful not to constrict or deform the upper end of the bay window (Scene 9.22).

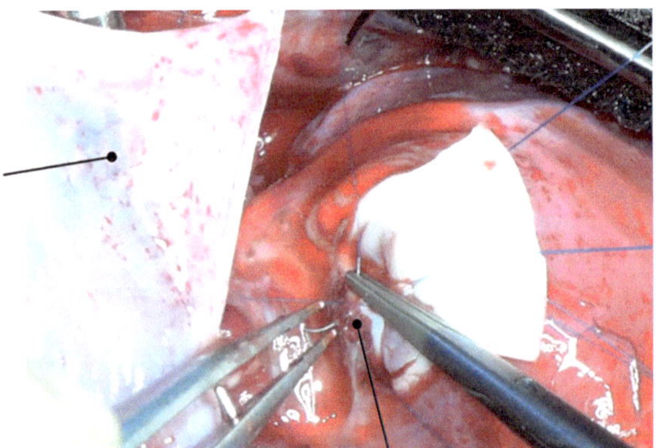

Scene 9.22 Repair of the coronary defects 1 (Video 10 min 46 s)

1. First, the defect of the coronary cuff is supplemented with an autologous pericardial patch.
2. The dorsal aspect of the posterior commissure is fastened to the center of the lower edge of the autologous pericardial patch with a U-shaped suture of 6-0 monofilament suture.
   - In the video case, the right coronary artery orifice was in close proximity to the commissure, so the commissure was sliced and removed from the wall, and the wall of the commissure was used as much as possible for the right coronary artery cuff. Therefore, very little wall remained at the base of the commissure (Scene 9.23).

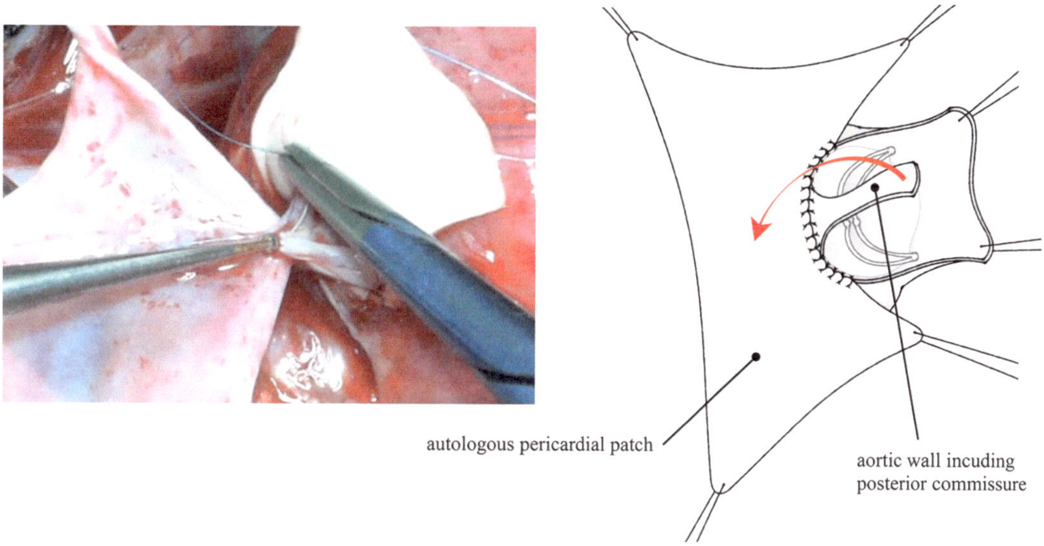

Scene 9.23 Repair of the coronary defects 2 (Video 11 min 26 s)

1 Anastomose the aortic wall including posterior commissure to the autologous pericardial patch (Scene 9.24).

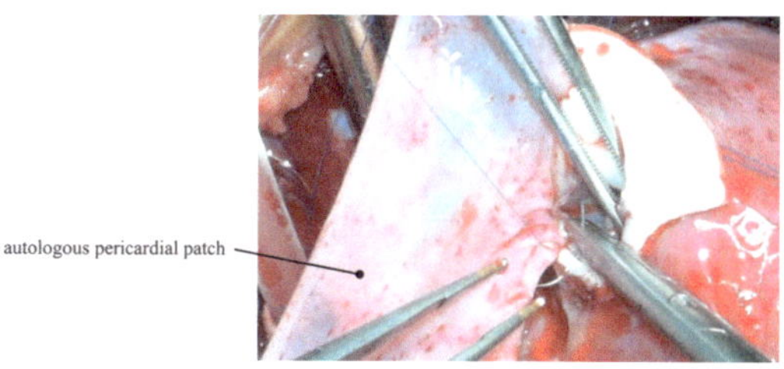

Scene 9.24 Repair of the coronary defects 3 (Video 11 min 54 s)

1 Anastomose the lower end of the autologous pericardial patch to the lower end of the coronary defect (aortic valve attachment site) with a continuous 6-0 monofilament suture.
- The suture should be kept away from the base of the aortic valve.
- The suture should include the surrounding adventitia to prevent bleeding (Scene 9.25).

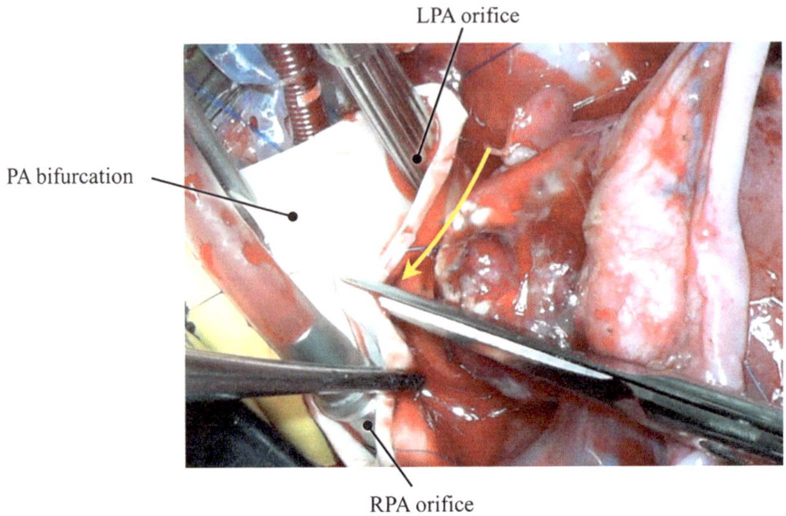

Scene 9.25 Longitudinal incision of the posterior wall of the pulmonary bifurcation (Video 15 min 39 s)

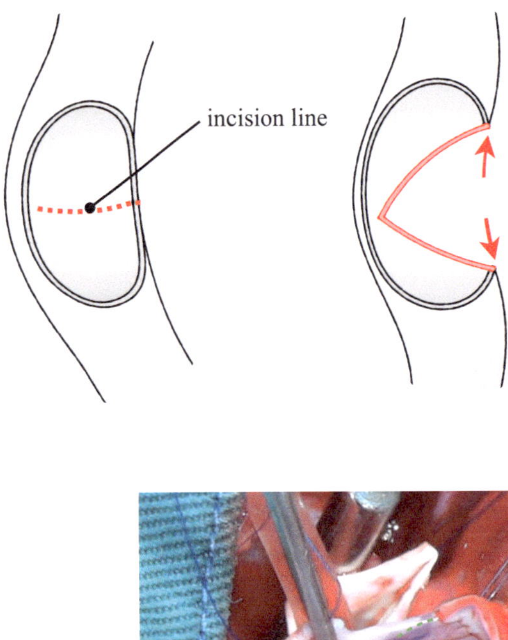

1 Incise the posterior wall of the pulmonary artery bifurcation vertically (*yellow allow*).
  - Incise from the inferior edge of the posterior wall at the center of the bifurcation, through the center of the right and left pulmonary artery orifices, to the anterior wall.
  - The anterior wall may be left approximately 10 mm (a sufficient incision allows for more expansion) (Scene 9.26).

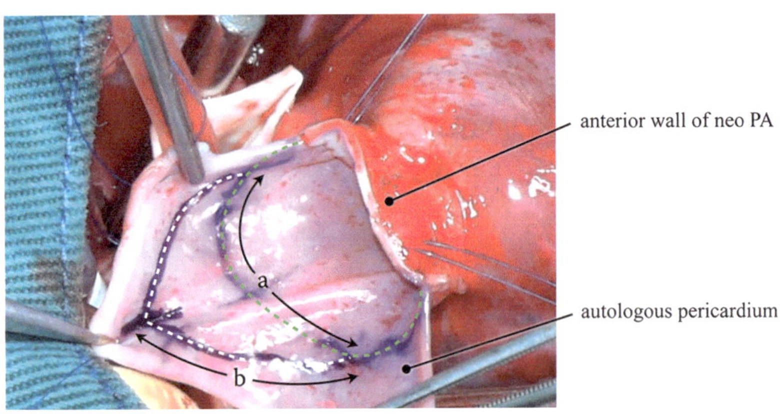

Scene 9.26 Trimming of the autologous pericardial patch (Video 16 min 11 s)

- Compensate the coronary defect and extend the long axis of the pulmonary artery bifurcation with a single fresh autologous pericardial patch.
    1. After suturing the lower half of the autologous pericardial patch to the coronary defect, the patch is marked so that the base of the pulmonary artery is cylindrical according to the height of the anterior wall of the new pulmonary artery (*green dashed line*).
    2. The width of the posterior wall (*a*) is then determined according to the length of the longitudinal extension of the pulmonary artery bifurcation.
    3. The shape of the autologous pericardial patch is determined according to the length of the incision line of the posterior wall of the pulmonary artery bifurcation (*white dashed line*).
    4. The incision length of the posterior wall of the pulmonary artery will be the length of *b* (the autologous pericardial patch should be slightly longer than the incision line).

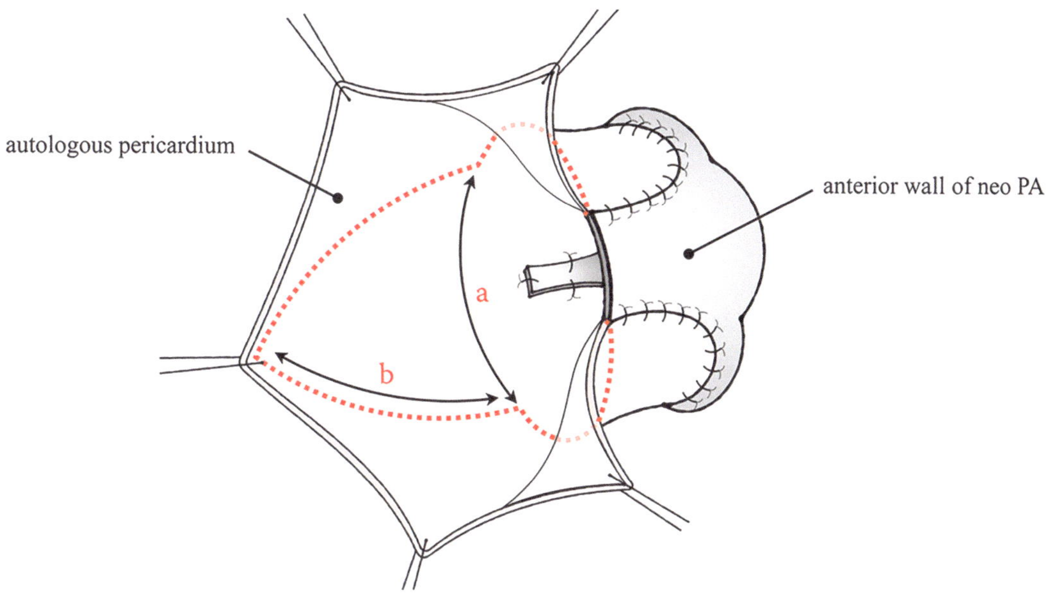

- The posterior wall width (*a*) of the autologous pericardium determines the longitudinal extension distance of the pulmonary artery bifurcation.
- As the length increases, the posterior wall width (*a*) increases.
- The length of *b* is the incision length of the posterior wall of the pulmonary artery (the autologous pericardium side should be trimmed slightly longer).
- The pericardium is harvested in advance in a large rectangular shape (Scene 9.27).

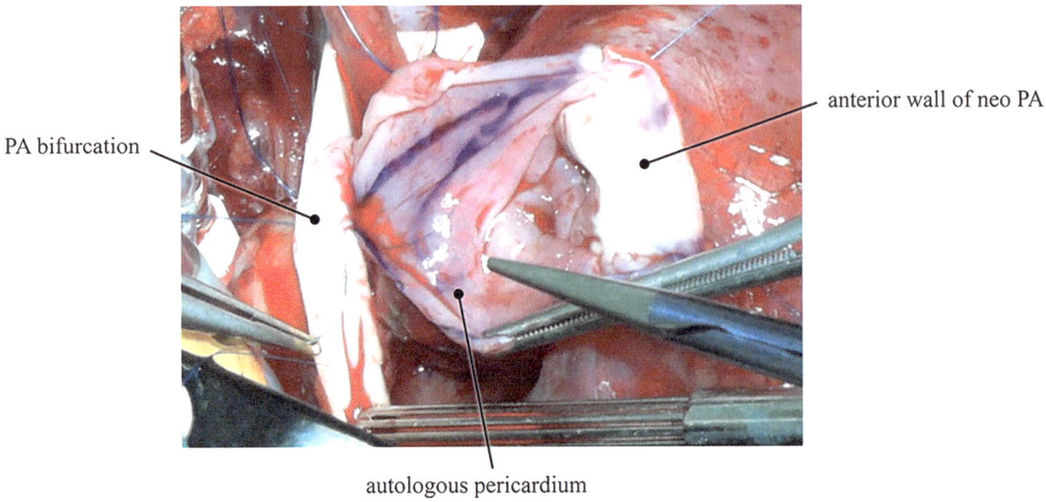

Scene 9.27 Pericardial patch supplementation to the pulmonary bifurcation 1 (Video 16 min 38 s)

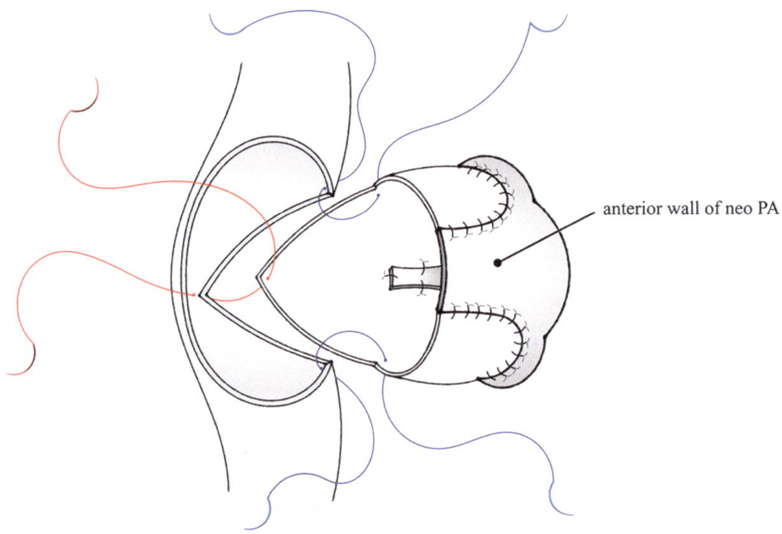

1 The apex of the pericardium is aligned with the leading edge of the pulmonary artery bifurcation incision, and anastomosis is proceeded from this site with a continuous suture of 7-0 or 6-0 monofilament suture (Scene 9.28).

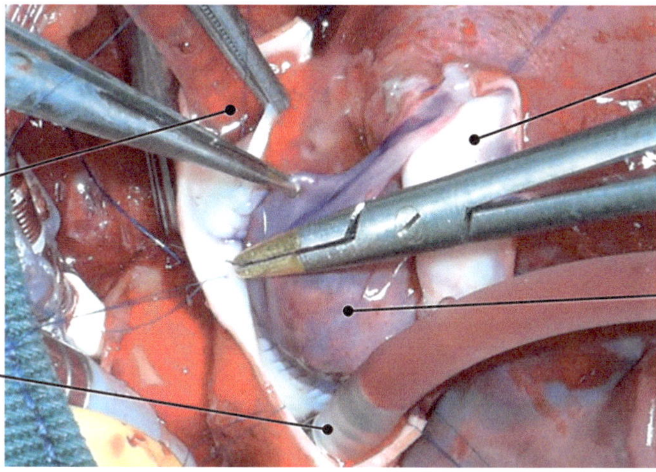

Scene 9.28 Pericardial patch supplementation to the pulmonary bifurcation 2 (Video 18 min 07 s)

1 Anastomose an autologous pericardial patch to the pulmonary artery bifurcation longitudinal incision with a continuous 6-0 monofilament suture (Figures *a-b* and *a-c* below).

- Be careful not to shrink the right and left pulmonary artery openings (Figures *a-b* and *a-c* below) due to the purse-string effect.

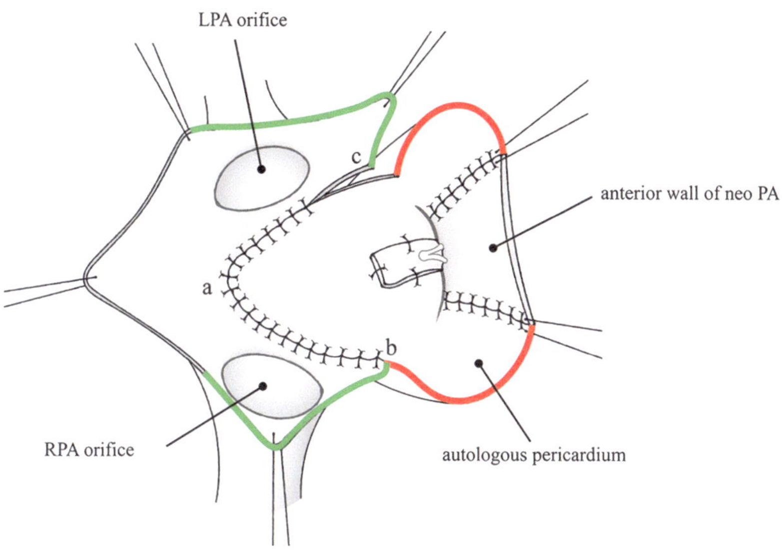

2 Anastomose the lateral wall of the pulmonary artery bifurcation (*green line*) to the autologous pericardial patch and anastomose the anterior wall to the proximal part of the neo pulmonary artery (anterior wall of the old aorta).

- When suturing the lateral wall of the pulmonary artery bifurcation (*green line*) to the autologous pericardial patch (*red line*), be careful not to shrink the pulmonary artery side (*green line*) (if this area is sutured, it will cause bifurcation stenosis) (Scene 9.29).

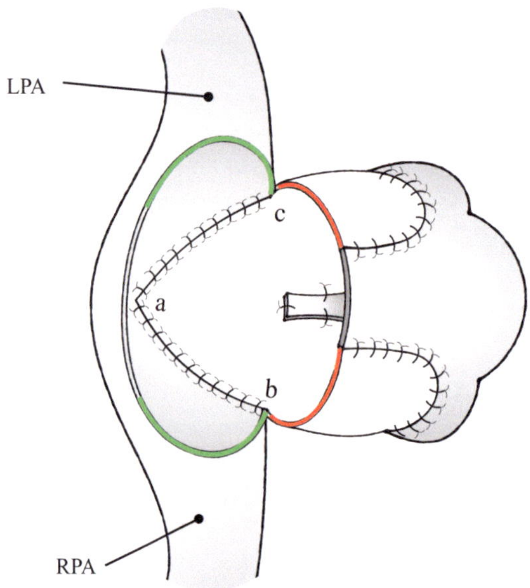

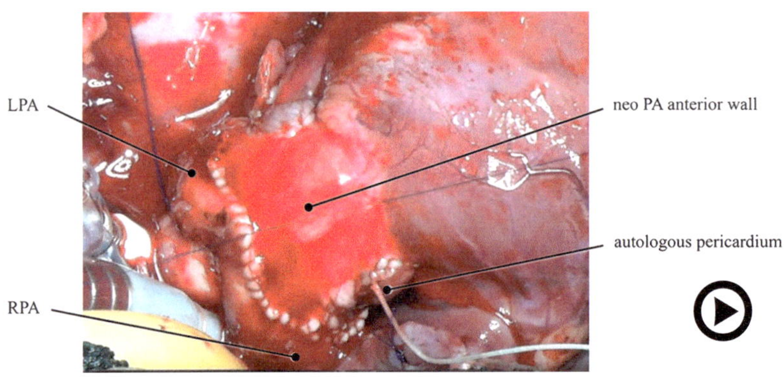

Scene 9.29 Completion of arterial switch operation (Video 20 min 41 s) (▶ https://doi.org/10.1007/000-hkg)

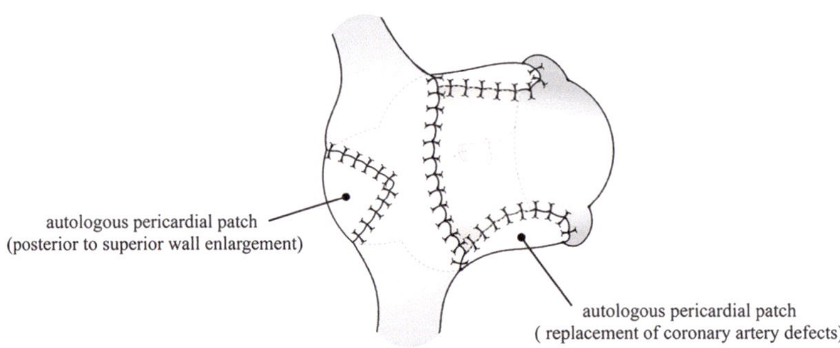

1 The pulmonary artery bifurcation is sufficiently extended longitudinally by the autologous pericardial patch.

2 After completion of the anastomosis, check for overstretching of the pulmonary artery to the left and right pulmonary hilum.

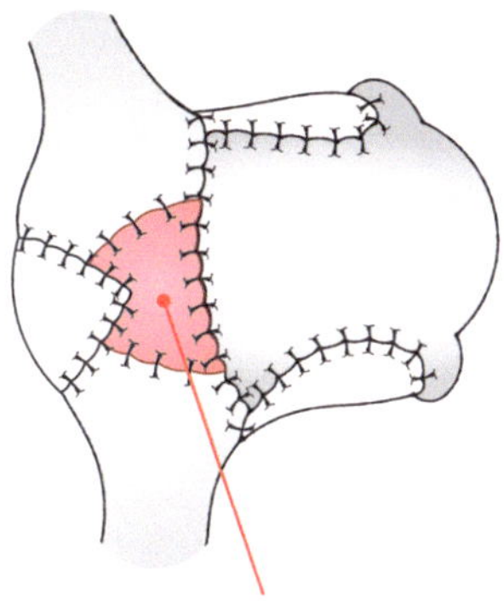

additional autologous pericardial patch (anterior wall augmentation)

- If overstretch remains in the anterior wall of the pulmonary artery, an additional patch is placed anterior to the bifurcation.

References

Original Jatene Method

Jatene AD, Fontes VF, Paulista PP, et al. Successful anatomic correction of transposition of the great vessels. A preliminary report. Arq Bras Cardiol. 1975;28:461–4.

Jatene AD, Fontes VF, Paulista PP, et al. Anatomic correction of transposition of the great vessels. J Thoarac Cardiovasc Surg. 1976;72:364–70.

Lecompte's Maneuver

Lecompte Y, Zannini L, Hazan E, Jarreau MM. Anatomic correction or transposition of the great arteries. J Thorne Cardiovasc Surg. 1981;82:629–6310.

Mee Method

Asou T, Karl TR, Pawade A, Mee RB. Arterial switch: translocation of the intramural coronary artery. Ann Thorac Surg. 1994;57:461–5.

Aubert Method

Aubert J, Pannetier A, Couvelly P, et al. Transposition of the great arteries: new technique for anatomical correction. Br Heart J. 1978;40:204–8.

Imai Method

Kawada M, Imai Y, Kurosawa H, et al. Modification of the Aubert operation. Nippon Kyobu Geka Gakkai Zasshi. 1989;37:1723.

Koshiyama H, Nagashima M, Matsumura G, et al. Arterial switch operation with and without coronary relocation for intramural corom1ry artery. Ann Thorac Surg. 2016;102:1353–9.

Coronary Artery: Shaher Classification

Shaher RM, Puddu GC. Coronary arterial anatomy in compete transposition of the great vessels. Am J Cardiol. 1966;17:355–61.

Coronary Artery: Leiden Classification

Gittenberger-de Groot AC, Sauer U, Oppenheimer-Dekker A, Quaegebeur J. Coronary arterial anatomy in transposition of the great arteries: a morphologic study. Pediatr Cardiol. 1983;4:15–24.

Gittenberger-de Groot AC, Koenraadt WMC, Bartelings MM, et al. Coding of coronary arterial origin and branching in congenital heart disease: the modified Leiden Convention. J Thorac Cardiovasc Surg. 2018;156:2260–9.

Coronary Artery: Yacoub Classification

Yacoub MH, Radley-Smith R. Anatomy of the coronary arteries in transposition of the great arteries and methods for their transfer in anatomical correction. Thorax. 1978;33:418–24.

Trap Door Method

Mee RBB. The arterial switch operation. In: Stark J, de Leval M, editors. Surgery for congenital heart defects. 2nd ed. WB Saunders; 1994. p. 483–500.

Bay-Window Method

Yamagishi M, Shunto K, Fujiwara K, et al. "Bay window" technique for the arterial switch operation of the transposition of the great arteries with complex coronary arteries. Ann Thorac Surg. 2003;75:1768–74.

Yashima M, Yamagishi M, Yaku H. Long-term results of bay window technique for coronary translocation in the arterial switch operation. World J Pediatr Congential Heart Surg. 2019;10:151–6.

Pulmonary Artery Reconstruction: Longitudinal Extension Method

Hongu H, Yamagishi M, Maeda Y, et al. Alternative pulmonary artery reconstruction technique in the arterial switch operation. Eur J Cardiothorac Surg. 2021;60:98–104.

Transposition of the Great Arteries (TGA) and Transposition Type Double Outlet Right Ventricle (TGA Type DORV) with Left Ventricular Outflow Obstruction (LVOTO)

10

1 Morphological Characteristics of TGA and TGA Type DORV with LVOTO

1. *d-TGA (II),*
2. *TGA type DORV (false Taussig-Bing).*
3. *Transitional type between false Taussig-Bing and [SDL} DORV.*

In these cases of TGA or TGA type DORV combined with left LVOTO (pulmonary valve stenosis, subvalvular stenosis), Rastelli, REV, and aortic translocation surgery are indicated instead of arterial switch surgery (Figs. 10.1 and 10.2).

The morphological characteristics of each type are described as follows.

1.1 d-TGA (II) with LVOTO

- Pulmonary artery: left posterior, aortic valve: right anterior.
- Pulmonary artery valve overrides on ventricular septum.
- VSD is present below the pulmonary artery valve.
- Pulmonary artery and mitral valve are continuous (fibrous continuity).
- Pulmonary artery overrides on ventricular septum more than 50%, but because pulmonary artery and mitral valve are continuous, diagnosis is TGA (II), not DORV (false Taussig-Bing).
- There is concern that the right ventricular effective volume is reduced by the intraventricular conduit.

Supplementary Information The online version contains supplementary material available at https://doi.org/10.1007/978-981-96-6194-7_10. The videos can be accessed individually by clicking the DOI link in the accompanying figure caption or by scanning this link with the SN More Media App.

M. Yamagishi, *Surgical Treatment of Congenital Heart Disease*,
https://doi.org/10.1007/978-981-96-6194-7_10

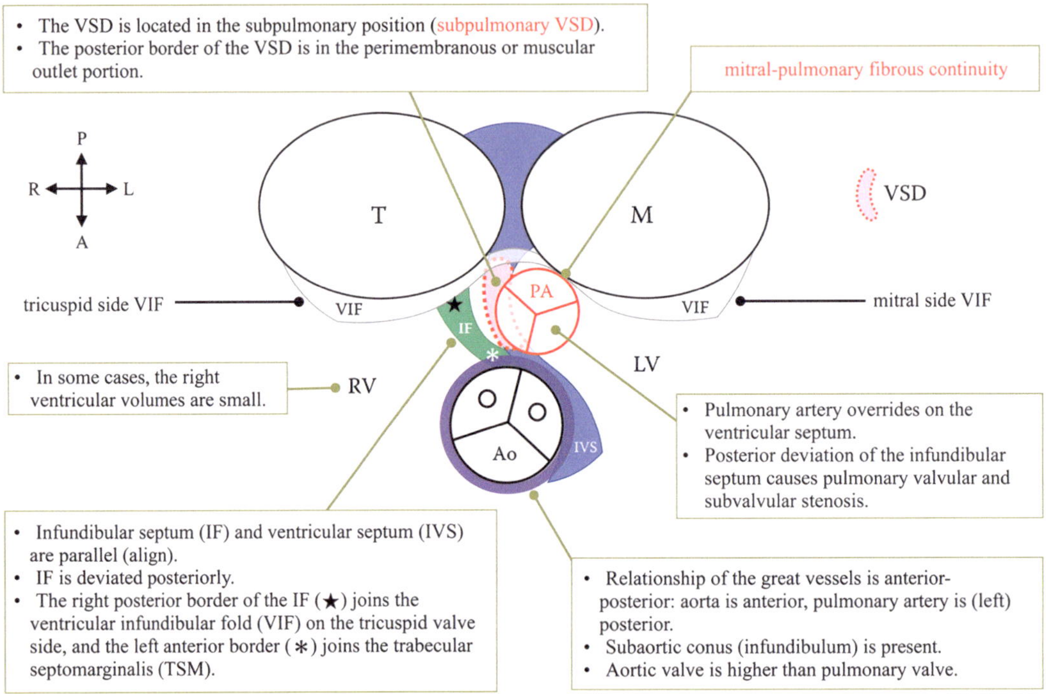

Fig. 10.1 Morphological characteristics of d-TGA (II) with LVOTO

Fig. 10.2 CT image of d-TGA (II) with LVOTO

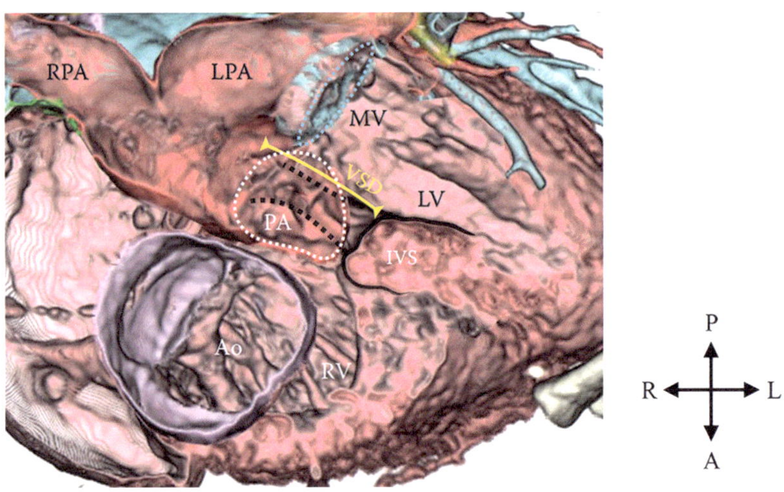

1.2 TGA Type DORV (False Taussig-Bing) with LVOTO

The morphology of false Taussig-Bing is similar to that of d-TGA (II), but a ventriculo-infundibular fold (VIF) appears between the pulmonary and mitral valves and the fibrous continuity disappears. In addition, more than 50% of the pulmonary arteries override on the ventricular septum, which fulfills the diagnostic criteria for DORV. The degree of pulmonary valve overriding varies, and in some cases, the pulmonary valve completely originates from the right ventricle (Figs. 10.3 and 10.4).

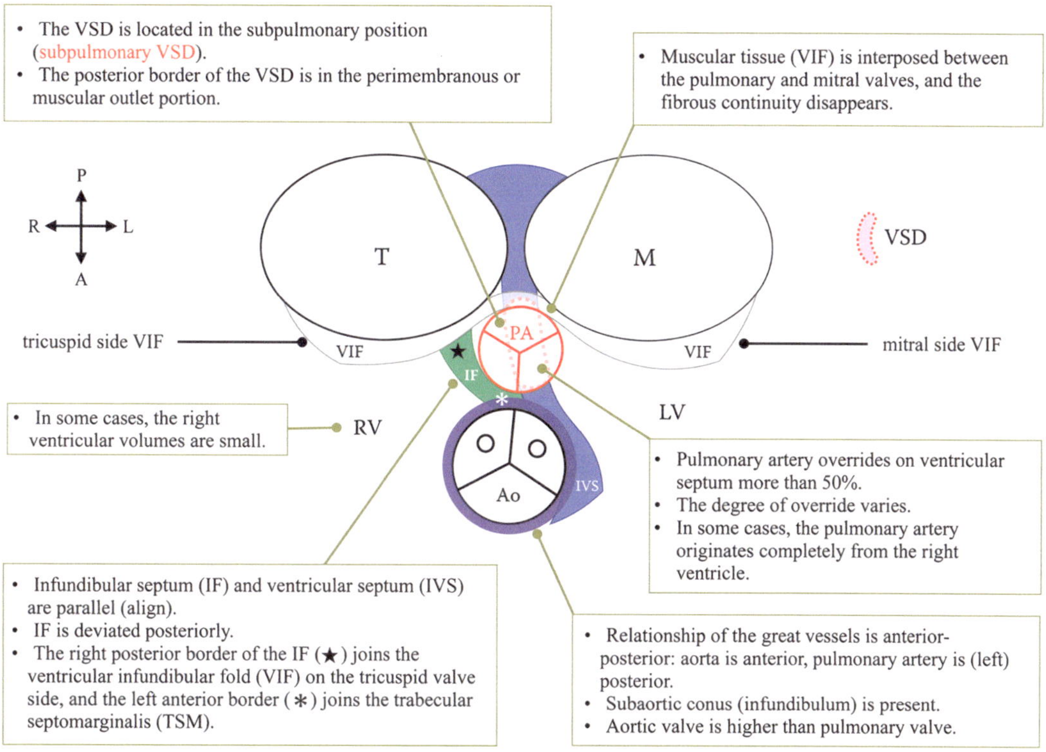

Fig. 10.3 Morphological characteristics of false Taussig-Bing with LVOTO

Fig. 10.4 CT image of false Taussig-Bing with LVOTO

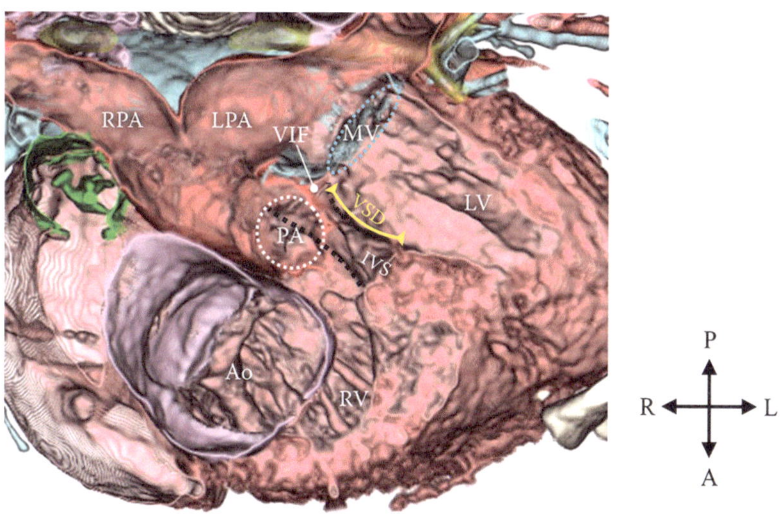

- Pulmonary artery valve: posterior, more than 50% overriding on ventricular septum; aortic valve: anterior.
- Pulmonary artery valve is further deviated to the right than in d-TGA (II), the fibrous continuity between the pulmonary artery valve and mitral valve is severed, and muscular tissue (VIF) appears (fulfilling the diagnostic criteria for DORV).
- VSD is present below the pulmonary valve, but slightly anteriorly deviated.
- Aortic valve is originates completely from right ventricle.
- VSD is large enough but far from the aortic valve.

In false Taussig-Bing, the VSD is located below the posterior pulmonary valve (subpulmonary VSD). Because the aortic valve is located anteriorly, a long intraventricular conduit must be created in the right ventricle to divert intraventricular blood flow from the VSD to the aortic valve. The infundibular septum (IF) is parallel to the interventricular septum (IVS) and provides a barrier to blood flow from the VSD to the aortic valve. The chordae tendineae and papillary muscles of the tricuspid valve also obstruct the intraventricular conduit (Fig. 10.5).

■ *Intracardiac configuration viewed from the right ventricular side*

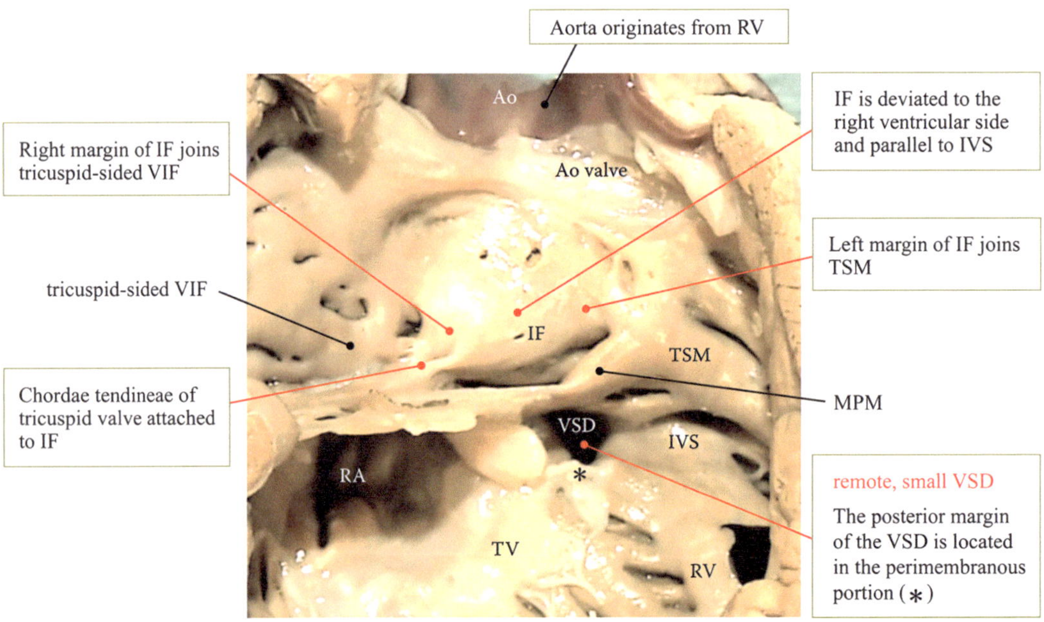

Fig. 10.5 Heart specimen of false Taussig-Bing with LVOTO

■ *Intracardiac configuration viewed from the left ventricular side*

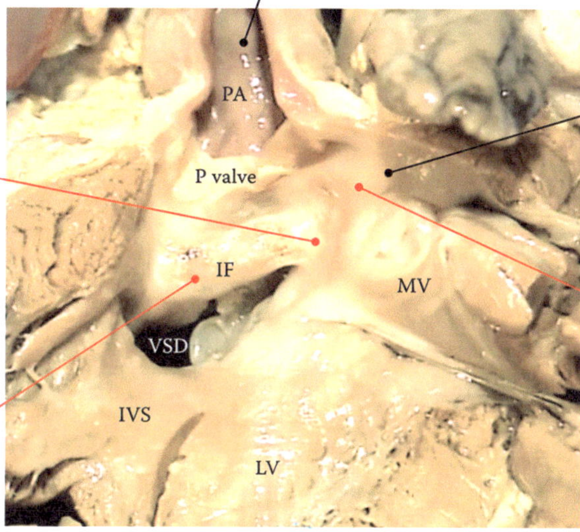

Ao aorta, *Ao valve* aortic valve, *PA* pulmonary artery, *P valve* pulmonary valve, *IF* infundibular septum, *TSM* trabecular septomarginalis, *VIF* ventriculo-infundibular septum, *IVS* interventricular septum, *VSD* ventricular septal defect, *TV* tricuspid valve, *MV* mitral valve, *RV* right ventricle, *LV* left ventricle, *RA* right atrium, *MPM* medial papillary muscle

1.3 Transitional Type Between False Taussig-Bing and [SDL} DORV with LVOTO

In the transitional forms of false Taussig-Bing and {SDL}DORV, the aorta also rides on the ventricular septum. The VSD is extended anteriorly below the aortic valve, but the posterior part of the VSD still exists below the pulmonary valve (doubly committed VSD). In the transitional type, in which the VSD is anteriorly deviated but mainly exists below the pulmonary valve, aortic translocation operations can be performed to transpose the aortic valve posteriorly to secure straight blood flow pathway from the left ventricle to the aortic valve (Figs. 10.6 and 10.7).

- Pulmonary artery: deviated to the right and becomes right posteriorly.
- Aortic valve: slightly deviated to the left and closer to the IVS.
- Pulmonary valve overrides on the ventricular septum, but is further deviated to the right than in d-TGA (II), with muscular tissue (VIF) interposed between the pulmonary valve and mitral valve (fulfilling the diagnostic criteria for DORV).
- VSD is present below the pulmonary valve but is extended anteriorly.
- The aorta originates completely from the right ventricle.

1.4 Morphological Checkpoints for Selecting the Appropriate Surgical Procedure

In order to determine the appropriate procedure, the items listed below should be checked (Fig. 10.8).

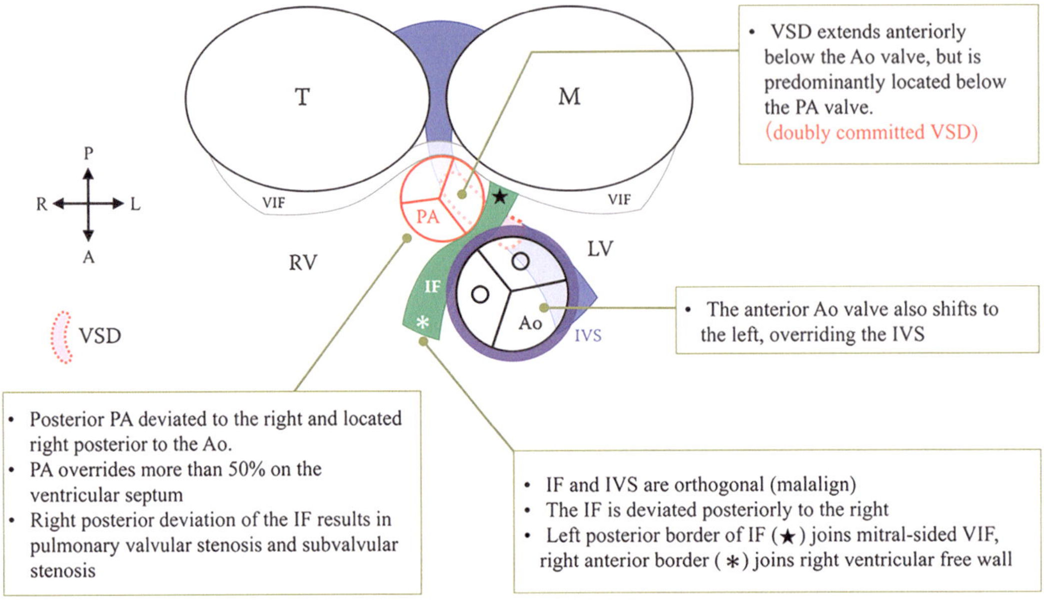

Fig. 10.6 Morphological characteristics of transitional type between false Taussig-Bing and [SDL} DORV with LVOTO

Fig. 10.7 CT image of transitional type between false Taussig-Bing and [SDL} DORV with LVOTO

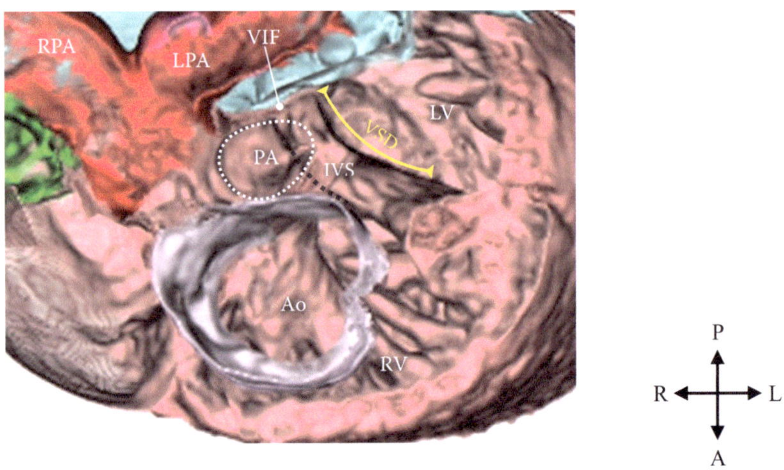

relationship of great arteries

- antero-posterior, side-by-side, right oblique, left oblique

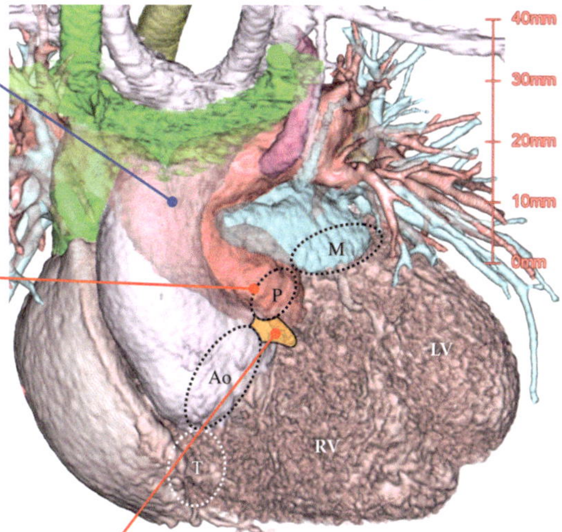

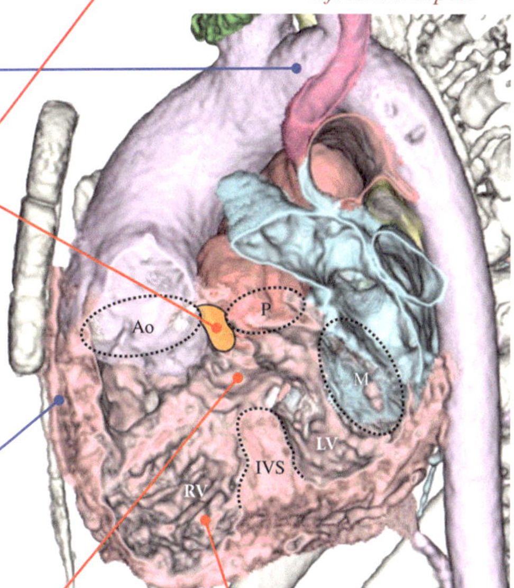

pulmonary artery

- presence or absence of bifurcation stenosis, peripheral stenosis (presence or absence of BT shunt anastomotic stenosis)
- growth degree (PA index)
- bifurcation morphology
- main pulmonary artery morphology

pulmonary valve, subpulmonary area

- valve morphology (valve leaflet)
- degree of annular stenosis
- presence or absence of subvalvular stenosis
- whether and to what degree there is overriding on the ventricular septum

coronary arteries

- origin, running pattern
- presence or absence of running anterior to the right ventricular outflow tract
- presence or absence of running posterior to the pulmonary annulus

aortic arch

- presence or absence of coarctation and interruption

infundibular septum

- relationship to ventricular septum (parallel, orthogonal)
- length (with or without extension toward the apex)
- What tissues do the two edges of the funnel septum connect ?
  ventriculoinfundibular fold: VIF (tricuspid and mitral)
  trabecular septomarginalis: TSM
  right ventricular free wall, etc.
- presence or absence of chordae tendineae of the tricuspid valve to the infundibular septum

right ventricular outflow tract

- space behind anterior chest wall
  Is there room for an extracardiac conduit ?
- Coronary artery right ventricular branch
  Is there space in the anterior wall of the right ventricle to create an opening for an extracardiac conduit ?

ventricular septal defect

- location: is the posterior margin a membranous septum or a muscular septum?
- size: Is it large enough to serve as a left ventricular outflow tract ? Is there a need for enlargement?
- direction of extension (anterior, apical)
- relationship to infundibular septum
- What is its relationship (distance) to the semilunar valve?
- Type of VSD: subpulmonary VSD, doubly committed VSD, subaortic VSD, remote VSD

right ventricular morphology

- right ventricular volume
  degree of postoperative decrease in effective right ventricular volume (residual right ventricular volume)
- Intracardiac conduit
  route setting
  Can it be anastomosed to the right ventricular inner wall (trabeculation)?

Fig. 10.8 Morphological checkpoints

2 Conventional Procedures

In patients with left ventricular outflow tract stenosis (LVOTO) is combined with complete transposition of the great vessels (TGA) or transposition type of double outlet right ventricle (DORV), arterial switch operation using the pulmonary valve for the body circulation cannot be applied except for very mild pulmonary valve stenosis.

Conventional operations for TGA and TGA type DORV with LVOTO include Rastelli operation and Réparation a l'étage ventriculaire (REV). Both procedures require intraventricular rerouting to direct blood flow from the left ventricle through the VSD to the aortic valve (Fig. 10.9).

2.1 Intraventricular Rerouting for TGA and TGA Type DORV

1 *Pathway of systemic blood flow (intraventricular conduit)*
- Blood flow through the VSD is directed toward the inner wall of the intracardiac conduit and bends toward the aortic valve after hitting the inner wall of the conduit.
- This may cause turbulence and large energy losses in the conduit.
- If the intracardiac conduit is folded, turbulent flow may cause thrombus formation and intimal thickening.
- The conduit patch must be trimmed to prevent twisting or folding of the long conduit.
- The presence of papillary muscles, chordae tendineae, or other structures along the anastomotic route of the intracardiac conduit from the VSD to the aortic valve should be checked.
- If the chordae tendineae of the tricuspid valve are attached to the infundibular septum, they should be cut at the base and reconstructed by suturing the chordae tendineae to the conduit wall after construction

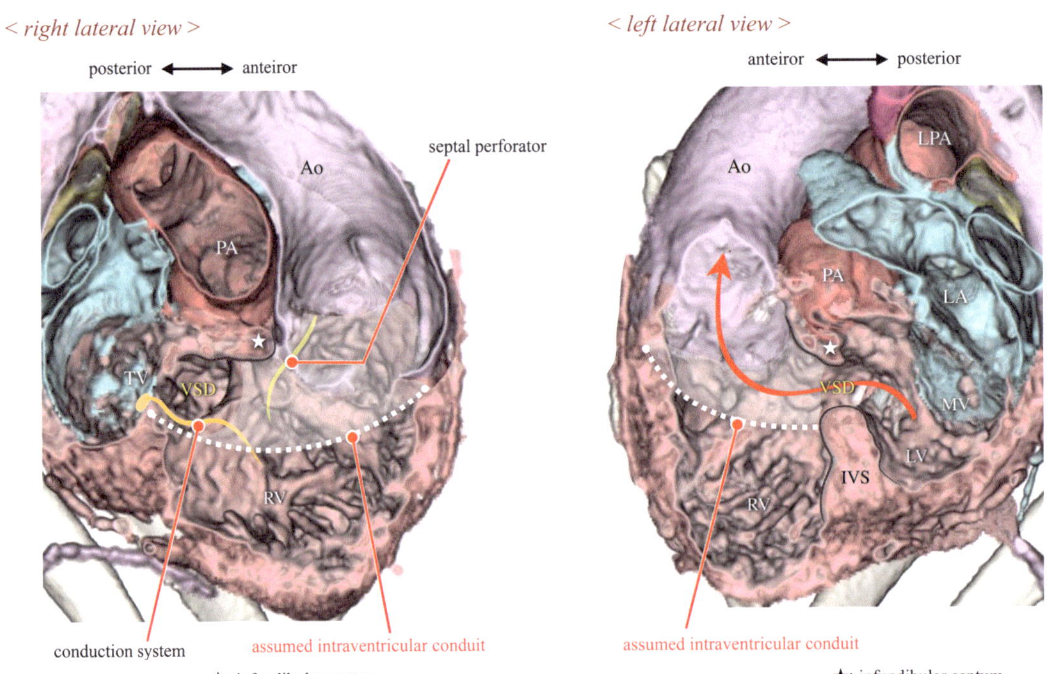

Fig. 10.9 Intraventricular rerouting

of the intraventricular conduit (it is important to confirm that no tricuspid regurgitation has occurred at this time).
- Because the right ventricular trabeculation is rough, care must be taken to avoid leaks when anastomosing the intraventricular conduit to the inner wall of the right ventricle (especially the area along the aortic annulus and the free wall of the right ventricle).

2 *Material of intraventricular conduit*
- Intraventricular conduits are better with flat patches than with curved prosthetic grafts.
- Dacron prosthetic grafts may cause intimal hyperplasia, and heterogeneous pericardium may cause calcification.
- An ePTFE patch is the preferred material for the intraventricular conduit.

3 *Enlargement of VSD*
- The VSD serves as the left ventricular outflow tract and must be enlarged in the case of a narrow VSD.
- The VSD cannot be enlarged posteriorly because the conduction system runs behind the VSD (on the inflow side).
- In some cases, the VSD cannot be enlarged sufficiently anteriorly because of the presence of coronary artery septal branches.
- In cases that require VSD enlargement, the infundibular septum, which obstructs blood flow, should be resected first.
- Since the pulmonary artery is cut and closed, there is no need to consider damage to the pulmonary valve caused by resection of the infundibular septum.
- The infundibular septum is parallel to the ventricular septum and is perpendicular to the direction of blood flow to provide a barrier to blood flow from the left ventricle through the VSD.

4 *Right ventricular volume*
- Small right ventricular volumes are seen in some cases.
- An intraventricular conduit further reduces the effective right ventricular volume. After an intraventricular conduit is placed, a residual right ventricular volume of approximately 70% of normal is required.

2.2 Conventional Procedure: Rastelli Operation

An intraventricular rerouting procedure of blood flow is performed to create a blood flow pathway from the left ventricle to the aortic valve (left ventricular outflow tract) via the VSD.

The right ventricular pulmonary artery is reconstructed using an extracardiac conduit (prosthetic valved conduit, homograft, etc.) (Figs. 10.10, 10.11, and 10.12).

1 Intraventricular conduit creates a left ventricular outflow tract through the VSD to the aortic valve (intraventricular rerouting).
2 The space below the pulmonary valve is also part of the left ventricular outflow tract.

Fig. 10.10 Schematic diagram of Rastelli operation

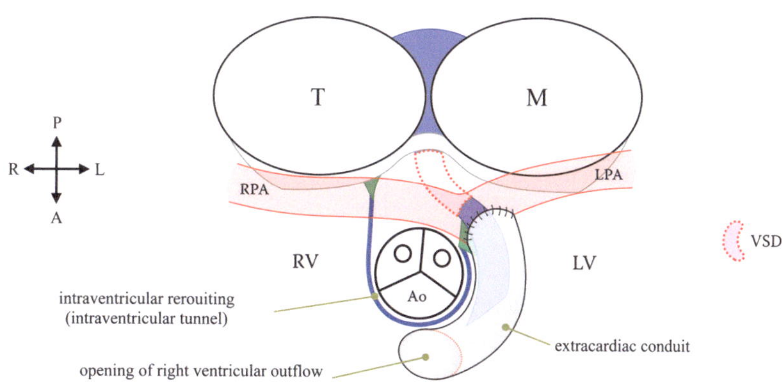

Opening of right ventricular outflow

- The opening for conduit anastomosis should always be created at the right ventricular outflow portion, not the inflow portion.
- Ensure that there are no major coronary arteries (left anterior descending, right ventricular) running to the site of the opening.
- The thickened myocardial bundle in the right ventricular outflow tract is to be resected, so any coronary artery that may be perfusing the thickened myocardial bundle may be cut off.

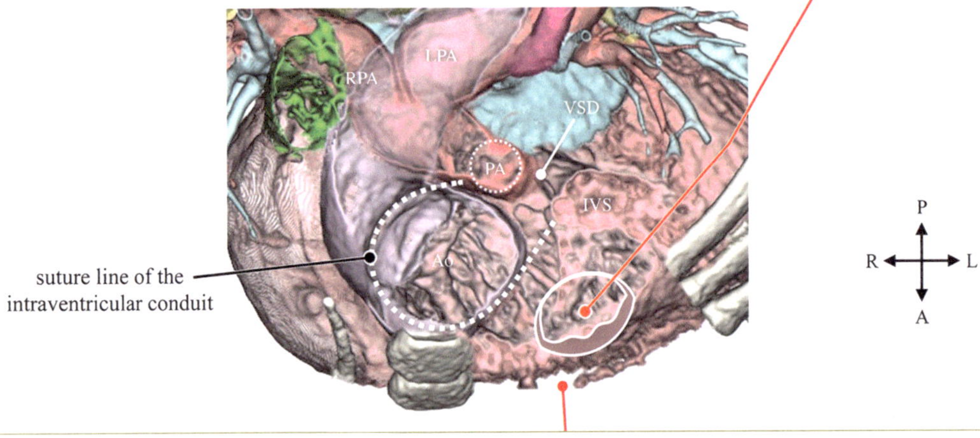

Space behind anterior chest wall

- Sufficient space is required between the right ventricular outflow tract and the anterior chest wall for an extracardic conduit, but the space behind anterior chest wall is narrow due to the anterior aorta.
- The possibility of compression of the conduit from the anterior chest wall must be considered.

Fig. 10.11 CT image and assumed suture line of the intraventricular conduit and RV opening

3 The main pulmonary artery is transected at its origin.
4 The right ventricular outflow tract is incised longitudinally.
5 An extracardiac conduit is used to create a blood channel between the right ventricular outflow tract opening and the pulmonary artery bifurcation.

2.3 Conventional Procedure: Réparation a l'étage Ventriculaire (REV)

The left ventricular outflow tract (left ventricular outflow tract) is created from the left ventricle to the aortic valve via the VSD by intraventricular rerouting of blood flow. Anterior transposition of the pulmonary artery and direct anastomosis between the right ventricle and the pulmonary artery (to maintain autologous tissue continuity of the posterior wall of the pulmonary artery) (Figs. 10.13, 10.14, and 10.15).

1 Intraventricular blood flow diversion is the same as the Rastelli procedure.
2 The aorta is once cut off and the pulmonary artery is transposed anteriorly.
3 The posterior wall of the anteriorly transposed pulmonary artery bifurcation is anastomosed directly to the right ventricular outflow tract orifice.
4 The anterior surface of the right ventricular outflow tract is enlarged using a monocuspid patch.
5 Use of a conduit can be avoided, but the anteriorly translocated pulmonary artery bifurca-

Assumed RV-PA extracardiac conduit

- When using a conduit with a bulging sinus, the valve (sinus) should be positioned closer to the pulmonary artery bifurcation to avoid compression from the anterior chest wall.
- In cases where compression from the anterior thoracic wall is a concern, consider a smaller diameter conduit.
- To preserve right ventricular function and avoid blood flow energy loss, the right ventricular orifice should always be located in the outflow tract, not in the right ventricular inlet or trabecular portion.

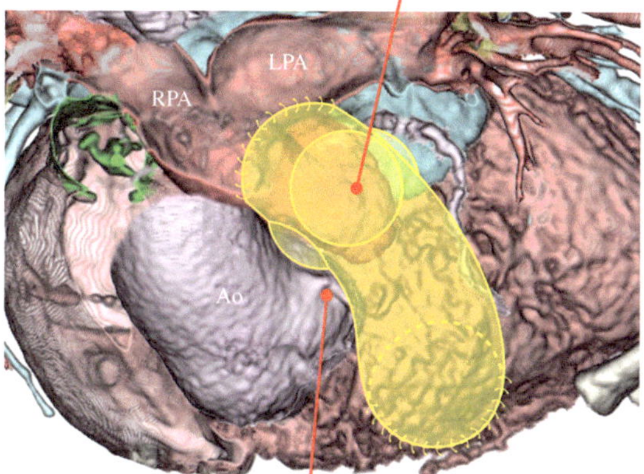

Origin of the right coronary artery

- In cases where the origin of the right coronary artery is on the left side of the aorta, care should be taken to avoid compression of the origin of the right coronary artery by a conduit.

Fig. 10.12 CT image and assumed RV-PA extracardiac conduit

Fig. 10.13 Schematic diagram of REV operation

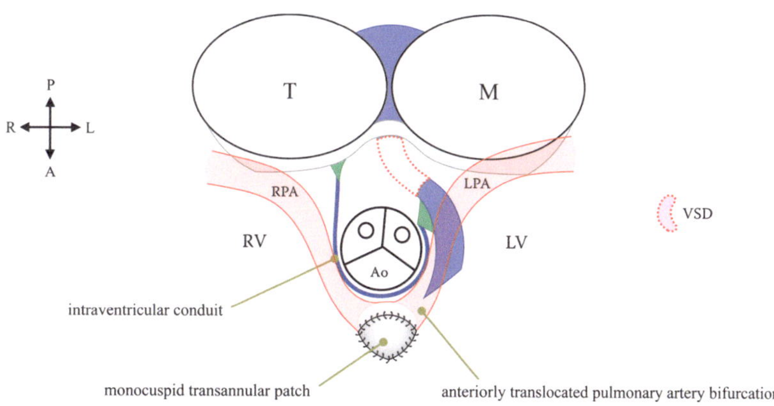

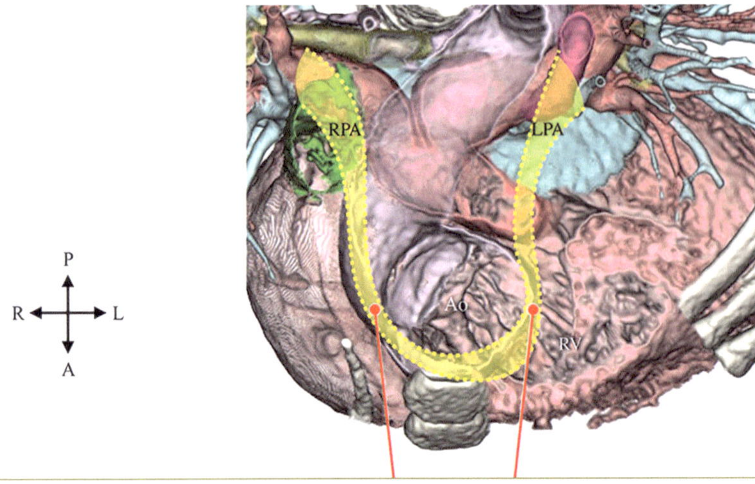

Right and left pulmonary arteries

- An anteriorly located aorta is often dilated due to increased aortic flow caused by decreased pulmonary-to-body blood flow ratio.
- Therefore, if the pulmonary artery bifurcation is transposed anteriorly, as in the assumed line, there is concern that the left and right pulmonary arteries may be hyperextended, resulting in stenosis.

Fig. 10.14 CT image and assumed right and left pulmonary arteries after REV operation

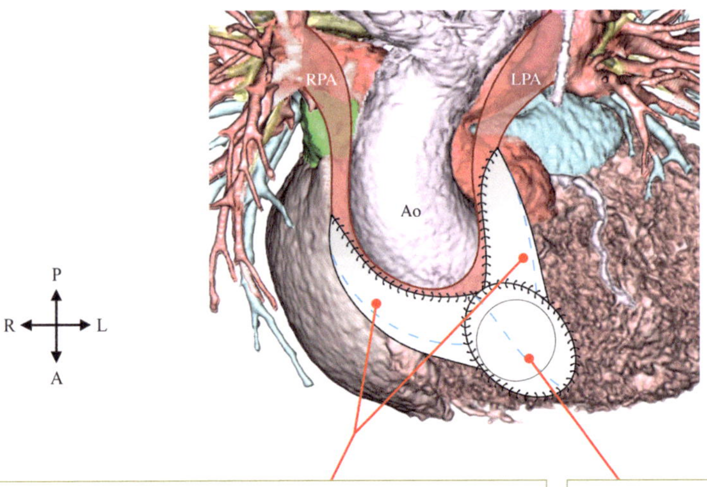

Augmentation of right and left pulmonary arteries

- To avoid stenosis, the right and left pulmonary arteries from the bifurcation to the peripheral pulmonary arteries should be augmented with a supplement such as autologous pericardium.
- Pulmonary bifurcation augmentation allows short-axis widening, but not long-axis extension, so late restenosis should be considered.

Augmentation of RVOT anterior wall

- Autologous tissue continuity of the posterior wall can be reconstructed, but the anterior wall must be augmented with a monocuspid transannular patch.

Fig. 10.15 Bilateral PA augmentation and RVOT reconstruction

tion (left and right pulmonary arteries) is hyperextended by the remaining posterior large aorta.

ESSENTIALS Problems of Rastelli Operation and REV

1. Intraventricular rerouting may be difficult in patients with remote VSD or small VSD. In particular, perimembranous inlet VSD cases localized to the ventricular inflow portion require a long, oversized intraventricular conduit into the right ventricle, which greatly reduces the remaining effective right ventricular volume as well as the concern of intraventricular conduit stenosis (left ventricular outflow tract stenosis). Suturing to the intraventricular conduit may be difficult because the right ventricular wall has a rough trabecular structure.
2. In this group of patients, the infundibular septum is parallel to the ventricular septum, which makes the infundibular septum orthogonal to the left ventricular outflow tract from the VSD to the aortic valve, thus creating a barrier to blood flow. In some cases, the chordae tendineae of the tricuspid valve attach to the infundibular septum.
3. After intraventricular rerouting, left ventricular outflow tract from the VSD to the aortic valve is a tortuous path for blood flow. Turbulent blood flow in the intracardiac conduit causes energy loss and increased shear stress on the conduit wall, which may lead to intimal hyperplasia and stenosis.
4. A residual right ventricular volume of at least 70% of normal is essential to maintain right ventricular function after surgery. If Rastelli or REV surgery is indicated, the reduction in residual effective right ventricular volume due to an additional intraventricular conduit should be considered. Biventricular repair of the hypoplastic right ventricle by both conventional techniques is difficult because of the small volume of the right ventricle in some cases.
5. The Rastelli procedure uses an extracardiac conduit for right ventricular outflow tract reconstruction, leaving the possibility of reoperation due to conduit stenosis. Although the REV procedure preserves autologous tissue continuity, there is concern about stenosis of the pulmonary artery bifurcation due to the anterior transposition of the aorta and hyperextension of the left and right pulmonary arteries. Because the pulmonary valve cannot be preserved, pulmonary regurgitation is also a problem.

3 Aortic Translocation

In contrast to conventional operations, aortic translocations (Nikaidoh operation, half-turned truncal switch operation) were developed. Aortic translocation is a procedure in which the aortic valve is moved into the outflow tract of the left ventricle. Although the aorta overrides on the ventricular septum postoperatively, the reconstructed left ventricular outflow tract is almost straight, and the remaining VSD can be closed with an almost flat patch. Because it does not use the VSD as the sole left ventricular outflow tract, it can be adapted to remote VSD and small VSD cases. The left ventricular outflow tract occupies a smaller volume of the right ventricle, so the effective volume of the right ventricle is not greatly reduced, and it can be applied to a hypoplastic right ventricle.

Aortic translocation operation is a useful technique to achieve ideal hemodynamics (Fig. 10.16).

3.1 Nikaidoh Operation

Only the aortic valve is harvested and the pulmonary valve is resected without preserving the pulmonary valve. There are two methods: *par-*

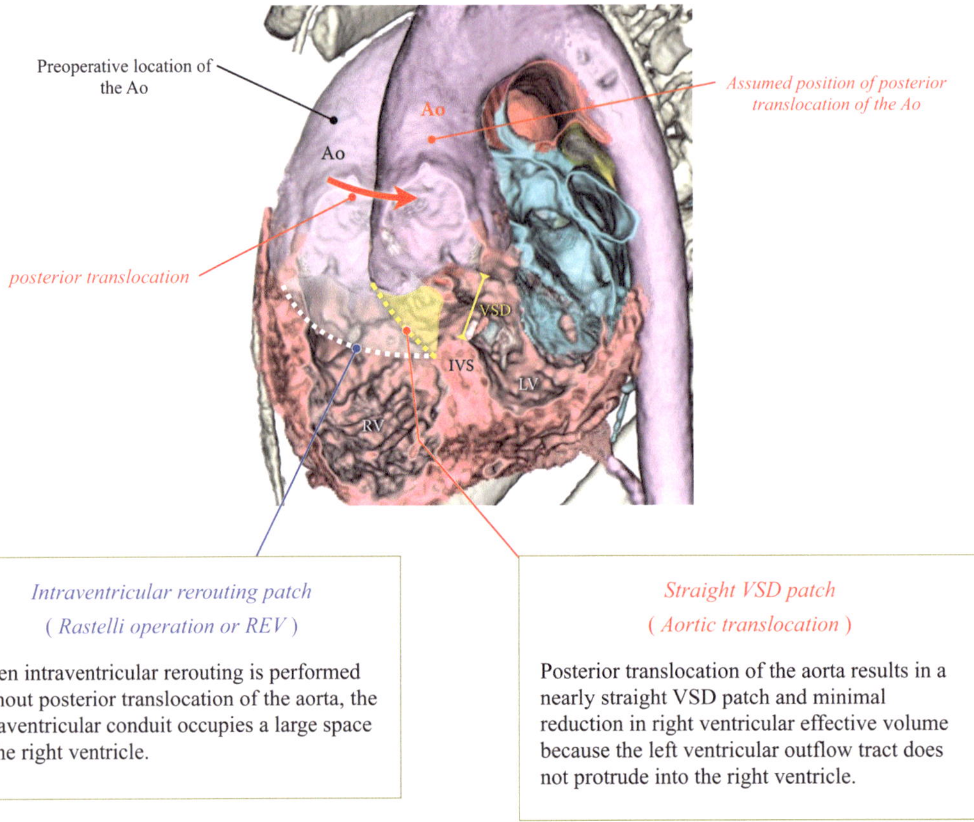

Fig. 10.16 Assumed CT image of posterior translocation of the aorta

allel translocation, in which the aortic valve is moved backward with the coronary artery attached to the aorta, or *pivot translocation*, in which the right coronary artery is removed once and the left coronary artery is rotated around its origin.

Pivot translocation requires reconstruction of the right coronary artery and supplementation of the defect. A monocuspid patch or other supplement is required for the right ventricular outflow tract.

In the original method, the pulmonary artery is reconstructed posterior to the aorta, but the bifurcation can be moved anteriorly (Figs. 10.17 and 10.18).

- Parallel translocation is performed with both coronary arteries intact.
- Incising around the aortic valve at the origin of the coronary artery is difficult because the coronary arteries are not resected.
- In cases of severe stenosis, the aortic valve is posteriorly translocated a short distance, so the coronary arteries are not stretched too far, but care should be taken to avoid overstretching.
- In cases of mild to moderate stenosis, the posterior translocation distance of the aortic valve is longer, so overstretching of the coronary artery is inevitable. Therefore, parallel translocation should be avoided in cases of mild to moderate stenosis.

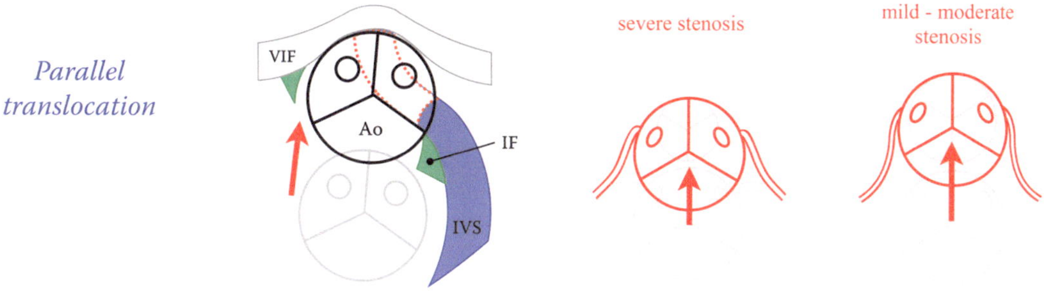

Fig. 10.17 Nikaidoh operation—parallel translocation and pivot translocation

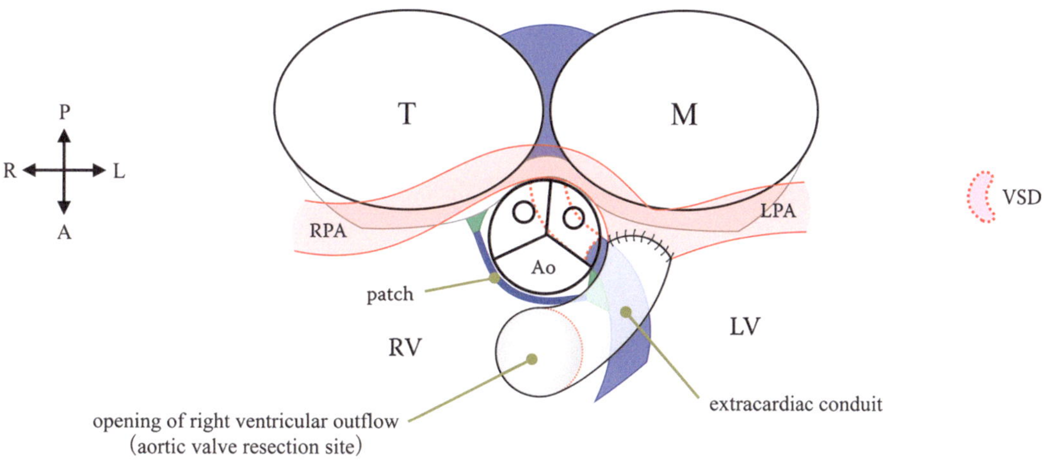

Fig. 10.18 Nikaidoh operation—RVOT reconstruction

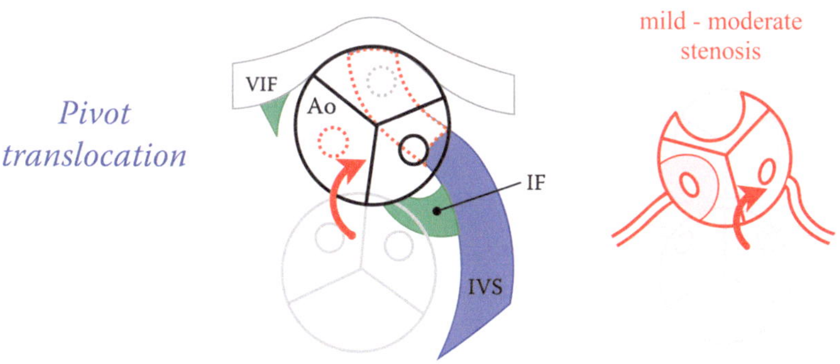

- The resected aortic valve is rotated, leaving intact the left coronary artery and a subaortic muscle bar and infundibular septum beneath the left coronary artery origin.
- Note the deformation of the aortic valve (left coronary apex) during rotation.
- The right coronary artery is once resected and anastomosed to the rotated aortic wall. The right coronary artery should be replaced with a prosthetic material.
- This procedure can be used in cases of mild to moderate stenosis.

A large intraventricular conduit is not required for posterior translocation of the aortic valve.

The aortic valve rests on the ventricular septum. The left ventricular outflow tract is straightened.

The pulmonary artery bifurcation and right ventricular outflow tract orifice (aortic valve resection site) are reconstructed with a monocuspid patch or extracardiac conduit.

This technique can be used for mild to moderate stenosis.

3.2 Half-Turned Truncal Switch Operation

The aortic and pulmonary valves are harvested as a truncal block and the truncal block is rotated 180°. Both the right and left coronary arteries are resected, and after rotation of the truncal block, the coronary artery is re-sutured to the contralateral coronary artery defect. The aorta is translocated posteriorly and the pulmonary artery bifurcation is translocated anterior to the aorta. The pulmonary valve is sutured to the opening of the right ventricular outflow tract. In cases of moderate or severe pulmonary stenosis, a monocuspid patch is used to enlarge the pulmonary valve annulus. Pulmonary valve commissurotomy is performed for mild stenosis. The pulmonary valve annulus should be preserved (Figs. 10.19, 10.20, and 10.21).

- The aortic and pulmonary valves are resected as a single truncal block and rotated 180°.
- Both coronary arteries are resected and re-anastomosed to the contralateral coronary artery defect after 180° rotation of the truncal block.
- In the disease group for which this technique is indicated, the ventricular septum and infundibular septum are in parallel, allowing for 180° rotation.
- This procedure also utilizes the pulmonary valve.
- Care must be taken to avoid damage to the atrioventricular valve when harvesting the truncal block.
- In cases of severe pulmonary stenosis, the distance of posterior translocation of the aortic valve is short.
- The resected coronary button corresponds to the contralateral coronary artery defect rotated 180°.

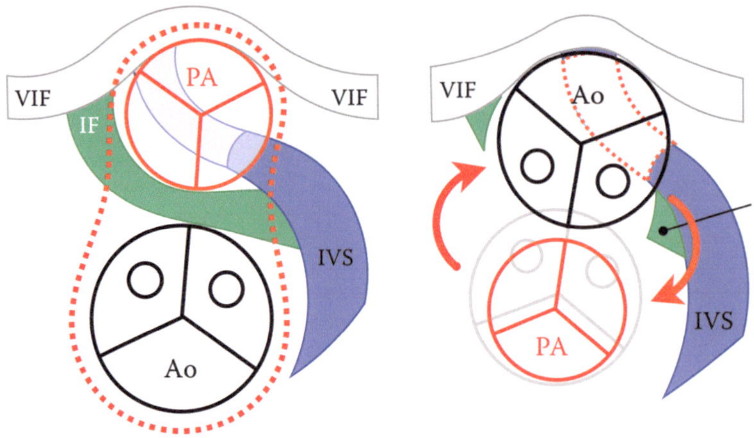

Fig. 10.19 Half-turned truncal switch operation

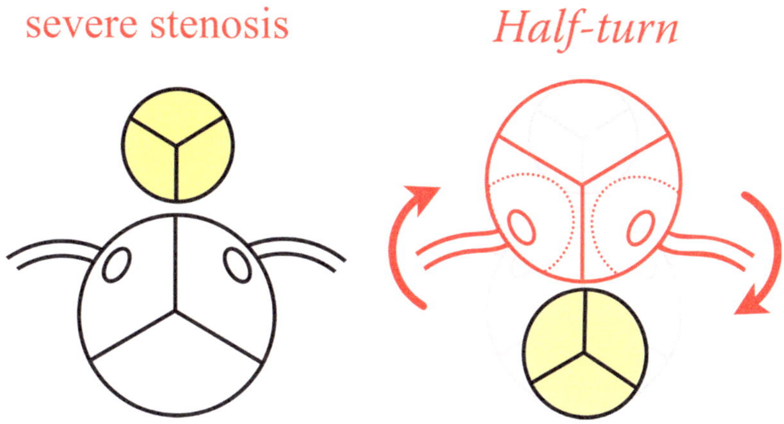

Fig. 10.20 Degree of pulmonary stenosis and half-turned truncal switch operation

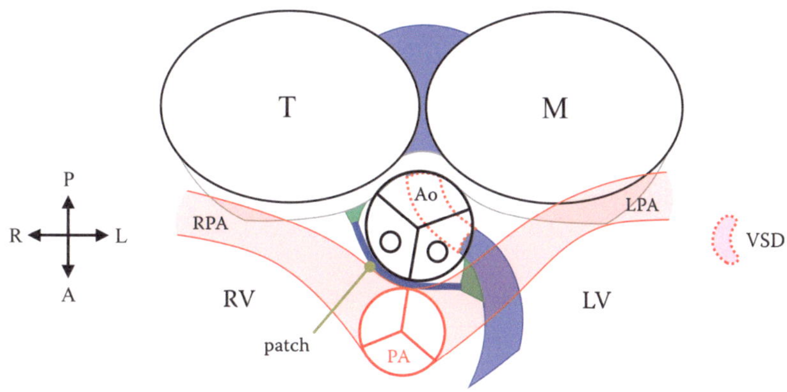

Fig. 10.21 Pulmonary artery reconstruction of half-turned truncal switch operation

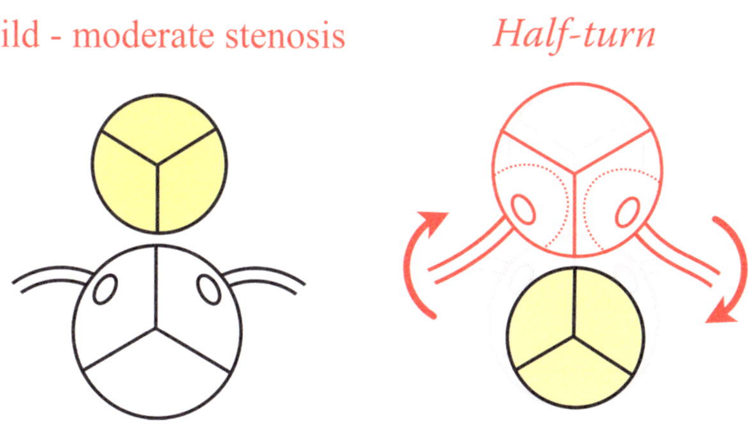

- In cases of mild to moderate pulmonary stenosis, the distance of posterior translocation of the aortic valve is long.
- In such cases, the coronary button can be anastomosed to the contralateral coronary artery defect without causing overstretching or bending of the coronary artery.
- Posterior translocation of the aortic valve is performed and the pulmonary valve (bifurcation) is also translocated anterior to the aorta.
- The aortic valve is anastomosed to the left ventricular outflow tract.
- The pulmonary artery bifurcation is anastomosed to the inverted pulmonary artery root.
- A pulmonary commissurotomy is performed for mild stenosis and augmented with a monocuspid transannular patch for moderate or severe stenosis.

3.3 Coronary Arteries and Aortic Translocation

The following table indicates whether aortic translocation (Nikaidoh and half-turned truncal switch operation) is indicated based on the coronary artery pattern. The key point is whether the aortic valve or truncal block (aortic valve and pulmonary valve as one block) can be resected and anastomosed.

Major coronary artery patterns are shown below. The frequency of coronary artery patterns indicates that aortic translocation is indicated in more than 70% of patients with this disease group (Fig. 10.22).

1 *Normal coronary artery*

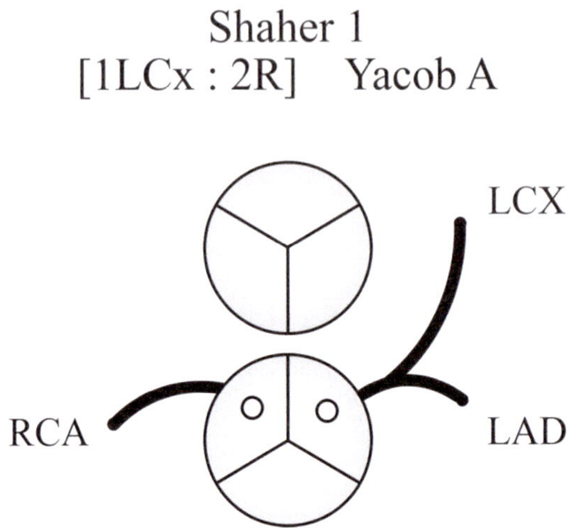

Fig. 10.22 Coronary artery pattern and indication for aortic translocation

- Both Nikaidoh and half-turned truncal switch operation are applicable.
- In cases of mild pulmonary stenosis, the pivot method should be considered in the Nikaidoh operation because of the longer posterior translocation distance of the aorta.
- *Nikaidoh operation: applicable.*
- *Half-turned truncal switch operation: applicable.*

2 *Left coronary artery runs behind pulmonary artery.*

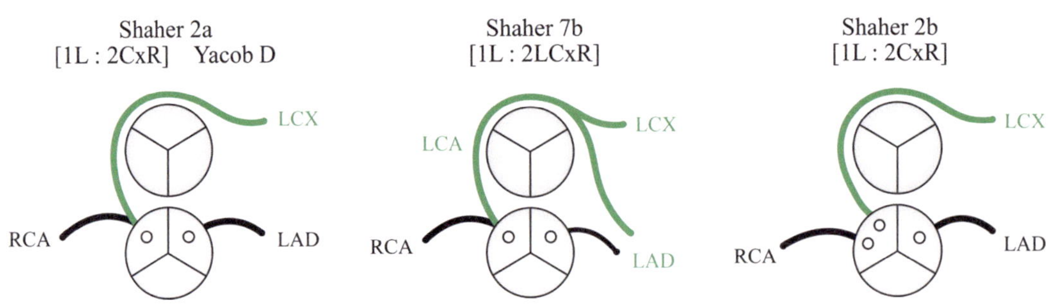

- The left coronary artery (main trunk or left circumflex) runs behind the pulmonary annulus.
- In the half-turned truncal switch operation, the coronary artery must be 2–3 mm from the base of the pulmonary artery when the truncal block is removed.
- The Nikaidoh procedure is applicable even if the coronary artery is close to the base of the pulmonary artery because the pulmonary artery is not used.
- Nikaidoh operation: *applicable.*
- Half-turned truncal switch operation: *applicable, but requires careful assessment.*

3 *Right coronary artery runs in front of the right ventricular outflow tract.*

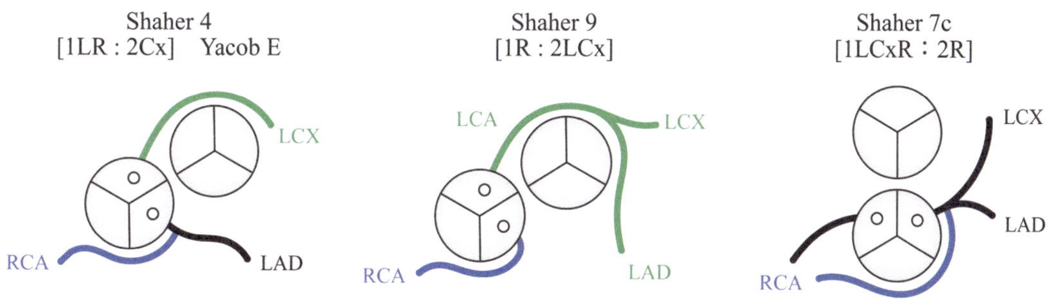

- Right coronary artery runs in front of the right ventricular outflow tract.
- The right ventricular outflow tract opening may need to be enlarged when reconstructing the new pulmonary artery, making aortic translocation a prudent choice.
- May be applicable in cases where the coronary artery runs far enough away from the right ventricular outflow tract opening.
- Nikaidoh operation: *not applicable.*
- Half-turned truncal switch operation: *not applicable.*

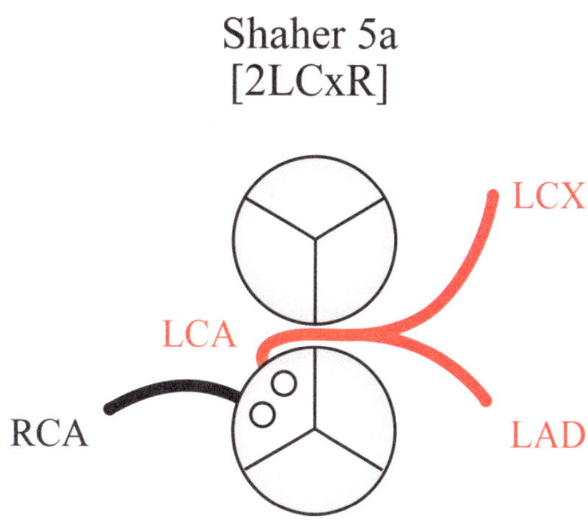

4 *Left coronary artery run between both great arteries.*

- Left coronary artery runs between both great arteries.
- Both Nikaidoh and half-turned truncal switch operations are contraindicated in this pattern.
- Nikaidoh operation: *not applicable.*
- Half-turned truncal switch operation: *not applicable.*

ESSENTIALS Procedure Selection Based on Degree of Pulmonary Stenosis

Degree of pulmonary stenosis	Atresia	Moderate	Mild - Moderate	Mild	Trivial
PA/Ao diameter ratio	0 *1	< 0.3 *2	0.3 - 0.5 *3	0.5 - 0.8 *4	> 0.8 *5
Rastelli operation	○	○	△	×	×
REV	×	○	△	×	×
Nikaidoh operation	×	○	△	△	×
Half-turned truncal switch operation	×	○	○	○	○

*1 All patients with pulmonary atresia are candidates for the Rastelli procedure.

*2 All techniques are indicated in cases of severe stenosis with a pulmonary artery to aortic annulus diameter ratio (PA/Ao diameter ratio) < 0.3. The Nikaidoh procedure is a good indication in cases of severe stenosis with a small posterior translocation distance due to coronary artery problems.

*3 All procedures are indicated even in patients with moderate stenosis with a PA/Ao diameter ratio of 0.3–0.5. Rastelli operation and REV do not involve posterior translocation of the aorta, which results in a narrow space in the right ventricular outflow tract in front of the aorta. Nikaidoh operation requires a longer posterior translocation distance, which may result in coronary overstretching. Therefore, these three procedures are not absolutely indicated.

*4 The Rastelli and REV procedures are not suitable for patients with mild stenosis with a PA/Ao diameter ratio of 0.5–0.8, because they require a longer intraventricular conduit, and the Nikaidoh procedure is associated with a greater risk of coronary overstretching. Half-turned truncal switch operation can be performed without problems.

*5 Half-turned truncal switch operation is only indicated for patients with very mild stenosis with a PA/Ao diameter ratio > 0.8. Arterial switch surgery is also indicated in patients with good pulmonary valve characteristics and uncomplicated subvalvular stenosis.

ESSENTIALS Summary of the Advantages and Disadvantages of Each Technique

Procedures	*Advantages*	*Disadvantages*
Rastelli operttion	• Easier surgery	• Stenosis of the intraventricular conduit • Decreased effective right ventricular volume • Extracardiac conduit stenosis
REV	• Relatively easy surgery • Avoids the use of extracardiac conduits	• Stenosis of the intraventricular conduit • Decreased effective right ventricular volume • Stenosis of the pulmonary artery bifurcation
Nikaidoh operation	• Straight left ventricular outflow tract • Right ventricular effective volume is maintained	• High degree of difficulty • Risk of coronary insufficiency • Pulmonary regurgitation (compensating material required) • Pulmonary artery bifurcation stenosis • (Aortic regurgitation)
Half-turned truncal switch operation	• Straight left ventricular outflow tract • Right ventricular effective volume is maintained • Avoids the use of extracardiac conduits	• High degree of difficulty • (Aortic regurgitation) • (Mitral regurgitation)

4 Surgical Procedure of Half-Turned Truncal Switch Operation (Figs. 10.23 and 10.24)

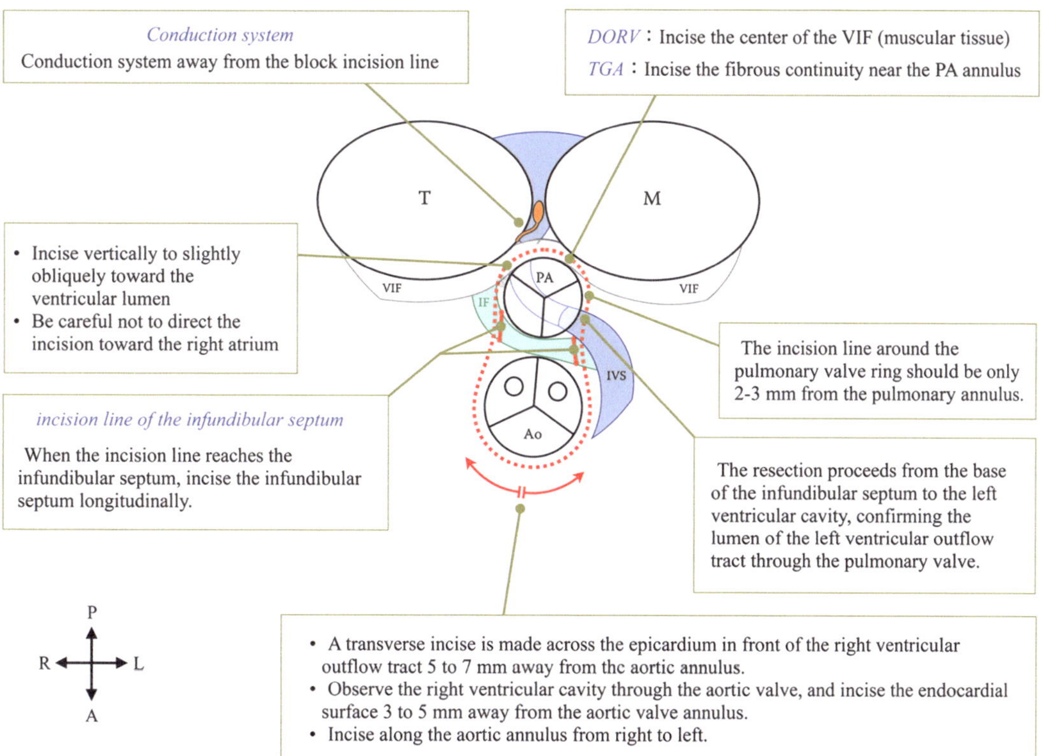

Fig. 10.23 Incision line and surrounding tissues

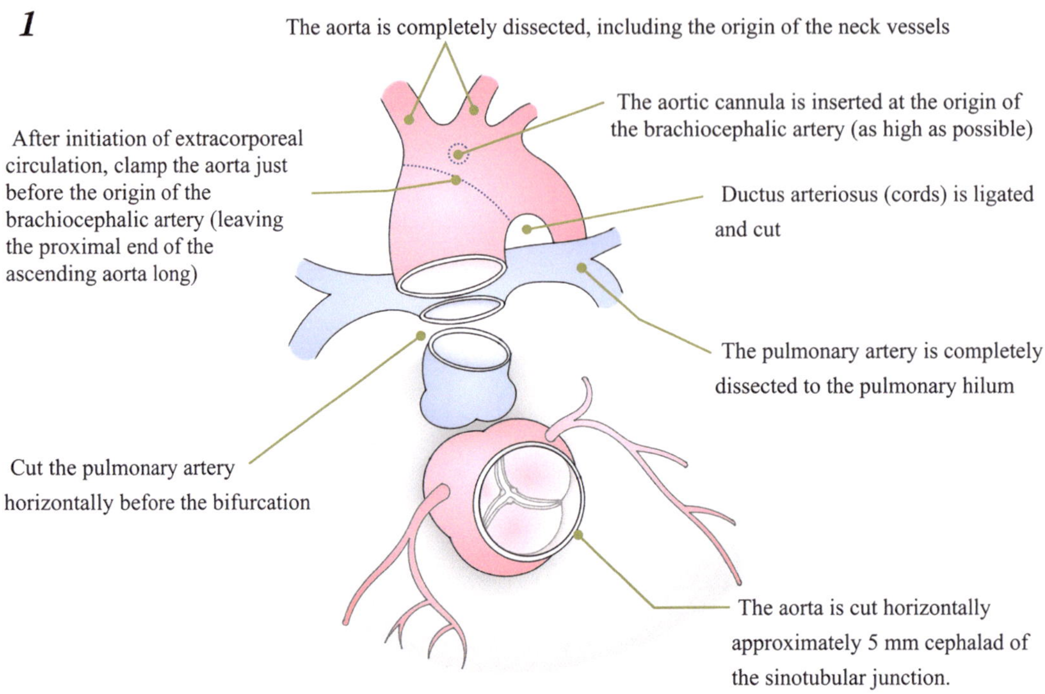

Fig. 10.24 Surgical procedure of half-turned truncal operation

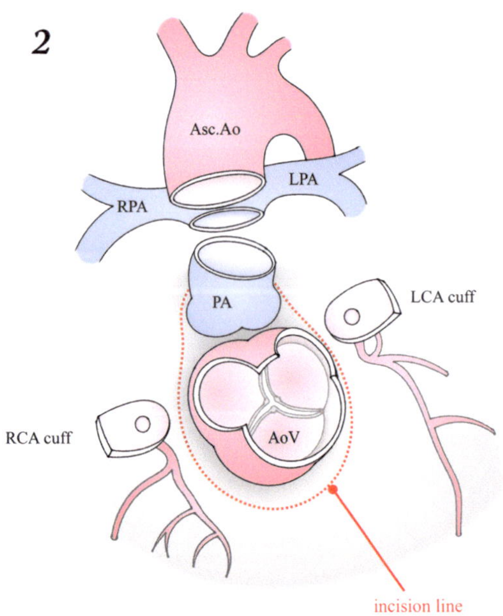

- Make a U-shaped incision in the aortic wall and harvest the coronary artery cuff.
- Both coronary cuffs should be as close to the same size as possible.
- The truncal block incision line passes just below the origin of the coronary artery, so the left and right coronary arteries should be dissected approximately 10 mm distal to the origin.

3

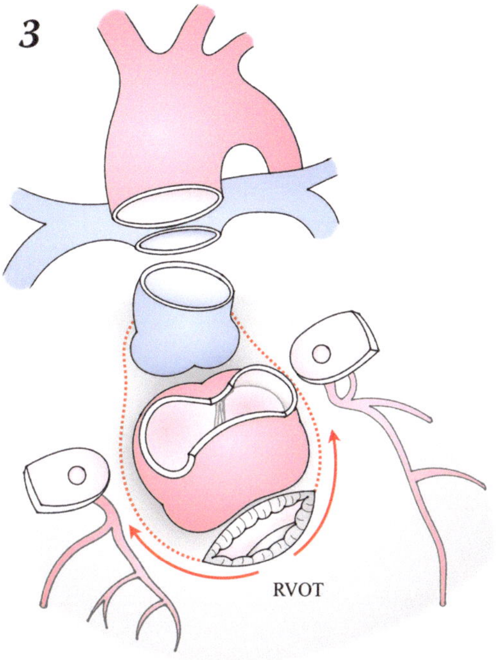

4

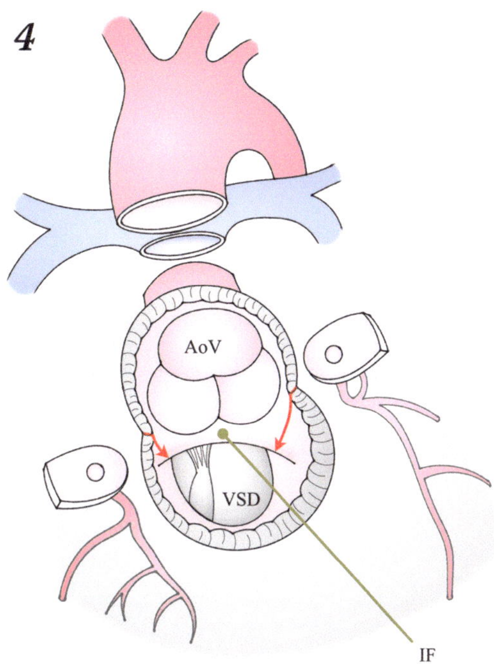

- Pierce the anterior surface of the right ventricular outflow tract 5 mm away from the aortic valve annulus to the endocardial surface with a scalpel (pointed blade).
- While viewing the right ventricular cavity through the aortic valve, ensure that the tip of the scalpel is away from the aortic valve attachments.
- Using this hole as a guide, incise the right ventricular outflow tract from right to left with a surgical scissors.
- The endocardial surface incision line should be made 3–5 mm away from the aortic valve attachment.
- Once the right ventricular outflow tract incision reaches the right and left infundibular septum, incise the infundibular septum vertically toward the left and right upper margins of the VSD.
- Because the myocardium of the right ventricular outflow tract is thick, it is best to incise the epicardial and endocardial sides separately.

- The incision line of the truncal block on the epicardial side should be approximately 5 mm from the margins of the semilunar valve.

5

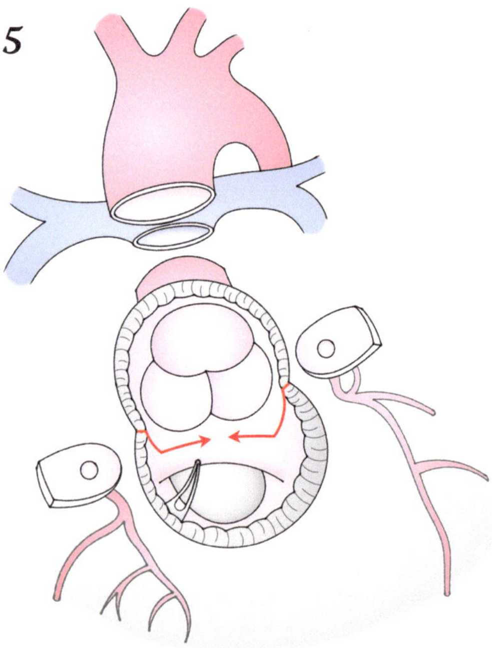

- If the infundibular septum is extended apexward and the distance to the VSD is long (remote VSD case), the infundibular septum can be incised longitudinally to the midpoint and then transversely.
- However, the remaining infundibular septal bridge should be resected because it causes left ventricular outflow tract stenosis.
- If the tricuspid chordae are attached to the infundibular septum, they should be cut at their attachment to the septum and anastomosed to the VSD patch for reconstruction.

6

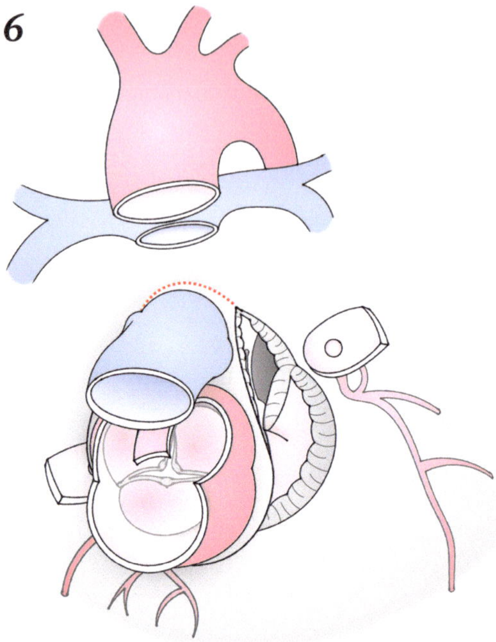

- When the incision reaches the space between the mitral annulus and the pulmonary annulus, make an incision along the pulmonary annulus near the pulmonary valve attachment so as not to damage the mitral annulus.
- While checking the left ventricular cavity through the infundibular septum incision and the pulmonary artery valve, use a scalpel (sharp blade) to penetrate the left ventricular cavity.
- Using this hole as a guide, incise along the pulmonary annulus from right to left.

7

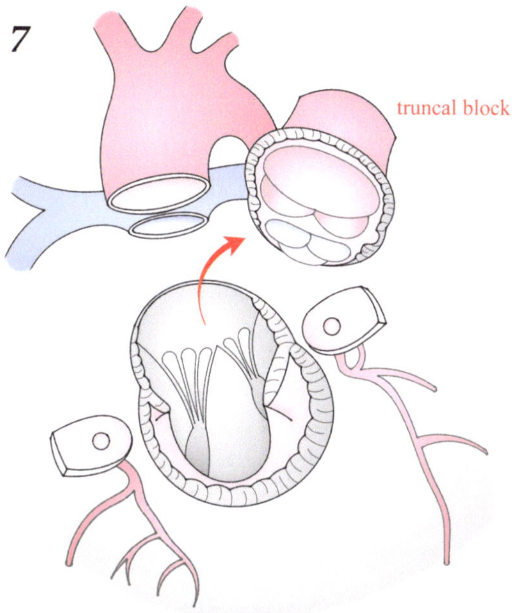

- Harvest the truncal block containing the aortic and pulmonary valves.
- Check pulmonary valve characteristics and measure the pulmonary annular diameter.
- If a pulmonary valve commissurotomy can ensure a pulmonary annulus to normal ratio of approximately 80% (Z value = −2.0), the annulus should be preserved.

8 *Trimming of the VSD patch*

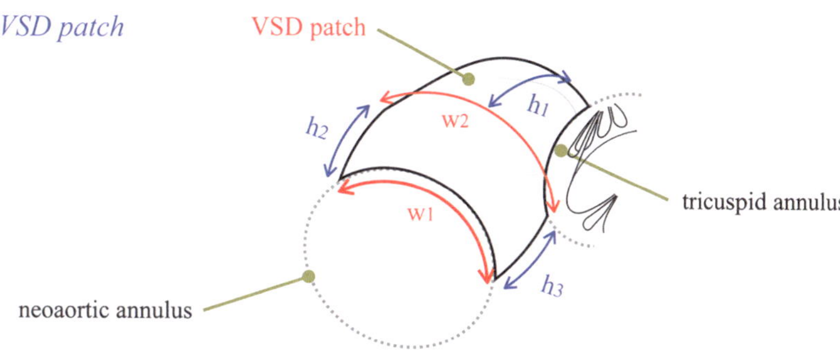

- The length of the upper edge of the VSD patch (W1) is determined from the difference between the circumference of the aortic annulus and the circumference of the left ventricular outflow tract.
- For the remote VSD, determine the height (h1) and width (w2) of the patch so that the patch is dome-shaped from the lower edge of the VSD to the upper edge of the tricuspid annulus.
- Note that w2 should be lengthened to avoid narrowing the left ventricular outflow tract and to allow the patch to bulge.
- Determine the distance from the upper margin of the tricuspid annulus to the aortic annulus (h3), the height of the contralateral side (h2), and the width of the upper margin of the patch (w1), respectively.

9

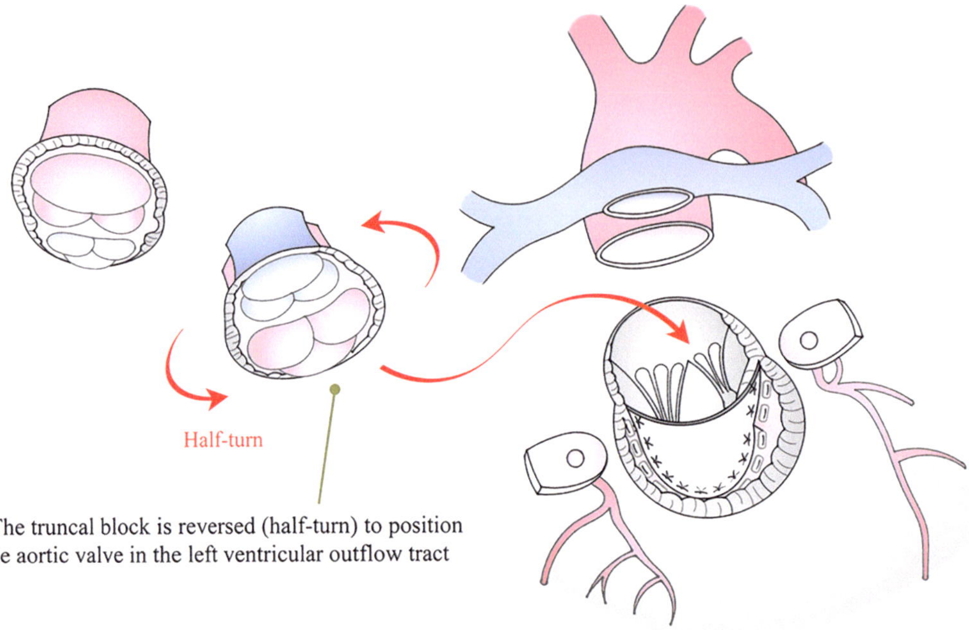

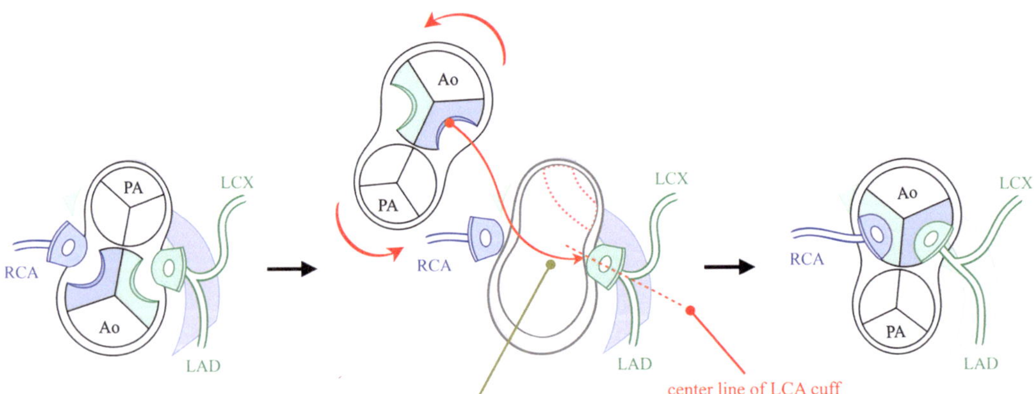

1. First, determine the suture position of the half-turned truncal block.
   - Align the bottom edge (center point) of the right coronary artery defect with the left coronary artery cuff (on the center line of the coronary artery orifice).
2. After determining the truncal block suture position on the left coronary cuff side, determine the truncal block suture position on the right coronary cuff side.
   - Align the bottom edge (center point) of the left coronary artery defect with the right coronary artery cuff (on the center line of the coronary artery orifice).

ESSENTIALS Degree of Overriding of the Aorta and VSD Patch Configuration

TGA

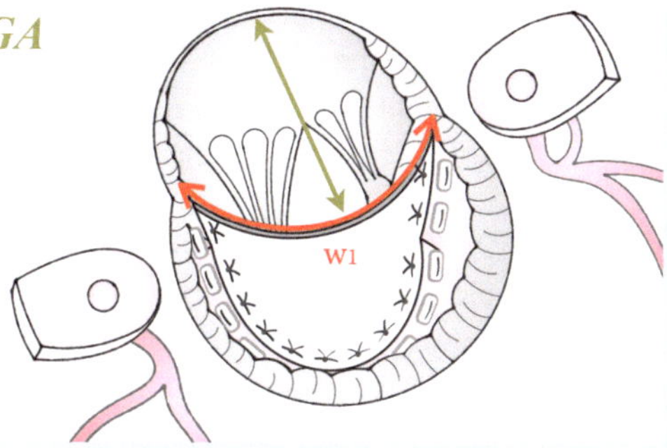

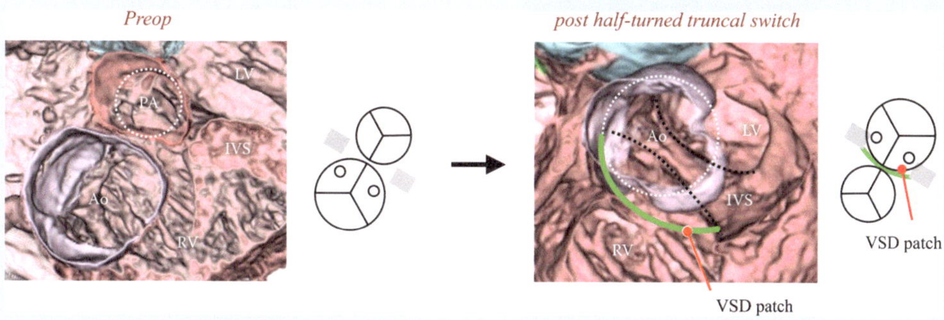

DORV

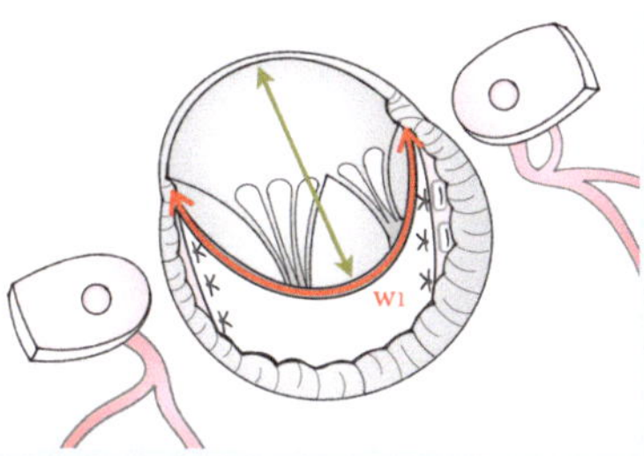

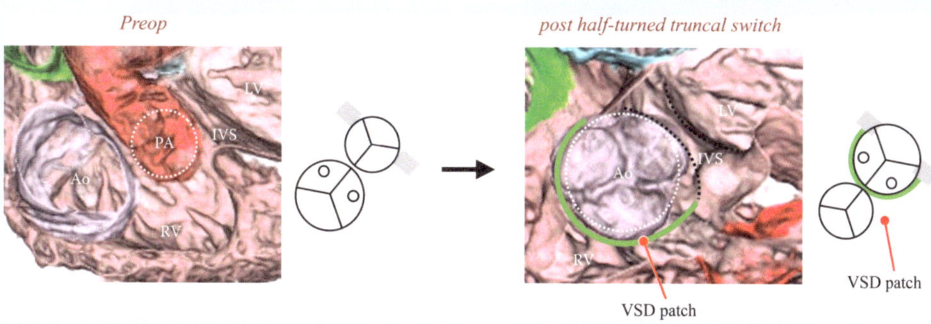

10

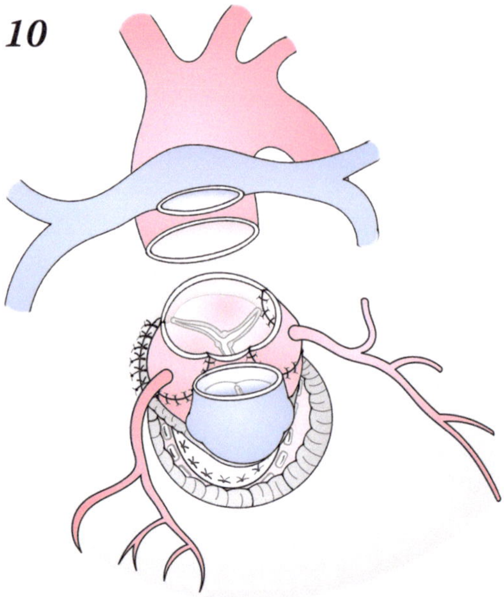

- Anastomose the aortic annulus to the left ventricular outflow tract and the superior margin of the VSD patch.
- Residual infundibular septum stumps on the truncal block side are resected except for those used for suturing the VSD patch.
- After anastomosis of the truncal block to the left ventricular outflow tract, a coronary cuff is sutured to the corresponding aortic wall defect.

11

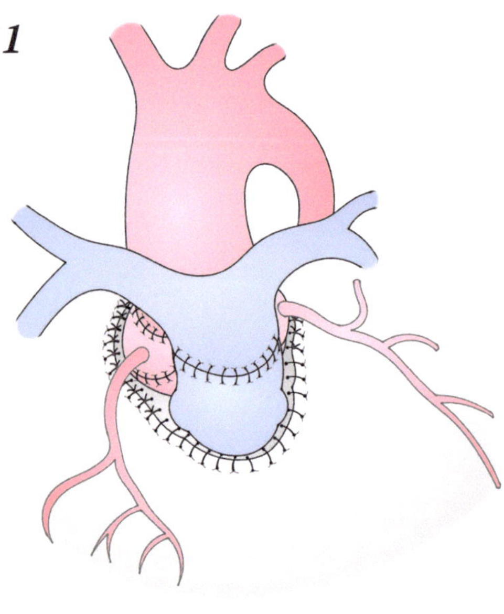

- In cases of mild to moderate pulmonary stenosis with preserved leaflet mobility and pulmonary annular diameter of at least 80% of normal (Z value −2.0) can be secured by commissurotomy, the pulmonary annulus is preserved and the truncal block pulmonary annulus is anastomosed directly to the right ventricular outflow tract opening.
- Because of the difference in diameter between the right ventricular outflow tract opening and the truncal block pulmonary annulus, the right ventricular outflow tract opening side is sutured with a constricted suture.
- Avoid the use of supplemental materials as much as possible.

12

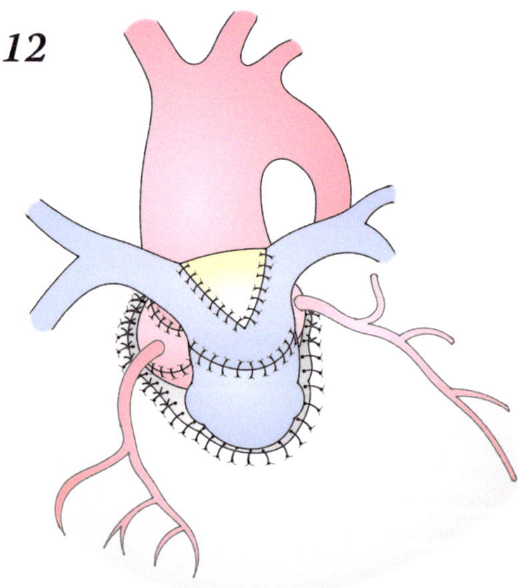

- If tension appears to be present at the anteriorly displaced pulmonary artery bifurcation or the right and left pulmonary arteries, a longitudinal incision is made cephalad of the bifurcation and the incision is augmented with an autologous pericardial patch to release tension in the longitudinal axial direction of the pulmonary artery.

13

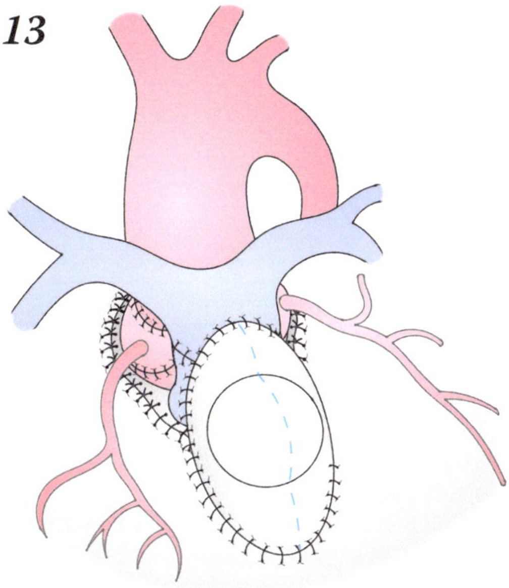

- In cases of moderate to severe pulmonary valve stenosis and narrow valve annulus, a longitudinal incision is made in the anterior aspect of the anterior translocated pulmonary artery and right ventricular outflow tract, and the right ventricular outflow tract is enlarged with a monocuspid patch.

5 Half-Turned Truncal Switch Operation (Surgical Video) (Fig. 10.25)

Case

- Age: 1 year 6 months old.
- Body weight: 7.9 kg.
- Diagnosis: TGA type DORV (false Taussig-Bing), perimembranous outlet VSD, PS.
- Coronary artery pattern: Shaher type 1 (Yacoub type A).
- Pulmonary annular diameter = 9.1 mm (85% of normal value).
- Aortic annular diameter = 14 mm.
- Pulmonary/aortic annular diameter ratio = 0.65.
- LV-PA pressure gradient = 76 mmHg.

< cephalic view >

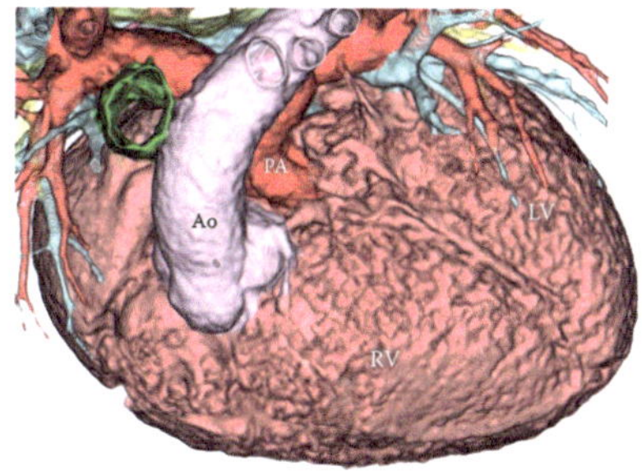

Fig. 10.25 Preoperative CT images

- Aorta is located anterior to the right and pulmonary artery posterior to the left.

< cephalic view, horizontal cross-section >

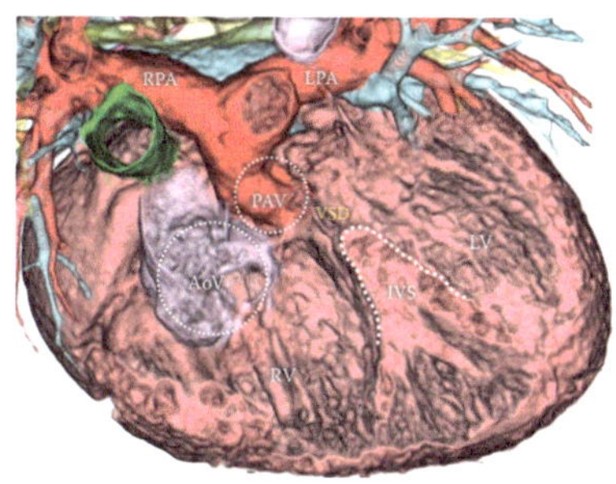

- VSD is present below the pulmonary artery valve.
- Pulmonary valve originates from the right ventricle more than 50% of its annulus.
- If a blood flow pathway from the VSD to the aortic valve is to be created, it must pass under the pulmonary artery valve and a large intraventricular route must be created in the right ventricle. For this reason, intraventricular rerouting was considered inappropriate in this case.

< left lateral view >

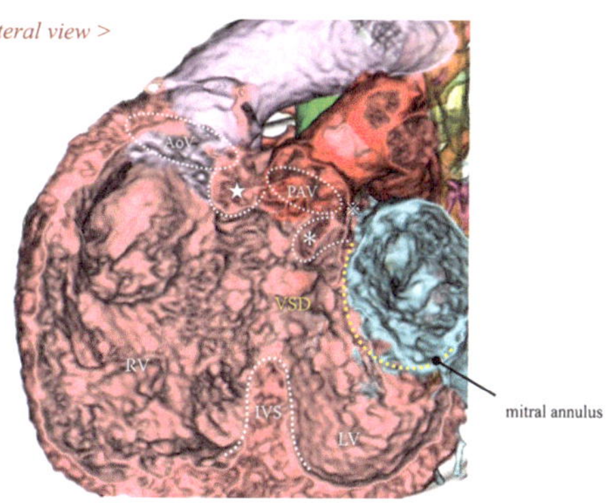

- The VSD is located below the pulmonary valve.
- Muscular bundle is present between the upper border of the VSD (*).
- The ventriculo-infundibular fold (※) of the muscular bundle is interposed between the mitral annulus (yellow dotted line) and the pulmonary valve (PAV).
- Infundibular septum (★) is present between aortic valve (AoV) and PAV.
- Because of the long distance from the VSD to the AoV, the effective right ventricular volume is significantly reduced when an intracardiac conduit is constructed in the right ventricle.

< coronal cross-section >

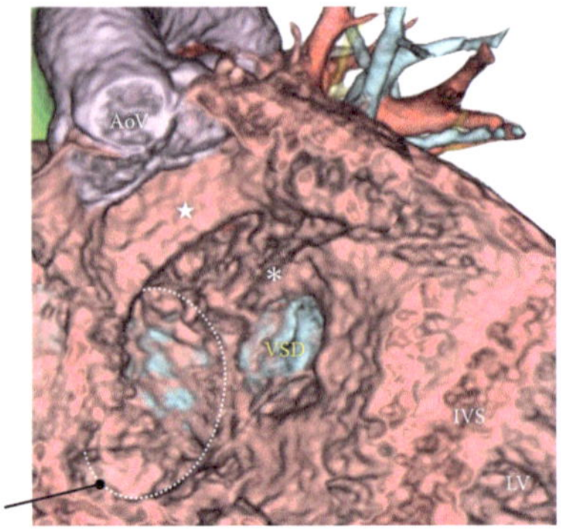

- The VSD is located in the perimembranous portion and is remote from both semilunar valves (remote VSD).
- Infundibular septum (★) and interventricular septum (IVS) are parallel.
- Muscular septum is present at the superior border of the VSD (*).
- The infundibular septum is orthogonal to the pathway from the left ventricle (LV) through the VSD to the AoV, creating a barrier to the blood flow pathway (Scene 10.1).

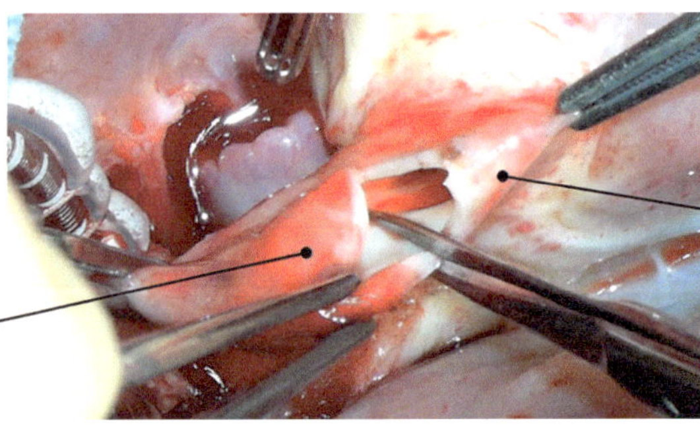

Scene 10.1 Transect of the ascending aorta (Video 0 min 05 s)

1. Insert the cannula into the aorta as high as possible (near the origin of the brachiocephalic artery).
2. Start extracorporeal circulation, clamp the aorta, and arrest the heart.
3. The second and subsequent infusions of cardioplegia are injected retrograde from the coronary sinus.

- The aorta is transected approximately 5 mm superior to the sinotubular junction.
- The origin of the left and right coronary arteries is confirmed prior to transection.
- Unlike the arterial switch procedure, it is not necessary to transect too high (Scene 10.2).

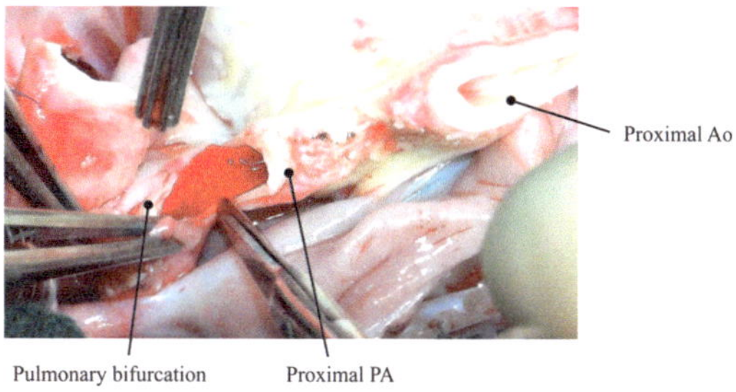

Scene 10.2 Transect of the pulmonary artery (Video 0 min 26 s)

1. Cut the main pulmonary artery before the pulmonary artery bifurcation.
   - In cases with a narrow main pulmonary artery, the main pulmonary artery is cut at an angle to allow easy access to the reversed pulmonary artery wall (posterior wall side).
   - During reconstruction, the narrow pulmonary annulus is incised and a monocuspid transannular patch is supplemented (Scene 10.3).

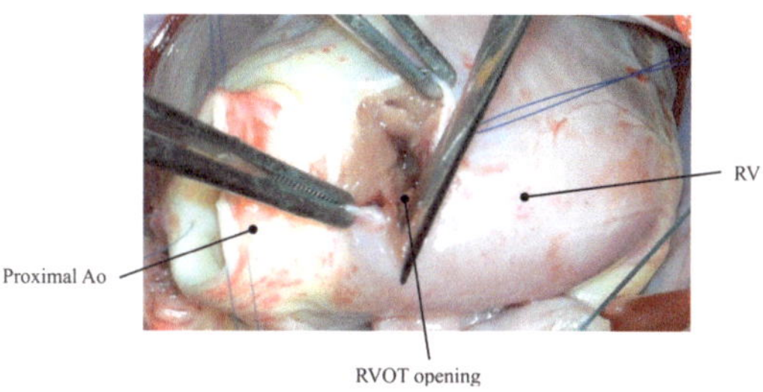

Scene 10.3 Transverse incision of right ventricular outflow tract (Video 1 min 00 s)

1 Verify the valve ring attachment through the aortic valve and incise the right ventricular outflow tract transversely approximately 5 mm below the aortic valve ring (Scene 10.4).

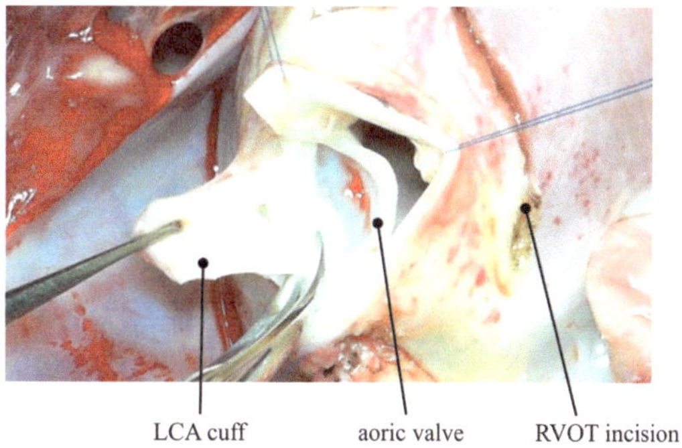

Scene 10.4 Harvest of left coronary cuff (Video 2 min 28 s)

1. Harvest the left coronary cuff in a U-shape.
   - To harvest the truncal block, incise along the aortic valve annulus and dissect 5–7 mm from the origin of the coronary artery.
   - The coronary cuff may be harvested before incising the right ventricular outflow tract (Scene 10.5).

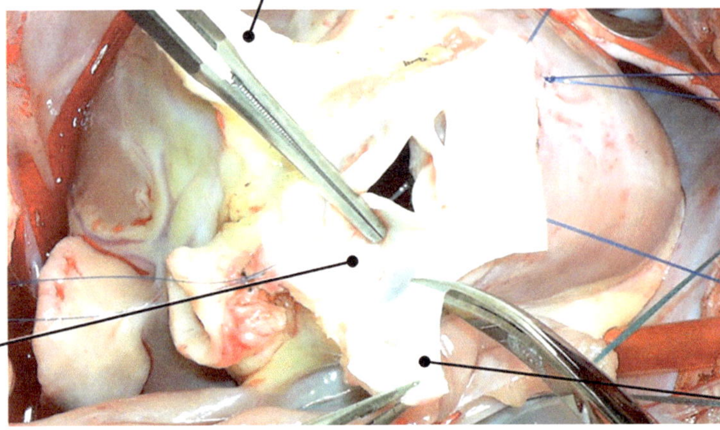

Scene 10.5 Harvest of right coronary cuff (Video 3 min 24 s)

1 Harvest the right coronary cuff in a U-shape.
  - As with the left coronary artery, dissect 5–7 mm from the origin of the coronary artery (Video 10.6).

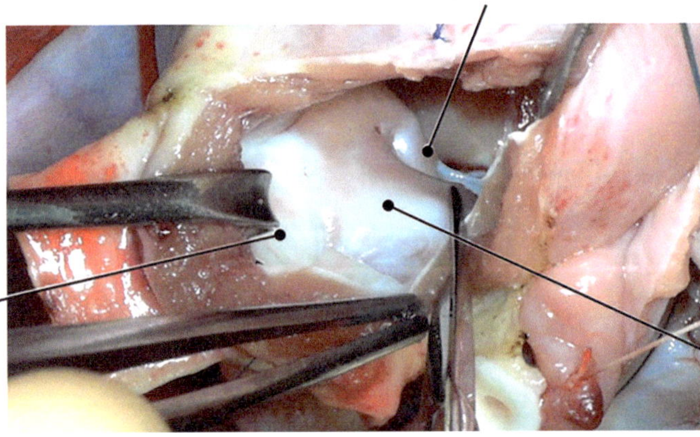

Scene 10.6 Harvest of truncal block 1 (Video 4 min 14 s)

1 Transverse incision is made on the right side of the right ventricular outflow tract.
2 While confirming the aortic annulus through the right ventricular incision, proceed with the transverse incision of the right ventricular outflow tract.
3 Incise along the aortic annulus to the ventricular septum approximately 3 mm from the aortic annulus.
  - In cases of false Taussig-Bing (DORV), the tricuspid annulus may be close to the aortic annulus, so be careful to keep the incision line away from the tricuspid annulus.
  - If there is a tricuspid chordae attached to the infundibular septum, temporarily cut the chordae at the base (the tricuspid chordae is reconstructed after patch closure of the ventricular septal defect) (Scene 10.7).

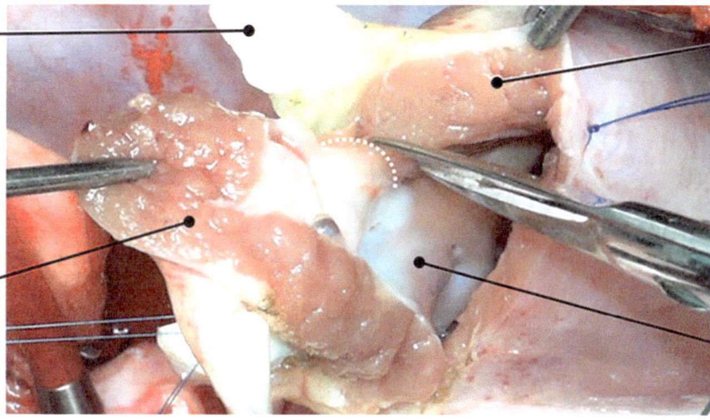

Scene 10.7 Harvest of truncal block 2 (Video 4 min 57 s)

1. Continue the transverse incision on the left side of the right ventricular outflow tract.
   - Incise the upper right ventricular wall midway between the left coronary artery origin and the aortic annulus (white dotted line).
   - Be careful not to incise too close to the origin of the coronary artery (Scene 10.8).

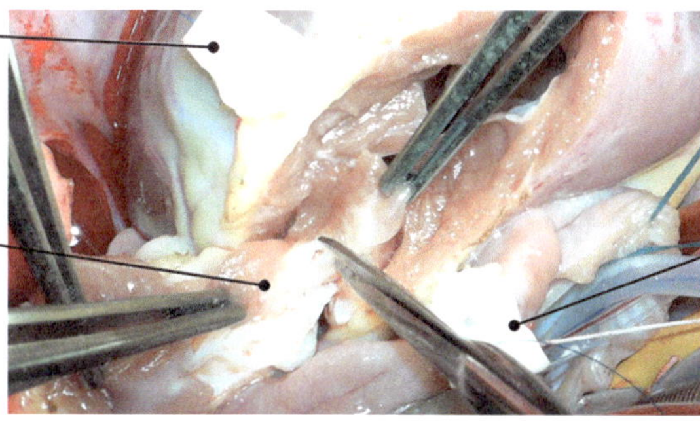

Scene 10.8 Harvest of truncal block 3 (Video 6 min 17 s)

1. Incise the dorsal side of the pulmonary artery annulus along the annulus.
   - In this case, the pulmonary artery originates almost entirely from the right ventricle, and there is no risk of damaging the mitral valve by incising around the pulmonary annulus because there is a muscle bundle (ventricular septal wall and VIF at the top of the VSD) between the pulmonary annulus and the mitral annulus.
   - However, even in cases of false Taussig-Bing, if the muscular bundle (VIF) between the pulmonary artery and the mitral valve is thin, care must be taken not to damage the mitral valve when incising in this area.
   - In cases of DORV with a thin VIF, incise at the midpoint of the VIF.
   - In cases of TGA with fibrous continuity, incise the fibrous continuity (slightly closer to the pulmonary annulus) (Scene 10.9).

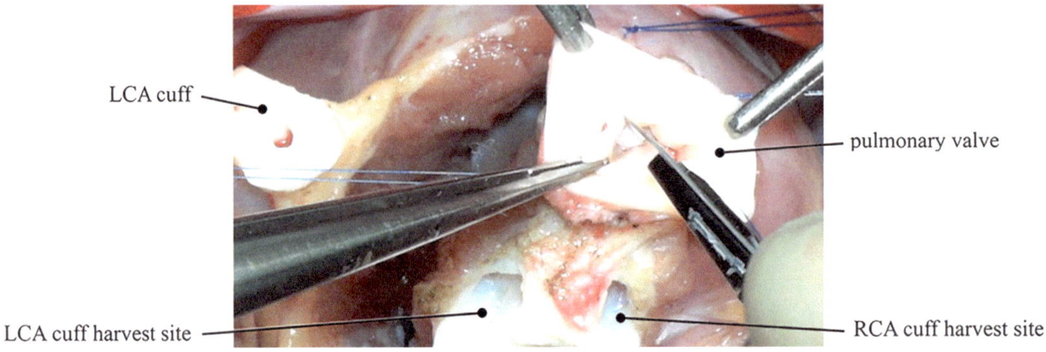

Scene 10.9 Pulmonary commissurotomy (Video 6 min 39 s)

1 Confirm the caliber and morphology of the harvested pulmonary valve.
2 If a commissurotomy can be performed to preserve the pulmonary annulus with a ratio of 80% or greater to normal, the annulus should be preserved.
   - If preservation of the annulus is not possible, incise the annulus and expand the annulus and right ventricular outflow tract by supplementing with a monocuspid patch.
   - In half-turned cases, the pulmonary commissure is not always located in the mid-anterior position (e.g., in cases of a bicuspid valve with a transverse split).
   - In such cases, even if the right ventricular outflow tract is off-center, the commissure should be incised as much as possible to preserve autologous valve function (Scene 10.10).

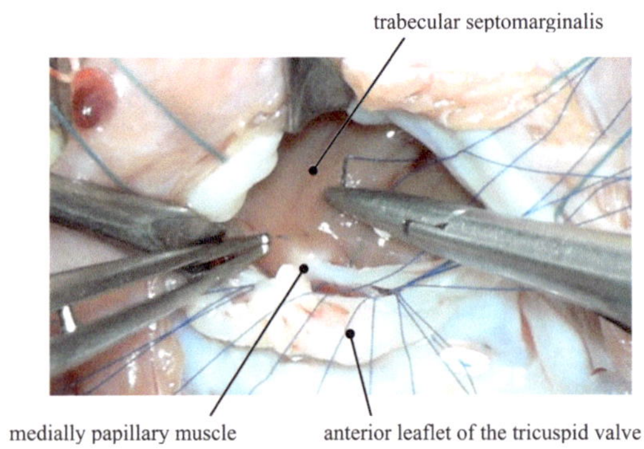

Scene 10.10 VSD closure 1 (Video 6 min 59 s)

- Because the posterior margin of the VSD in this case is located in the inflow area (around the membranous area) and the view of the posterior margin of the VSD from the right ventricular outflow tract opening is poor, VSD closure of the posterior margin is performed through the tricuspid valve.
  1. 5-0 monofilament sutures with pledgets are placed around the postero-inferior margin of the VSD.
  2. The lower half of the oval ePTFE patch, trimmed to a longer diameter, is anastomosed to the postero-inferior margin of the VSD.
  3. The upper half of the ePTFE patch is pulled through the right ventricular outflow tract opening.

POINT

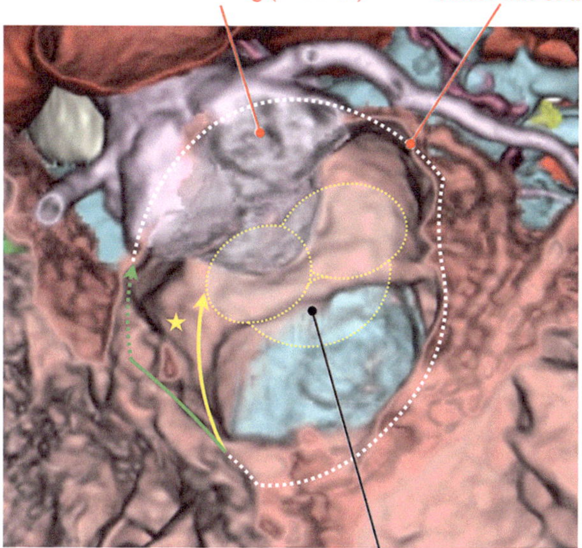

- In cases of TGA and DORV with mild overriding of the pulmonary valve, the aortic valve is largely posteriorly translocated to the left ventricular side after half-turning of the truncal block (*yellow dashed line*).
- In such cases, the patch suture line at the posterior margin of the VSD can be sutured in the direction of the VIF (*yellow* ★) without much use of the tricuspid annulus, as shown by the yellow arrow.

- In cases such as the present one, in which both great arteries originate entirely from the right ventricle, the pulmonary valve is also deviated to the right ventricular side to a large extent, so that the aortic valve does not shift dorsally much after half-turning.
- Therefore, the VSD patch will bulge to the right ventricular side.
- In such cases, in order to ensure a wide left ventricular outflow tract (so that the VSD patch does not protrude below the aortic valve), the annulus of the anterior leaflet of the tricuspid valve must be used for VSD closure for a long distance (*green solid line*), and then the patch suture line must be directed toward the aortic valve (*green dashed line*) (Scene 10.11).

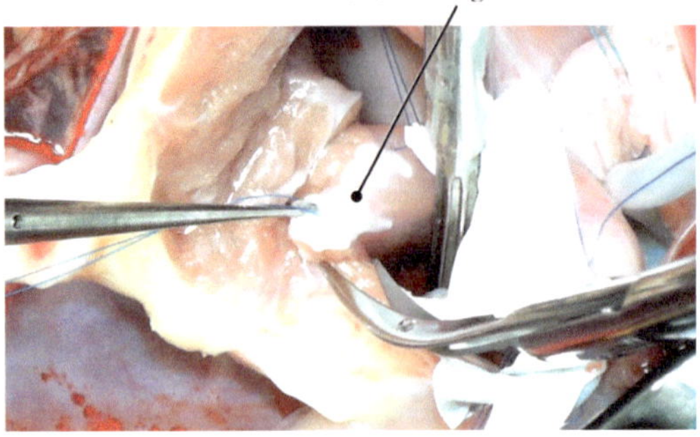

Scene 10.11 VSD enlargement (Video 9 min 40 s)

- Since the VSD was rather small in this case, the anterior margin of the VSD, where the conduction system and coronary septal branches were absent, was resected, and the VSD was enlarged.
  1. The myocardium is resected from the superior margin to the anterior margin of the VSD.
  2. The infundibular septal fragment and the enlarged anterior margin of the VSD are anastomosed to reconstruct continuity from the anterior margin of the ventricular septum to the right ventricular outflow tract opening (Scene 10.12).

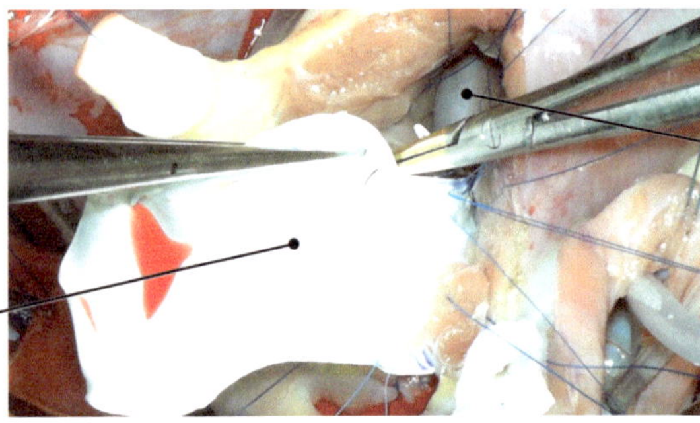

Scene 10.12 VSD closure 2 (Video 10 min 11 s)

1 The ePTFE patch is pulled through the right ventricular outflow tract opening and sutured to the VSD margins.

2 The upper edge of the excess patch is trimmed (Scene 10.13).

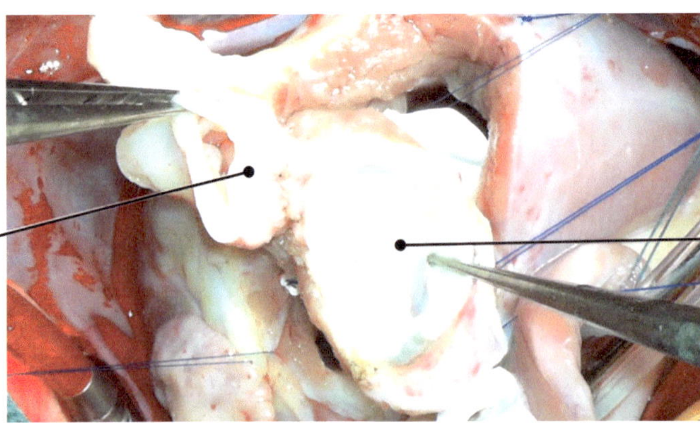

Scene 10.13 Half-turn of the truncal block (Video 13 min 54 s)

1 Rotate the truncal block a half turn to position the aortic valve over the left ventricular outflow tract.
2 Fine-tune the position of the truncal block so that the defect harvested from the right coronary artery corresponds to the origin of the left coronary artery and the defect harvested from the left coronary artery corresponds to the origin of the right coronary artery.

- In a normal coronary artery pattern (Shaher type 1), the left coronary artery origin has fewer degrees of freedom than the right coronary artery origin (due to the bifurcation of the circumflex branch).
- Therefore, priority should be given to positioning the truncal block according to the left coronary artery origin (Scene 10.14).

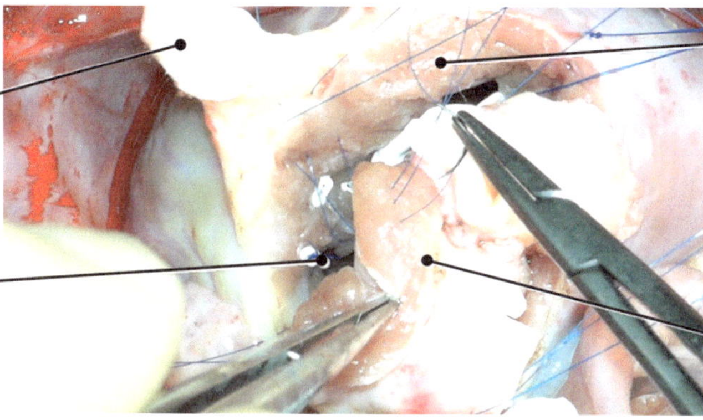

Scene 10.14 Anastomosis of the truncal block (Ao annulus) 1 (Video 14 min 56 s)

1 Anastomose the rotated truncal block half-turn with interrupted 6-0 monofilament suture (5-0 monofilament suture will tear the myocardium).
2 First, sutures are placed in the central region of the right coronary artery defect on the side of the truncal block and to the left ventricular outflow tract cross-section just below the origin of the left coronary artery.
3 The truncal block side is sutured to the lower half of the myocardial cut surface so that the truncal block is anastomosed slightly higher than the left ventricular outflow tract cross-section.

- The left ventricular outflow tract opening is sutured to the upper half of the cross section.
- In cases with anterior-posterior relationships of the great arteries, the aortic valve is higher than the pulmonary valve because of the presence of the infundibulum under the aortic valve.
- If the truncal block is rotated half-turn and the aortic annulus is anastomosed at the same level as the pulmonary annulus (left ventricular outflow tract cross-section), the coronary artery defect opening is lower than before half-turning, and the coronary artery origin anastomosed to the defect opening may bend.

POINT

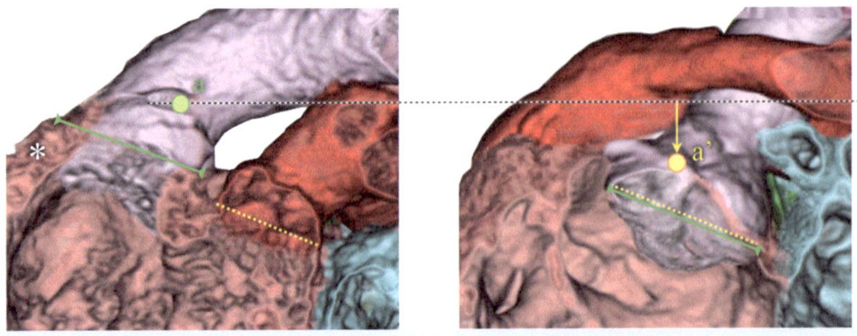

- Due to the presence of an infundibulum beneath the aortic valve (*), the aortic annulus (*green solid line*) is positioned higher than the pulmonary annulus (yellow dotted line) in TGA and TGA type DORV (a: left coronary artery orifice).
- An imaginary view is shown when the aortic annulus (*green solid line*) is sutured to the original pulmonary artery annulus (*yellow dashed line*) by image processing.
- The position of the left coronary artery orifice (*a'*) is significantly lower and there is concern that the reconstructed left coronary origin may bend downward.

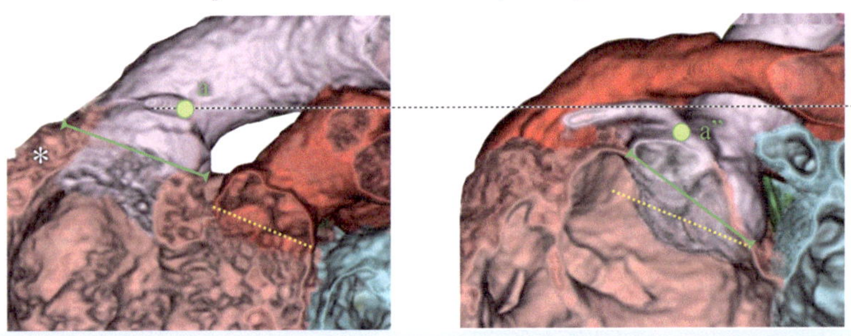

- In this case, the aortic annulus (*green solid line*) near the left coronary orifice is sutured higher than the original pulmonary annulus (*yellow dashed line*), so that the implanted left coronary orifice (a″) does not differ significantly from the original height (*black dotted line*) (Scene 10.15).

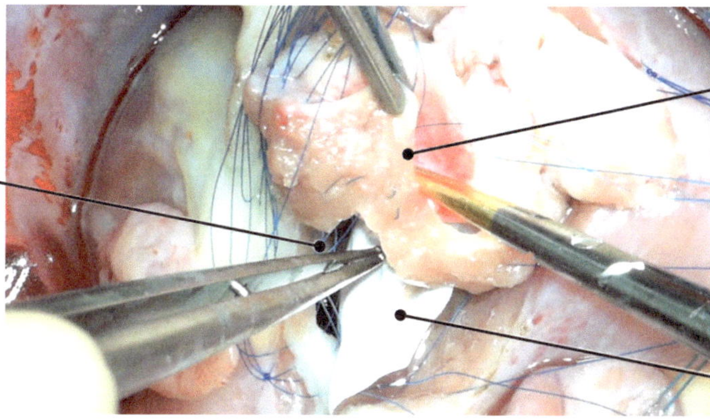

Scene 10.15 Anastomosis of the truncal block (Ao annulus) 2 (Video 14 min 56 s)

1 The truncal block is anastomosed posterior to the left ventricular outflow tract with interrupted 6-0 monofilament suture.
   - Because of the thin wall thickness of the VIF or the mitral-pulmonary fibrosis continuity, the truncal block is sutured at the same level as the cross section of the orifice.
   - In DORV cases where the myocardial bundle of the VIF is thin, or in TGA cases where there is fibrous continuity between the mitral and pulmonary valves, sutures are placed with care to avoid damaging the mitral valve (Scene 10.16).

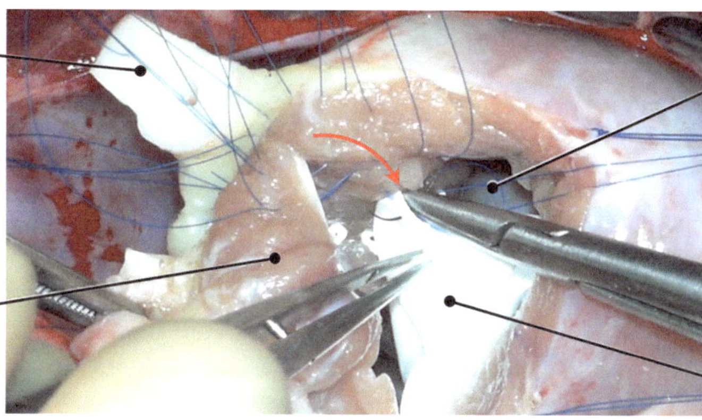

Scene 10.16 Anastomosis of the truncal block (Ao annulus) 3 (Video 18 min 57 s)

1 Anastomose the truncal block to the left ventricular outflow tract section anterior to the left coronary artery origin.
2 The suture line is lowered downward (toward the VSD patch) as it advances anteriorly (*red arrow*).
3 At the left edge of the upper border of the VSD patch, a 6-0 monofilament suture with a pledget is placed over the septal cross section, VSD patch, and truncal block (this area is prone to leakage) (Scene 10.17).

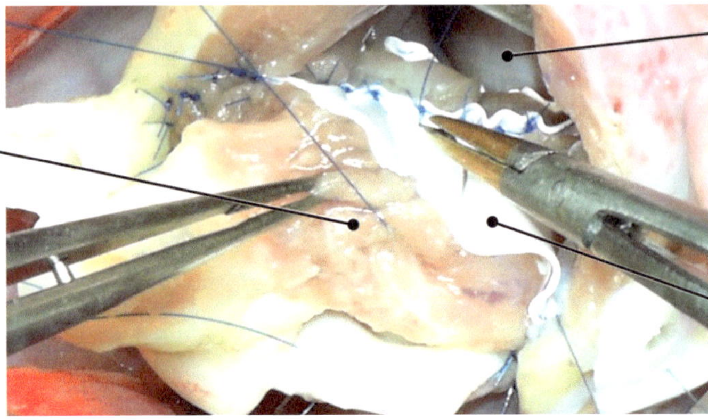

Scene 10.17 Anastomosis VSD patch to the truncal block (Video 21 min 57 s)

1. Trim the upper edge of the VSD patch to fit the truncal block.
2. Resect the excess myocardium of the infundibular septum, leaving a seam allowance for the VSD patch so as not to induce right ventricular outflow tract stenosis.
3. Anastomose the VSD patch to the infundibular septum with a continuous 6-0 monofilament suture.
   - If the infundibular septum is fragile, use a mattress suture of 6-0 monofilament with a pledget (Scene 10.18).

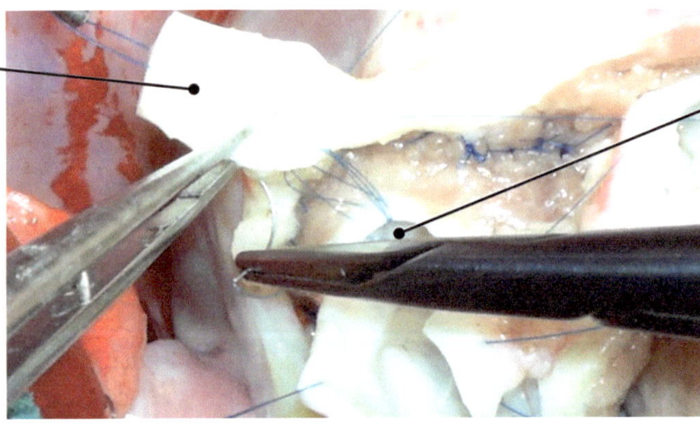

Scene 10.18 LCA reconstruction (Video 26 min 06 s)

1. Anastomose the left coronary cuff to the right coronary artery defect (coronary artery cuff harvest site) with a continuous 6-0 monofilament suture.
   - If the defect is located low, the anterior wall of the ascending aorta is harvested and added to the lower part of the defect (Scenes 10.19 and 10.20).
   - In this case, the truncal block was anastomosed slightly higher, and the height of the defect opening and the height of the left coronary cuff were appropriate, so that the ascending aortic wall was not needed to be supplemented to the lower part of the defect opening (Scene 10.19).

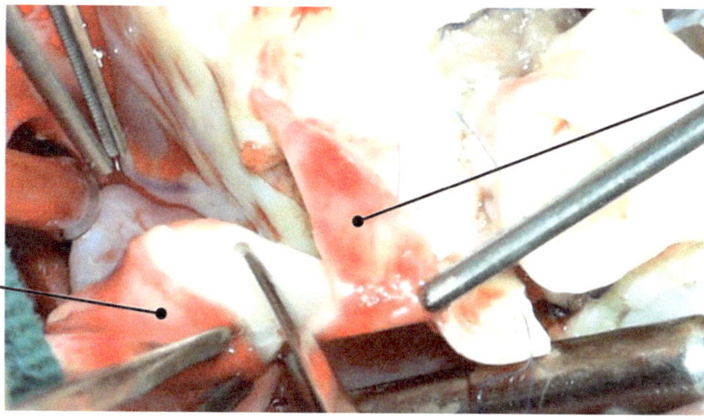

Scene 10.19 Harvest of ascending aortic wall (Video 30 min 35 s)

- The proximal end of the aorta is shifted posteriorly by the half-turn, resulting in dorsal backbending of the ascending aorta when the aorta is reconstructed.
- The backbending results in an excess anterior wall of the ascending aorta corresponding to the proximal aortic cross-section.

1. The excess anterior wall of the ascending aorta is resected in a crescent shape (Scene 10.20).

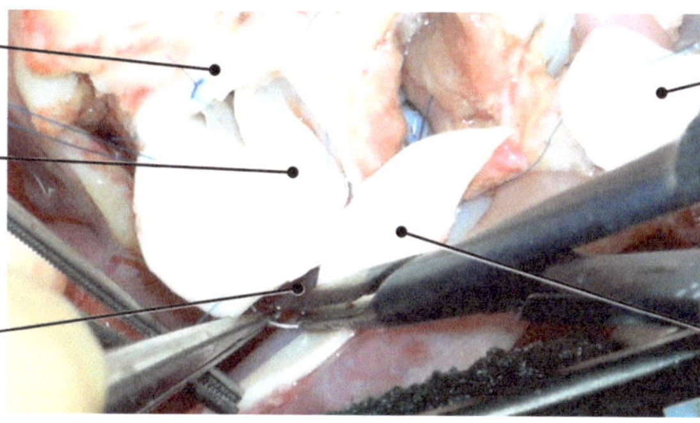

Scene 10.20 RCA reconstruction 1 (Video 30 min 53 s)

1. Although the height of the aortic wall defect (left coronary cuff harvest site) and the right pulmonary artery cuff match, the right coronary artery may be slightly overstretched, so the crescent-shaped anterior ascending aortic wall patch is anastomosed to the bottom of the aortic wall defect with a continuous 6-0 monofilament suture.
2. Trim the anterior margin of the appended ascending aortic wall patch in an arc to match the distance to the base of the right coronary cuff.
   - Trimming only the anterior margin of the ascending aortic wall in an arc maintains the angle of the right coronary cuff (similar effect to the trap-door technique) (Scene 10.21).

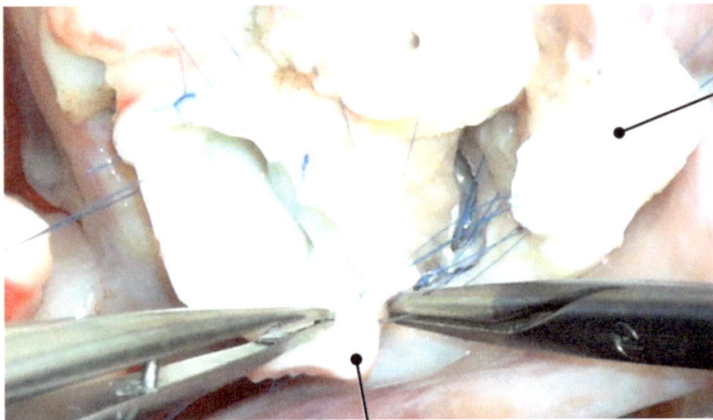

Scene 10.21 RCA reconstruction 2 (Video 34 min 10 s)

1. The right coronary cuff is anastomosed with a continuous 6-0 monofilament suture to the left coronary cuff harvest site, which is supplemented by the crescent-shaped ascending aortic wall patch (Scene 10.22).

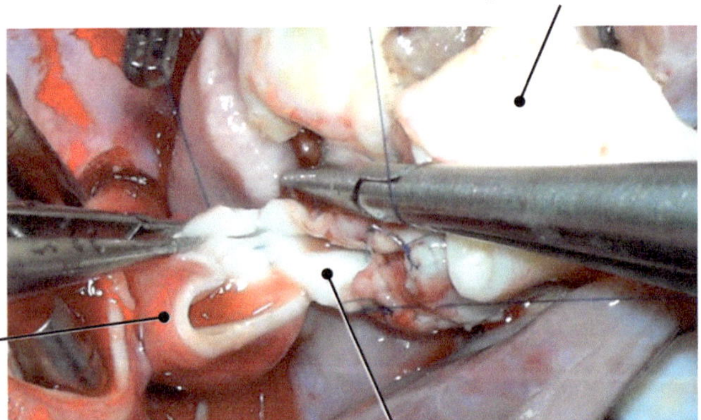

Scene 10.22 Reconstruction of the ascending aorta (Video 37 min 55 s)

1. Translocate the pulmonary artery bifurcation anterior to the ascending aorta.
2. The dorsally displaced ascending aorta and the half-turned proximal aortic stump are anastomosed end-to-end with a continuous 6-0 monofilament suture (Scene 10.23).

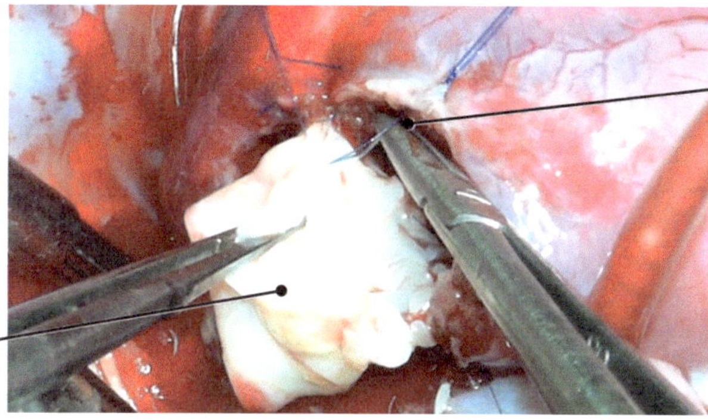

Scene 10.23 RVOT reconstruction (Video 41 min 36 s)

1. Release the aortic clamp and restart heart beating.
2. Anastomose the pulmonary annulus to the right ventricular outflow tract opening with a continuous 6-0 monofilament suture.
   - Perform a mitral regurgitation test (water test) before releasing the aortic occluder, and if regurgitation is confirmed, an additional commissuroplasty of the posteromedial commissure near the anastomosed aortic annulus should be performed.
   - The aortic annular marginal myocardium of the truncal block posterior to the pulmonary annulus is anastomosed to the right ventricular outflow tract cross-section and the right ventricular outflow tract should be pulled transversely.
   - Because the diameter of the right ventricular outflow tract opening is often larger than the diameter of the pulmonary annulus, the anastomosis is performed while adjusting the stitch width between the pulmonary annulus side and the right ventricular opening side (Scene 10.24).

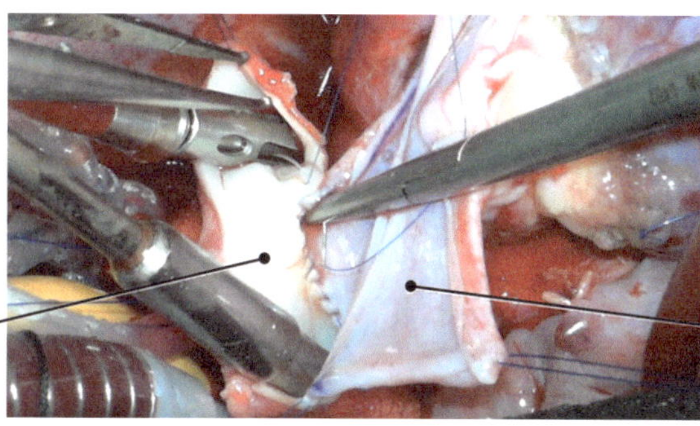

Scene 10.24 Main pulmonary artery reconstruction 1 (Video 49 min 06 s)

1. Make a longitudinal Incision at the anteriorly displaced pulmonary artery bifurcation from the dorsal aspect (the aspect in contact with the ascending aorta) to the cephalic side.
2. The dorsal wall of the main pulmonary artery is also incised longitudinally.
3. The autologous pericardium is sutured to the incised wall of the pulmonary artery bifurcation and the dorsal wall of the main pulmonary artery with continuous 6-0 monofilament suture to reconstruct the continuity of the posterior pulmonary artery wall and to extend the

right and left pulmonary arteries longitudinally.

- As in the longitudinal extension method for arterial switch surgery, the anteriorly translocated left and right pulmonary arteries are extended longitudinally to prevent overstretching.
- Compared to the REV in which the ascending aorta is not posteriorly translocated, in the half-turned truncal switch operation, the ascending aorta is also posteriorly translocated, which prevents overstretching of the anteriorly displaced pulmonary bifurcation, but some extension is inevitable, so the longitudinal extension method is also useful in half-turned truncal switch operation (Scene 10.25).

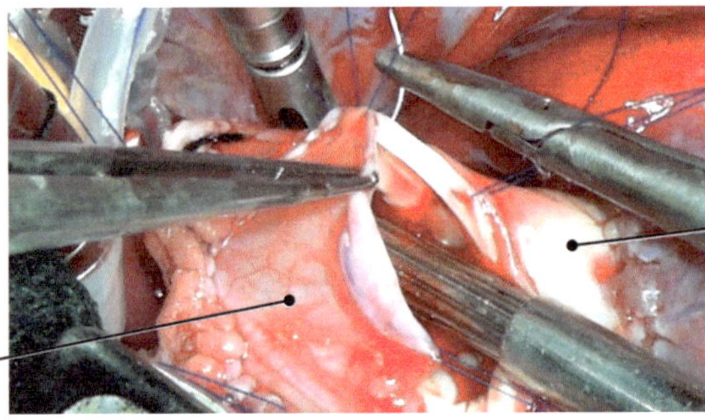

Scene 10.25 Main pulmonary artery reconstruction 2 (Video 55 min 22 s)

1. Another autologous pericardial patch is anastomosed to the anterior wall of the main pulmonary artery using a continuous 6-0 monofilament suture, and the anterior wall of the pulmonary artery is also augmented.

- Even if the longitudinal extension of the posterior wall is not necessary, the anterior wall of the pulmonary artery should be augmented as much as possible (Scene 10.26).

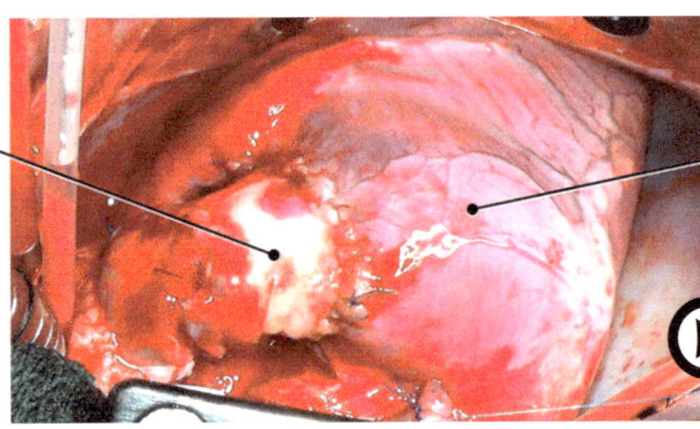

Scene 10.26 Completion of the half-turned truncal switch operation (Video 59 min 21 s) (▶ https://doi.org/10.1007/000-hkh)

- Complete the half-turned truncal switch procedure.
- Check for overstretching of the pulmonary artery bifurcation and right and left pulmonary arteries.

SPOTLIGHT CT Images After the Half-Turned Truncal Switch Operation

< left lateral view >

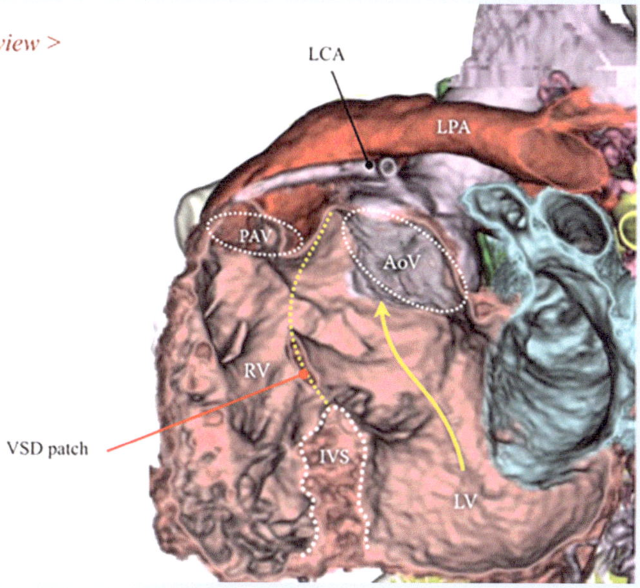

< cephalic view, horizontal cross-section >

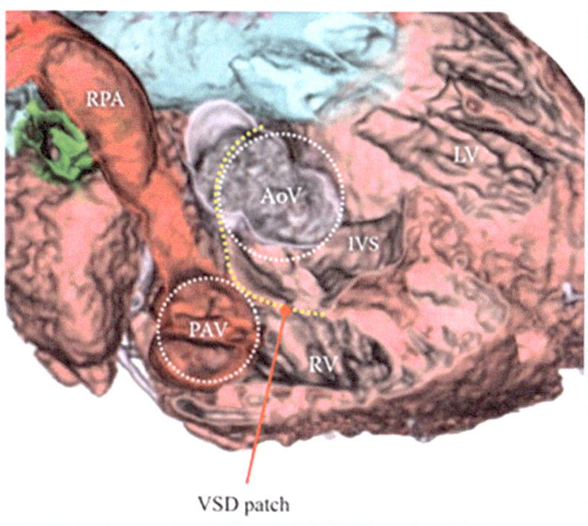

- The aorta is posteriorly translocated and the pulmonary artery is in anteriorly translocated.
- The pulmonary annulus is enlarged by commissurotomy.
- There is no stenosis of the right or left pulmonary artery.
- Since the pulmonary artery originated almost entirely from the right ventricle preoperatively, the aortic valve is slightly overridden on the interventricular septum postoperatively, but the left ventricular outflow tract (*yellow arrow*) is almost straight.
- The VSD closure patch is only partially visible on the CT, but it is almost flat and the right ventricular effective volume is secured.
- The left coronary artery is not bent, overstretched, or stenosed.

References

Nikaidoh Operation

Nikaidoh H. Aortic translocation and biventricular outflow tract reconstruction: a new surgical repair for transposition of the great arteries associated with ventricular septal defect and pulmonary stenosis. J Thorac Cardiovasc Surg. 1984;88:365–72.

Half-Turned Truncal Switch Operation

Yamagishi M, Shuntoh K, Matsushita T, Fujiwara K, Shinkawa T, Miyazaki T, Kitamura N. Half-turned truncal switch operation for complete transposition of the great arteries with ventricular septal defect and pulmonary stenosis. J Thorac Cardiovasc Surg. 2003;125:966–8.

Nomura K, Yamagishi M, Yamamoto Y, Ko Y. Half-turned truncal switch operation for single coronary in a patient with transposition of the great artery and pulmonary stenosis. J Thorac Cardiovasc Surg. 2017;154:268–70.

Hongu H, Yamagishi M, Miyazaki T, Maeda Y, Taniguchi S, Asada S, Fujita S, Yaku H. Late results of half-turned truncal switch operation for transposition of the great arteries. Ann Thorac Surg. 2018;106:1421–8.

Hongu H, Yamagishi M, Maeda Y, Itatani K, Asada S, Fujita S, Nakatsuji H, Yaku H. Comparison of half-turned truncal switch and conventional operations. Interact Cardiovasc Thorac Surg. 2021;33:101–9.

Asada S, Yamagishi M, Oda S, Maeda Y, Fujita S, Hongu H, Yamashita E, Nakatsuji H, Nagase T, Nakai R, Hayashi T. Modified half-turned truncal switch operation for posterior transposition of the great arteries with left ventricular outflow tract obstruction. JTCVS Tech. 2023;20:138–42.

Congenital Aortic Stenosis (AS), Aortic Regurgitation (AR)

11

1 Surgery for Congenital Aortic Valve Disease

1.1 Treatment Strategy

Congenital aortic stenosis (AS) includes valvular stenosis, subvalvular stenosis, combined valvular and subvalvular stenosis, and supravalvular stenosis. In valvular stenosis, bicuspid valves with a raphe, a remnant of valve insufficiency, are more frequent. In bicuspid valve cases, turbulent blood flow through the valve orifice results in thickening of the valve leaflets, decreased mobility, and consequent worsening of aortic regurgitation (AR), as well as enlargement of the ST junction and dilatation of the ascending aorta.

- *Critical AS (Neonatal Severe Aortic Stenosis)*
  Critical AS (severe cases presenting with heart failure symptoms in the neonatal period or infancy) may be accompanied by endocardial fibroelastosis (EFE), left ventricular hypoplasia, mitral valve disease (hypoplasia, regurgitation), etc. In these most severe cases, biventricular repair is often difficult, and a single ventricle repair (Fontan circulation by staged surgery) must be pursued.
- *Biventricular Repair*
  In cases with left ventricular or mitral valve morphology amenable to biventricular repair, catheter intervention (percutaneous aortic balloon angioplasty) or surgical aortic commissurotomy is indicated. The aortic valve leaflets are fragile in the neonatal period and early infancy, and some cases present with mucous degeneration. Surgical repair after balloon angioplasty is difficult because the aortic valve leaflets are ruptured during balloon angioplasty, not at the commissure, and aortic regurgitation is inevitable. Therefore, catheterization is indicated only for high-risk surgical cases, such as low-birth-weight infants or patients with severe heart failure, and in cases where left ventricular function is preserved, it is preferable to accurately incise the commissure by surgical intervention. Catheter intervention and surgery for aortic valves in the neonatal period and infancy are considered lifesaving first-line treatments. Future surgical reintervention is mandatory.

In this disease, not only valvular stenosis but also narrow valve annulus and subvalvular stenosis may be present. In cases of severe narrow valve annulus or subvalvular stenosis with aortic coarctation or interruption, biventricular repair is indicated by the Yasui procedure, which uses a dual pathway between the

Supplementary Information The online version contains supplementary material available at https://doi.org/10.1007/978-981-96-6194-7_11. The videos can be accessed individually by clicking the DOI link in the accompanying figure caption or by scanning this link with the SN More Media App.

M. Yamagishi, *Surgical Treatment of Congenital Heart Disease*,
https://doi.org/10.1007/978-981-96-6194-7_11

aortic and pulmonary valves for the systemic circulation.

On the other hand, in some patients with tricuspid aortic valve who underwent commissurotomy in neonatal or early infancy, annular enlargement (growth) and subvalvular stenosis may decrease. In such patients, staged surgical repair with annular and subvalvular enlargement is indicated instead of the Yasui procedure.

- *Surgical Strategy*
  Surgical treatment for cases that develop after infancy and for cases of exacerbation of AS or AR after first-stage surgery may include the following treatment strategies.

1. *Valvuloplasty*
   In children, the valve leaflet is fragile and the lesions themselves are diverse, limiting the techniques available for valvuloplasty. In many cases, the aortic valve is cannot be formed using only the autologous aortic valve leaflet, so it is necessary to use either autologous pericardium or a heterologous pericardium for valve tissue augmentation. In young children, it is not possible to reinforce the annulus or sinus of Valsalva with prosthetic vessels due to growth problems.

   In children, even with valvuloplasty, it is inevitable that valve regurgitation and stenosis will worsen as the child grows. In such cases, reoperation (Ross operation or prosthetic valve replacement) should be considered at an appropriate age. However, valvuloplasty is a useful treatment option as an emergency evacuation until reoperation.
2. *Prosthetic Valve Replacement*
   In pediatric patients, large-diameter prosthetic valves cannot be selected due to their physique. The smallest diameter of existing prosthetic valves (mechanical valves) is 17.4 mm. If this diameter cannot be used, or if an adult-sized valve is selected for an older child, annular enlargement (Konno procedure) is required.

   Reoperation is mandatory if a smaller diameter prosthetic valve is selected. Early deterioration of bioprosthetic valves has been reported in children, and bioprosthetic valves are not an option except in special cases. Mechanical valves require anticoagulation, but anticoagulation (warfarin) can be difficult to control in children. Bleeding complications are a concern due to the higher incidence of trauma compared to adults. Fetal effects are a concern in female patients.
3. *Prosthetic Valve Replacement with Aortic Annulus Enlargement (Konno Operation)*
   A longitudinal incision is made from the annulus to the left anterior to the aortic annulus through the ventricular septum in an apical direction, as well as an incision anterior to the right ventricular outflow tract. In cases of subvalvular aortic stenosis, the subvalvular stenosis can be repaired simultaneously.

   After suturing a large-diameter prosthetic valve, patches are placed in the ventricular septum, anterior wall of the aortic root, and right ventricular outflow tract. In the original Konno operation, the ventricular septal patch and the anterior wall of the aortic root are replaced with the same patch, and the right ventricular outflow tract is replaced with an extended patch consisting of two layers of the ventricular septal patch and the patch.

   The Konno operation is a revolutionary technique that allows three-dimensional enlargement of not only the aortic valve annulus, but also the left ventricular outflow tract. By adjusting the width of the expansion according to the size of the prosthetic valve to be implanted, it is possible to implant a prosthetic valve two to three sizes larger in diameter. The Konno operation can enlarge the valve annulus more significantly than other enlargement techniques such as the Nicks procedure. The Konno procedure is useful not only for children, but also for patients of all ages with a narrow aortic valve annulus.
4. *Ross Operation (Autolougous Pulmonary Valve Implantation to the Aortic Annulus).*
   The Ross operation was developed to overcome the problems of artificial valves, such as the need for anticoagulation therapy and durability. An autologous pulmonary valve (autograft) is harvested and implanted at the aortic annulus. The right ventricular outflow tract is

reconstructed with a homograft or prosthetic valve graft.

Autologous pulmonary valves implanted in the aortic valve position have growth potential and do not require anticoagulation therapy. This makes it a useful procedure for children and young patients, especially women of childbearing potential. The superiority of the Ross operation over mechanical valve replacement in terms of thromboembolic complications and cardiac and valve-related mortality has been reported, as well as better outcomes after the Ross operation than after biological valve replacement in terms of survival and avoided reoperation.

< *Merit of Ross Operation* >

- No need for anticoagulation therapy: No anticoagulation therapy is required from the acute postoperative period as no artificial valve is used.
- Growth potential: Growth of the pulmonary artery autograft is allowed as the patient grows.
- Pregnancy and delivery possible: No need for anticoagulation, thus avoiding the effects of warfarin on the fetus.

< *Problems of Ross Operation* >

- Difficulty: More difficult procedure than prosthetic valve replacement.
- Aortic root dilatation: In some cases, the new aortic root (the part of the pulmonary artery autograft) enlarges during the later period. In adolescents, when growth factors do not need to be taken into consideration, aortic root reinforcement with artificial grafts is effective for neo-aortic root dilation.
- Neo-aortic valve (pulmonary autograft) dysfunction: due to enlargement of the aortic root (ST junction) and histological fragility of the valve leaflets, regurgitation lesions may occur in the later period.
- Development of right ventricular outflow tract stenosis and pulmonary regurgitation: valved prosthesis (conduit) must be replaced with a larger diameter conduit as the patient grows.

5. *Ross-Konno Operation (Ross Operation with Aortic Annular Enlargement)*
   The narrow aortic annulus is enlarged by the Konno operation, and autologous pulmonary artery autograft is implanted into the enlarged aortic annulus. The incised ventricular septum is closed with a patch or by replacing the right ventricular outflow tract anterior wall flap that was resected with the autograft. This technique is useful for small infants and children who cannot have an artificial valve inserted, and anticoagulation therapy can be avoided.
6. *Modified Konno Operation (Preservation of Aortic Annulus and Enlargement of Subaortic Left Ventricular Outflow Tract)*
   This procedure is indicated for patients with subvalvular aortic stenosis without aortic valve or annulus involvement. The subvalvular stenosis is removed (widening of the left ventricular outflow tract) while preserving the aortic valve annulus. The stenotic lesion is identified through the aortic valve, and the ventricular septum at the site of the stenosis is incised from the right ventricular side to enlarge the prosthetic patch. This technique is useful in cases of severe stenosis that cannot be eliminated by incising the left ventricular outflow tract alone.

1.2 Anatomy of the Periaortic Valve and Right Ventricular Outflow Tract (Fig. 11.1)

- The aortic and pulmonary valve annuli are not in the same plane.
- In normal hearts, there is a muscular infundibulum beneath the pulmonary valve, and the pulmonary valve is positioned higher than the aortic valve.
- The left anterior descending branch runs in close proximity to the dorsal aspect of the main pulmonary artery (pulmonary valve annulus).

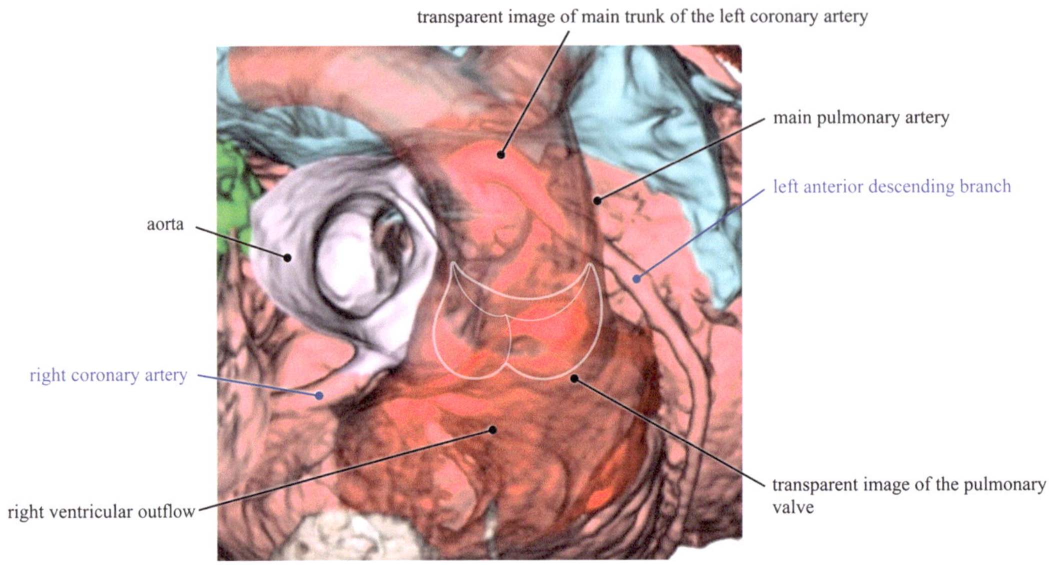

Fig. 11.1 CT images of periaortic valve and right ventricular outflow tract

< horizontal cross-section at aortic valve annulus level >

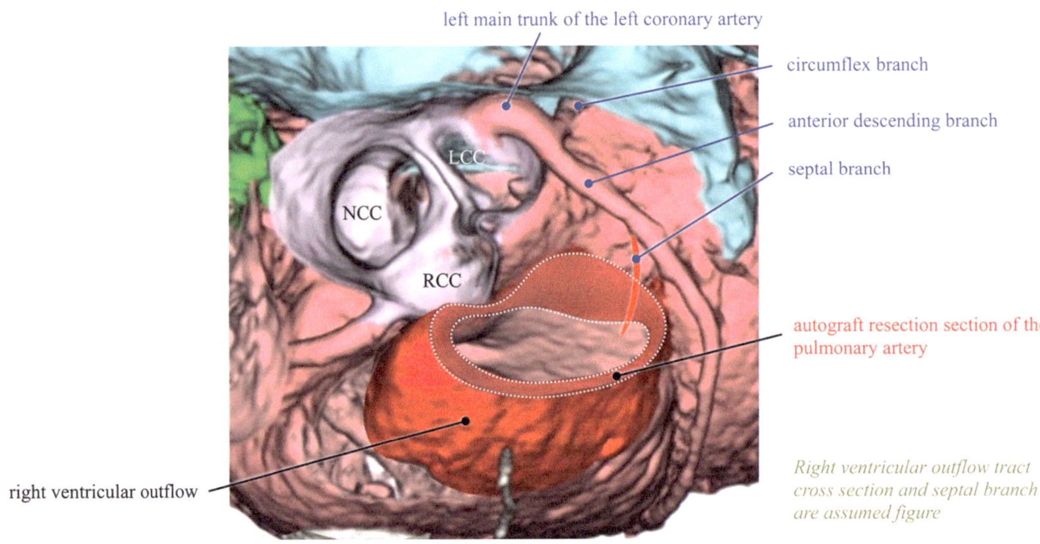

- The left coronary artery originates from the left dorsal coronary cusp (LCC) of the aorta and immediately bifurcates into a circumflex branch.
- The left anterior descending branch runs close to the dorsal aspect of the main pulmonary artery (pulmonary valve annulus).
- The degree of proximity between the pulmonary valve annulus and the anterior descending branch varies depending on the case.
- The septal branch bifurcates from the anterior descending branch on the left dorsal surface of the right ventricular outflow tract and passes within the ventricular septum.
- The septal branch is in close proximity to the autograft resection section of the pulmonary artery.
- The right dorsal aspect of the pulmonary artery autograft transection is adjacent to the right coronary cusp (RCC) of the aorta.

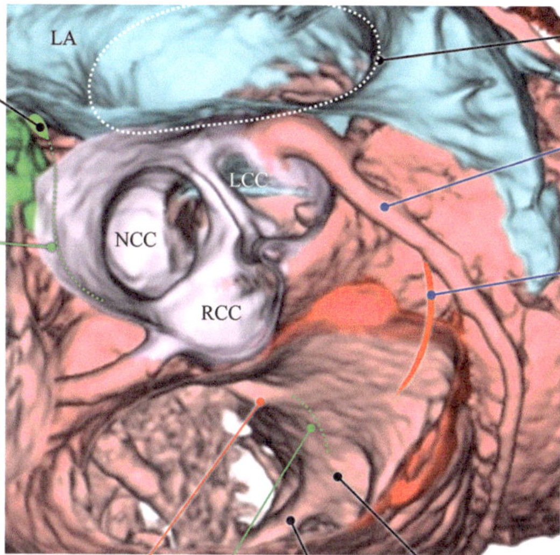

- The right dorsal side of the right ventricular outflow tract is proximal to the right coronary cusp (RCC) of the aortic valve.
- The left anterior descending branch runs dorsal to the right ventricular outflow tract, branches off the septal branch, and descends on the left side of the right ventricular outflow tract toward the apex.
- The main conduction bundle is closest to the aortic valve annulus anterior to the noncoronary cusp (NCC) and descends toward the apex.
- The medially papillary muscle (MPM) attaches to the right ventricular side surface of the ventricular septum, caudal to the right coronary artery.
- The conduction system (right bundle branch: RBB) runs beneath the endocardium at the base of the MPM toward the base of the anterior papillary muscle (APM).

< frontal cross-section >

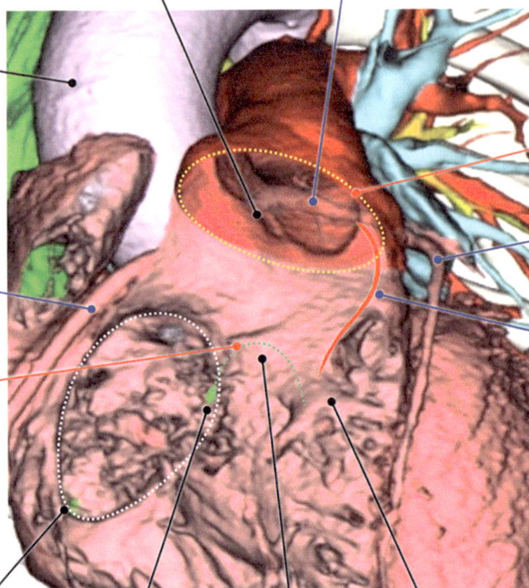

- The conduction system branches off the right bundle branch at the base of the medially papillary muscle and runs rightward in the trabecular septomarginalis toward the base of the anterior papillary muscle.

< left lateral cross-section >

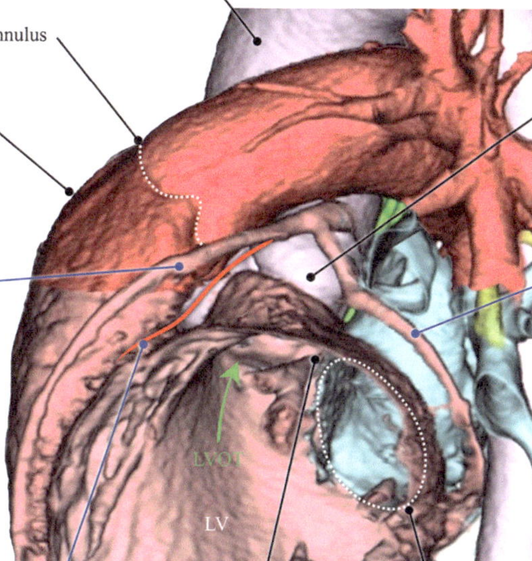

infundibulum

- In the normal heart, an infundubulum (muscular tissue) exists under the pulmonary valve annulus, and the pulmonary valve annulus is higher (cephalic) than the aortic valve annulus.

left anterior descending branch

- The left anterior descending branch runs dorsal to the main pulmonary artery (pulmonary valve annulus).
- The degree of proximity between the pulmonary artery and the anterior descending branch varies depending on the case.
- When harvesting the pulmonary artery autograft, the relationship between the left anterior descending branch, the pulmonary artery, and the pulmonary valve annulus should be confirmed preoperatively.

septal branch

- The septal branch branches from the anterior descending branch dorsal to the main pulmonary artery and runs within the ventricular septum.

< dorsal cross-section >

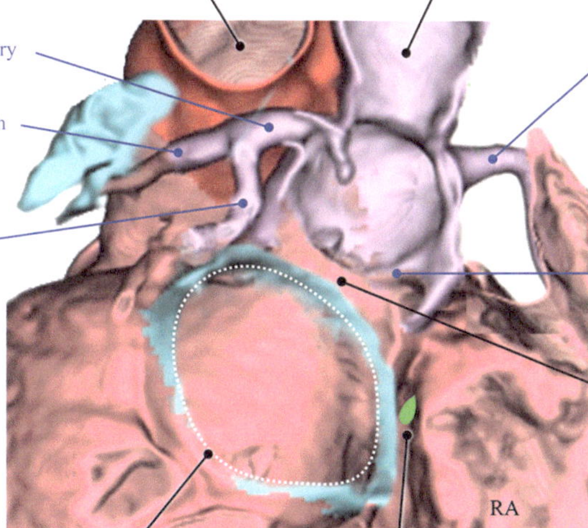

aortic-mitral fibrous continuity

- In the normal heart, the aortic and mitral valve annuli are fibrinously connected.

2 Ross Operation

2.1 Procedure of the Ross Operation (Fig. 11.2)

1. After initiation of extracorporeal circulation, harvest the pulmonary artery autograft with the heart beating.
   - Insert a flexible suction tube from the right atrium to the right ventricle to maintain good visual field.
2. Sew a traction suture to the anterior surface of the pulmonary artery (anterior and posterior to the incision line).
   - The incision line should be near the midpoint between the sino-tubular (ST) junction and the bifurcation (the ST junction of the pulmonary artery may be unclear).
   - The incision should be approximately 10 mm higher than the ST junction (it need not be too cephalad).
3. Transect the pulmonary artery.
4. Insert forceps transpulmonary through the pulmonary artery opening to identify the incision site below the pulmonary artery valve.
5. Make a transverse incision through the pulmonary artery, taking care not to damage the pulmonary valve commissure, and create a guide hole for incision of the pulmonary artery.

Fig. 11.2 Procedure of the Ross operation

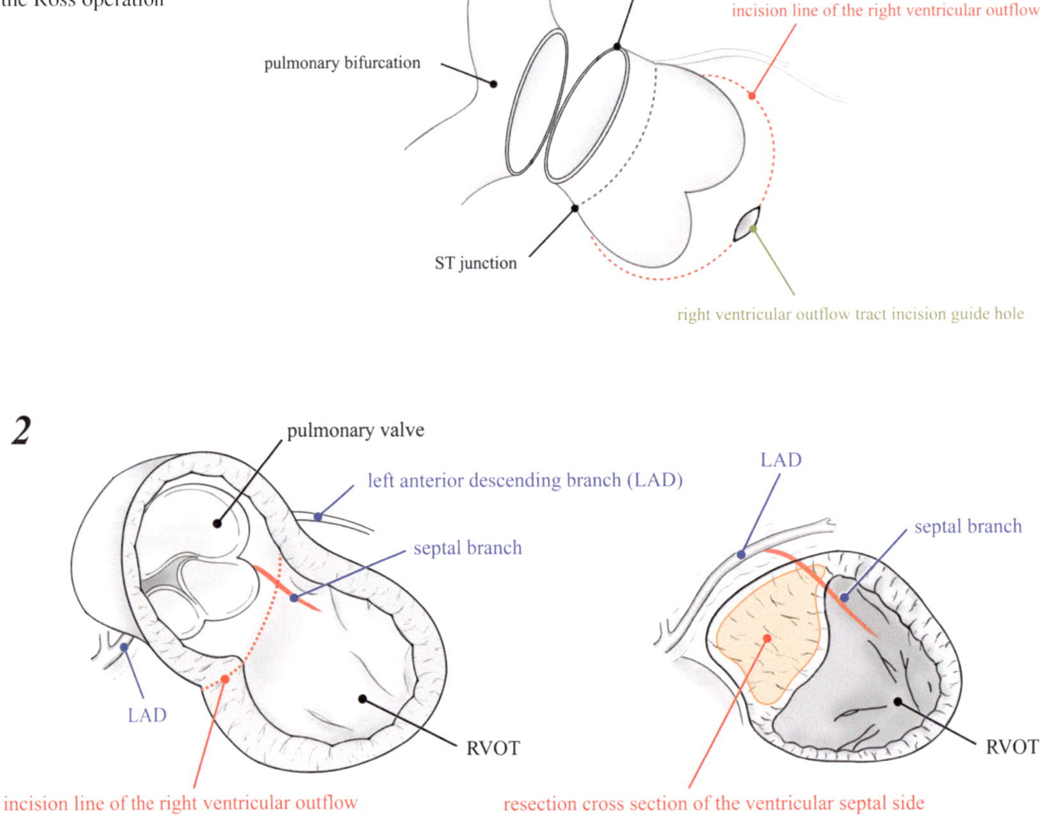

1. Starting from the incision guide hole, incise the anterior and lateral walls of the right ventricular outflow tract (RVOT) parallel to the pulmonary valve annulus approximately 3–5 mm from the valve annulus.
   • Bleeding from small vessels on the incision surface is stopped as needed.
2. The posterior wall (ventricular septal aspect) is also incised along the sinus of Valsalva with a shear knife parallel to the valve annulus.
   • The anterior descending branch of the coronary artery runs behind and to the left of the incision (the pulmonary and coronary arteries are separated by fibrous and fatty tissue).
   • The septal branch of the coronary artery runs in the myocardium on the left dorsal side of the incision, so incise and dissect this area to avoid damaging the septal branch.
   • The pulmonary artery autograft can be harvested with the heart beating, but incision of the posterior wall can be done after cardiac arrest (however, bleeding sites from small vessels are easier to identify with the heart beating).
   • Bleeding at this site is difficult to control after right ventricular outflow tract reconstruction.

3 Anastomosis of the Pericardial Patch to the Ventricular Septal Transection Site

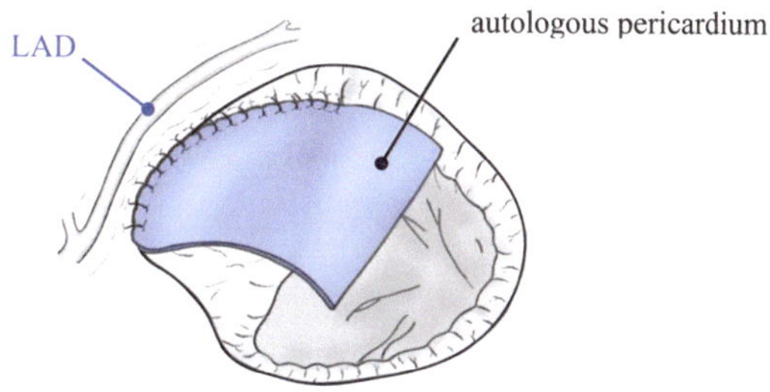

• The transected area is covered with autologous pericardium.
• The anastomosis is started from the dorsal aspect of the transected surface.

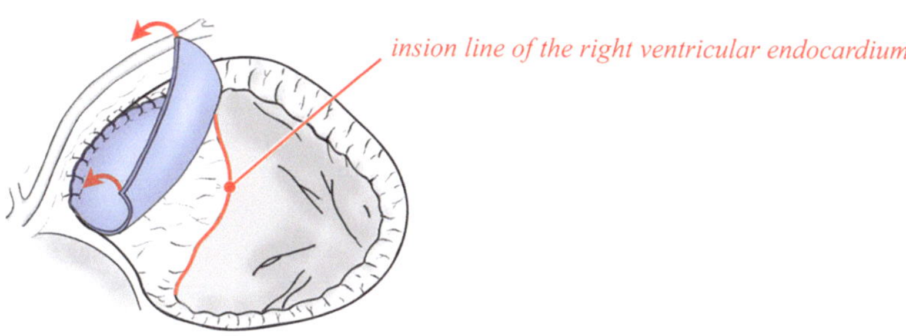

• Fold back the autologous pericardium at the right ventricular endocardial incision line (*red line*).

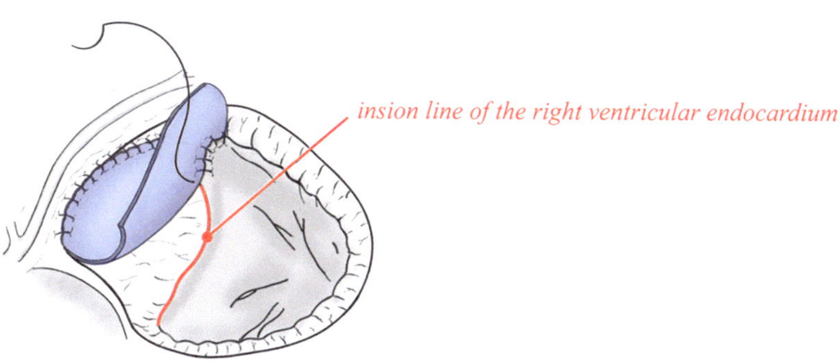

- The folded edge of the autologous pericardium is anastomosed to the endocardial incision line (*red line*).

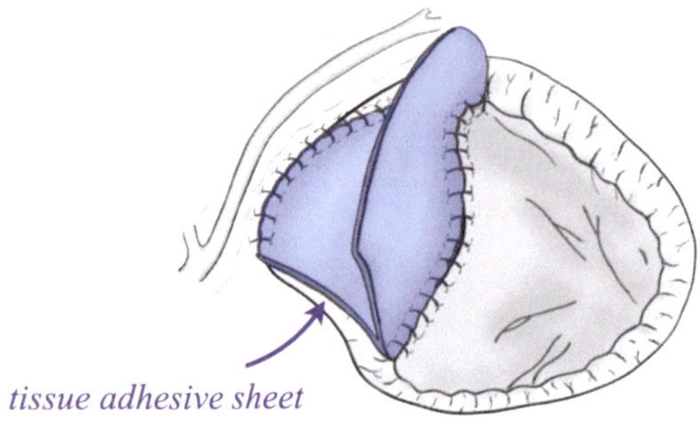

- Insert a tissue adhesive sheet between the autologous pericardium and the cut surface.

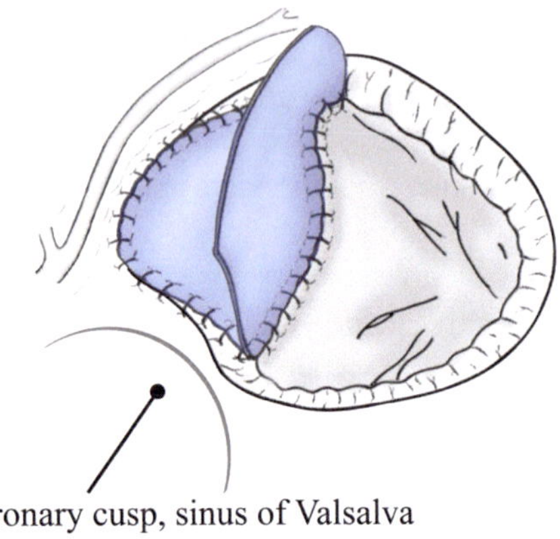

- The right edge of the autologous pericardium is also sutured to the cut surface (note that this area is adjacent to the aortic wall).

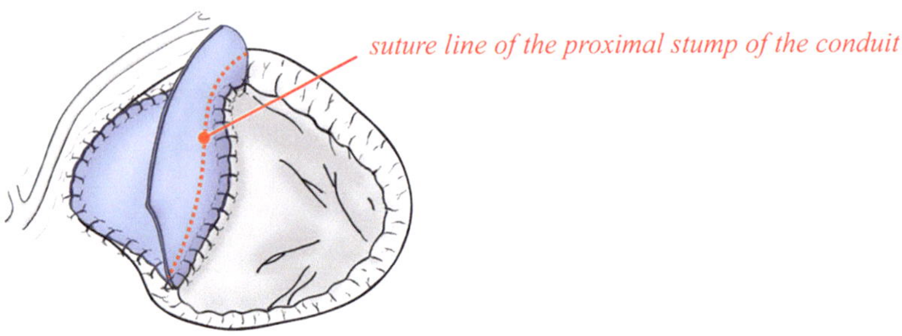

- The posterior wall of the proximal stump of the right ventricular-pulmonary artery conduit anastomoses to the autologous pericardium (*red dashed line*).

4

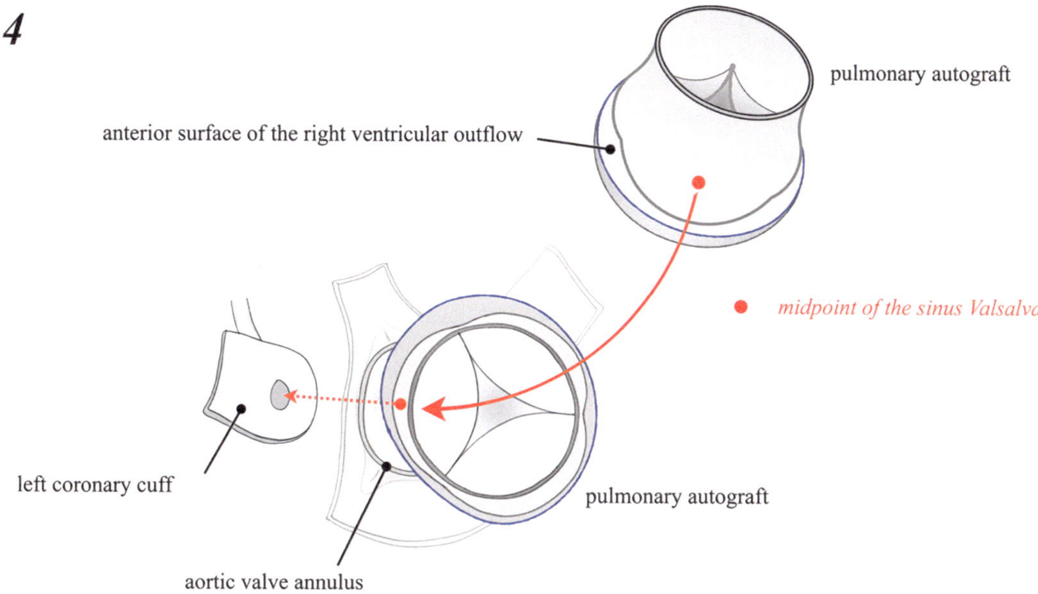

1. Place the pulmonary artery autograft in the position of the aortic valve.
2. The middle of the sinus in the anterior right ventricular outflow tract is replaced relative to the left coronary cuff to reinforce the site of aortic valve-mitral valve fibrous continuity with the anterior right ventricular myocardium.

- Position and angle the pulmonary artery autograft so that the sinus center is relative to the left coronary artery orifice, rather than aligning the commissure.
- The aortic commissure may not be in its normal position in cases such as bicuspid valve cases, so it is not an indicator for positioning.

5 *Mattress suture reinforced with an autologous pericardial strip*

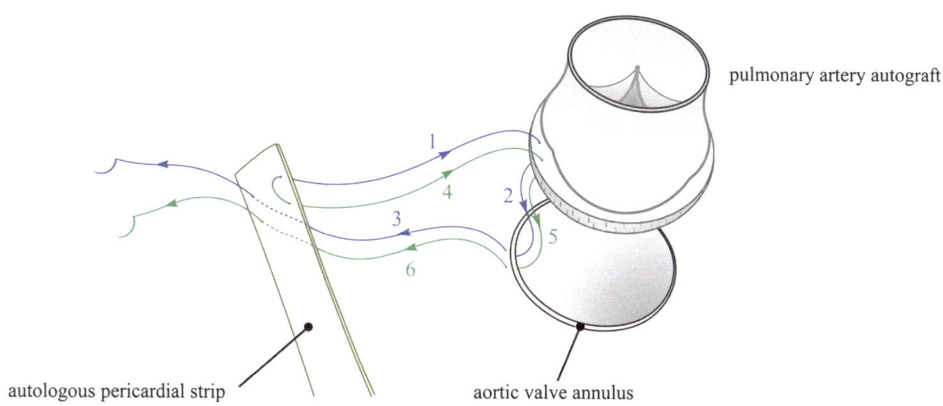

- Mattress suture of autologous pericardial strips, pulmonary artery autograft, and aortic valve annulus with 5–0 monofilament suture:
  1. Autologous pericardium strip → pulmonary artery autograft(*outside* → *inside*)
  2. Pulmonary artery autograft → aortic valve annulus(*inside* → *outside*)
  3. Aortic valve annulus → autologous pericardium strip
- In the same manner, mattress suture with a suture needle on the contralateral side of the same suture:
  4. Autologous pericardium strip → pulmonary artery autograft(*inside* → *outside*).
  5. Pulmonary artery autograft → aortic valve annulus(*inside* → *outside*).
  6. Aortic valve annulus → autologous pericardium strip.
- Sutures may be applied in the order of aortic valve annulus to pulmonary artery autograft:

(a) *Autologous pericardium strip → pulmonary artery autograft.*

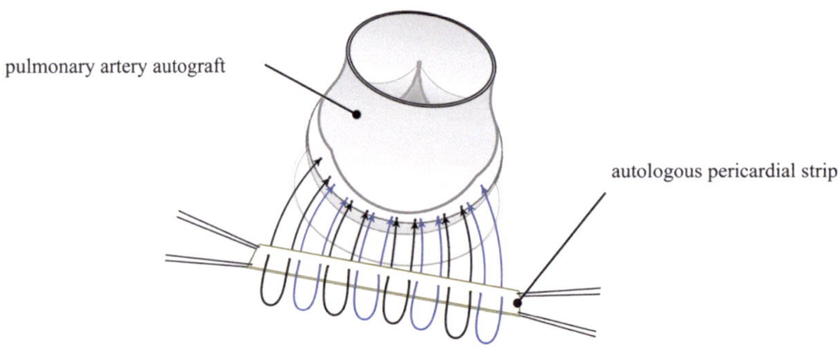

(b) *Pulmonary artery autograft → aortic valve annulus → autologous pericardium strip.*

- In this figure, all sutures are drawn separately for the (a) and (b) techniques for convenience, but in reality, the mattress sutures are performed one by one from (a) and (b) in this order.

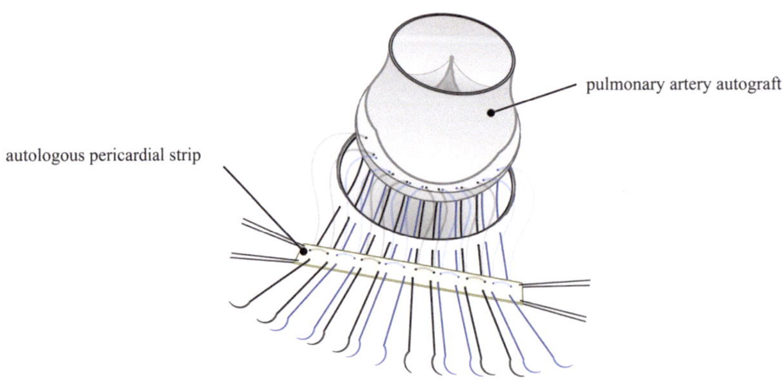

- One autologous pericardial strip is used in each sinus (total of three autologous pericardial strips).

6

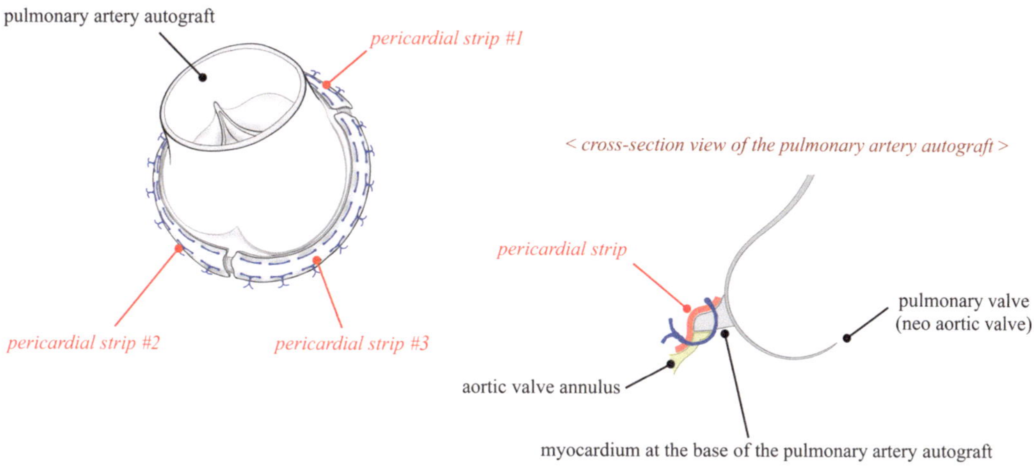

1. Ligate the mattress suture and anastomose the pulmonary artery autograft to the aortic valve annulus.
   - These suture-reinforced mattress sutures with autologous pericardium cover the entire circumference of the anastomosis between the pulmonary artery autograft and the aortic valve annulus.
   - This prevents bleeding as well as reinforcing the valve annulus.
   - Excessive protrusion (elevation) of the anastomosis site is eliminated. This effect prevents the valve annulus anastomosis from pushing up the coronary artery and causing coronary artery stenosis.

7

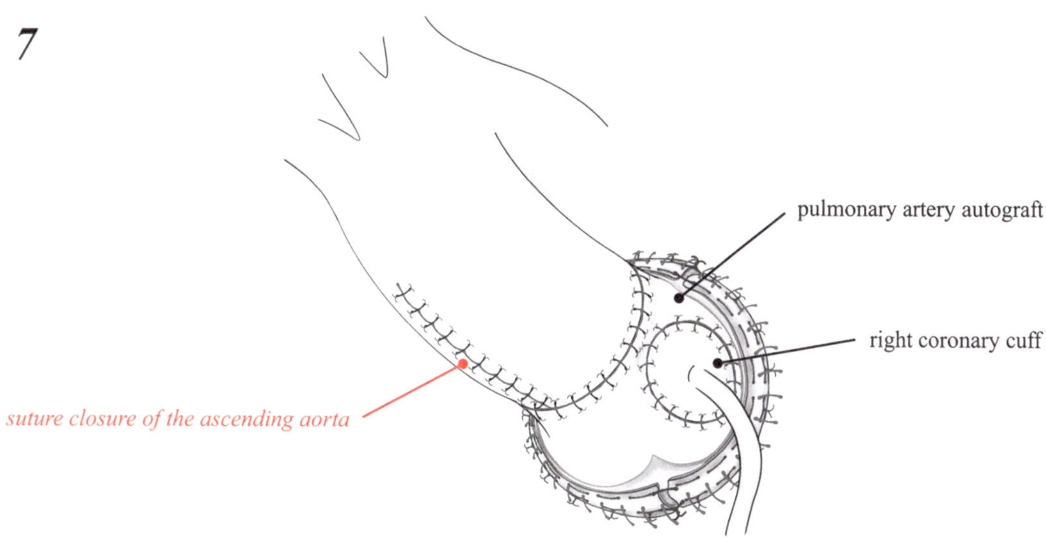

1. Punch-out the pulmonary artery autograft wall and anastomose the left and right coronary artery cuffs with a continuous 6-0 monofilament suture.
   - In the Ross procedure, the coronary cuffs are anastomosed in the sinus of Valsalva (proximal to the ST junction) of the pulmonary artery autograft.
2. If the ascending aorta is enlarged, a spindle-shaped resection is performed on the greater curvature side and suture closure is performed to reduce the transverse diameter.
3. The pulmonary artery autograft and ascending aorta are anastomosed end-to-end with a continuous 5-0 monofilament suture.
   - Because the pulmonary artery autograft is thin and fragile, the base of the pulmonary artery autograft should not be left long.
   - Anastomose with the ascending aorta just above the ST junction of the pulmonary artery autograft.

8

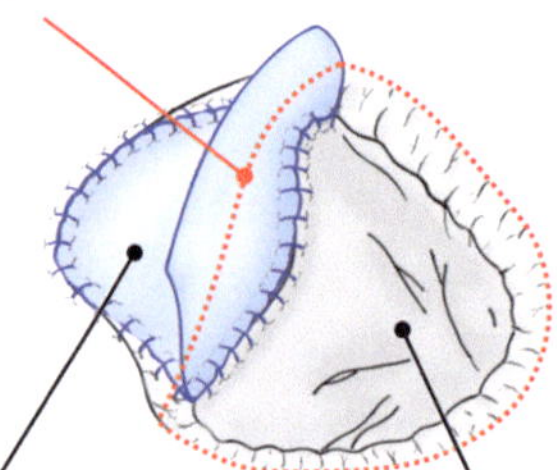

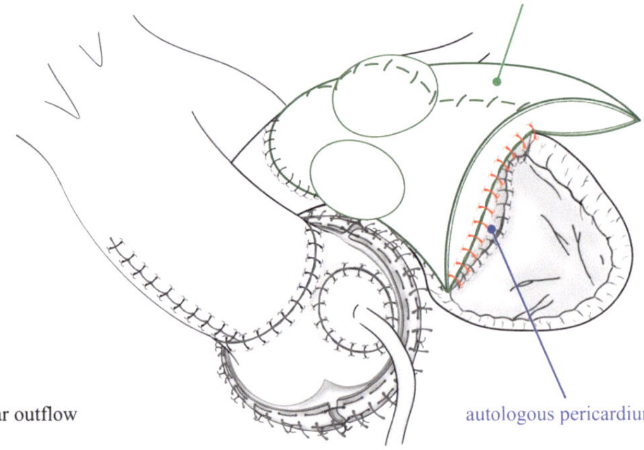

1. The folded surface of the autologous pericardium covering the pulmonary artery autograft resection section is used as the suture line (*left figure: red dashed line*) for the valved right ventricular-pulmonary artery conduit.
   - The posterior wall of the valved conduit is anastomosed only to the folded autocardium, not to the septal cross section. Avoid direct anastomosis of the valved conduit to the vulnerable septal cross section.
2. Anastomose the distal end of the conduit to the pulmonary artery bifurcation with a continuous ePTFE CV-6 or CV-5 suture (W.L. Gore & Associates, Inc.).
3. After anastomosing the distal end of the valved conduit, measure the distance between the pulmonary artery bifurcation and the posterior wall of the right ventricular outflow tract opening (autologous pericardial patch) to determine the length of the small curvature side of the valved conduit.
4. Anastomose the posterior wall of the valved conduit to the autologous pericardium with a continuous ePTFE CV-5 suture.
5. Anastomose the lateral and anterior walls of the valved conduit to the right ventricular outflow tract opening myocardium with continuous ePTFE CV-4 suture.

2.2 Ross Operation (Surgical Video) (Ross, Scene 1)

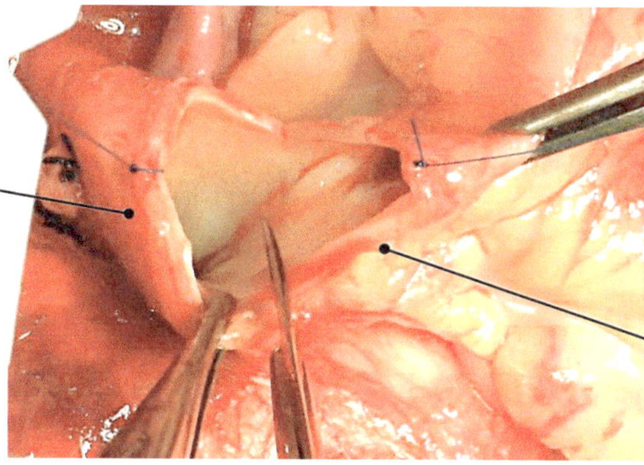

Ross, Scene 1 Harvest of the pulmonary artery autograft 1 (Video 00 min 05 s)

1. After initiation of extracorporeal circulation, harvest pulmonary artery autograft under heart beating.
   - Insert a flexible suction tube from the right atrium to the right ventricle to maintain good visual field.
2. Sew a traction suture in front of the main pulmonary artery (anterior and posterior to the incision line).
   - The incision line is midpoint between the ST junction and the bifurcation.
   - The incision should be approximately 10 mm higher than the ST junction (not too cephalad).
3. Incise the pulmonary artery transverse to the commissure at least 5 mm away from the commissure, taking care not to damage the pulmonary valve commissure (Ross, Scene 2).

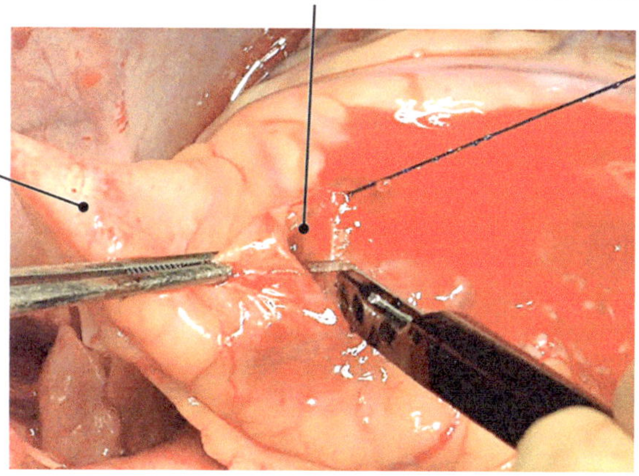

Ross, Scene 2 Harvest of the pulmonary artery autograft 2 (Video 00 min 35 s)

1. To avoid damage to the pulmonary valve, right-angle forceps are inserted through the main pulmonary artery incision to below the valve, and the incision line is positioned by palpating the tip.

- Make a transverse incision in the right ventricular outflow tract so as not to damage the pulmonary valve annulus.
- The incision site should be at least 10–15 mm caudal to the valve annulus (Ross, Scene 3).

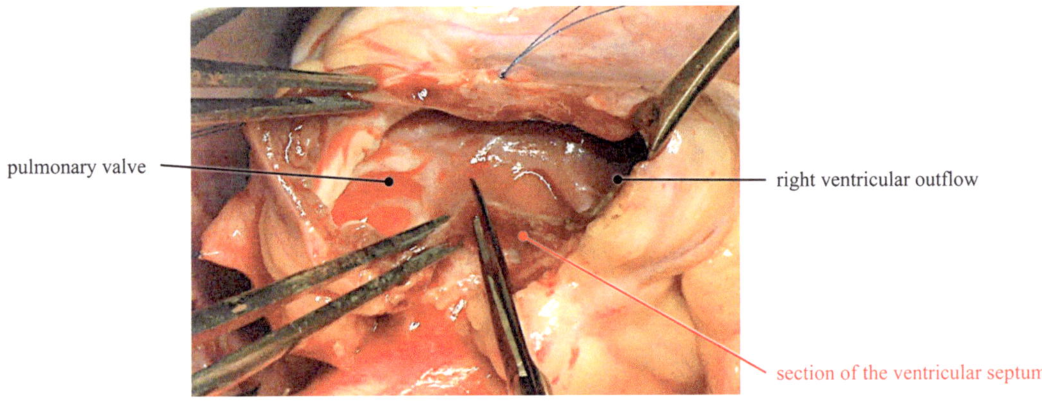

Ross, Scene 3 Harvest of the pulmonary artery autograft 3 (Scene 02 min 12 s)

1. Make a transverse incision 5 mm below the dorsal pulmonary valve annulus along the annulus.
2. The incision is made by inserting a straight scissors into the cross section in a slightly obliquely sloping manner.

- Because the anterior descending coronary artery is located in the dorsal fat tissue, be careful not to damage the coronary artery.

< Section of the Ventricular Septum >

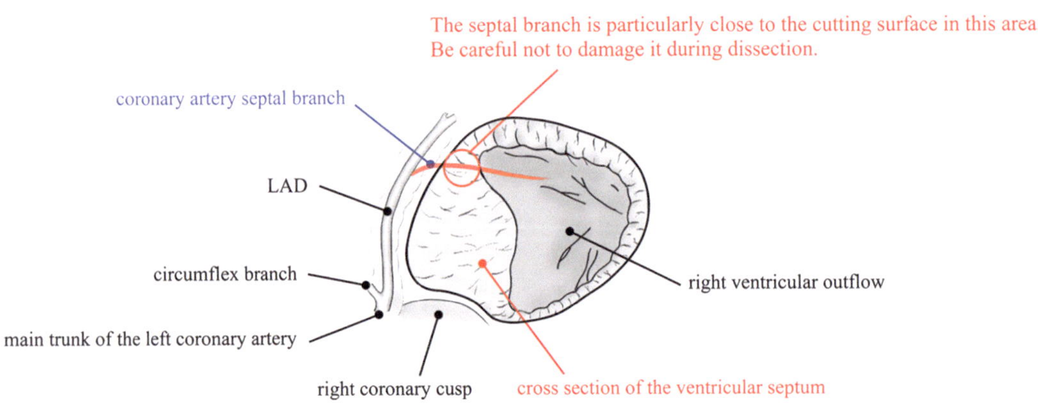

- The left main coronary artery and circumflex branch are separated from the pulmonary artery autograft transection, but the anterior descending branch is proximal to the transection aspect.
- The right side of the septal transection aspect is adjacent to the aorta (right coronary cusp, sinus of Valsalva).

< Incision Line of the Pulmonary Autograft >

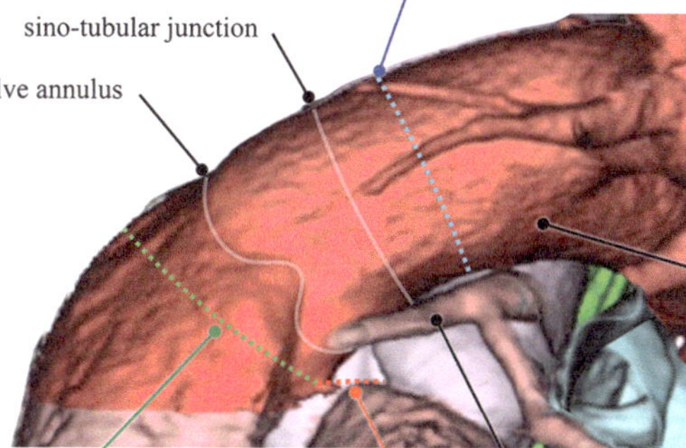

- *Incision line of the right ventricular outflow.* Start the incision on the anterior surface at least 10–15 mm caudal to the valve annulus. While viewing the lumen through the incision, incise along the valve annulus at a distance of approximately 5 mm from the annulus.
- *Incision line of the ventricular septum.* Slightly oblique to the anterior and lateral sections of the right ventricular outflow tract (*green dashed line*). Note the proximity to the left anterior descending branch (Ross, Scene 4).

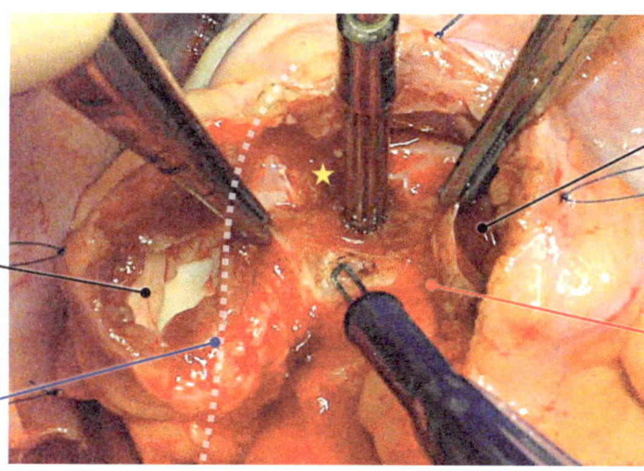

Ross, Scene 4 Harvest of the pulmonary artery autograft 4 (Video 02 min 44 s)

1. Incise the myocardium below the pulmonary valve (ventricular septum).
   - The anterior descending branch of the left coronary artery runs in the adipose tissue on the dorsal surface of the septum (white dotted line).
   - Because of the close proximity of the anterior descending branch, extreme care must be taken to dissect the dorsal adipose tissue and connective tissue.
   - The septal branch of the coronary artery is located near the anterior dorsal surface of the section (★), so care must be taken when dissecting it (Ross, Scene 5).

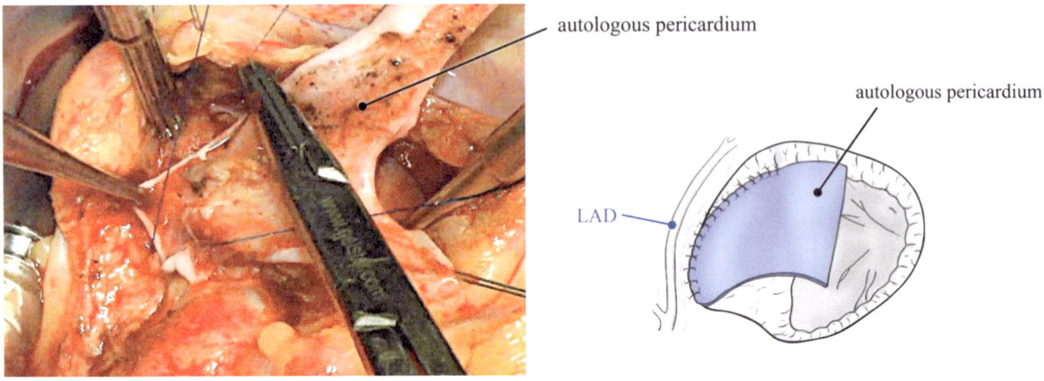

Ross, Scene 5 Harvest of the pulmonary artery autograft 5 (Video 06 min 31 s)

1. The section of ventricular septum is covered with fresh autologous pericardium to prevent re-bleeding and to reinforce the anastomosis of the right ventricular-pulmonary conduit.
   - When anastomosing the autologous pericardium on the dorsal side, care should be taken not to injure the anterior descending branch of the left coronary artery (LAD).
   - If the autologous pericardium anastomosis causes tension on the epicardium and coronary artery stenosis, the epicardium is dissected around the coronary artery to relieve the tension on the epicardium (Ross, Scene 6).

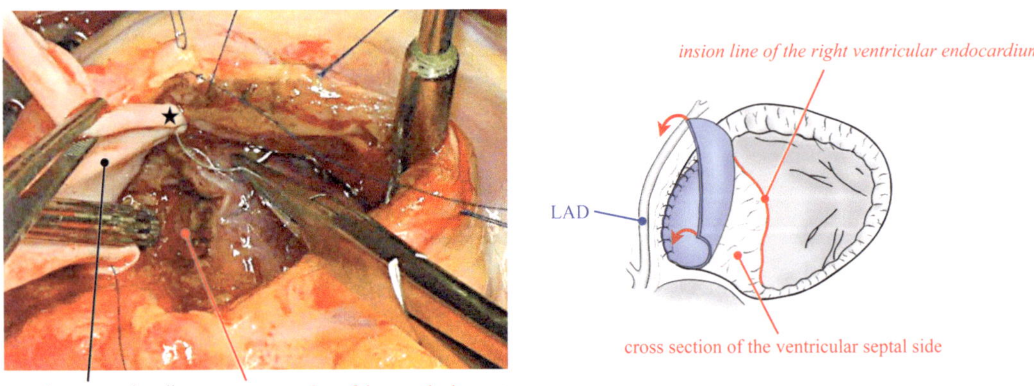

Ross, Scene 6 Harvest of the pulmonary artery autograft 6 (Video 07 min 52 s)

1. Once the autologous pericardium is anastomosed left anterior to the incision surface (★), fold back the pericardium (Ross, Scene 7).

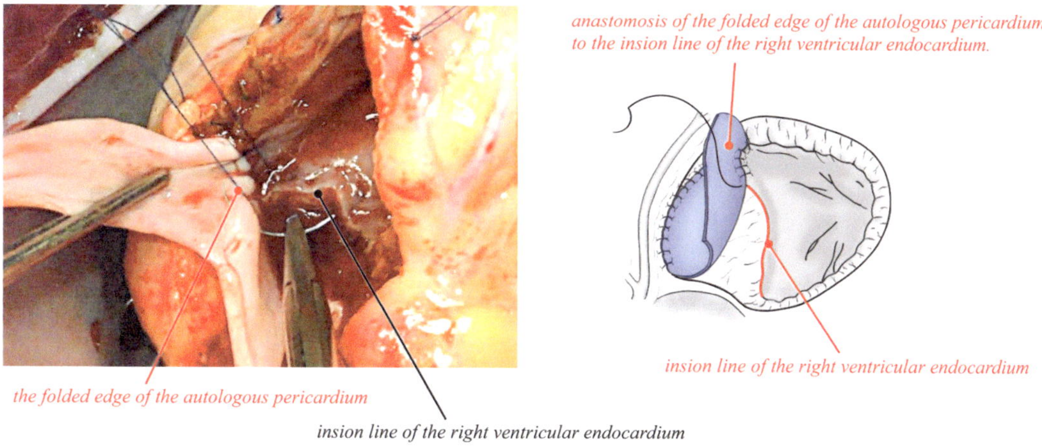

Ross, Scene 7 Covering of ventricular septal cross-section 1 (Video 09 min 00 s)

1. The folded edge of the autologous pericardium is anastomosed to the insion line of the right ventricular endocardium (Ross, Scene 8).

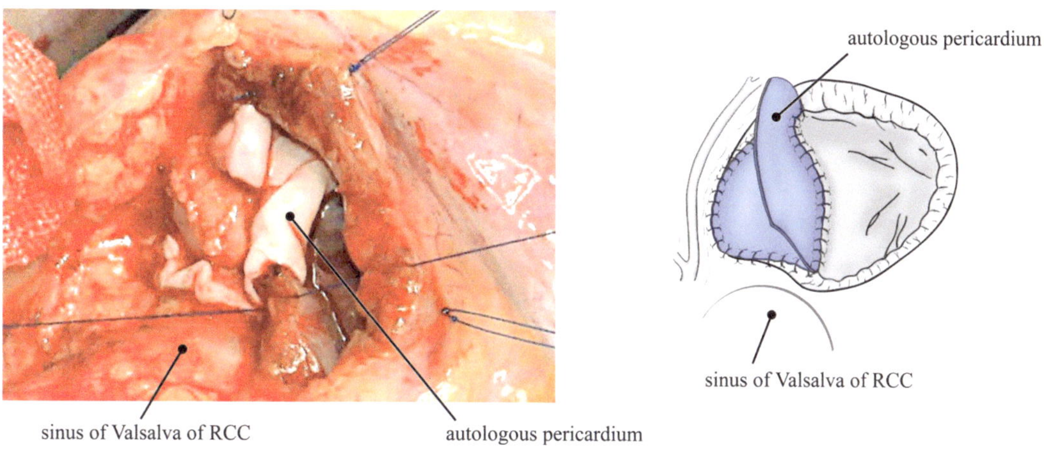

Ross, Scene 8 Covering of ventricular septal cross-section 2 (Video 10 min 06 s)

1. Insert the tissue adhesive sheet between the pericardium and the cross section and anastomose around the entire circumference of the ventricular septal cross section.

- Since the right side of the cross section is in close proximity to the sinus of Valsalva of the right coronary cusp (RCC), care should be taken not to damage the aortic wall (Ross, Scene 9).

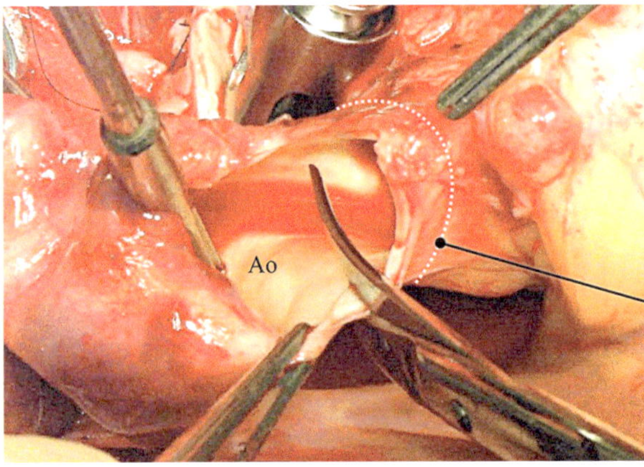

Ross, Scene 9 Transection of the ascending aorta (Video 12 min 22 s)

1. Clamp the aorta just before the brachiocephalic artery bifurcation and induce cardiac arrest.
2. Transect the aorta just above the ST junction (white dashed line).
   - Care should be taken with the site of origin of the coronary artery (especially in cases of high take-off coronary artery) (Ross, Scene 10).

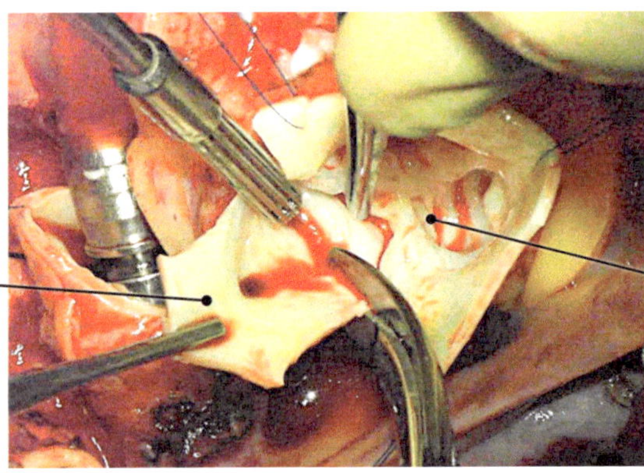

Ross, Scene 10 Harvest of LCC cuff (Video 12 min 45 s)

1. Incise the aortic wall of the left coronary artery origin in a U-shape and harvest the coronary cuff.
   - The coronary cuff should be large (excise the entire aortic wall of the sinus).
   - If the coronary artery orifice is close to the valve commissure, such as in the case of a bicuspid aortic valve, dissect the commissure first and harvest a large coronary cuff.
   - Dissect around the origin of the coronary artery with electric scalpel (Ross, Scene 11).

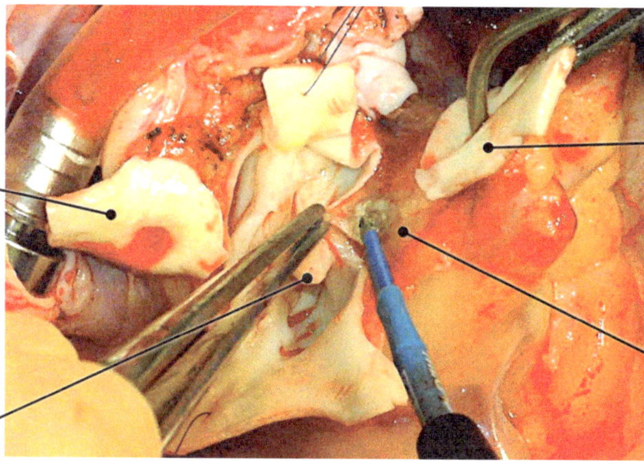

Ross, Scene 11 Harvest of RCC cuff (Video 13 min 47 s)

1. The aortic wall of the right coronary artery origin is also incised in a U-shape to harvest the coronary button.

- The area around the coronary artery origin is dissected with electric scalpel (Ross, Scene 12).

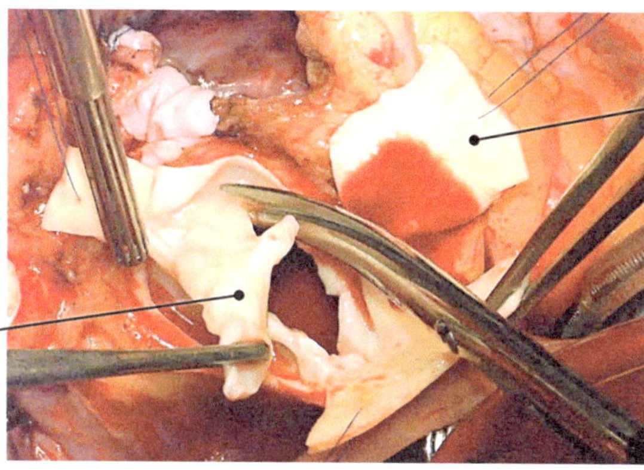

Ross, Scene 12 Resection of the aortic valve (Video 14 min 28 s)

1. Resect the aortic valve (bicuspid valve in this case) (Ross, Scene 13).

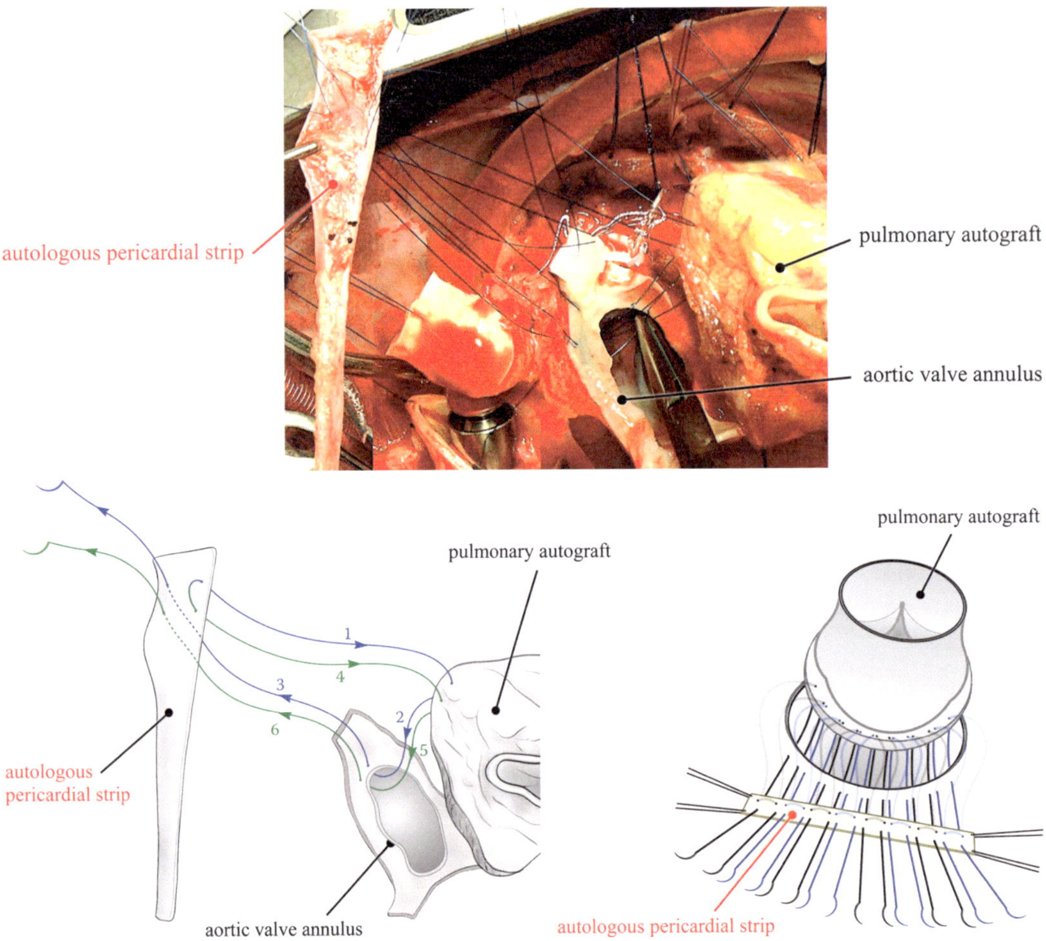

Ross, Scene 13 Anastomosis of the pulmonary autograft 1 (Video 15 min 05 s)

1. Pulmonary autograft anastomosis.
2. Prepare three strips of autologous pericardium (one for each sinus).
3. Apply a 5-0 monofilament suture from autologous pericardium → pulmonary artery autograft → aortic valve annulus → autologous pericardium.
4. The other side of the suture is also placed in a U-shaped mattress pattern: autologous pericardium → pulmonary artery autograft → aortic valve annulus → autologous pericardium.
5. Apply approximately 10–15 U-shaped mattress sutures to each sinus.
6. Perform the same suture at three sinuses (Ross, Scene 14).

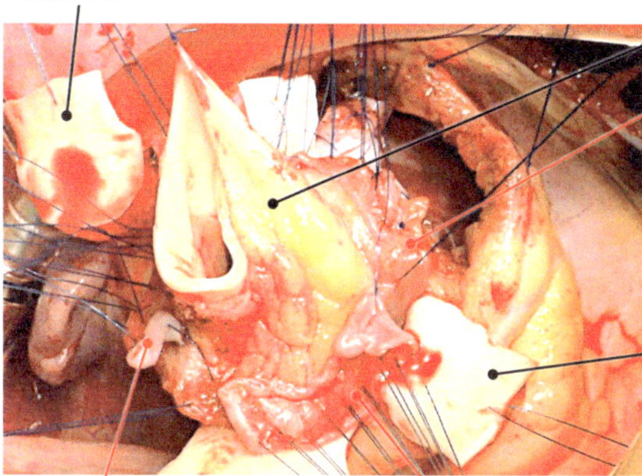

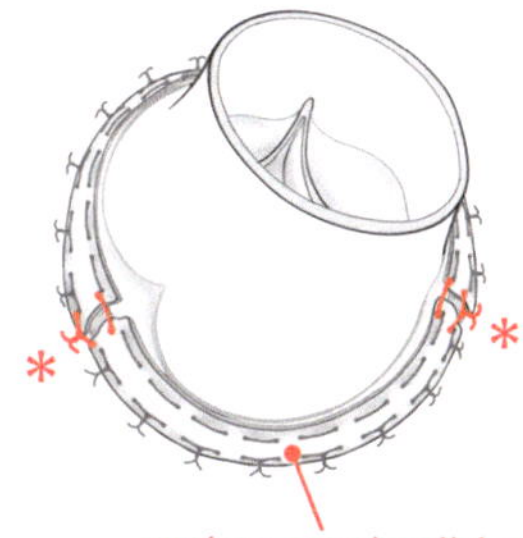

Ross, Scene 14 Anastomosis of the pulmonary autograft 2 (Scene 22 min 08 s)

1. Position the pulmonary valve autograft on the aortic valve annulus and ligate the mattress sutures.
2. To reinforce the valve annulus circumferentially, the three pericardial strips are tied together (*) (Ross, Scene 15).

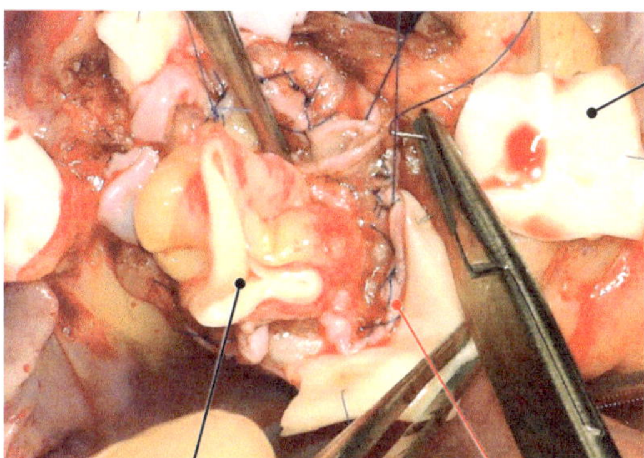

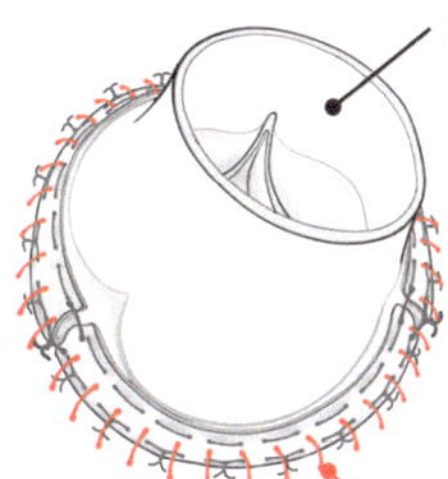

Ross, Scene 15 Reinforcement of pulmonary autograft anastomosis (Video 23 min 42 s)

1. Pericardial strips are sutured around the circumference of the left ventricular outflow tract with a continuous 4-0 monofilament suture to prevent bleeding and to reinforce the anastomosis (*right figure*) (Ross, Scene 16).

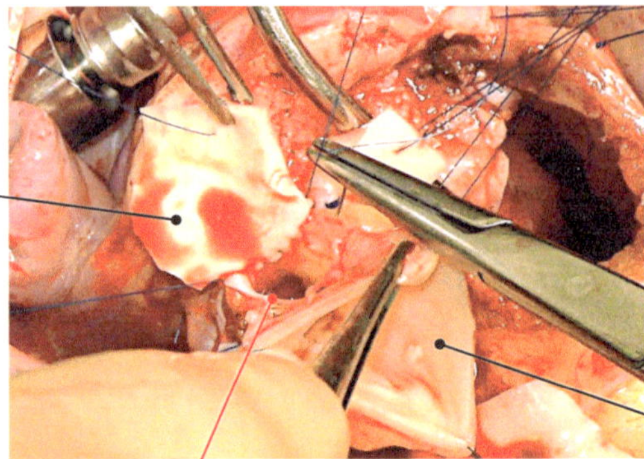

Ross, Scene 16 Anastomosis of the LCC cuff (Video 25 min 22 s)

1. The sinus of Valsalva of the pulmonary autograft is resected circumferentially and the left coronary cuff is anastomosed to the created opening with a continuous 6-0 monofilament suture.
2. Trim the upper edge of the LCC cuff to match the circular opening created in the pulmonary autograft wall after anastomosing the bottom half of the cuff (Ross, Scene 17).

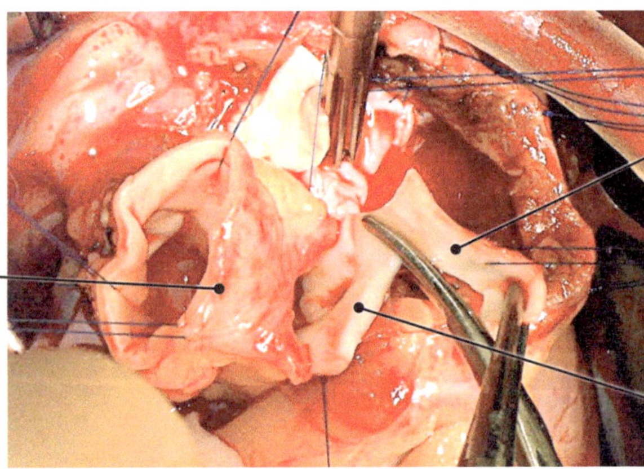

Ross, Scene 17 Anastomosis of the RCC cuff (Video 30 min 28 s)

1. Anastomose the RCC cuff in the same manner.
2. Trim the upper edge of the RCC cuff to match the circular opening created in the pulmonary autograft wall after anastomosing the bottom half of the cuff (Ross, Scene 18).

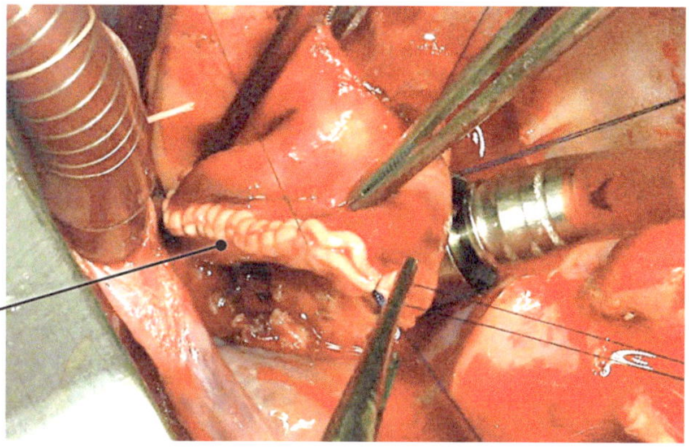

Ross, Scene 18 Plication of the ascending aorta (Video 34 min 39 s)

1. Spindle resection of the greater curvature side of the dilated ascending aorta.
2. Anastomose the incision longitudinally and plicate the aorta.

- This plication is not necessary (to be considered depending on the degree of enlargement of the ascending aorta).
- In adolescents and adults, the ascending aorta may be externally wrapped with an artificial graft (Ross, Scene 19).

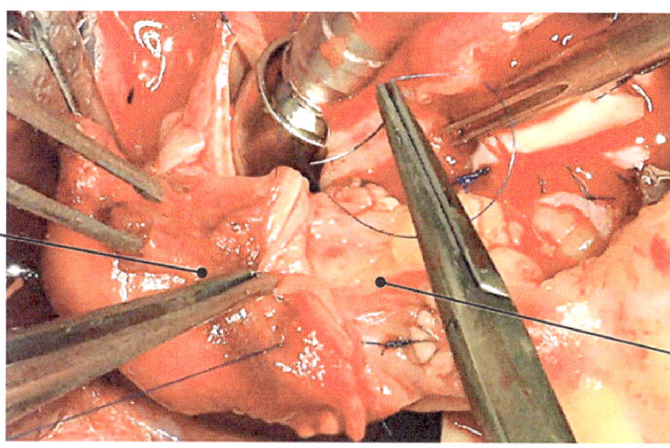

Ross, Scene 19 Ascending aorta-pulmonary autograft anastomosis (Video 38 min 20 s)

1. The pulmonary artery autograft is anastomosed to the ascending aorta in an end-to-end fashion with horizontal mattress 5-0 monofilament sutures and a continuous 5-0 monofilament suture.
   - If the pulmonary autograft stump has a long excess margin, an additional excess portion of the pulmonary autograft is resected near the ST junction (just above the coronary cuff suture) to remove as much of the weak pulmonary artery wall as possible (Ross, Scene 20).

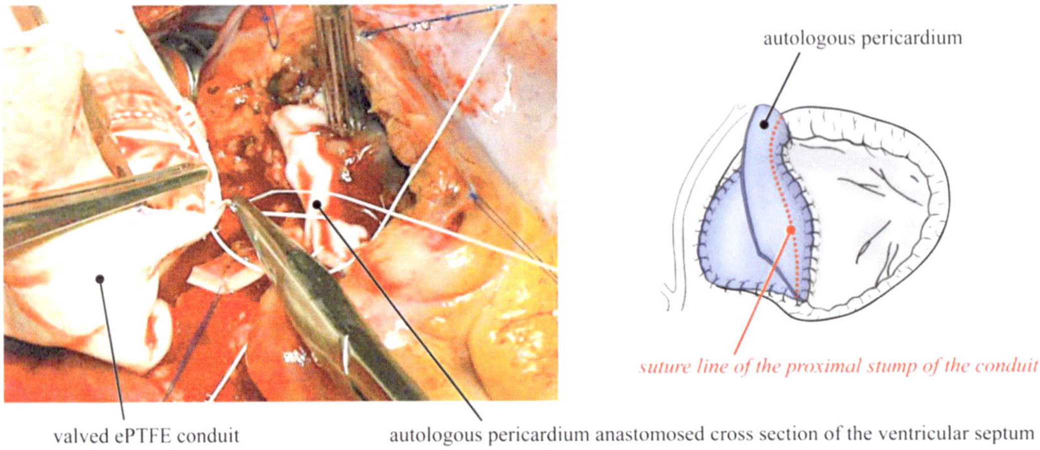

Ross, Scene 20 Anastomosis of valved ePTFE conduit 1 (Video 44 min 03 s)

1. The distal side of the right ventricular-pulmonary artery conduit (tricuspid valved ePTFE conduit) is anastomosed to the opening of the pulmonary artery bifurcation with a continuous ePTFE CV-6 suture.
2. The dorsal wall of the proximal end of the conduit and the right ventricular outflow tract is anastomosed to the autologous pericardium, which is filled at the cross section of the ventricular septum.
   - The use of autologous pericardium avoids cutting the myocardium.
   - In addition, the autologous pericardium is used to fine-tune the length of the lesser curvature conduit (Ross, Scene 21).

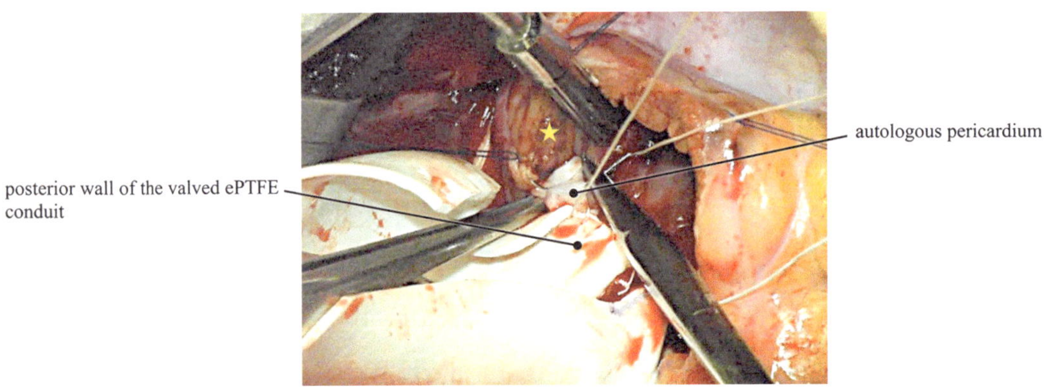

Ross, Scene 21 Anastomosis of valved ePTFE conduit 1 (Video 45 min 55 s)

1. The posterior wall of the proximal stump of the valved ePTFE conduit is anastomosed to the autologous pericardium (some myocardium may also be included in the suture).
2. The valved ePTFE conduit is anastomosed to the left end of the dorsal right ventricular outflow opening (★) including the pericardium as reinforcement because the myocardium is easily torn at this portion and the septal branch runs around this area.
   - Including the autologous pericardium in the anastomosis facilitates the transition of the suture line from the cross section of the ventricular septum (endocardial side) to the right ventricular outflow opening (epicardial side) (Scene 11.22).

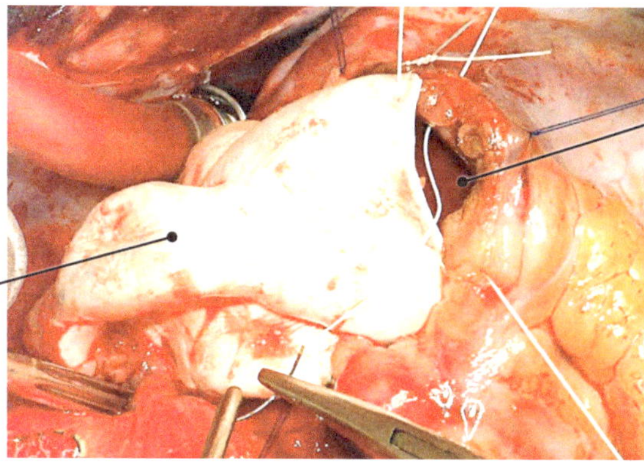

Ross, Scene 22 Anastomosis of valved ePTFE conduit 3 (Video 47 min 08 s) (▶ https://doi.org/10.1007/000-hkk)

1. Anastomose the proximal end of the right ventricular-pulmonary artery conduit to the right ventricular outflow opening using a continuous ePTFE CV-5 suture (CV-4 suture in adolescents and adults).
   - If the conduit is twisted or too long, do not hesitate to remove the lateral and anterior wall sutures, trim the conduit, and re-suture.
   - The length of the greater curvature side (anterior aspect) of the conduit should be shorter in the Ross procedure than in the Rastelli procedure (because the anterior aspect of the right ventricular outflow tract is not incised longitudinally in the Ross procedure).

3 Konno Operation

3.1 Anatomy of the Aortic Annulus, Both Ventricular Outflow, and Ventricular Septum (Fig. 11.3)

- Noncoronary cusp (NCC) present on the right dorsal side.
- Right coronary cusp (RCC) is present anteriorly, with the right coronary artery originating from and running along the tricuspid annulus.
- Left coronary cusp (LCC) is located posteriorly on the left side, where the left main coronary artery originates.

< horizontal cross-section at aortic valve annulus >

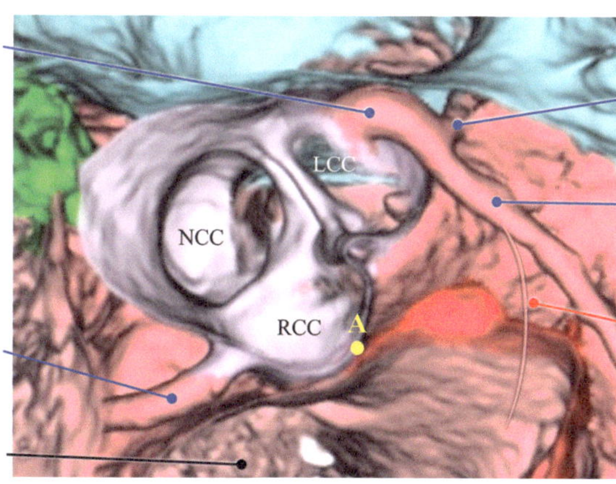

Fig. 11.3 Anatomy of the aortic root and right ventricular outflow

- An anterior descending branch (LAD) runs dorsal to the right ventricular outflow tract after branching off the circumflex branch (may be in close proximity to the right ventricular outflow tract in some cases).
- The septal branch branches on the left dorsal side of the right ventricular outflow tract (the location of the branch depends on the case).
- LAD runs to the left of the right ventricular outflow tract toward the apex (in proximity to the right ventricular outflow tract).
- The point to the left of the right coronary artery orifice and to the right of the RCC-LCC commissure is the starting point for incising the valve annulus in the Konno procedure (point (A)).
- Note, however, that the commissure may not be in its normal position in cases of congenital arterial valve stenosis or bicuspid aortic valve.

< horizontal cross-section at aortic valve annulus, lower level >

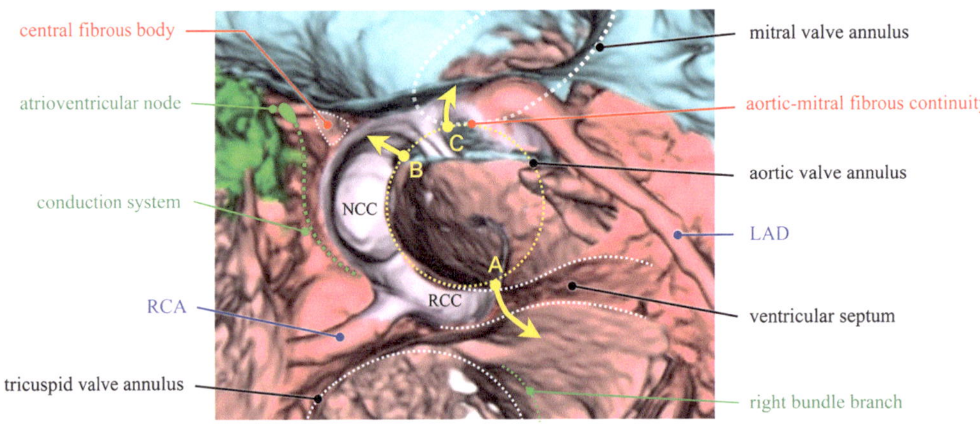

Point A: Start point of the incision in the Konno procedure.

- The aortic valve annulus near the RCC-NCC commissure is the starting point of the incision (point (A)).
- From point (A), the ventricular septum is incised toward the apex.
- If the incision is closer to the left than point (A), the incision point is toward the ventricular septum.

Point B: Start point of the incision in the Nicks procedure.

- Incise to the right of the NCC-LCC commissure toward the dorsal central fibrous body.

Point C: Start point of the incision in the Manougian procedure.

- Incise to the left of the LCC-NCC commissure toward the dorsal aortic valve-mitral annulus fibrosus continuity.
- Incise the mitral annulus and the anterior leaflet.

3.2 Incision in the Konno Procedure (Fig. 11.4)

1. *Longitudinal incision of the aorta.*

< horizontal cross-section >

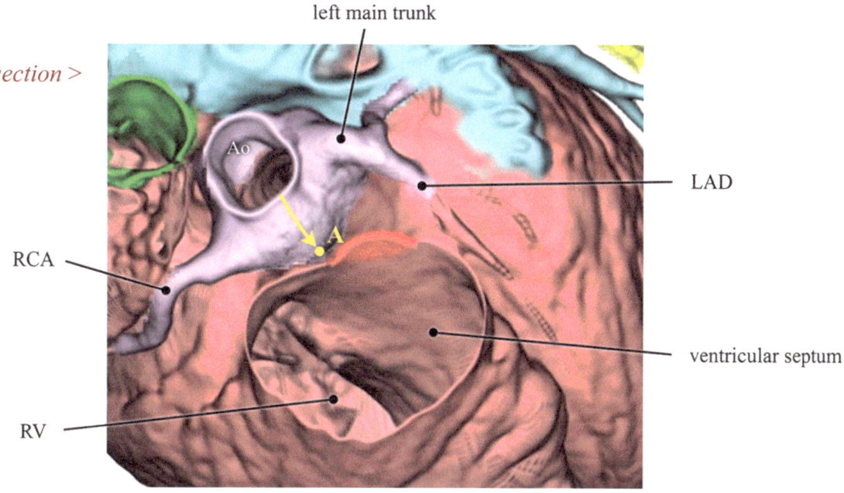

Fig. 11.4 Konno incision

1. For the Konno procedure (prosthetic valve implantation), the anterior wall of the ascending aorta is incised longitudinally.
2. For the Ross-Konno procedure (pulmonary artery autograft transplantation), the aorta is cut transversely just above the ST junction.
3. Incise the left side of the right coronary artery orifice (near the commissure of the right coronary cusp with the left coronary cusp) straight down to the aortic valve annulus (*yellow arrow*) (point (A)).
   - In cases such as bicuspid valves, the coronary artery orifice and commissure are not in the normal position, so the incision is made longitudinally as shown in the figure above.
   - When the incision is made closer to the left coronary artery orifice, point (A) is not directly over the right ventricular cavity, but in the ventricular septal cross section.
   - In the Ross-Konno procedure, the right ventricular outflow tract has already been opened by harvesting the pulmonary artery autograft, making it easy to determine the point (A).
2. *Transverse incision of the right ventricular outflow.*

< horizontal cross-section >

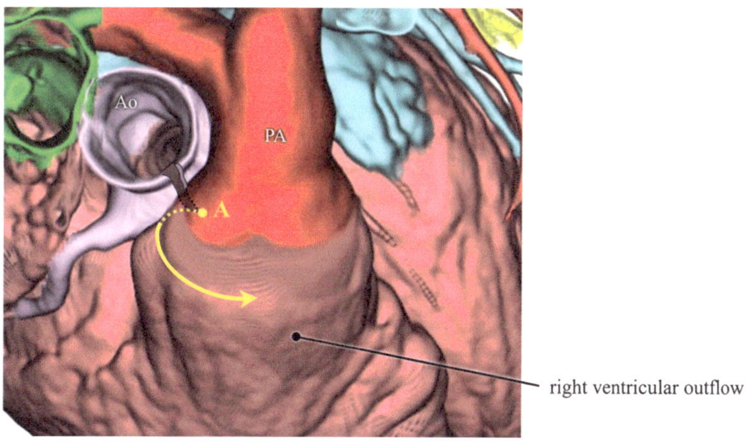

1. For the Konno procedure, make a transverse incision from point (A) through the right ventricular outflow tract parallel to the pulmonary valve annulus.
2. Make a transverse incision to the center of the right ventricular outflow tract (*yellow arrow*).

- The right ventricular outflow tract incision should be parallel to the pulmonary valve annulus and not toward the apex (to avoid distortion of the patch used for augmentation).
- In the Ross-Konno procedure, the right ventricular outflow tract is open at the time the pulmonary artery autograft is harvested, eliminating the need for an additional incision in the anterior wall of the right ventricle.

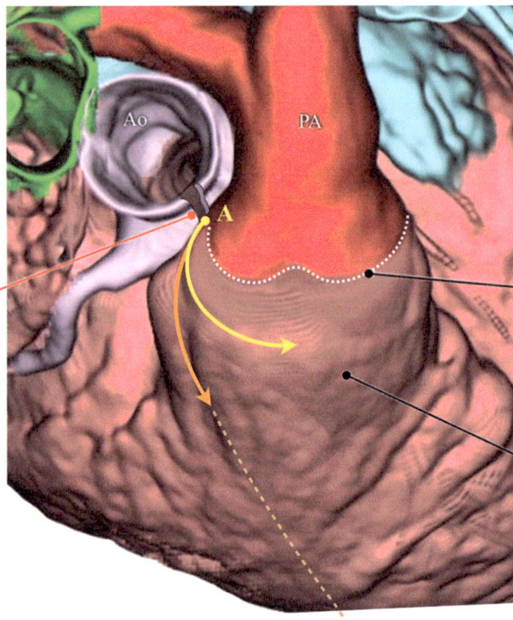

In the Konno procedure, the right ventricular anterior wall is incised after incision to the aortic valve annulus. The direction of this incision is important to reconstruct a well-defined right ventricular outflow tract.

- The incision of the right ventricular anterior wall should be made parallel to the pulmonary valve annulus (*yellow arrow*) and not toward the apex (white arrow).
- Incision toward the apex (*orange arrow*) may distort the right ventricular outflow patch replaced during reconstruction.

3. *Longitudinal incision of the ventricular septum.*

< horizontal cross-section >

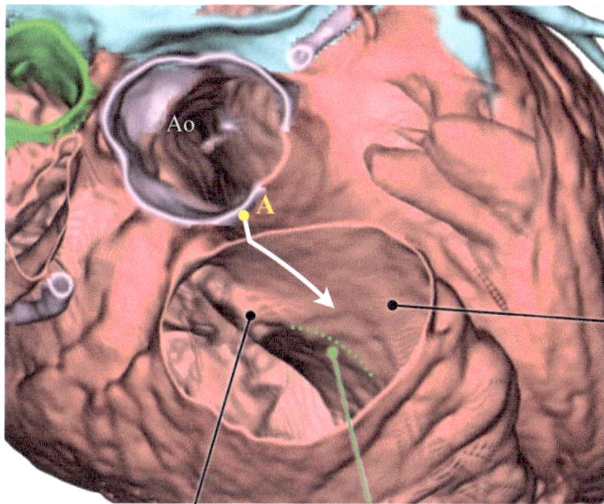

1. Incise the ventricular septum from point (A) toward the right ventricular apex (white arrow).
   - The right ventricular endocardial incision is directed approximately 5 mm anterior to the base of the medially papillary muscle.
   - Because the conduction system (*right bundle branch*) runs near the base of the medially papillary muscle, the incision line is moved away from the base of the medially papillary muscle to the left, leaving a seam allowance for the VSD patch.
   - The incision on the left ventricular endocardial side should be directed toward the base of the anterior papillary muscle of the mitral valve.
   - The incision on the left ventricular side should be slightly deeper than that on the right ventricular side.

4. *Incision lines of the right ventricular outflow and the ventricular septum.*

< coronal cross-section >

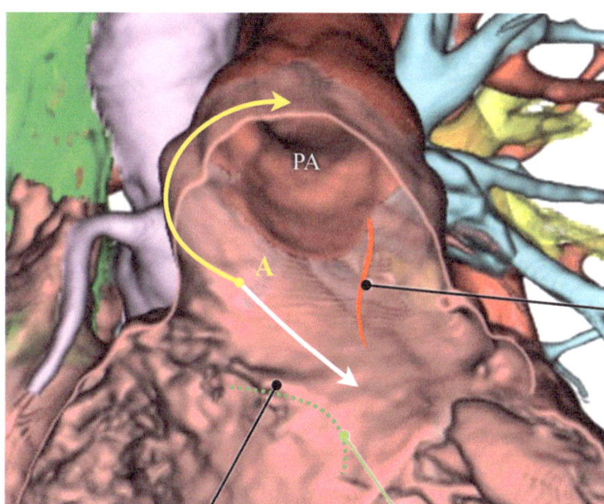

- Right ventricular outflow tract incision line (*yellow arrow*) and ventricular septal incision line (*white arrow*) viewed from coronal cross section.

1. The right ventricular outflow tract is incised parallel to the pulmonary valve annulus (*yellow arrow*).

2. The ventricular septal incision line (white arrow) is incised toward the left of the medially papillary muscle base.

- The conduction system (*right bundle branch: green dashed line*) runs near the base of the medially papillary muscle.
- The coronary septal branch (*red line*) runs anterior to the ventricular septal incision line.

5. *Incision lines of the ventricular septum.*

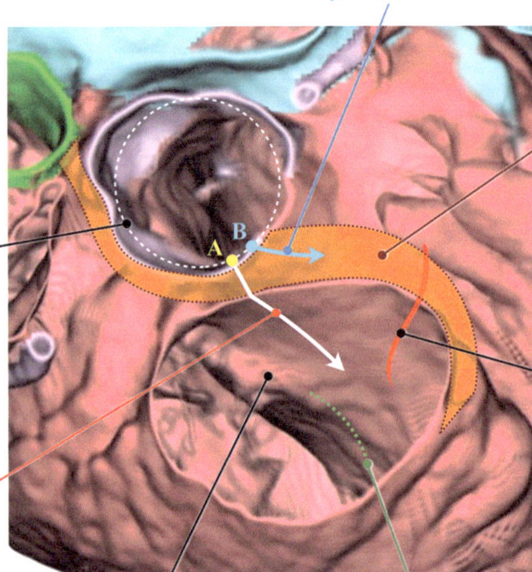

1. Incise the ventricular septum from the aortic valve annulus (point (A)) to the right ventricular apex (to the left of the base of the medially papillary muscle).
2. The length of the right ventricular incision is limited to near the base of the medially papillary muscle.
3. The incision on the left ventricular side is directed toward the base of the anterior papillary muscle and is deeper than the incision on the right ventricular side.
   - If the incision is directed toward the left, the coronary septal branch may be injured.
   - There is also a modified Konno incision that incises the ventricular septum, but the incision cannot be as deep, the valve annulus cannot be enlarged as much, and the patch suture line at the incised ventricular septum is more fragile (point (B), *light blue arrow*).

3.3 VSD Closure and Right Ventricular Outflow Reconstruction During the Konno Procedure (Fig. 11.5)

1. The suture for the closure of the ventricular septal defect is inserted into the right ventricular endocardium.
   - The base of the medially papillary muscle is in close proximity to the conduction system (right bundle branch), so the insertion point of the suture needle should be kept away from the base (*blue dashed line: suture needle insertion line*).
2. The suture needles pull out from the incised surface of the ventricular septum (*red dashed line: suture needle pull out line*).
   - If the suture needles stick out from the left ventricular endocardium, the patch will be sewn to the left ventricular endocardium side, and there is still a concern that this may cause subaortic stenosis.

Fig. 11.5 VSD closure and right ventricular outflow reconstruction during the Konno procedure

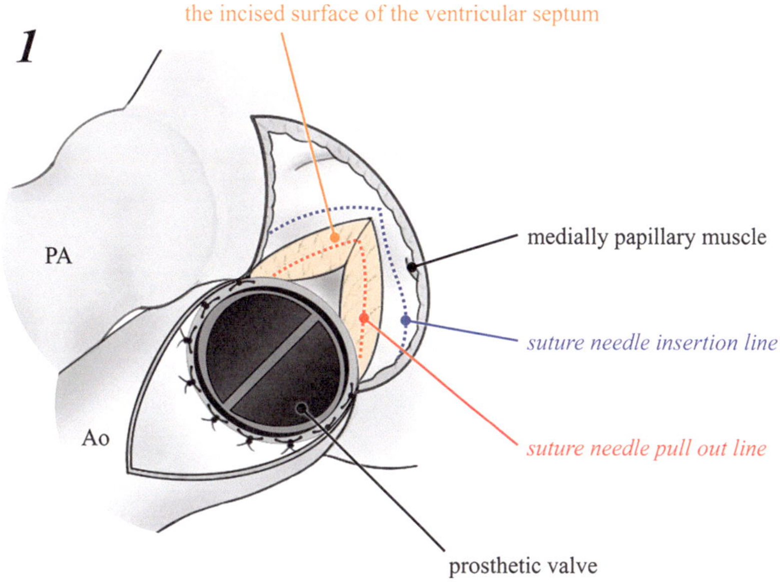

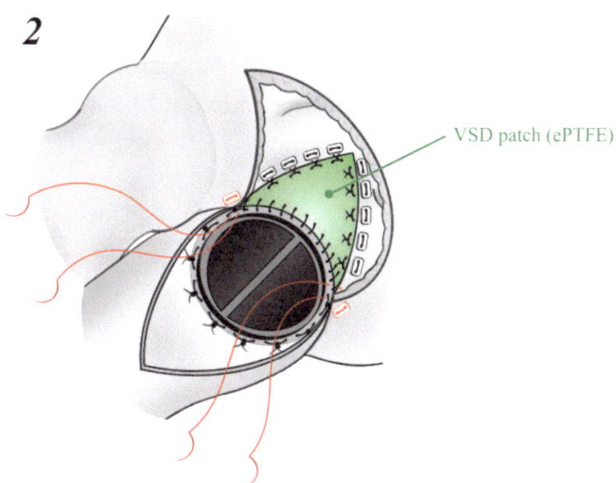

1. If the ventricular septal defect patch and the aortic root repair patch are separate patches, the ventricular septal defect should be closed before or after prosthetic valve implantation.
   - The upper edge of the ventricular septal defect is more easily sutured before prosthetic valve implantation.
   - If a separate patch is used, use an ePTFE patch for closure of the ventricular septal defect.
2. Anastomose the upper edge of the patch to the prosthetic valve cuff with a continuous 5-0 or 4-0 monofilament suture.
3. Reinforcement sutures (red pledget sutures) are placed at both ends of the upper edge of the ventricular septum to prevent bleeding.
   - The aortic root is enlarged using a Dacron graft patch.

3

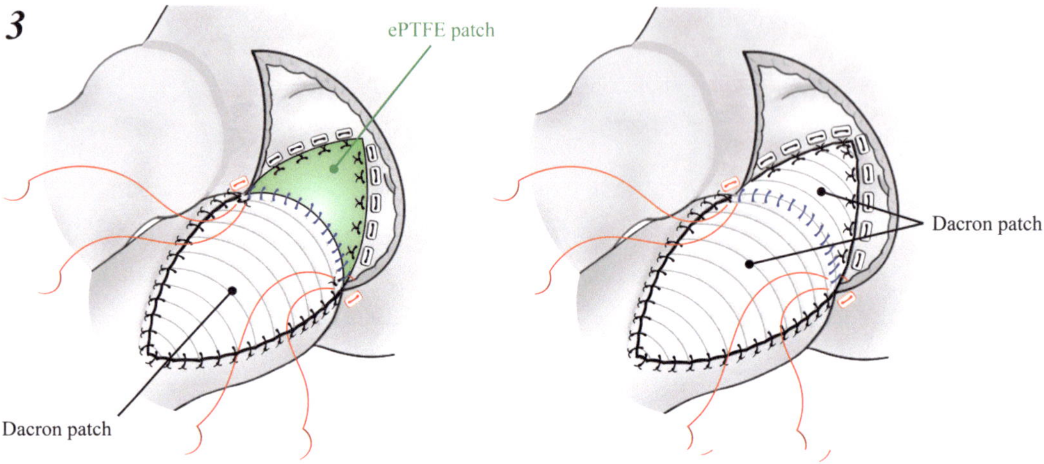

1. If the ventricular septal defect and aortic root are closed with a continuous patch, a Dacron prosthesis is used (right figure).
2. After the patch is sewn around the ventricular septal defect, patch trimming of the aortic root is performed.
   - If both the ventricular septum and aorta are shaped and trimmed first, the aortic patch may not fit the aortic wall defect after the ventricular septum is sewn.
3. Anastomose the prosthetic valve cuff to the Dacron prosthesis using a continuous 5-0 or 4-0 monofilament suture.
4. Apply a reinforcement suture (*red pledget suture*) to both ends of the superior edge of the ventricular septum to prevent bleeding.

4

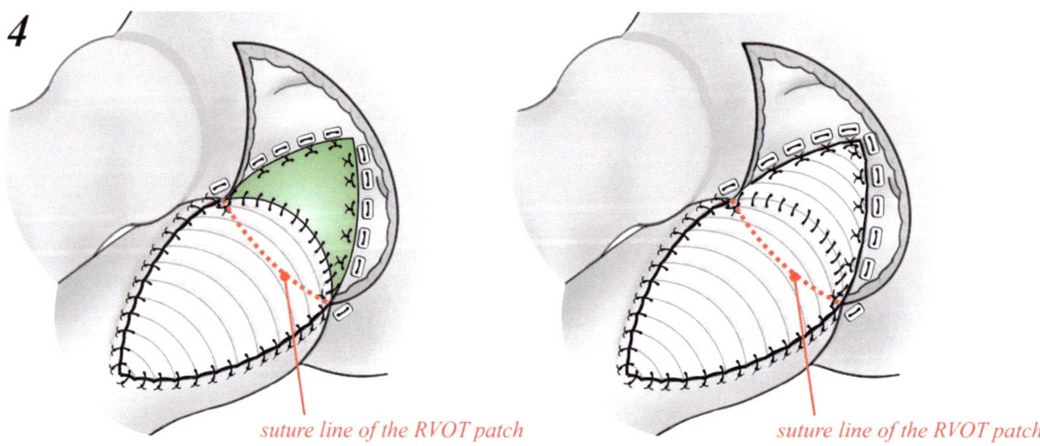

1. The right ventricular outflow tract (RVOT) patch is sewn to the Dacron graft cephalad (red dashed line) of the aortic valve annulus to which the prosthetic valve is sewn.
2. If the right ventricular outflow tract patch is sutured to the aortic valve annulus, distortion (folding) of the patch may occur.
3. The material used for the right ventricular outflow patch should be a flexible heterologous pericardium or ePTFE graft patch.

5

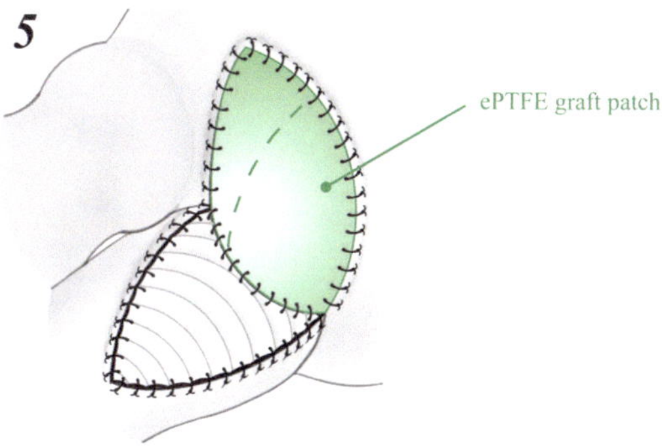

1. Trim the patch through the ePTFE graft according to the curvature of the right ventricular outflow tract and aortic wall.
2. Anastomose the ePTFE patch to the right ventricular outflow tract using an ePTFE CV-5 or CV-4 suture.
   - The aortic side of the patch is anastomosed more cephalad than the aortic valve annulus.

3.4 Demonstration of the Konno Procedure Using a Porcine Heart (Konno, Scene 1)

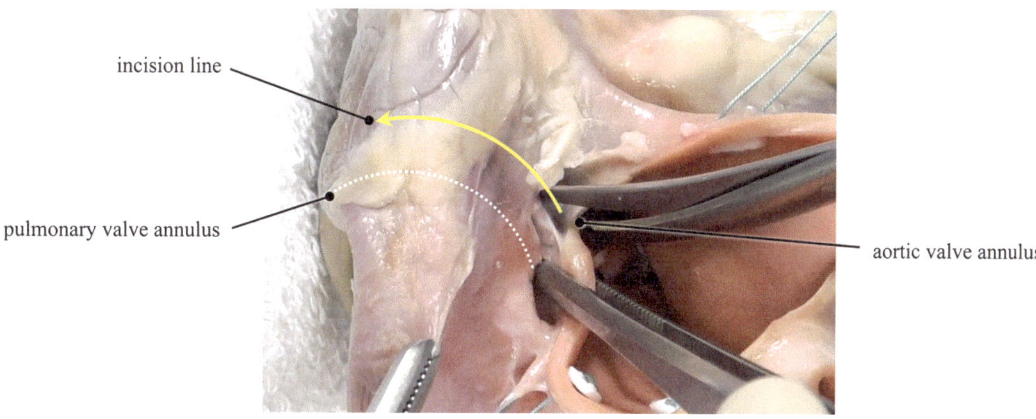

Konno, Scene 1 Incision of the right ventricular outflow tract (Video 0 min 08 s)

1. Incise the right ventricular outflow tract from the lowest point of the aortic incision (aortic valve annulus) parallel to the pulmonary valve annulus (*yellow arrow*).
   - Check the pulmonary valve through the right ventricular outflow tract opening, and incise the right ventricular outflow tract taking care not to damage the valve.
2. Incise approximately half the width of the right ventricular outflow tract (Konno, Scene 2).

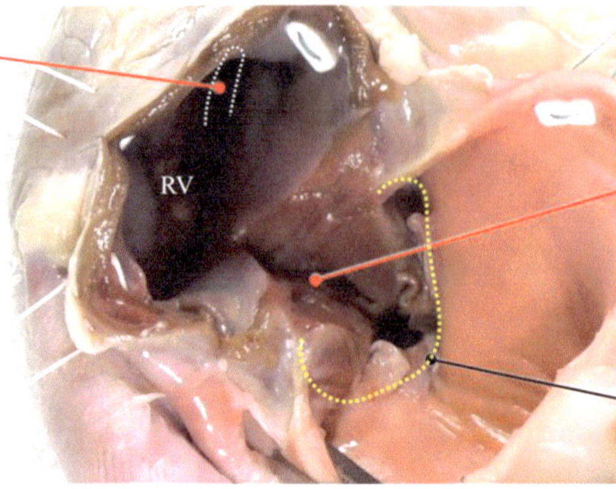

Konno, Scene 2 Incision of the ventricular septum (Video 0 min 54 s)

1. Incise from the aortic valve annulus (*yellow dashed line*) to the left of the base of the medially papillary muscle, looking into the right ventricular cavity.
   - The right ventricular side is incised near the base of the medially papillary muscle.
   - The left ventricular side is incised slightly deeper than the right ventricular side toward the anterior papillary muscle of the mitral valve (Konno, Scene 3).

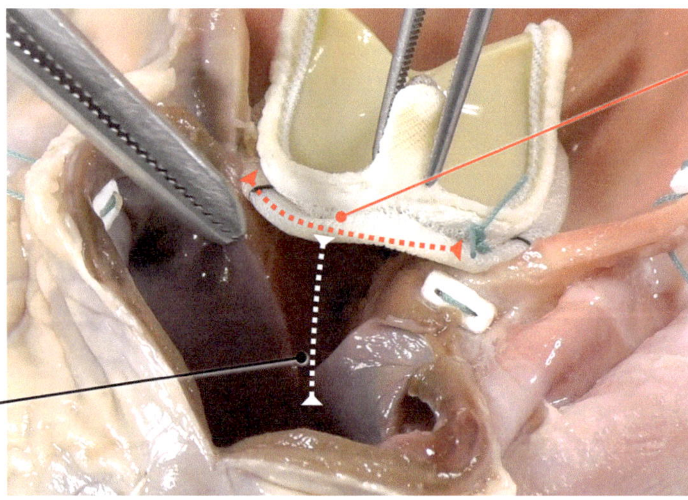

Konno, Scene 3 Shape of the patch to close the VSD (Video 1 min 12 s)

1. Determine the shape (width and depth) of the patch to close the ventricular septal defect.
   - The depth of the incision (white dashed line = patch length) should be equal to or slightly greater than the enlarged width of the valve annulus (*red dashed line = patch width*) (Konno, Scene 4).

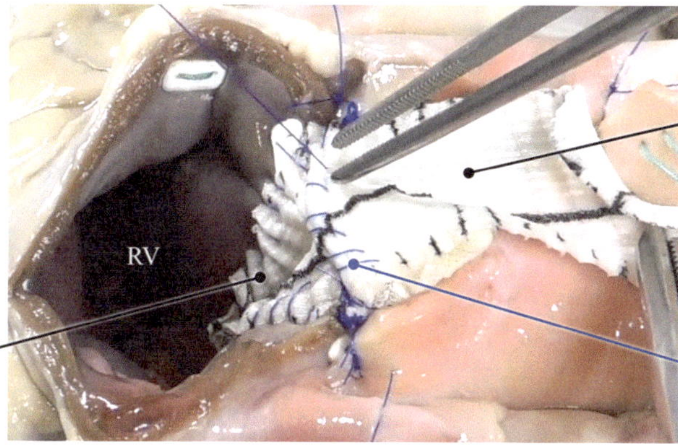

Konno, Scene 4 Repair of the VSD and anterior aortic wall (Video 5 min 53 s)

1. Dacron patch sewn onto prosthetic valve ring (cuff) using a continuous 4-0 monofilament suture.
   - Dacron patch closed with a continuous Dacron patch from the ventricular septal defect to the anterior wall of the aorta (Konno, Scene 5).

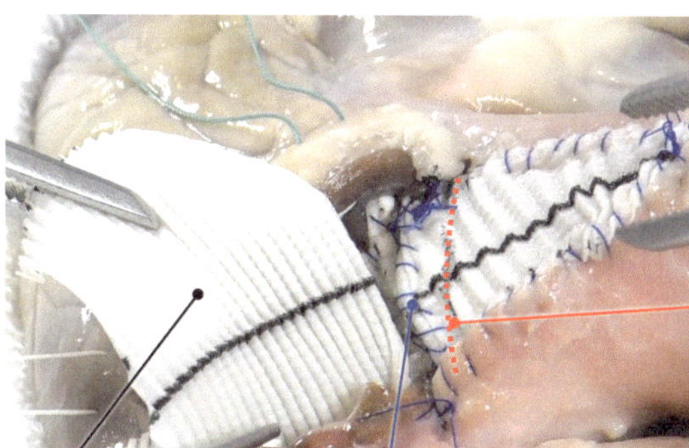

Konno, Scene 5 Repair of the right ventricular outflow tract 1 (Video 3 min 23 s)

1. Trim the right ventricular outflow tract patch (Dacron prosthesis is used in this case because of the demonstration surgery; ePTFE prosthesis wall is used in the clinical case).
   - The patch is triangular and tilted towards the outflow tract.
   - It is better to suture the patch to the anterior aortic wall first and then trim to the final shape.
   - The suture line (*red dashed line*) of the right ventricular outflow tract reconstruction patch should be cephalad of the aortic valve annulus (Konno, Scene 6).

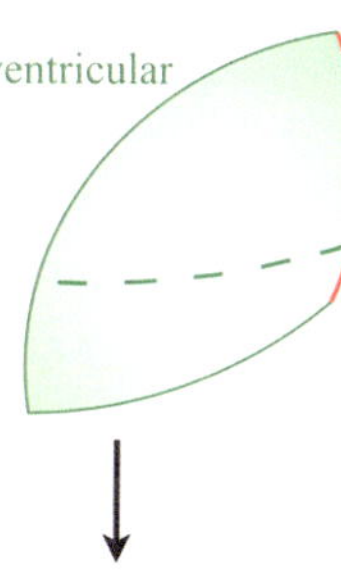

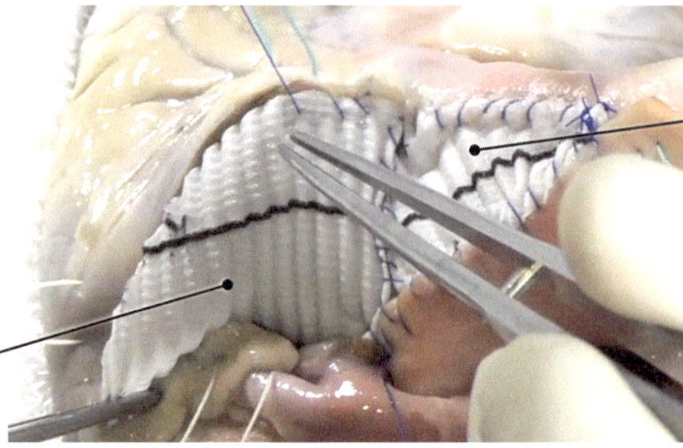

Konno, Scene 6 Repair of the right ventricular outflow tract 2 (Video 3 min 56 s)

1. Dacron vascular prosthesis anastomosed to the right ventricular outflow tract (ePTFE suture is used in clinical cases) (Konno, Scene 7).

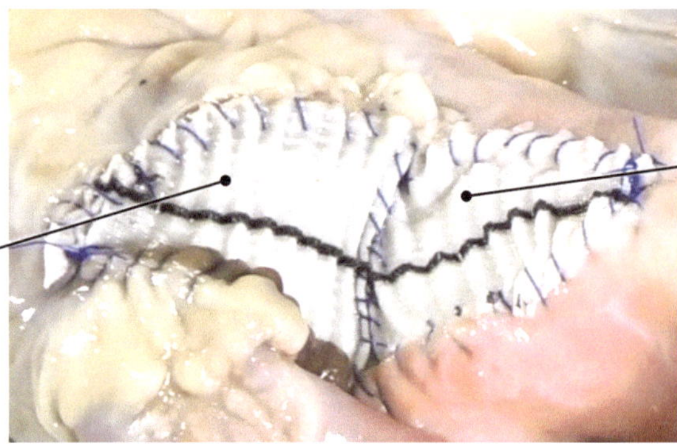

Konno, Scene 7 Completion of the Konno procedure (Video 4 min 07 s) (▶ https://doi.org/10.1007/000-hkj)

1. Completion of the Konno procedure

4 Ross-Konno Operation

In the Konno procedure, a prosthetic valve is implanted at the aortic valve position after the narrow aortic valve annulus is enlarged, whereas in the Ross-Konno procedure, a pulmonary valve autograft is implanted at the aortic valve position. The ventricular septal incision is closed with a patch or a resected right ventricular outflow tract anterior wall flap.

4.1 Ross-Konno Operation (Surgical Video)

Case

- Age: 2 years old.
- Diagnosis: Congenital valvular aortic stenosis, mild coarctation of the aorta.
- Percutaneous aortic balloon angioplasty at 2 and 3 months of age.
- Previous operation: Aortic valvuloplasty at 9 months and 1 year 10 months of age.
- Procedure: Ross-Konno operation and right ventricular outflow tract reconstruction (18 mm ePTFE valved conduit) (Ross-Konno, Scene 1).

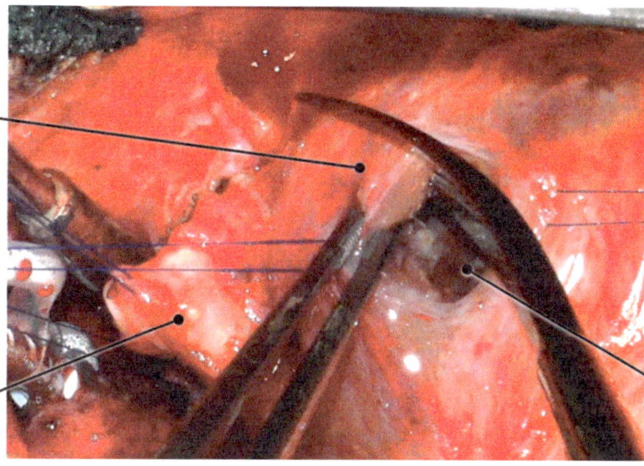

Ross-Konno, Scene 1 Harvest of the pulmonary autograft 1 (Video 0 min 42 s)

1. If the anterior wall of the right ventricular outflow tract is used as a flap patch for ventricular septal closure, incise the anterior wall 20 mm caudal to the pulmonary valve annulus.
2. From the incision, incise the anterior wall in a U-shape toward the right and left edges of the pulmonary valve annulus (Ross-Konno, Scene 2).

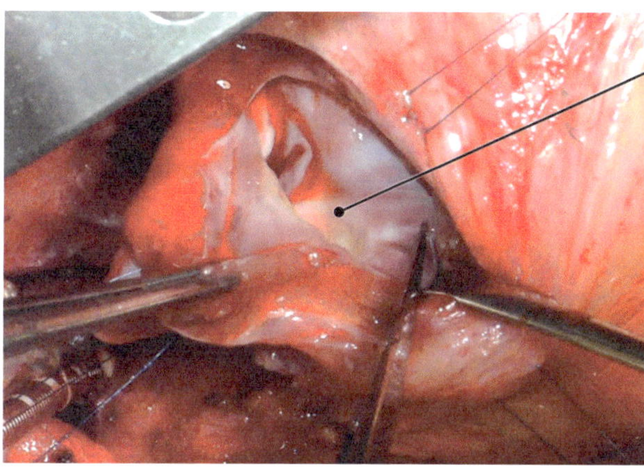

Ross-Konno, Scene 2 Harvest of the pulmonary autograft 2 (Video 1 min 21 s)

1. Incise the posterior wall (ventricular septal surface) along the pulmonary valve annulus and 5 mm below the dorsal valve annulus as in the Ross procedure.
2. The incision is made by inserting a straight scissors into the cross section in a slightly obliquely sliding manner.

- Because the anterior descending coronary artery lies within the dorsal fat tissue, care must be taken not to damage the coronary artery (Ross-Konno, Scene 3).

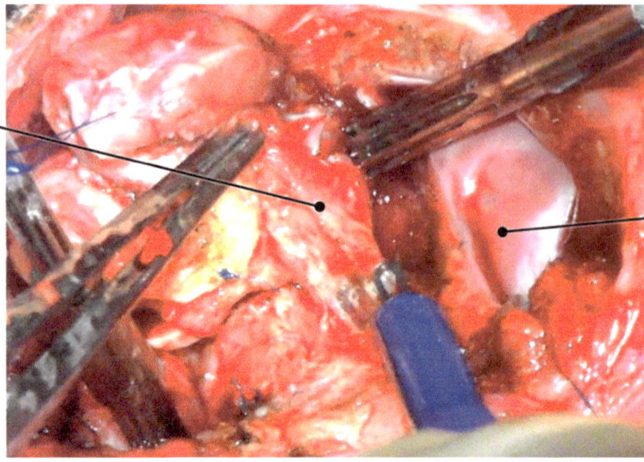

Ross-Konno, Scene 3 Harvest of the pulmonary autograft 3 (Video 2 min 11 s)

1. Incise the ventricular septal aspect (as in the Ross procedure) (Ross-Konno, Scene 4).

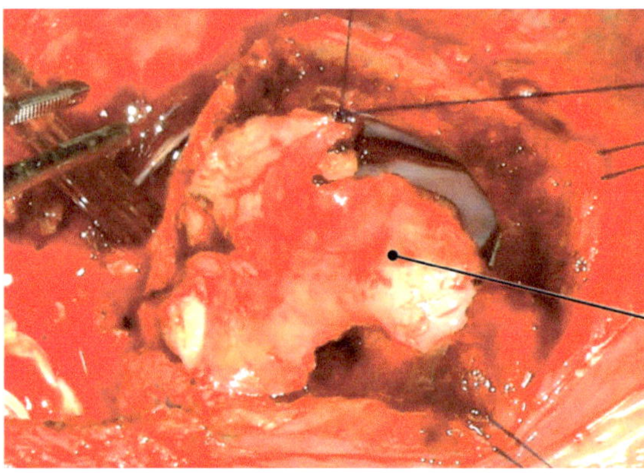

Ross-Konno, Scene 4 Anastomosis of the pericardial patch to the ventricular septal transection site (Video 6 min 05 s)

1. The septal section from which the pulmonary artery autograft is harvested is covered with autologous pericardium.
2. The pericardium on the right ventricular outflow tract side is used as the suture line for the ePTFE graft (Ross-Konno, Scene 5).

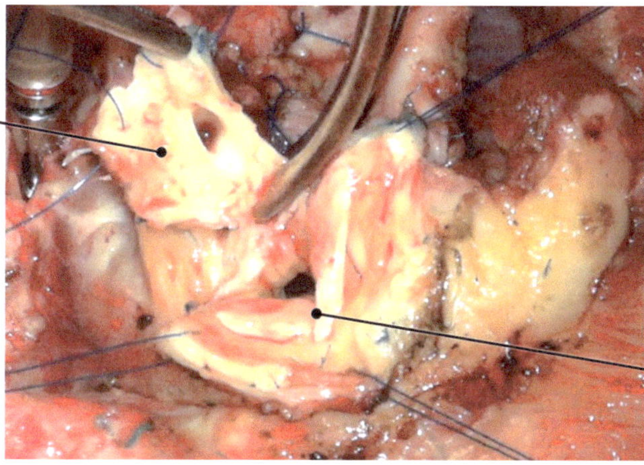

Ross-Konno, Scene 5 Harvest of the left coronary cuff (Video 9 min 05 s)

1. After resection of the aortic valve, the left coronary cusp is harvested from the aortic wall in a U-shaped fashion.
   - Since this is a reoperation case, the adherent tissue around the origin of the coronary artery is sufficiently dissected to obtain the mobility of the coronary button, taking care not to damage the coronary artery (Ross-Konno, Scene 6).

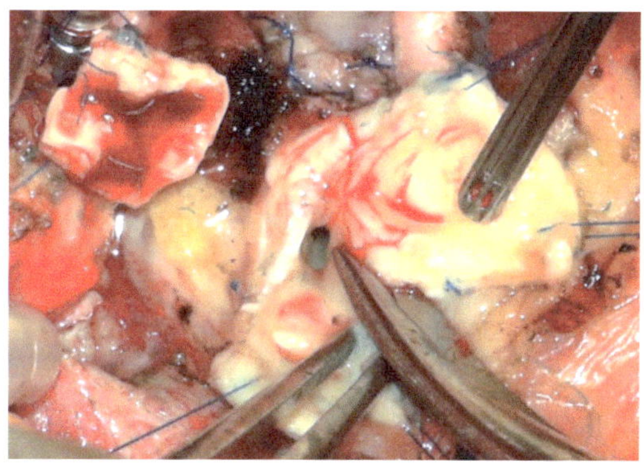

Ross-Konno, Scene 6 Harvest of the right coronary cuff (Video 10 min 00 s)

1. The right coronary cusp is harvested from the aortic wall in the same manner (Ross-Konno, Scene 7).

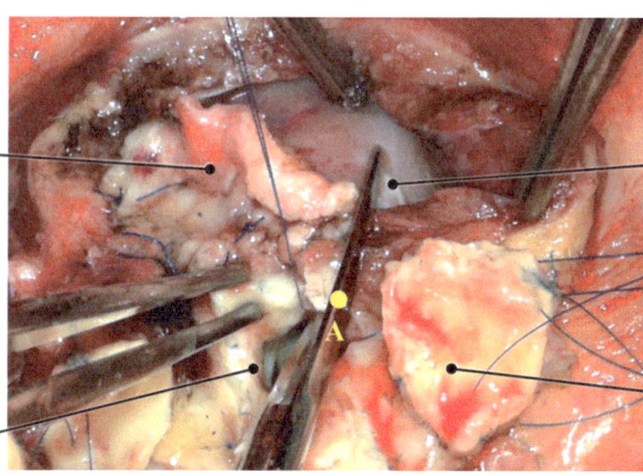

Ross-Konno, Scene 7 Konno incision 1 (Video 11 min 08 s)

1. Incise the ventricular septum (Konno incision) from the aortic valve annulus (point (A) in the figure above) to the left of the origin of the right coronary cusp and to the right of the autograft resection surface (autologous pericardium supplementation site) toward the right ventricular apex.

- The Konno incision is made toward the left at the base of the medially papillary muscle.
- The medially papillary muscle is located to the right of the incision line, and the coronary artery septal branch is located to the left.

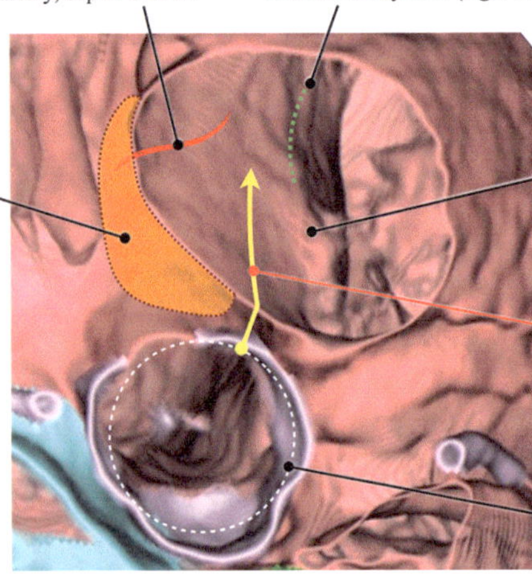

Konno incision of the ventricular septum

- Note that if the incision is directed to the left, the septal branch may be injured.
- The orientation of the septal incision is especially important when the anterior wall of the right ventricular outflow tract is filled in through the ventricular septal incision (to prevent torsion of the anterior wall of the flap) (Ross-Konno, Scene 8).

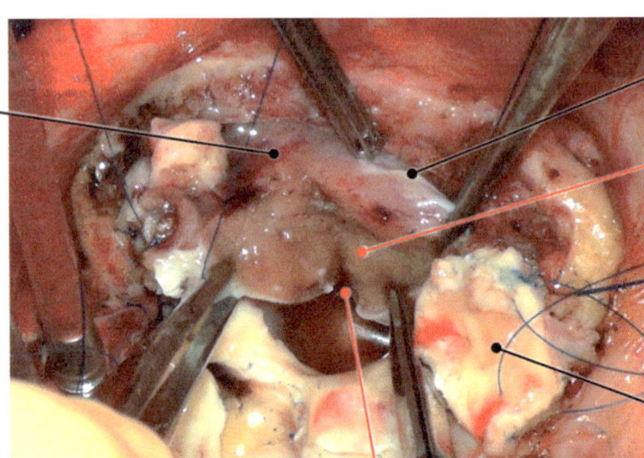

Ross-Konno, Scene 8 Konno incision 2 (Video 11 min 35 s)

1. The septal incision on the left ventricular side is made toward the base of the anterior papillary muscle, slightly deeper than on the right ventricular side (Ross-Konno, Scene 9).

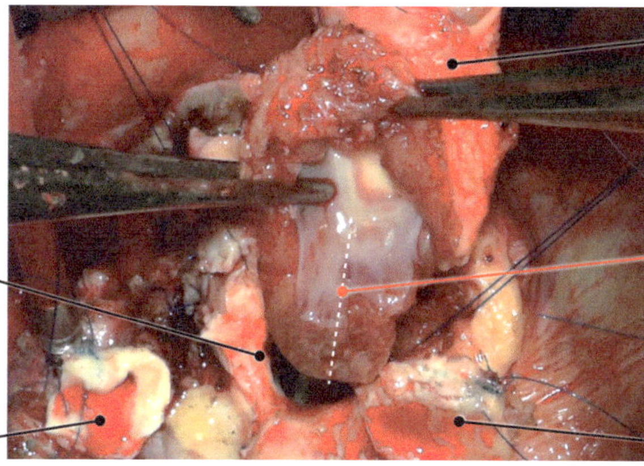

Ross-Konno, Scene 9 Positioning of the pulmonary artery autograft 1 (Video 12 min 21 s)

1. Position the pulmonary artery autograft so that the midline of the right ventricular outflow tract anterior wall flap corresponds to the midline of the ventricular septal incision.
- Be careful not to twist the anterior wall flap (Ross-Konno, Scene 10).

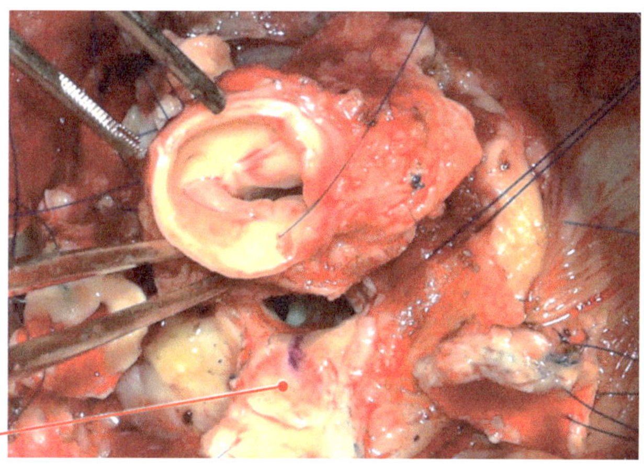

Ross-Konno, Scene 10 Positioning of the pulmonary artery autograft 2 (Video 12 min 35 s)

1. Mark the aortic valve annulus where the pulmonary artery autograft wall corresponds on the opposite side of the right ventricular outflow tract anterior wall flap.
   - When the pulmonary artery autograft is anastomosed at this position, make sure that the assumed anastomotic sites of the left and right coronary buttons do not correspond to (be in close proximity to) the pulmonary artery valve commissure.
- In case the anastomotic site corresponds to the pulmonary valve commissure, slightly adjust the angle of the pulmonary artery autograft.
- If the anterior wall flap and the ventricular septal incision are misaligned, trim the anterior wall flap.
- If the gap is too large, do not use an anterior wall flap and use an ePTFE patch to close the septal defect (Ross-Konno, Scene 11).

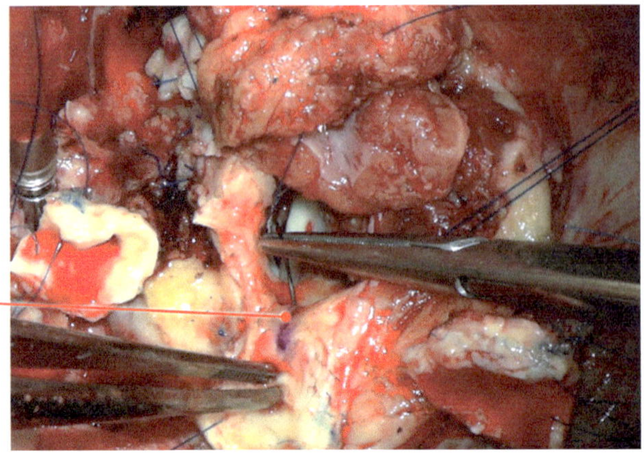

Ross-Konno, Scene 11 Anastomosis of the pulmonary artery autograft 1 (Video 12 min 48 s)

1. The pulmonary autograft was anastomosed to the aortic valve annulus using 5-0 monofilament mattress sutures.
   - In this case, the autologous pericardial strip was not used for reinforcement because of the presence of adhesive tissue around the pulmonary autograft.
   - First, a reference suture is anastomosed to the dorsal side of the aortic valve annulus (Ross-Konno, Scene 12).

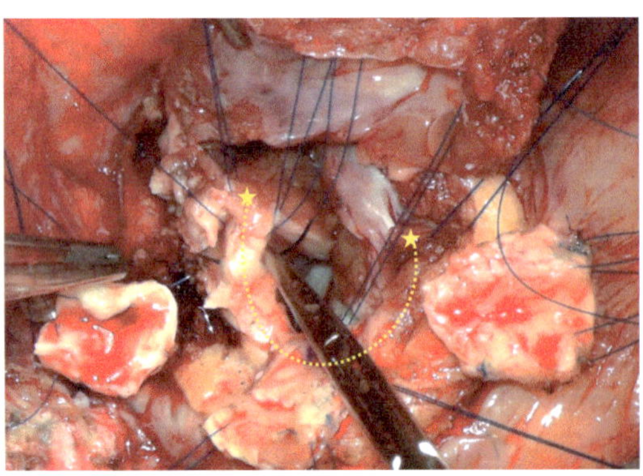

Ross-Konno, Scene 12 Anastomosis of the pulmonary artery autograft 2 (Video 13 min 19 s)

1. Similarly, anastomose the pulmonary autograft to the aortic valve annulus using 5-0 monofilament mattress sutures.
   - Anastomose the pulmonary autograft so that both ends of the base of the anterior wall flap of the pulmonary autograft (valve annulus) correspond to both ends (★) of the incised aortic valve annulus (*yellow dashed line*).
   - The suture width of the aortic valve annulus should be slightly smaller than that of the pulmonary autograft to prevent future enlargement of the pulmonary annulus (Ross-Konno, Scene 13).

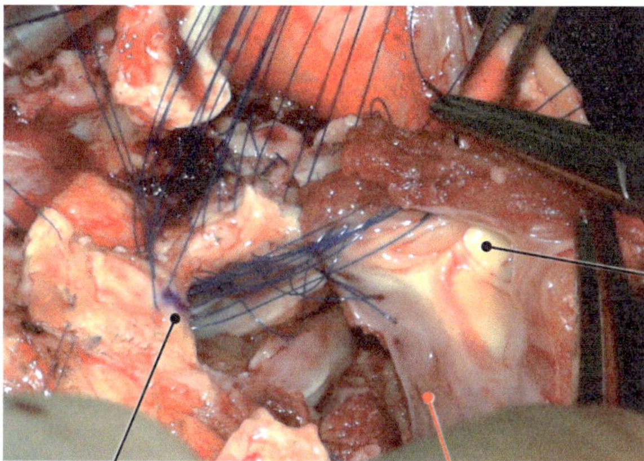

Ross-Konno, Scene 13 Anastomosis of the pulmonary artery autograft 3 (Video 14 min 35 s)

1. The posterior wall of the pulmonary autograft is anastomosed to the aortic valve annulus with 5-0 monofilament mattress sutures (Ross-Konno, Scene 14).

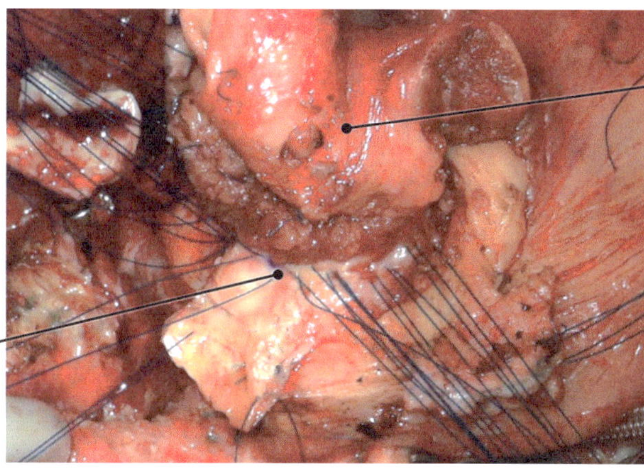

Ross-Konno, Scene 14 Anastomosis of the pulmonary artery autograft 4 (Video 16 min 04 s)

1. Apply the pulmonary artery autograft to the aortic valve annulus and ligate the sutures (Ross-Konno, Scene 15).

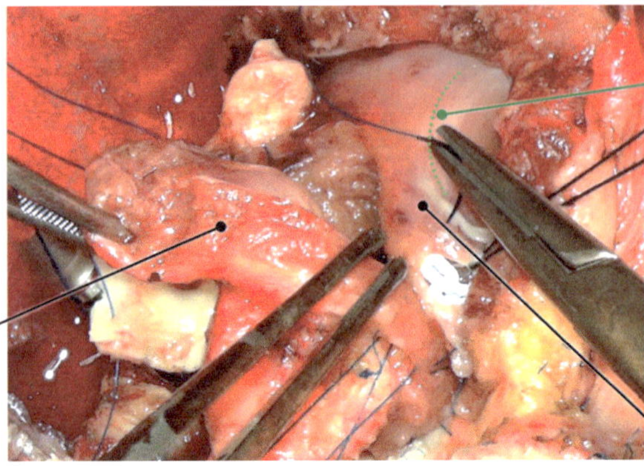

Ross-Konno, Scene 15 Anastomosis of the RV anterior wall flap 1 (Video 16 min 51 s)

1. Check that the anterior wall flap of the right ventricular outflow tract fits (is not misaligned) with the ventricular septal incision before starting suture.
   - If there is misalignment, it is necessary to trim the anterior wall flap.
2. Sew a 5-0 monofilament suture with pledget to the right side edge of the ventricular septal cross section and the anterior wall flap.
   - It is not necessary to be sutured in all layers of the ventricular septum.
   - Insert the suture needle into right ventricular endocardium and stab out to ventricular septal cross section and then insert to anterior wall flap (Ross-Konno, Scene 16).

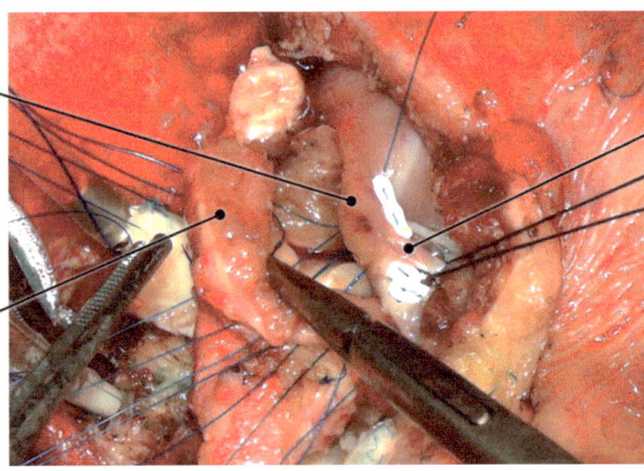

Ross-Konno, Scene 16 Anastomosis of the RV anterior wall flap 2 (Video 18 min 21 s)

1. Sutures are sewn to the ventricular septal cross section near the base of the medially papillary muscle, taking care not to damage the conduction system (right bundle branch) (Ross-Konno, Scene 17).

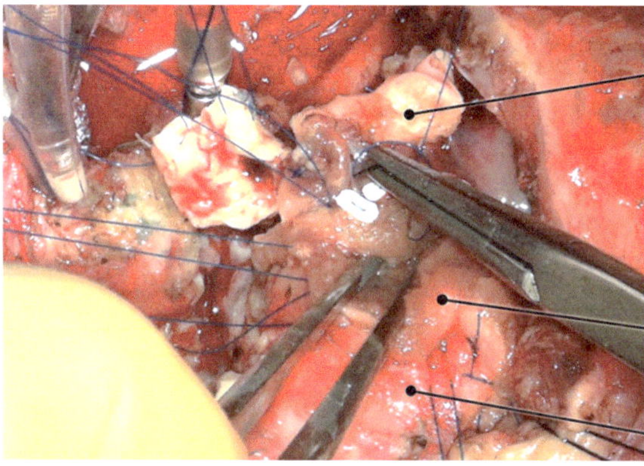

Ross-Konno, Scene 17 Anastomosis of the RV anterior wall flap 3 (Video 20 min 14 s)

1. The left edge of the anterior wall flap of the right ventricular outflow is sutured to the cross section of the ventricular septum (Ross-Konno, Scene 18).

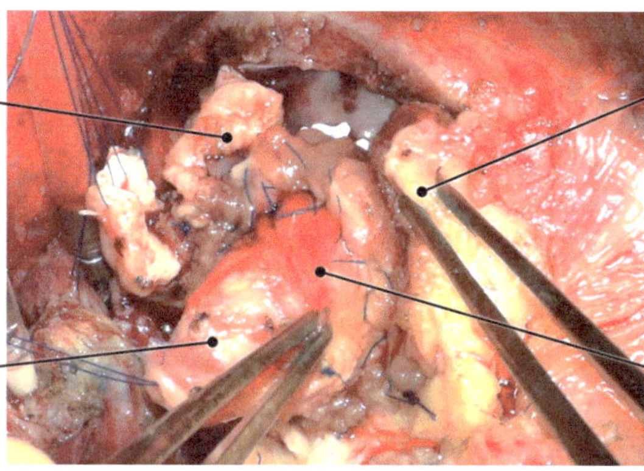

Ross-Konno, Scene 18 Anastomosis of the pulmonary autograf 1 (Video 22 min 21 s)

1. Pull the right side of the right ventricular outflow opening posteriorly to confirm that it can be anastomosed directly to the anterior wall flap.
   - In the Konno procedure, the right ventricular outflow opening is repaired by filling in the patch, but in the Ross-Konno procedure, the proximal end of the right ventricular-pulmonary artery conduit must be anastomosed to the left of the right ventricular outflow tract opening.
   - The right end of the right ventricular outflow tract incision may be closed with a patch or, as in this case, the right end of the large opening may be sutured to the anterior wall of the pulmonary artery autograft (Ross-Konno, Scene 19).

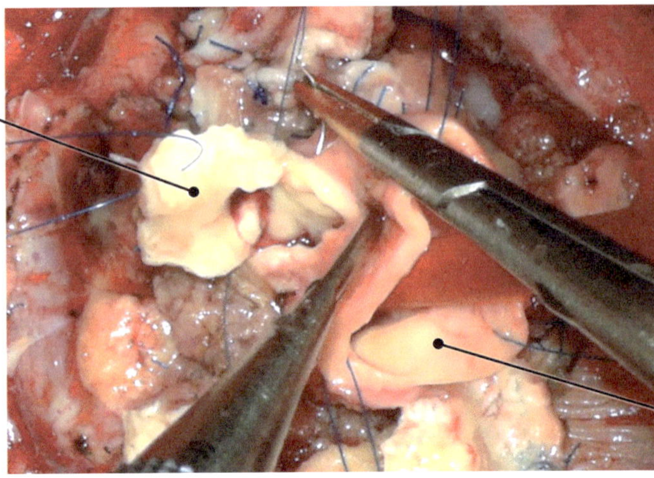

Ross-Konno, Scene 19 Anastomosis of LCA cuff (Video 25 min 07 s)

1. Circularly punch out the pulmonary artery autograft wall.
2. Anastomose the left coronary artery cuff to the pulmonary autograft opening with a continuous 6-0 monofilament suture (Ross-Konno, Scene 20).

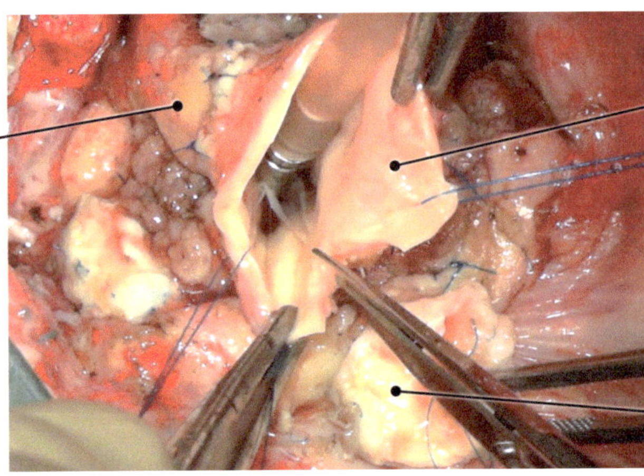

Ross-Konno, Scene 20 Anastomosis of RCA cuff (Video 28 min 22 s)

1. In this case, there was a commissure at the site of the right coronary cuff implantation and the mobility of the right coronary button was poor due to adhesion, so a longitudinal incision was made in the pulmonary autograft and the coronary artery was anastomosed higher than the sinus of Valsalva.
2. The lower half of the right coronary button is anastomosed to the pulmonary autograft incision with a continuous 6-0 monofilament suture (Ross-Konno, Scene 21).

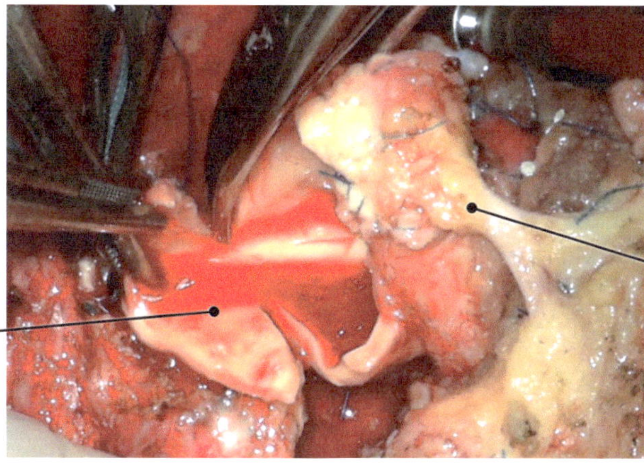

Ross-Konno, Scene 21 Trimming of the pulmonary autograft (Video 32 min 54 s)

1. Check the cross-sectional shape of the pulmonary artery autograft and ascending aorta, and trim the posterior wall of the pulmonary autograft to a spindle shape (Ross-Konno, Scene 22).

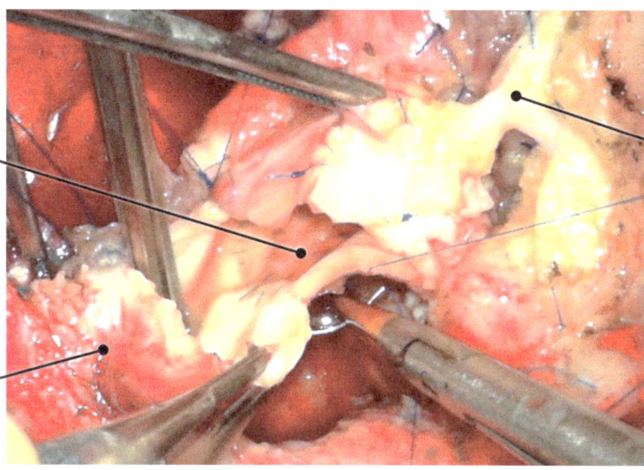

Ross-Konno, Scene 22 Ascending aorta-pulmonary autograft anastomosis (Video 34 min 06 s)

1. Anastomose the posterior wall of the proximal end of the ascending aorta to the posterior wall of the pulmonary autograft with a continuous 5-0 monofilament suture (Ross-Konno, Scene 23).

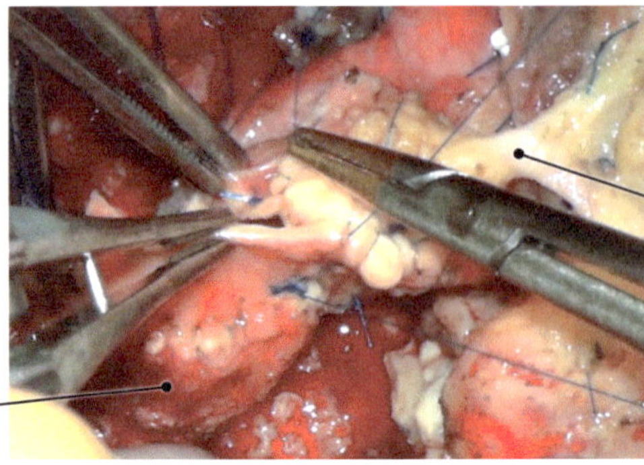

Ross-Konno, Scene 23 Repair of the anterior aortic wall (Video 35 min 19 s)

1. Fill in the resected spindle shape pulmonary autograft posterior wall patch and reconstruct the new aorta anterior wall (upper border of the right coronary button) (Ross-Konno, Scene 24).

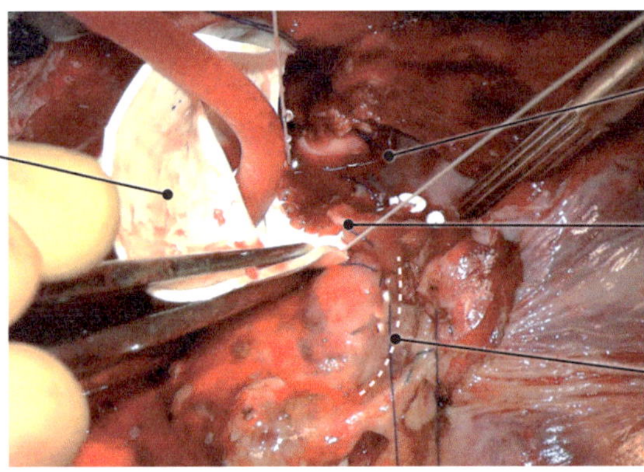

Ross-Konno, Scene 24 Right ventricular outflow tract reconstruction 1 (Video 37 min 44 s)

1. The distal end of the valved ePTFE conduit is anastomosed to the pulmonary artery bifurcation opening with a continuous ePTFE CV-6 or CV-5 suture.
2. The posterior wall of the proximal end of the valved ePTFE conduit is anastomosed to the autologous pericardium filled in at the ventricular septal cut surface with a continuous ePTFE CV-5 suture.
3. The right posterolateral wall of the ePTFE conduit is anastomosed to the anterior wall flap of the right ventricular outflow (Ross-Konno, Scene 25).

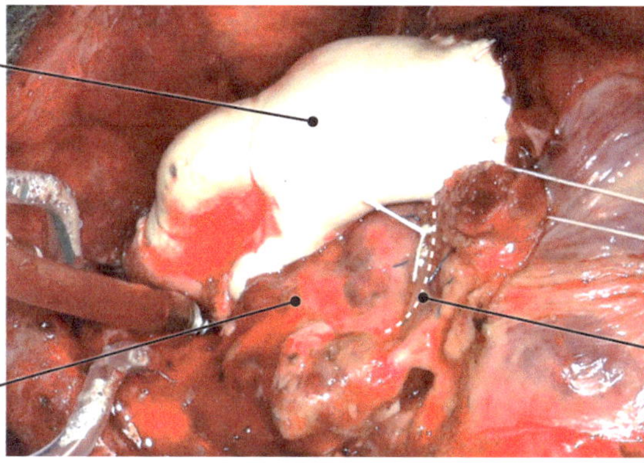

Ross-Konno, Scene 25 Right ventricular outflow tract reconstruction 2 (Video 38 min 29 s) (▶ https://doi.org/10.1007/000-hkm)

1. The proximal end of the valved ePTFE conduit was anastomosed to the right ventricular outflow tract opening, and reconstruction of the right ventricular outflow tract was completed.

- In this case, the right side of the right ventricular outflow tract opening was sutured directly to the pulmonary autograft.

SPOTLIGHT Modified Konno Operation for Subaortic Stenosis

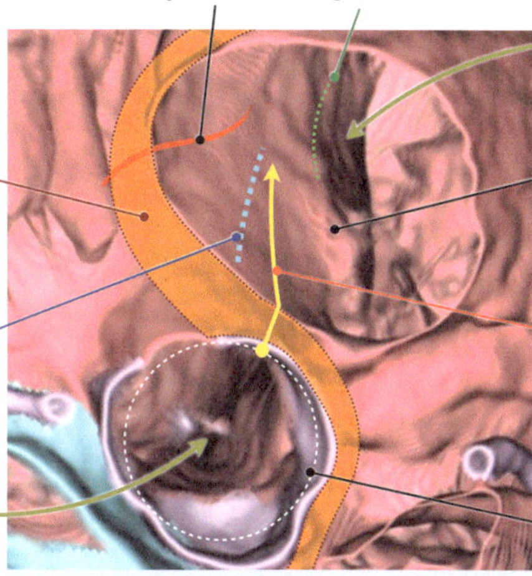

While approaching through the aortic incision and identifying the stenotic lesion site, make a longitudinal incision through the right ventricular outflow tract incision into the ventricular septum and enlarge the patch at the incision.

1. Incise the right ventricular outflow tract longitudinally.
2. Incise the ascending aorta, and insert forceps into the left ventricle via the aortic valve.
3. Indicate the site of stenosis with forceps inserted into the left ventricle.
4. Identify the incise site by palpating the forceps tip through the right ventricular outflow tract incision.

(continued)

5. Incise the ventricular septum to the left of the middle papillary muscle to the left ventricular cavity (*light blue dashed line*), and remove some of the myocardium.
6. Sew a patch over the incised ventricular septum to enlarge the subaortic valve (left ventricular outflow tract).
7. The right ventricular outflow tract incision is also patched and enlarged.

References

Yasui Operation for Severe Aortic Stenosis in Neonates

Yasui H, Kad H, Yonenaga K, Mitani A, Tomita Y, Iwao H, Yoshii K, Mizobuchi Y, Sugawara H. Primany repair of interrupted aortic arch and severe aortic stenosis in neonates. J Thorac Cardiovasc Surg. 1987;93:539–45.

Konno Operation (Narrow Aortic Valve Annular Enlargement)

Konno S, Imai Y, Iida Y, Nakajima M, Tatsuno K. A new method for prosthetic valve replacement in congenital aortic stenosis associated with hypoplasia of the aortic valve ring. J Thorac Cardiovasc Surg. 1975;70:909–17.

Ross Operation

Ross DN. Surgical reconstruction of the aortic valve. Lancet. 1963;1:571–4.

Ross DN. Replacement of aortic and mitral valves with a pulmonary autograft. Lancet. 1967;2:956–8.

Ross-Konno Operation

Reddy VM, Rajasinghe HA, Teitel DF, Haas GS, Hanley FL. Aortoventriculoplasty with the pulmonary autograft: the "Ross-Konno" procedure. J Thorac Cardiovasc Surg. 1996;111:158–65.

Modified Konno Operation (Release of Subaortic Valve Stenosis)

Vouhe PR. Valve-sparing konno and hypertrophic obstructive cardiomyopathy in children. Oper Tech Thorac Cardiovasc Surg. 2014;19:164–78.

Ebstein Disease

12

1 Morphology of Ebstein Disease

Ebstein disease is a disease associated with abnormal tricuspid valve morphology and right ventricular myocardial disease (dysplasia). The degree of tricuspid valve morphology varies, and depending on the degree, the clinical manifestations may include tricuspid regurgitation, stenosis, right ventricular hypofunction, and arrhythmias.

The tricuspid valve is undermined during the embryonic period when it is detached from the right ventricular myocardial wall. In this syndrome, this mechanism of undermining is inhibited by a lack of delamination, which results in the presence of an abnormal muscular bar and fibrous bridge between the valve leaflet and the inner wall. The absence of complete delamination results in the valve leaflet adhering to the right ventricular wall (plastering).

The septal leaflet and posterior leaflet have a high degree of delamination failure and plastering. The anterior leaflet is often large and sail-like, but in severe cases, the anterior leaflet may also have a defect due to delamination failure.

The tricuspid valve annulus falls closer to the apex than the original valve annulus (atrioventricular junction) due to plastering, forming a functional tricuspid valve annulus. The space between the true valve annulus and the functional annulus is called the right atrialized right ventricle, where wall thinning and fibrosis (Uhl's formation) occur, resulting in reduced contractility and enlargement of the right ventricle along with the true valve annulus (Fig. 12.1).

Ebstein disease has the following morphologic features, resulting in various degrees of tricuspid regurgitation, right atrial enlargement, right ventricular enlargement, cyanosis, circulatory failure, and supraventricular and ventricular arrhythmias.

Supplementary Information The online version contains supplementary material available at https://doi.org/10.1007/978-981-96-6194-7_12. The videos can be accessed individually by clicking the DOI link in the accompanying figure caption or by scanning this link with the SN More Media App.

M. Yamagishi, *Surgical Treatment of Congenital Heart Disease*,
https://doi.org/10.1007/978-981-96-6194-7_12

Anterior leaflet

- Large sail-like anterior leaflet
- The leaflets may have lacunae (defects).
- Tethered chordae tendineae attaching the edge of the leaflets may pull the leaflets toward the apex, restricting leaflet mobility.

Functional right ventricle

- The effective volume of the right ventricle with contractility is reduced.

Left ventricle

- Left ventricular hypoplasia may occur due to compression from the right ventricle.

Septal leaflet, Posterior leaflet

- Abnormal leaflet tissues are also seen in areas that are not plastering.
- Abnormal muscular bar or fibrous tissue (abnormal chrdae tendineae) between the leaflets and the right ventricular wall due to failure of delamination.

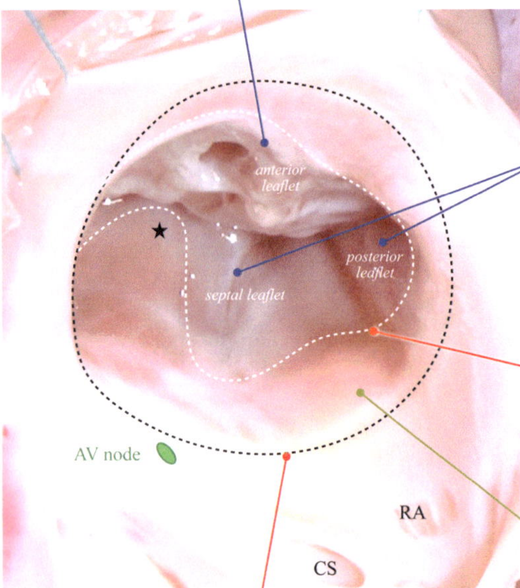

Functional tricuspid valve annulus

- Tricuspid annulus shifted downward toward the apex.
- The septal leaflet has the highest degree of deviation, followed by the posterior leaflet.
- At a point closer to the anterior leaflet, the functional annulus of the septal leaflet is deeply deviated apically (★).

True tricuspid valve annulus
(Right atrioventricular junction)

- True tricuspid valve annulus is enlarged due to tricuspid regurgitation.

Atrialized right ventricle

- Right ventricular wall between true and functional valve annulus
- Septal leaflet, posterior leaflet, and part of the anterior leaflet adhere to the inner wall of the ventricle.
- The right ventricle shows wall thinning and fibrosis (Uhl's) as well as lumen enlargement.

pulmonary valve

- In most cases, pulmonary valve morphology is normal.
- Right ventricular outflow tract stenosis may complicate some cases.
- Neonates with severe tricuspid regurgitation may present with functional pulmonary atresia during a period of physiologic pulmonary hypertension, which must be differentiated from organic pulmonary atresia.

lung

- In severe cases of newborns, the lungs are compressed by cardiomegaly and hypoplastic lungs are seen.

Fig. 12.1 Morphological characteristics

2 Surgical Strategy for Ebstein Disease

The onset of the syndrome varies from neonates to adults. Depending on the age (in months), the degree of morphological abnormality, and cardiac function, the surgical treatment strategy (surgical timing and procedure) varies widely. Severe cases that develop in the neonatal period are treated with the Starns procedure to close the tricuspid valve orifice, followed by single ventricle repair (Fontan procedure). The timing of surgery in cases that develop after infancy varies from case to case, but tricuspid valve repair should be performed before ventricular function deteriorates.

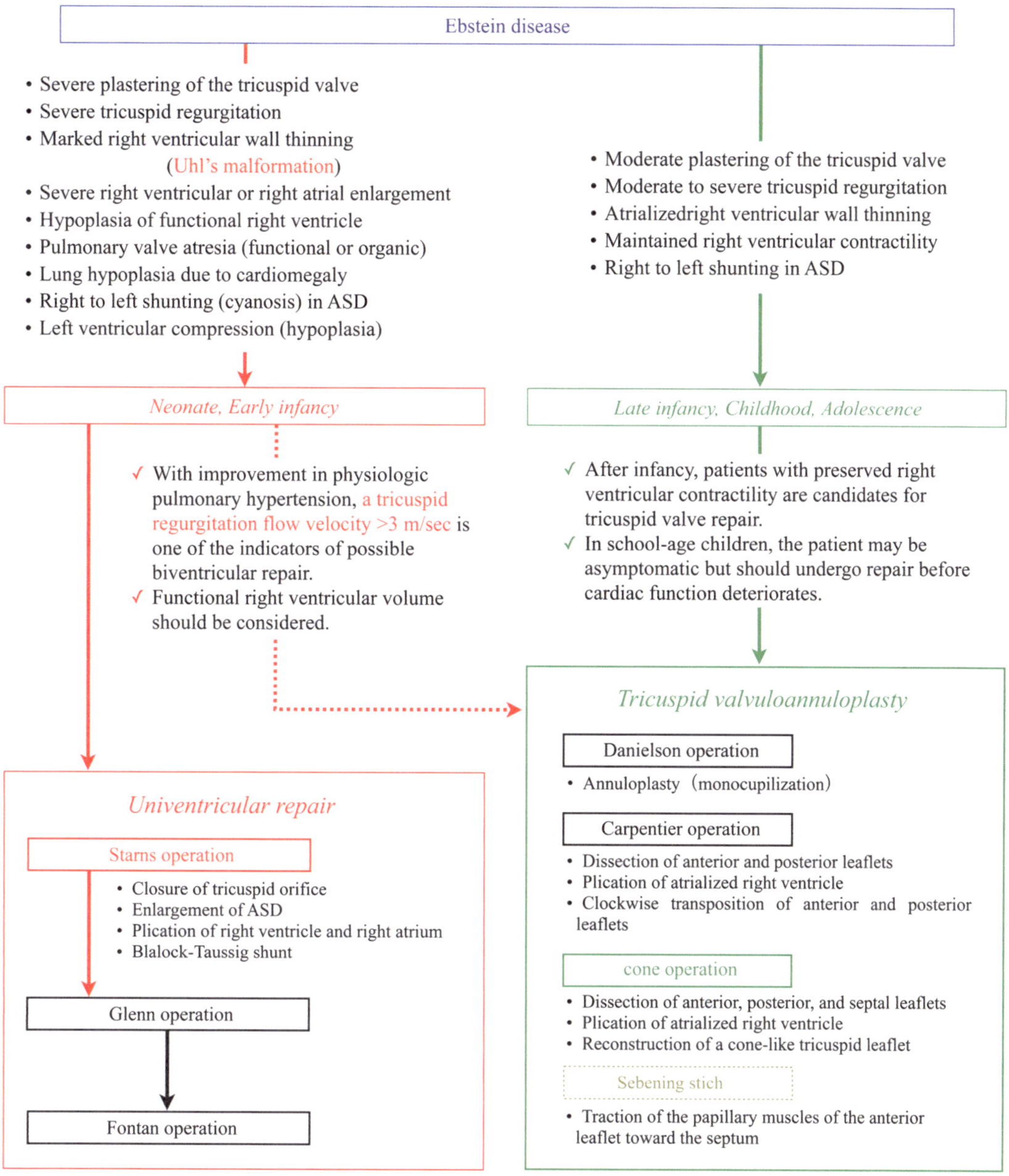

3 Cone Operation

The Carpentier procedure, in which the anterior and posterior leaflets are separated from their attachments and the septal leaflet is preserved, has been the mainstay of valvuloplasty for Ebstein's anomaly, but there is a possibility of residual tricuspid regurgitation from the septal leaflet. In contrast, in the cone operation, the anterior and posterior leaflets are separated as in the Carpentier procedure, and the septal leaflet is also separated to form a circumferential cone-shaped valve leaflet. The cone procedure is a variant of the Carpentier procedure, but has the

Fig. 12.2 Cone operation

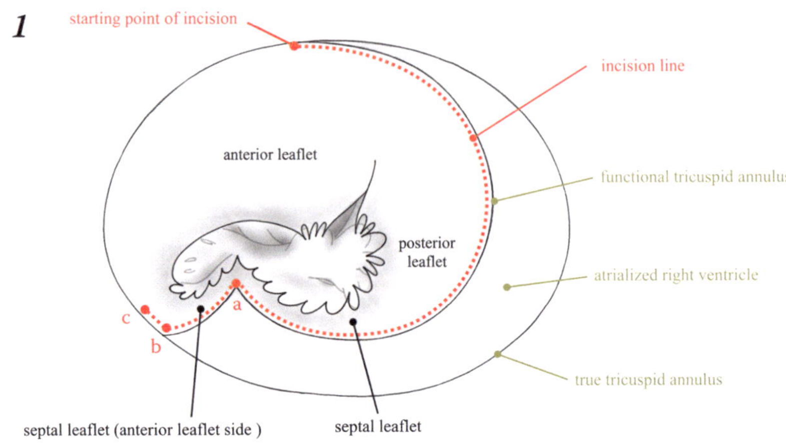

advantage of controlling residual tricuspid regurgitation because the septal leaflet is also included (Fig. 12.2).

1. Begin the leaflet incision at the 11–12 o'clock position of the functional tricuspid annulus.
2. The incision line should be 1–2 mm from the apex attachment.
3. Incise the septal leaflet of the anterior leaflet side at its attachment (a–b).
4. Once the incision is made to the valve ring, the anterior leaflet is also incised approximately 5 mm (b–c).
   - This additional incision (b–c) improves the bulging of the septal apex and sutures the valve ring.

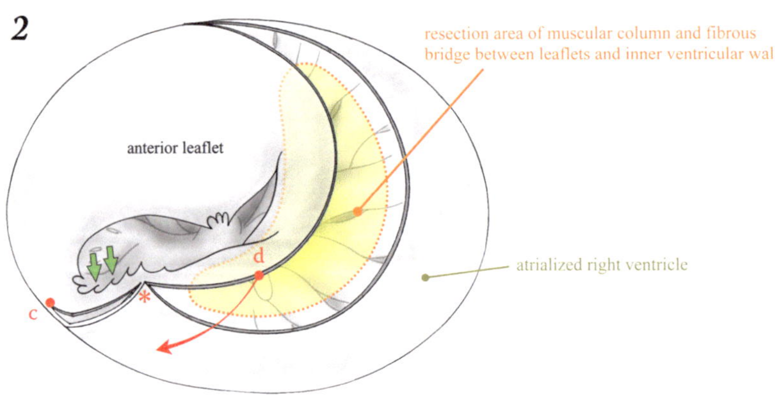

1. The incisions at the valve leaflet attachment of the septal apex may be contiguous (*).
2. Excise the muscle column and fibrous bridge attached to the valve leaflet, excluding the chordae tendineae attached to the valve leaflet edge.
   - If, when the incised septal leaflet (d) is transposed to point (c), even the chordae tendineae attaching to the edge of the valve leaflet are under tethered to the valve leaflet, it is necessary to cut off part of the chordae tendineae, leaving the main chordae tendineae.
   - In particular, since tethering of the septal leaflet of the anterior leaflet side often occurs, the chordae tendineae at the edge of the valve leaflet (*green arrow*) should be partially transected and the anterior leaflet-septal leaflet commissure closed with interrupted 6-0 monofilament sutures.

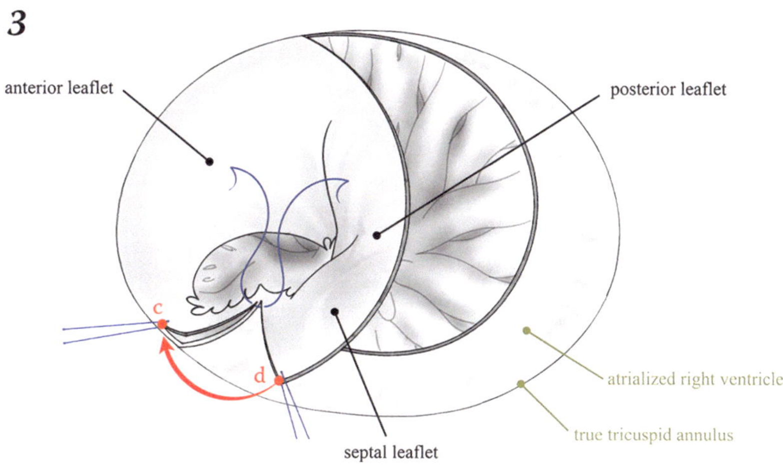

1. The edge of the septal leaflet (d) corresponds to point (c).
2. Suture the septal leaflet incisions with interrupted 6-0 monofilament sutures.

- Apply traction sutures to points (c) and (d).
- Suture the septal leaflets from the apex side.
- The septal leaflets are sutured tightly because of the tension on the suture.

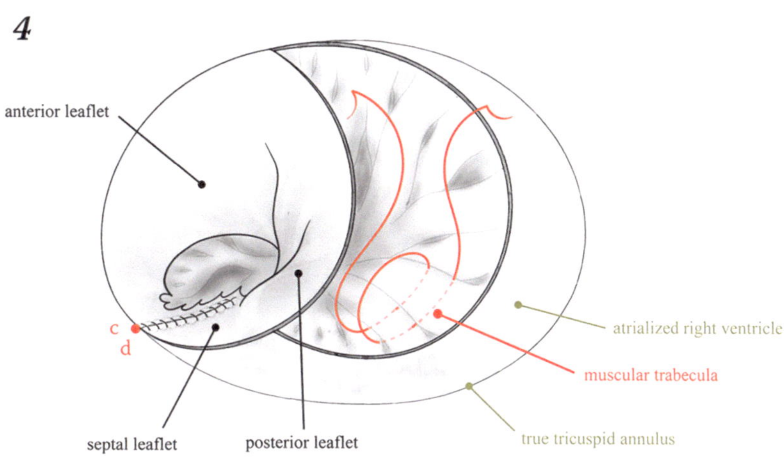

1. Measurement of the valve orifice diameter (transverse cone diameter) after suturing the septal leaflets.
2. Plication of the tricuspid annulus is performed with Z-sutures of 5-0 monofilament suture at the muscular trabecula below the septal-posterior commissure.
   - Be careful not to pass the suture through all layers (note the thin wall thickness).
   - Observe the epicardial surface prior to suture ligation to ensure that there is no coronary artery damage or bending.

- Approximately two Z-sutures on the ventricular side and one suture on the right atrialized right ventricle.
- In older children and adults, U-shaped 4-0 monofilament sutures with pledget may be used.
- Do not place sutures on the right atrium above the true tricuspid annulus.

5

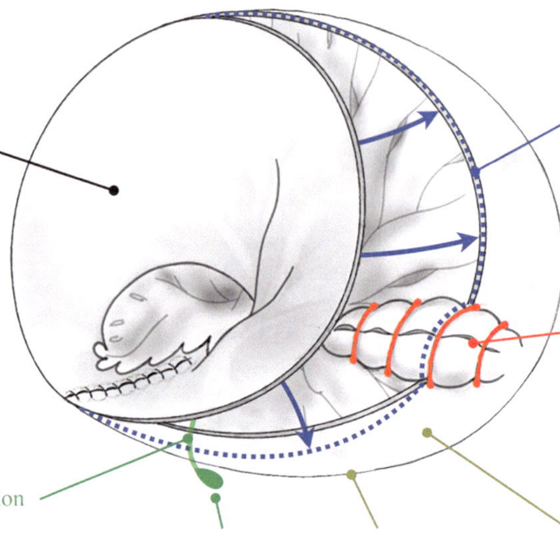

1. Ligate sutures for annular plication suture.
2. Check the coronary artery damage and bending again from the epicardial surface.
   - The suture line of the valve leaflets is indicated by the blue dotted line.
   - Anastomose the valve leaflets with a 6-0 monofilament suture.
   - Suture the leaflet near the atrioventricular node and the conduction pathway, suturing only the endocardium.
   - Suturing higher than the AV node has been reported, but higher sutures may result in tethering of the septal leaflet.

6

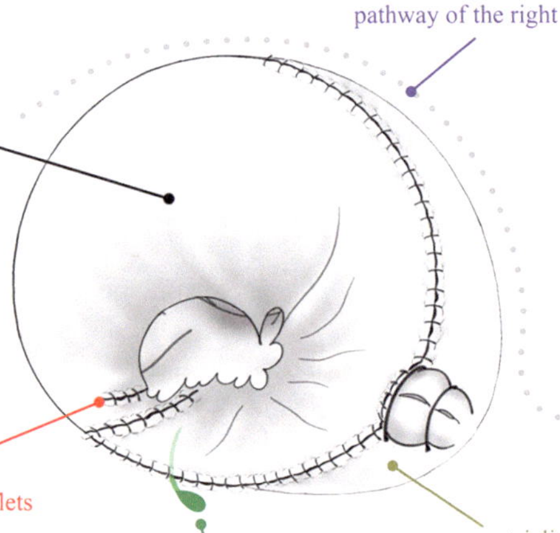

1. Perform a water test after suturing the valve leaflet to check for residual regurgitation.
2. If regurgitation remains at the anterior leaflet-septal leaflet commissure, cut the chordae tendineae that are preventing the septal leaflet from floating, and suture the anterior leaflet-septal leaflet commissure.

- In children, a growth-inhibiting prosthetic valve ring is not necessary.

Case Modified Cone Operation in Cases with Small Septal and Posterior Leaflets

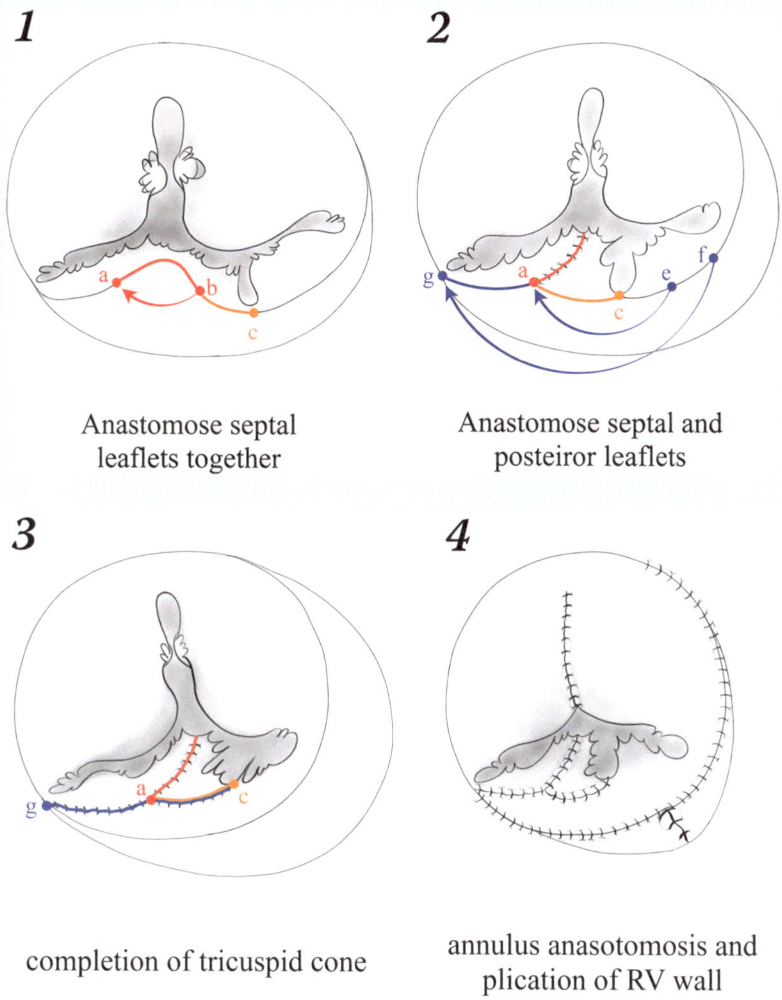

4 Cone Operation for 1-Year-Old Infant (Surgical Video)

Case 12.1

- 1-year-old infant
- Ebstein disease, severe tricuspid regurgitation, PFO
- *Operation*: Cone operation, right ventricular outflow reconstruction using 10 mm tricuspid ePTFE conduit, plication of the right atrial wall (Case 12.1, Scene 1)

Case 12.1, Scene 1 Exposure of tricuspid valve (Video 0 min 10 s)

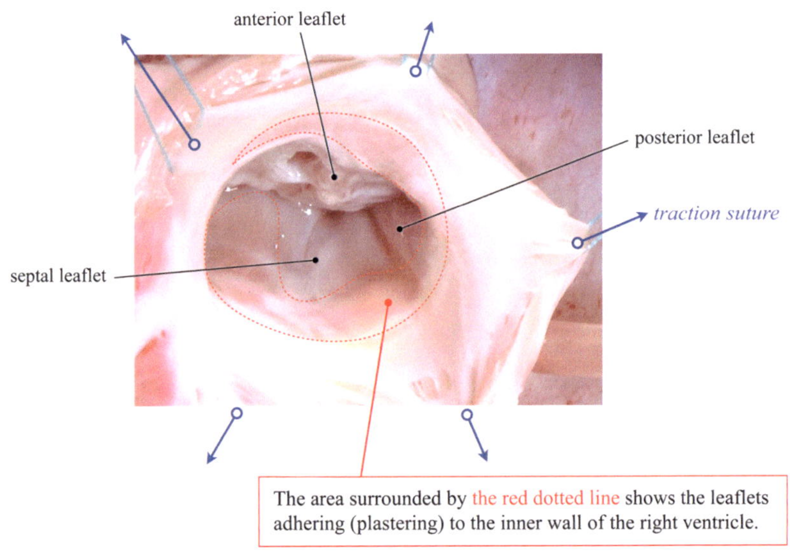

1. Some traction sutures (O→) are placed on the right atrial wall to hold the valve annulus in a shape-retaining state (Case 12.1, Scene 2).

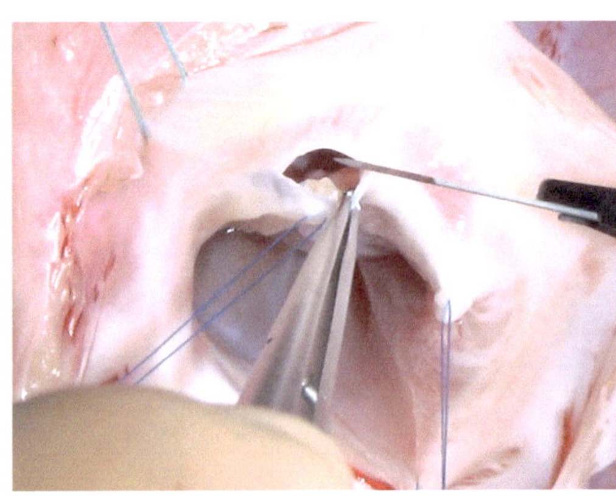

Case 12.1, Scene 2 Incise tricuspid annulus (Video 0 min 23 s)

1. 6-0 monofilament traction sutures are placed medial to the incision line to maintain the leaflet in an extended shape.
2. Incise the anterior leaflet attachment site (11–12 o'clock) with a sharp blade parallel to the leaflet, approximately 2 mm from the valve annulus (Case 12.1, Scene 3).

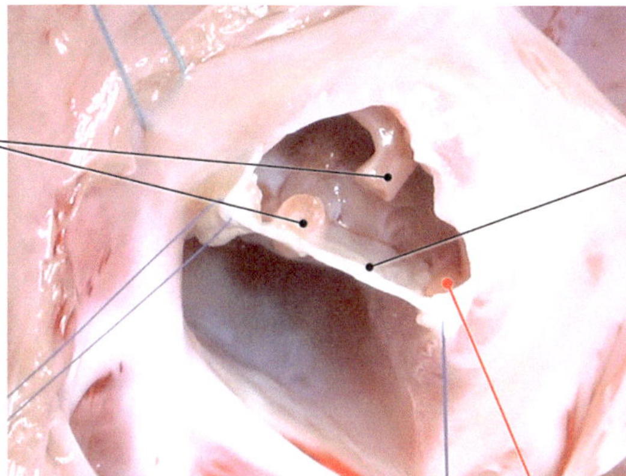

Case 12.1, Scene 3 Incise muscular bundle (Video 0 min 35 s)

1. Muscular columns are seen between the leaflet and the right ventricular wall.
   - The muscular columns are directly attached to the leaflet with no chordae tendineae in between.
   - Except for this muscular column, the anterior leaflet is well delaminated and the anterior leaflet is floating away from the right ventricular wall.
2. The muscular columns are cut close to the leaflet (Case 12.1, Scene 4).

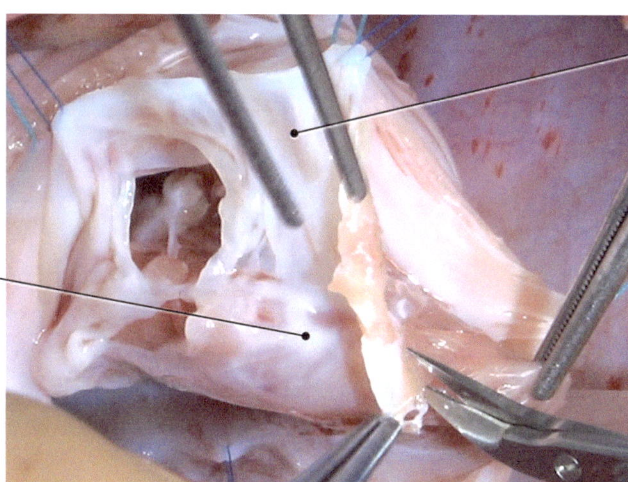

Case 12.1, Scene 4 Dissection of posterior leaflet (Video 2 min 03 s)

1. Dissect the posterior leaflet adherent to the right ventricular inner wall.
   - If the leaflet is perforated during dissection, it is repaired.
   - Delamination may be observed during the dissection process, and the valve leaflet and inner wall may not adhere to each other (Case 12.1, Scene 5).

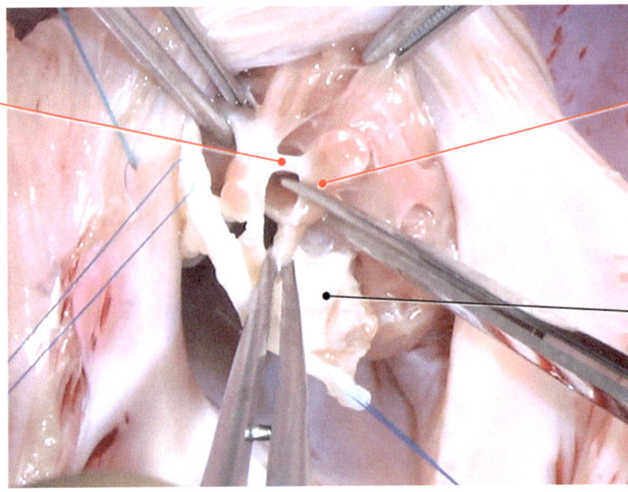

Case 12.1, Scene 5 Dissection of fibrous bridge and muscular bar (Video 3 min 09 s)

- Due to delamination failure, there is a large amount of muscular columns and fibrous bridges extending from the right ventricular cavity to the leaflets, restricting the leaflets of the valve.

1. The muscular columns and fibrous bridges are completely transected, leaving the chordae tendineae attached to the edge of the leaflet (Case 12.1, Scene 6).

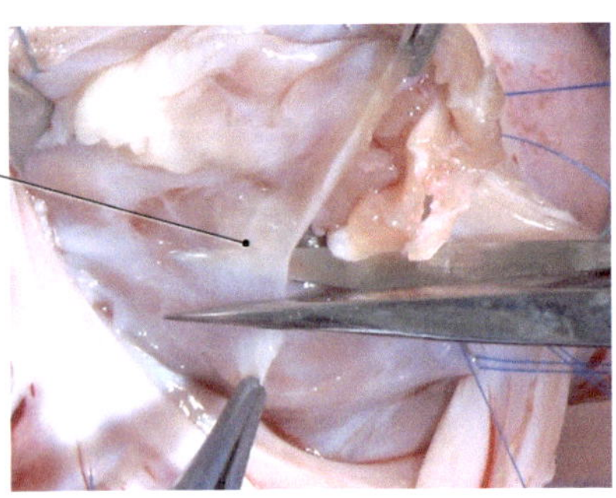

Case 12.1, Scene 6 Dissection of septal leaflet 1 (Video 6 min 02 s)

1. Incise the base of the septal leaflet (functional tricuspid annulus) that is plastered to the inner wall by sliding the surgical scissors (Case 12.1, Scene 7).

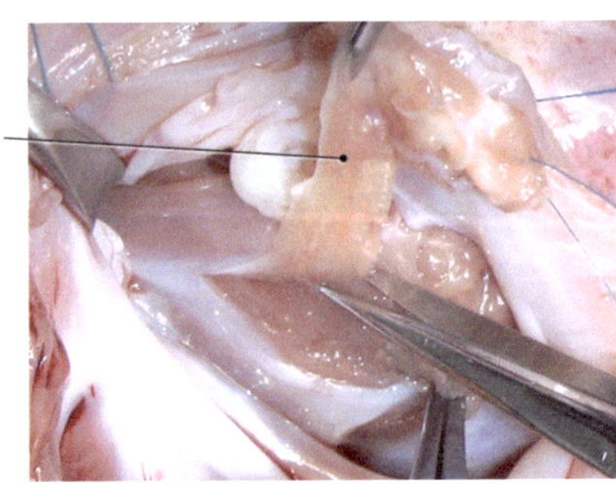

Case 12.1, Scene 7 Dissection of septal leaflet 2 (Video 6 min 14 s)

1. In a similar manner, dissect the septal leaflet that is being plastered (Case 12.1, Scene 8).

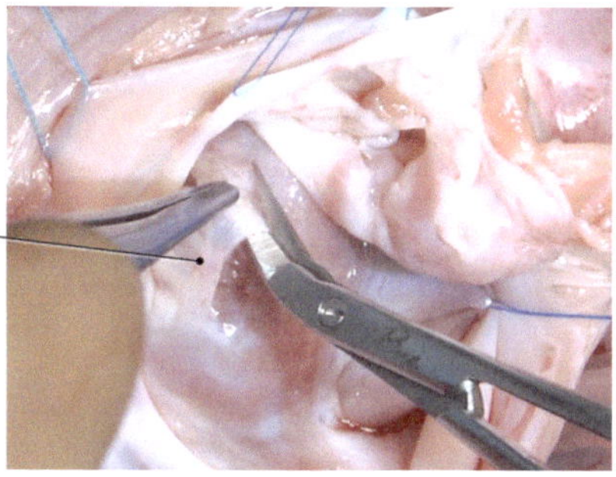

Case 12.1, Scene 8 Dissection of septal leaflet 3 (Video 6 min 33 s)

1. Incise the septal leaflet attachment on the anterior leaflet side to the true annulus.
   - Because the septal leaflet on the anterior leaflet side is small and does not float well, any chordae tendineae that may cause tethering should be removed, leaving the chordae tendineae attached to the leaflet edge.
   - After incision of the septal leaflet attachment to the valve annulus, the anterior annulus may be incised counterclockwise approximately 5 mm.
   - By incising the anterior leaflet attachment to the valve annulus, the distance to suture the leaflet longitudinally can be increased and a larger leaflet can be created.
   - In addition, the circumference of the valve annulus will be smaller when the cone is created by incising the anterior leaflet annulus (plication effect) (Case 12.1, Scene 9).

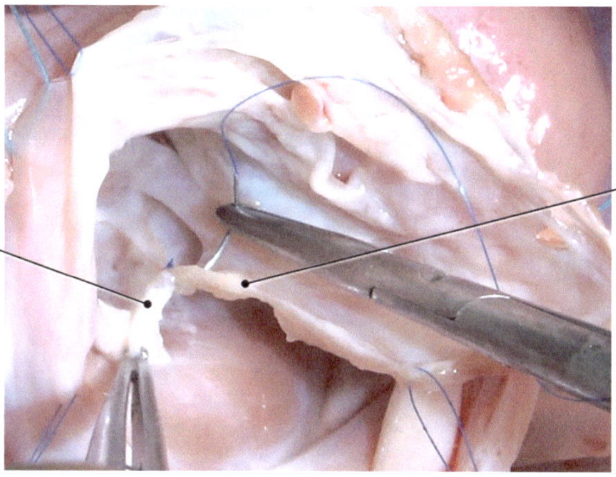

Case 12.1, Scene 9 Anastomosis between anterior and septal leaflets (Video 7 min 04 s)

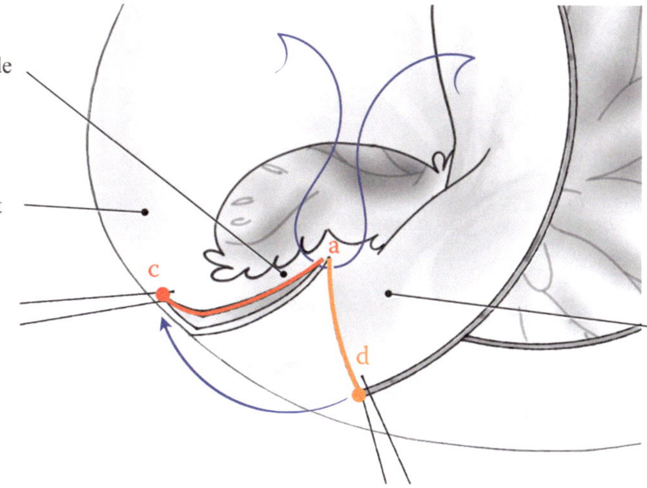

1. Dislocate the incised surface (a–d) of the posterior leaflet side septal leaflet to the left and meet the incised surface (a–c) of the anterior leaflet side septal leaflet (dislocate point (d) to point (c)).
2. Anastomose the incised surfaces from the apex with interrupted 6-0 monofilament sutures (Case 12.1, Scene 10).

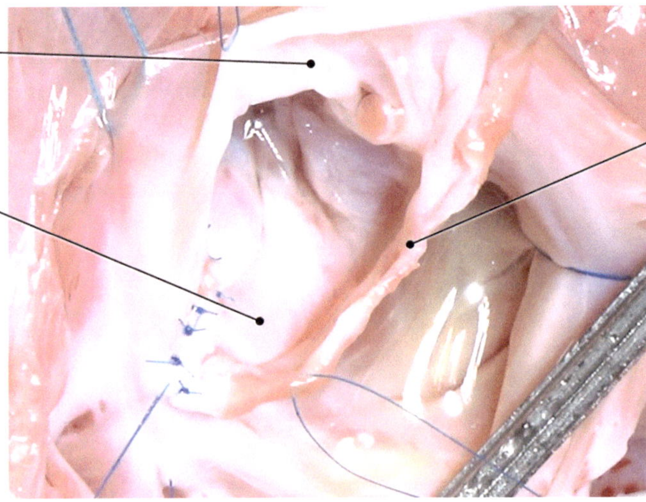

Case 12.1, Scene 10 Anastomosis between anterior and posterior leaflet side septal leaflets (Video7 min 33 s)

1. Suture the posterior side and anterior side septal leaflets longitudinally to the true valve annulus.

- This longitudinal joining of the leaflets allows for the formation of a circumferential leaflet (creation of a cone) (Case 12.1, Scene 11).

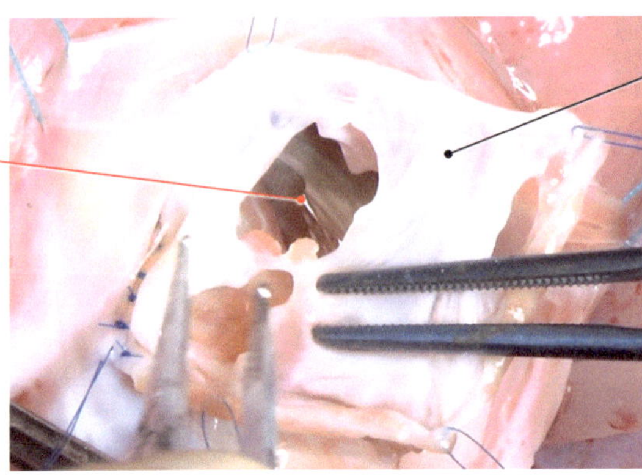

Case 12.1, Scene 11 Lacunare at anterior leaflet (Video 8 min 03 s)

- A large lacunae presents on the anterior leaflet (Case 12.1, Scene 12).

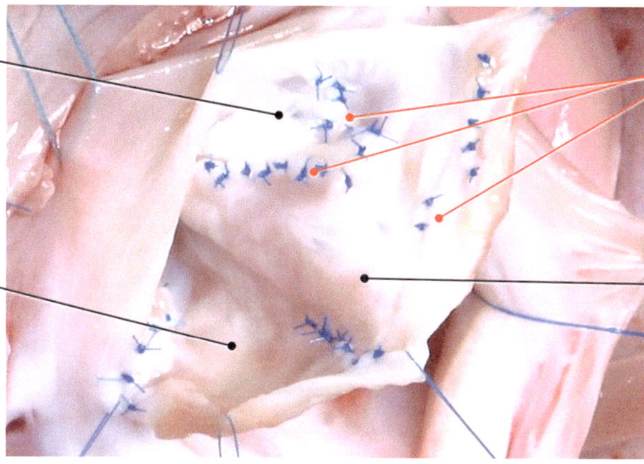

Case 12.1, Scene 12 Suture closure of lacunare (Video 8 min 11 s)

1. The lacunae are closed longitudinally with interrupted 6-0 monofilament sutures not to reduce the longitudinal length of the leaflet as much as possible.

   - Once the cone-like leaflet is created, the ventricular side of the leaflet should be checked for residual muscular column or fibrous bridge that could limit the mobility of the leaflet or contribute to tethering, and any remaining tissue should be completely transected.
   - Chordae tendineae at the leaflet edge should be preserved, but those that may contribute to tethering should be transected.
   - If the leaflet edge is attached to the ventricular wall in a curtain-like fashion, some small longitudinal incises should be made at the coaptation zone of the leaflet (creation of fenestrations) (Case 12.1, Scene 13).

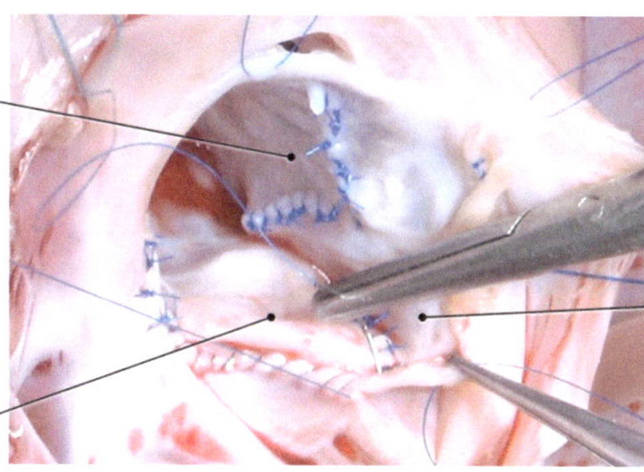

Case 12.1, Scene 13 Anastomosis of septal leaflet to the true annulus (Video 9 min 13 s)

1. The septal leaflet is anastomosed to the true valve annulus with a continuous 6-0 monofilament suture.
2. In areas where the atrioventricular conduction passes, only the endocardium is sutured thinly on the ventricular side.
3. The septal leaflet is anastomosed just below the orifice of the coronary sinus.

- The septal leaflet is sutured to the ventricular septal surface before plication of the annulus, since the ventricular septal surface is not involved in the plication and the circumference of the cone annulus corresponding to the ventricular septal surface (cone annulus) should be preserved.

- The width of the ventricular annulus plication is determined by the circumference of the cone annulus remaining after suturing the septal leaflet to the septal surface (Case 12.1, Scene 14).

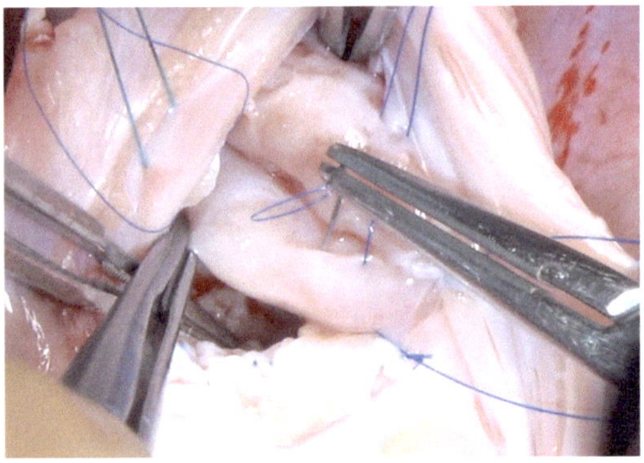

Case 12.1, Scene 14 Plication of ventricular wall (Video 11 min 17 s)

1. Plicate the right ventricle and right atrialized right ventricle longitudinally.
    - Determine the width of the true valve annulus suture to match the created cone diameter.
    - Using the longitudinal trabeculation, suture 3–4 Z-sutures with 5-0 monofilament thread.
    - Insert the suture needle from the endocardial surface to the midpoint of the right ventricular wall (do not insert the needle too deeply).
    - Visually check from the epicardial surface to make sure that the right coronary artery (RCA) is not damaged or in close proximity to the RCA.
    - After suture ligation, continue to check for bending of the RCA by viewing from the epicardial surface.
    - Be careful to close the atrialized right ventricular side so that the suture lumen does not remain tunnel-like.
    - After suture ligation, measure the diameter of the new valve annulus and confirm that it matches the cone diameter (Case 12.1, Scene 15).

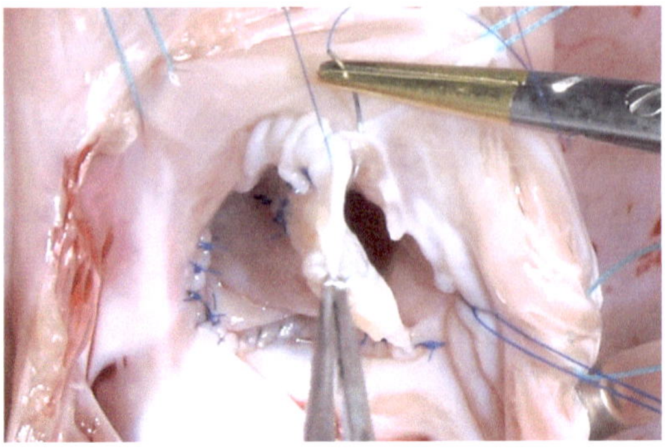

Case 12.1, Scene 15 Anastomosis of anterior leaflet to the true annulus (Video 12 min 34 s)

1. The remaining cone valve annulus is anastomosed with a continuous 6-0 monofilament suture (Case 12.1, Scene 16).

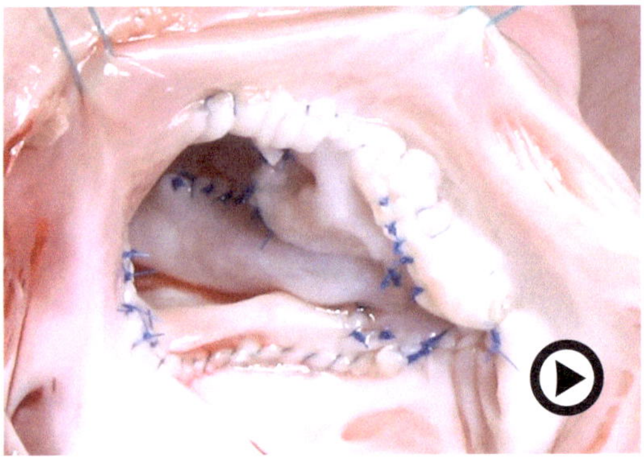

Case 12.1, Scene 16 Completion of cone operation (Video 15 min 57 s) (▶ https://doi.org/10.1007/000-hkp)

1. Completion of cone operation.
2. Water test to confirm residual regurgitation.
    - Residual regurgitation may occur at the commissure between the anterior leaflet and septal leaflet.
    - In this case, first transect any chordae tendineae that are interfering with the floating of the septal leaflet.
    - Partial closure of the commissure is performed with several interrupted 6-0 monofilament sutures.
    - In patients with impaired right ventricular function, leave the PFO (ASD) open or only partially closed.
    - In pediatric patients, do not use a prosthetic valve ring.

5 Cone Operation for 1-Month-Old Infant (Surgical Video)

Case 12.2

- One-month-old infant.
- Ebstein disease, severe TR, anatomic pulmonary atresia.
- Intraoperatively, the decision was made to perform a cone operation if valvulo-annuloplasty was possible and Starns operation if not.
- The patient had mild myxoid degeneration of the apex, but the mobility of the anterior apex was good, and the area of the anterior apex was considered usable, although not large.
- Plastering of the posterior leaflet and septal leaflet was observed, but the mobility of the remaining leaflet was preserved, so cone operation was chosen.
- *Operation*: Cone operation, right ventricular outflow reconstruction using 10 mm tricuspid ePTFE conduit, plication of the right atrial wall (Case 12.2, Scene 1).

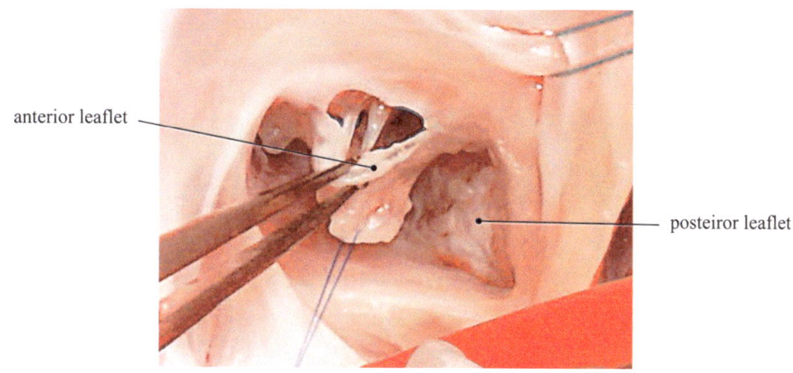

Case 12.2, Scene 1 Incise tricuspid annulus (Video 0 min 12 s)

1. Traction valve leaflet with several 6-0 monofilament sutures.
2. Incise the anterior leaflet attachment site (11–12 o'clock) parallel to the valve annulus with a pointed blade, approximately 1 mm away from the annulus.
3. Excise all fibrous tissue and chordae tendineae that restrict floating of the leaflet, except for the chordae tendineae attached to the leaflet edge.
   - Because of the fragility of the leaflet, a traction suture is applied and the incision is made precisely while extending the leaflet, taking care not to damage the leaflet (Case 12.2, Scene 2).

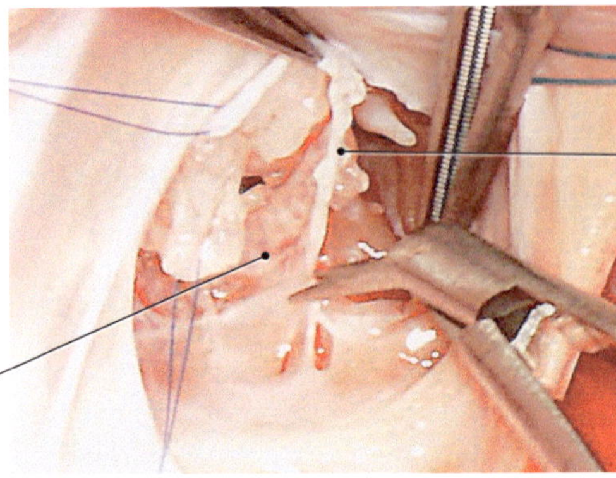

Case 12.2, Scene 2 Dissection of posterior and septal leaflets (Video 1 min 40 s)

1. Incise the attachment of the posterior leaflet and septal leaflet to the inner wall of the right ventricle.
2. Resect the muscular columns and fibrous bridges from the right ventricular cavity to the leaflet (Case 12.2, Scene 3).

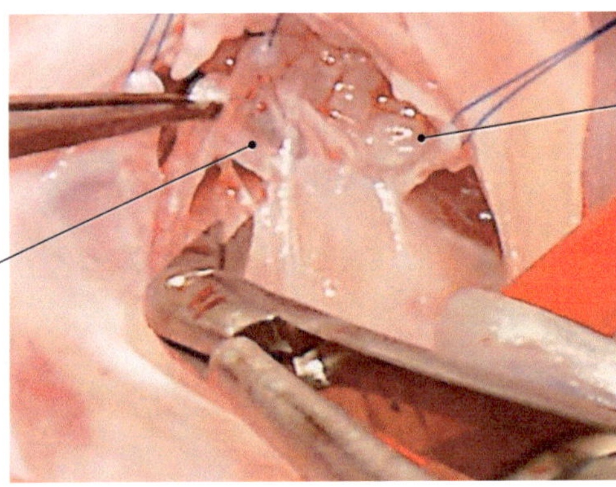

Case 12.2, Scene 3 Dissection of septal leaflet (Video 2 min 32 s)

1. Incise the attachment of anterior leaflet side septal leaflet (Case 12.2, Scene 4).

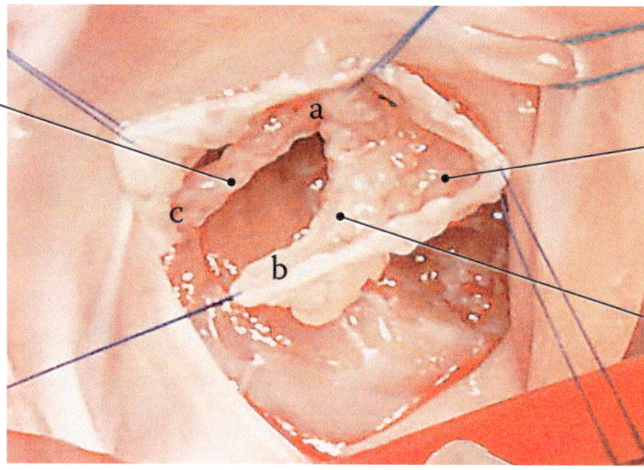

Case 12.2, Scene 4 Completion of dissection of tricuspid leaflets (Video 3 min 08 s)

1. Incision of each leaflet attachment and resection of muscle columns and fibrous bridges due to delamination failure are completed.
2. The incision surface of the posterior septal leaflet attachment (a–b) and the incision surface of the anterior septal leaflet attachment (a–c) are aligned (Case 12.2, Scene 5).

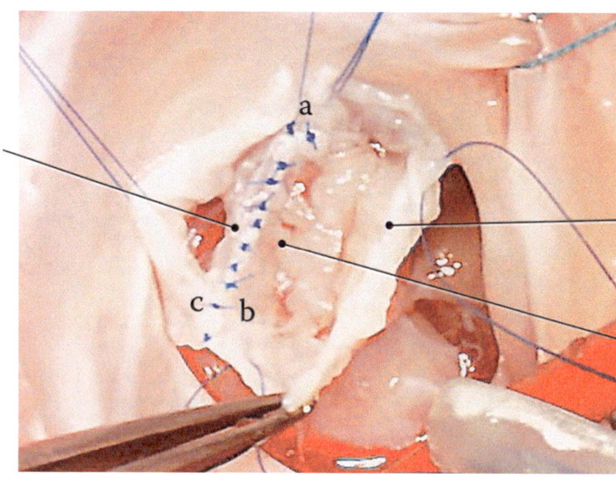

Case 12.2, Scene 5 Anastomosis between anterior and posterior leaflet side septal leaflets (Video 4 min 14 s)

1. Anastomose the incision surface of the posterior septal leaflet attachment (a–b) and the incision surface of the anterior septal leaflet attachment (a–c) with interrupted 6-0 monofilament suture.

- Because the leaflet tissue is myxomatous and very fragile, suture the leaflets carefully to avoid tearing the leaflets (Case 12.2, Scene 6).

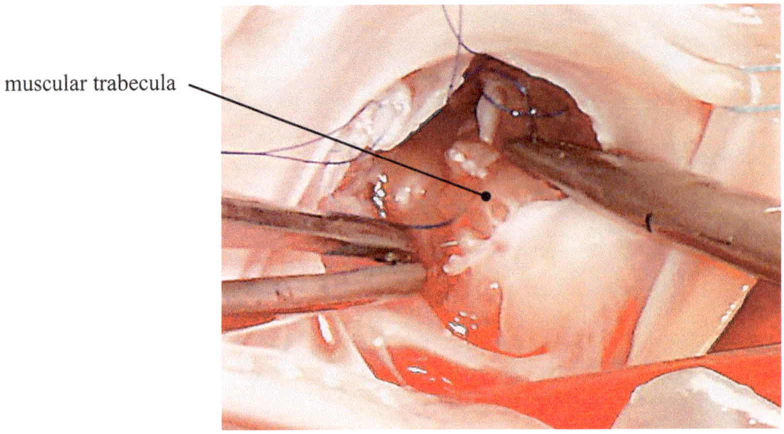

Case 12.2, Scene 6 Plication of ventricular wall (Video 5 min 24 s)

1. Plicate the right ventricle longitudinally with Z-sutures of 5-0 monofilament suture.
   - Check the right coronary artery (RCA) for damage and proximity to the RCA by viewing it from the epicardial surface.
   - After suture ligation, check for bending of the RCA by viewing from the epicardial surface (Case 12.2, Scene 7).

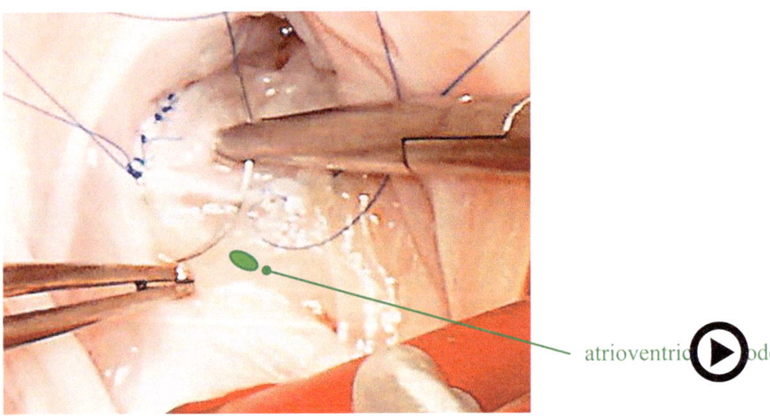

Case 12.2, Scene 7 Anastomosis of septal leaflet to the true annulus (Video 10 min 07 s) (▶ https://doi.org/10.1007/000-hkn)

1. The septal leaflet is anastomosed to the true valve annulus with a continuous 6-0 monofilament suture.
2. In areas where the atrioventricular conduction system passes, only the endocardium on the ventricular side is thinly sutured.

6 Reoperation: 5 Years After Cone Operation (Surgical Video)

Case 12.2 (Reoperation)

- Five years after cone operation in case 2, TR severe, right ventricular-pulmonary artery conduit stenosis.
- *Operation*: Tricuspid valve plication (commissural closure, anterior leaflet extension with autologous pericardium), right ventricular-pulmonary artery conduit replacement (20 mm diameter).

< prior cone operation >

The commissure between the anterior leaflet and the septal leaflet left open.

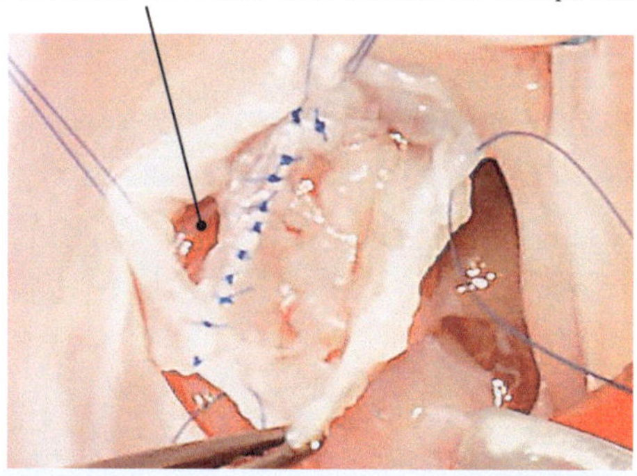

- The patient was an early infantile case, and suture closure of the commissure was not performed at the initial cone operation to ensure valve opening area (Case 12.2 (reop), Scene 1).

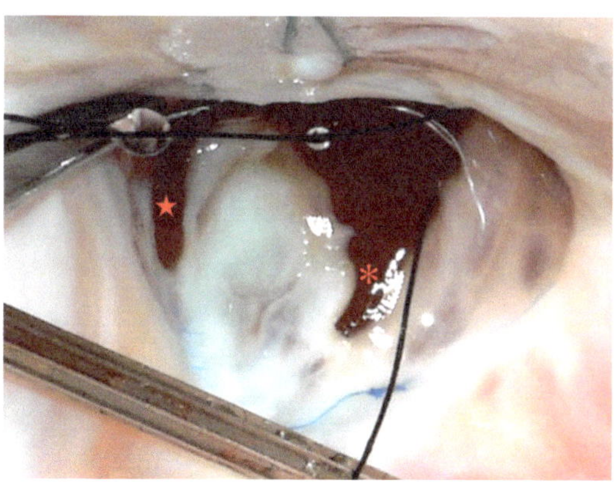

Case 12.2 (reop), Scene 1 Clefts of the tricuspid valve (Video 0 min 10 s)

- At the time of reoperation, the commissures between the anterior leaflet-septal leaflet (★) and the septal leaflet-posterior leaflet (*) are greatly widened. (The commissures were not closed in the previous cone operation).
- Since regurgitation from the commissure that was not closed during the late phase was exacerbated, a water test should be performed after completion of the cone, and (partial) closure of the commissure between the anterior leaflet and the septal leaflet should be considered to the extent that it does not become a stenosis (Case 12.2 (reop), Scene 2).

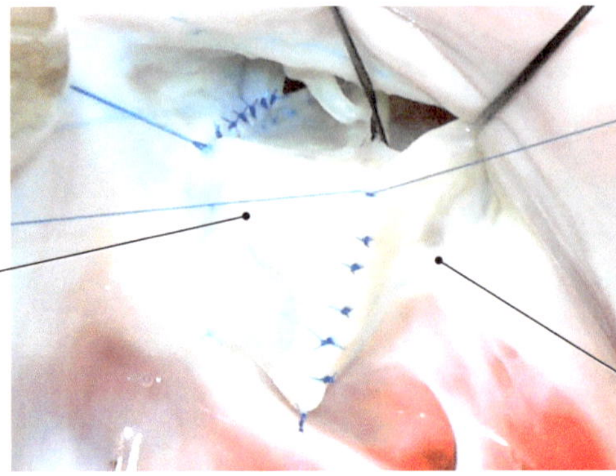

Case 12.2 (reop), Scene 2 Suture closure of the clefts (Video 2 min 12 s)

1. Both widened commissures are closed with interrupted 6-0 monofilament sutures (Case 12.2 (reop), Scene 3).

Case 12.2 (reop), Scene 3
Anastomosis of septal leaflet to the true annulus (Video 10 min 07 s)

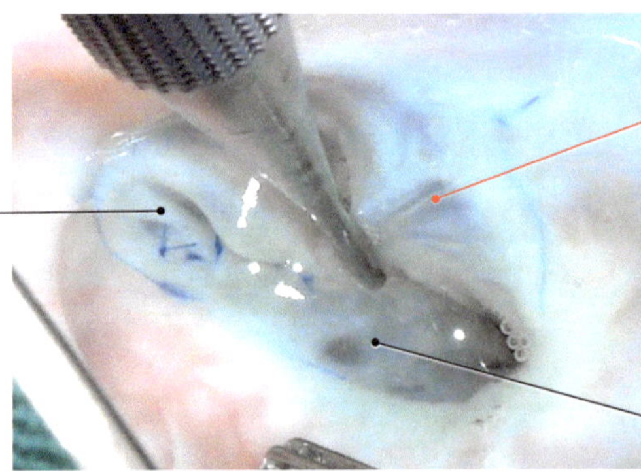

1. The water test is performed.
2. Because the area of the anterior leaflet is too small, no ballooning of the anterior leaflet is observed and the regurgitation is uncontrollable (Case 12.2 (reop), Scene 4).

Case 12.2 (reop), Scene 4 Residual tricuspid regurgitation (Video 2 min 40 s)

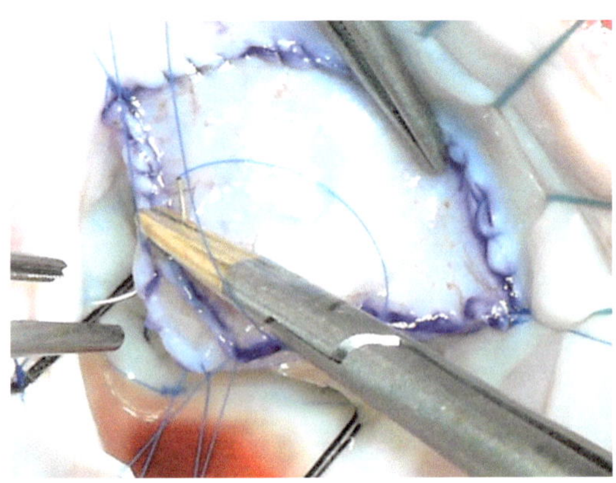

1. Incise the base of the anterior leaflet along the valve annulus.
   - The width of the incision is approximately the length of the leaflet base.
2. The anterior leaflet is extended by suturing an oval ethanol-treated autologous pericardium with a continuous 6-0 monofilament suture.
   - The longer diameter of the autologous pericardium should match the width of the anterior leaflet incision.
   - The short diameter is the distance from the valve annulus to the coaptation zone (Case 2 (reop), Scene 5).

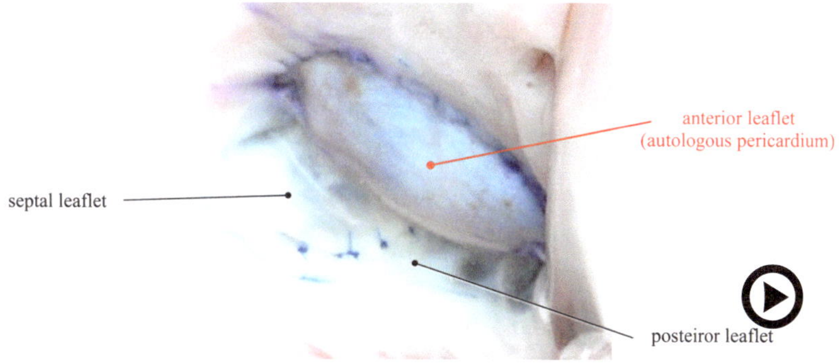

Case 12.2 (reop), Scene 5 Completion of tricuspid valvuloplasty (Video 8 min 50 s) (▶https://doi.org/10.1007/000-hkq)

- The water test showed good ballooning of the anterior leaflet.
- Tricuspid regurgitation disappeared.

References

Danielson Operation

Danielson GK, Maloney JD, Devloo RA. Surgical repair of Ebsstein's anomaly. Mayo Clin Proc. 1979;54:185–92.

Carpentier Classification, Carpentier Operation

Carpentier A, Chauvaud S, Mace L, Relland J, Mihaileanu S, Marino JP, Abry B, Guibourt P. A new reconstructive operation for Ebstein's anomaly of the tricuspid valve. J Thorac Cardiovasc Surg. 1988;96:92–101.

Starns Operation

Starns VA, Pitlick PT, Bernstein D, Griffin ML, Choy M, Shumway NE. Ebstein's anomaly appearing in the neonate. A new surgical approach. J Thorac Cardiovasc Surg. 1991;101:1082–7.

Sebening Stich

Augustin N, Schmidt-Habelmann P, Wottke M, Meisner H, Sebening F. Results after surgical repair of Ebstein's anomaly. Ann Thorac Surg. 1997;63:1650–6.

Cone Operation

da Silva JP, Baumgratz JF, da Fonseca L, Franchi SM, Lopes LM, Tavares GMP, Soares AM, Moreira LF, Barbero-Marcial M. The cone reconstruction of the tricuspid valve in Ebstein's anomaly. The operation: early and midterm results. J Thorac Cardiovasc Surg. 2007;133:215–23.
Dearani JA, Bacha E, da Silva JP. Cone reconstruction of the tricuspid valve foe Ebstein's anomaly: anatomic repair. Oper Tech Thorac Cardiovasc Surg. 2008;13:109–25.

Hypoplastic Left Heart Syndrome (HLHS) 13

1 Morphology and Hemodynamics of Hypoplastic Left Heart Syndrome

Hypoplastic left heart syndrome (HLHS) is defined as a disease with (1) normal macrovascular relationships (pulmonary artery: left anterior, aorta: right posterior), (2) atrioventricular valve is not a common atrioventricular valve, and (3) dysgenesis of the left heart system (hypoplastic left ventricle; closed, stenotic, or hypoplastic aortic and mitral valves; hypoplastic ascending aorta and hypoplasia of the ascending aorta and aortic arch).

HLHS-related malformations include atrioventricular septal defect with left ventricular hypoplasia resulting in a functional single ventricle, tricuspid valve closure with transposition of the great vessels, and left ventricular insertion of both atrioventricular valves with transposition of the great vessels.

These disease groups, including HLHS, are characterized by ductal-dependent systemic circulation (Fig. 13.1).

Supplementary Information The online version contains supplementary material available at https://doi.org/10.1007/978-981-96-6194-7_13. The videos can be accessed individually by clicking the DOI link in the accompanying figure caption or by scanning this link with the SN More Media App.

1.1 Morphology and Hemodynamics of Hypoplastic Left Heart Syndrome

Hemodynamics: Ductus-Dependent Systemic Circulation

- Blood flowing from the ductus arteriosus into the aorta maintains systemic circulation.
- Prostaglandin E1 opens the ductus arteriosus.
- Stenosis may occur in the pulmonary artery and aortic attachments of the ductus arteriosus.

Hemodynamics: Pulmonary Hypertension

- Pulmonary hypertension, pulmonary congestion, and increased right ventricular capacitance load are observed.
- When physiological pulmonary hypertension improves (days after birth), N2 is administered to decrease inhaled oxygen concentration (FiO_2 around 0.19) to decrease pulmonary blood flow and attempt to improve pulmonary congestion.

Morphology: Hypoplasia of the Aortic Arch

- Preoperative cerebral and coronary blood flow may be reduced in cases of severe hypoplasia.
- The branching morphology of the cervical vessels should also be considered.

M. Yamagishi, *Surgical Treatment of Congenital Heart Disease*,
https://doi.org/10.1007/978-981-96-6194-7_13

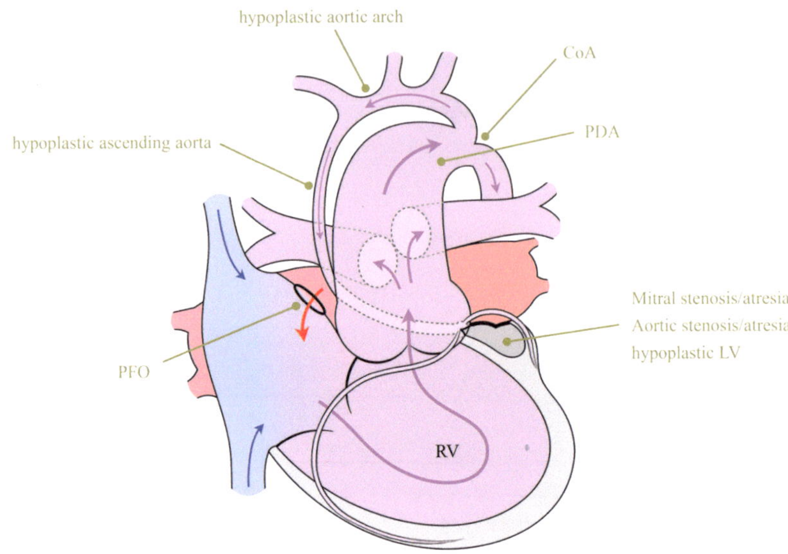

Fig. 13.1 Morphology and hemodynamics of HLHS

- The morphology (length) of the distal arch (isthmus) and the extent of ductus arteriosus invasion influence the anastomosis with the descending aorta.

Morphology: Hypoplasia of the Ascending Aorta

- Diameter of the ascending aorta is narrow because it serves only coronary blood flow.
- Diameter is often less than 3 mm in cases of aortic valve atresia and greater than 3 mm in cases of aortic valve stenosis.
- Blood flow is directed retrograde from the aortic arch to the sinus of Valsalva.
- The coronary arteries are perfused by retrograde blood flow from the ascending aorta.
- Variant HLHS cases also have retrograde blood flow in the ascending aorta.

Morphology: Coarctation of the Aorta

- Various degrees of stenosis (coarctation) complicate the condition.
- Ductus arteriosus tissue is present at the site of stenosis and distal to the aortic arch and descending aorta.

Morphology: Persistent Foramen Ovale

- Pulmonary venous blood flows through the foramen ovale (PFO) into the right atrium.
- The PFO can be narrow or rarely closed.
- Severe pulmonary hypertension is present in cases with a closed PFO.

Morphology: Mitral Stenosis/Atresia, Aortic Stenosis, Atresia

- Both valves show closure or stenosis, and a combination of the following is seen.
- In the case of aortic atresia (AA), there are more surgical procedures that can be performed with the heart beating.

mitral atresia(MA)+ aortic atresia(AA)

mitral atresia(MA)+ aortic stenosis(AS)

mitral stenosis(MS)+ aortic atresia(AA)

mitral stenosis(MS)+ aortic stenosis(AS)

Morphology: Left Ventricle

- Residual left ventricular volume is relatively large due to influx of blood into the left ventricle.
- Left ventricular intraventricular pressure may increase in MS+AA cases.
- In MA cases, residual left ventricular volume is small and slit-like, and the residual left ventricle does not compress the right ventricle.

Morphology: Tricuspid Valve, Right Ventricle

- Tricuspid valve morphology is often normal, but regurgitation may be present with right ventricular dilatation.
- Cases of right ventricular dilatation and reduced contractility are also seen.

ESSENTIALS Mitral Stenosis (MS) and Aortic Atresia (AA)

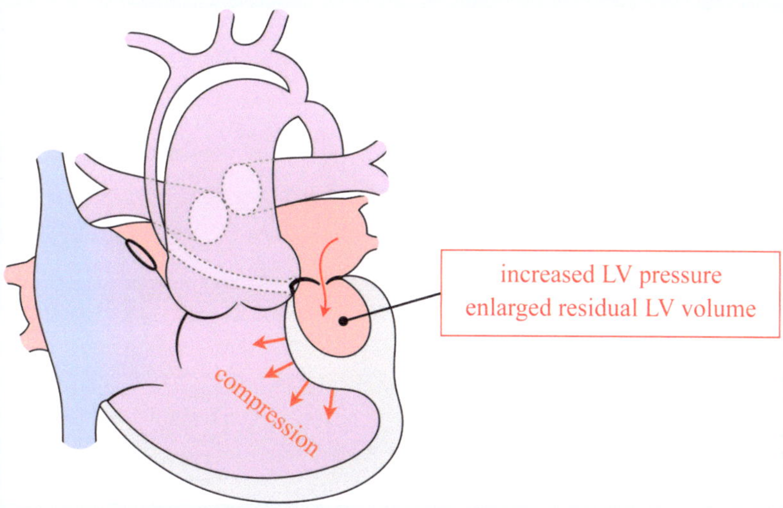

- Residual left ventricular volume is relatively large due to the presence of left ventricular inflow.
- In MS+AA cases, left ventricular pressure is increased, resulting in endocardial thickening (endocardial fibroelastosis), which may form a fistula with the coronary artery.
- Wall thickening, including in the ventricular septum, causes compression of the right ventricle, which greatly affects right ventricular function and prognosis.

1.2 Morphology and Hemodynamics of Hypoplastic Left Heart Syndrome

If HLHS is suspected at the time of fetal echocardiogram, planned delivery should be performed followed by surgical intervention. Consider balloon atrial septal septoplasty (BAS) immediately after birth in cases of narrow foramen ovale. Maintain patency of the patent ductus arteriosus with administration of Prostaglandin E1 (Fig. 13.2).

< check list by echocardiography >

PDA (presence of narrowing)
PFO (presence of narrowing)
Mitral valve (stenosis or atresia)
Aortic valve (stenosis or atresia)
Left ventricular volume
Ascending aorta (diameter, direction of blood flow)
Aortic arch (diameter, direction of blood flow)
Cervical vessels (branching)
Tricuspid valve (presence of regurgitation)
Pulmonary valve (presence of regurgitation)
Pulmonary veins (presence of anomalous drainage)
Trachea, bronchus (presence of stenosis)

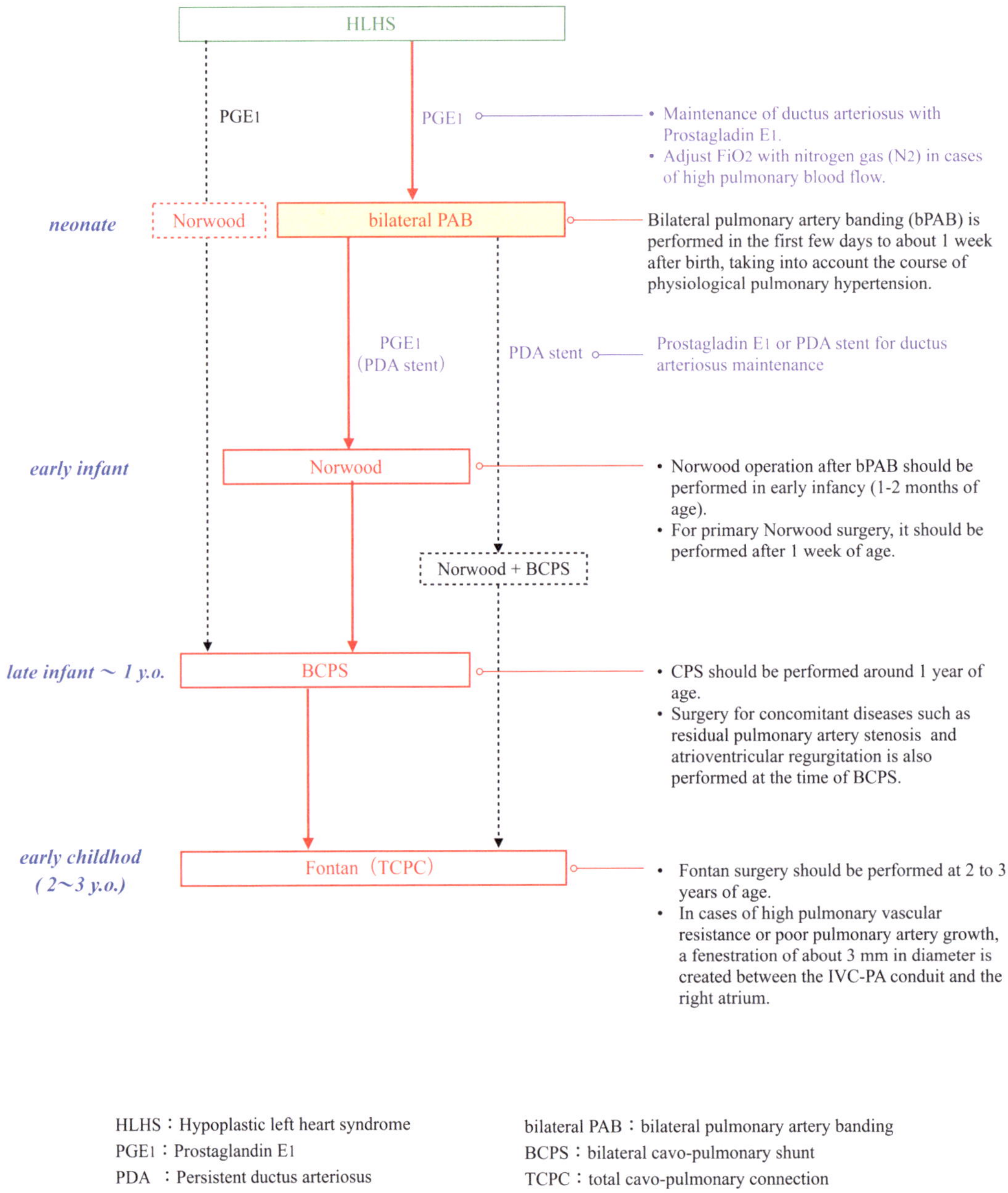

Fig. 13.2 Treatment strategy of HLHS

1.3 CT Findings of Hypoplastic Left Heart Syndrome

The morphology of the ascending aorta and aortic arch in this syndrome is highly variable. In general, the ascending aorta is narrow and the aortic arch is often hypoplastic, which is complicated by coarctation of the aorta. The main pulmonary artery is thicker, and the orifices of the right and left pulmonary arteries branching from the posterior wall are often in a vertical relationship. CT images of a typical case are shown below (Fig. 13.3).

- Normal relationship of the great arteries (left anterior pulmonary artery, right posterior aorta).
- The ascending aorta is very thin.
- Branching of neck vessels are normal in this case.
- The main pulmonary artery is very large and is connected to the ductus arteriosus.

* Site of right pulmonary artery banding

< right anterior view of the aorta>

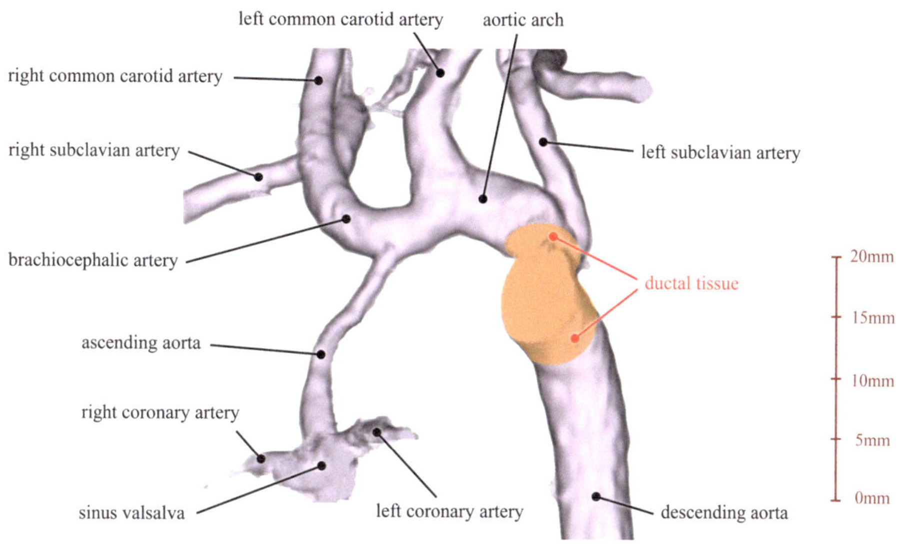

< anterior view >

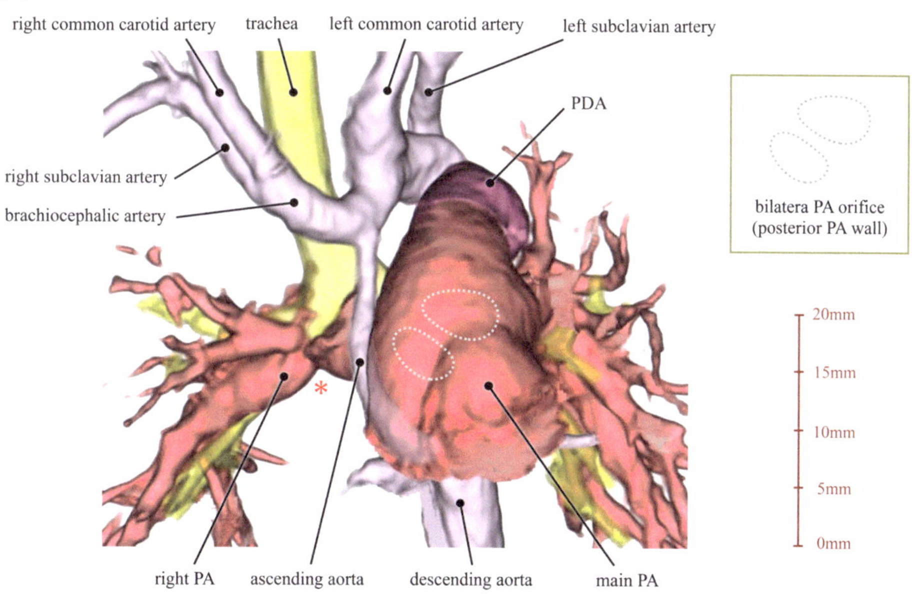

Fig. 13.3 CT findings of HLHS

- The ascending aorta is very thin, and the left and right coronary arteries originate from its sinus.
- The ductus arteriosus (orange area) widely extends into the distal aortic arch and descending aorta.
- In this case, the aortic stenosis is mild.
- The proximal side of the aortic arch is slightly narrow, while the distal side of the arch is only mildly hypoplastic.

< right lateral view >

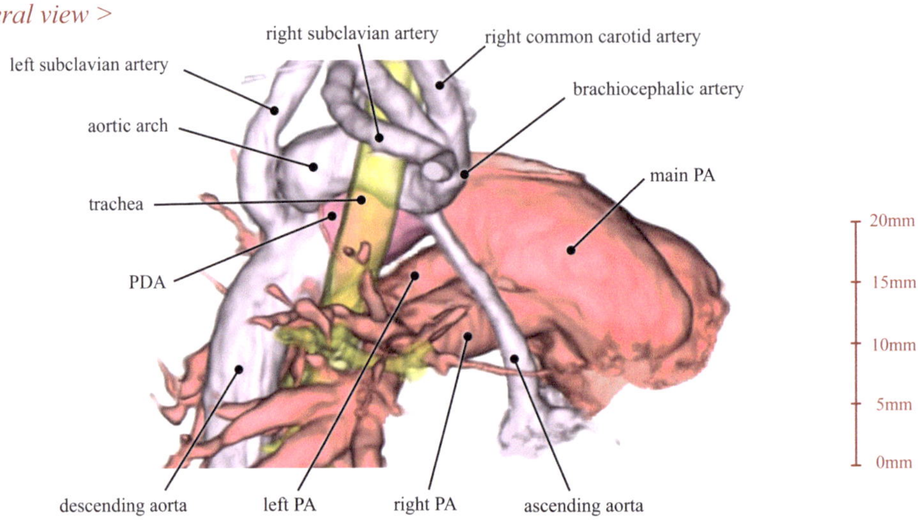

- The ascending aorta is very narrow and lies to the right posterior to the main pulmonary artery.
- The left and right pulmonary arteries originate dorsal to the main pulmonary artery.
- The left pulmonary artery originates slightly higher than the right pulmonary artery.

< left lateral view >

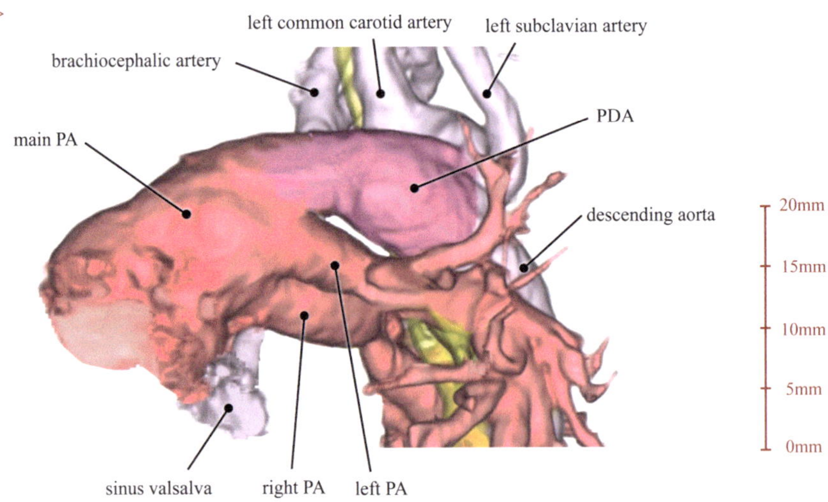

- The ductus arteriosus leads from the apex of the main pulmonary artery to the aortic arch and the descending aorta.
- The left and right pulmonary arteries originate dorsal to the main pulmonary artery.
- The left pulmonary artery originates slightly higher than the right pulmonary artery.

< dorsal view >

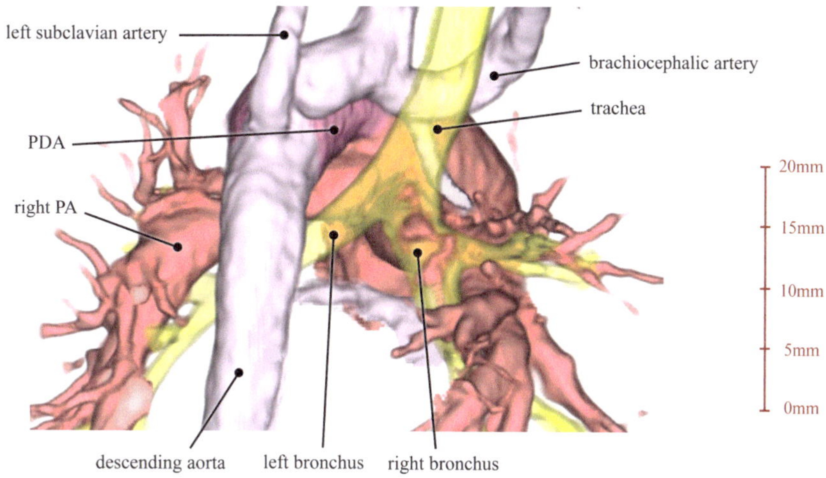

- The ductus arteriosus and the descending aorta pass over the left bronchus.

< cephalic view >

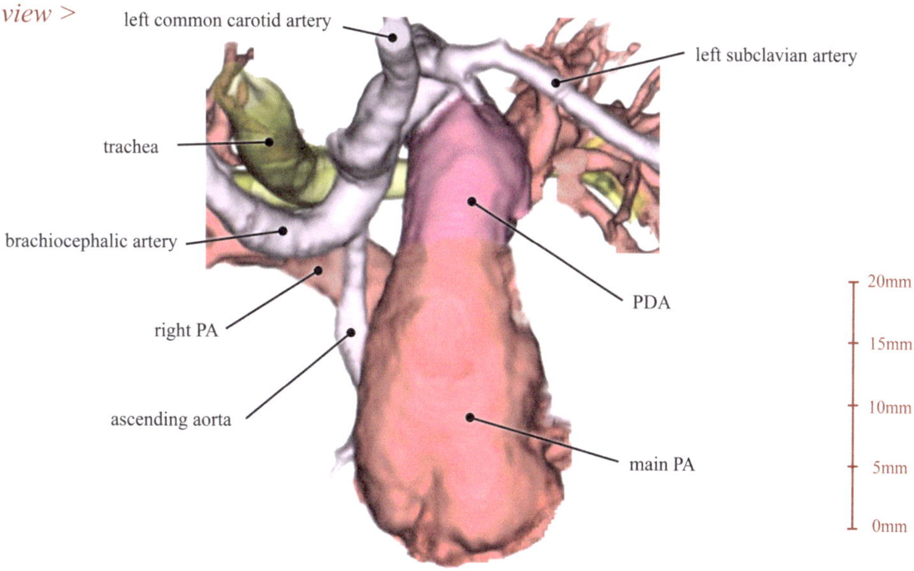

- The ductus arteriosus is connected to the main pulmonary artery by the same caliber, making it difficult to identify the border between the two vessels.

< cephalic view, horizontal cross-section of main PA, PDA removed >

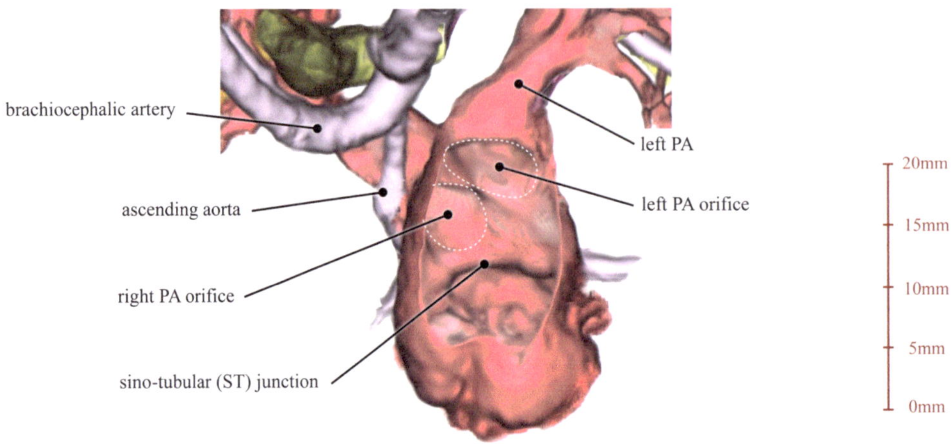

- Left and right pulmonary arteries originate from the posterior wall of the main pulmonary artery.
- Left and right pulmonary artery orifices are in close proximity.
- The left pulmonary artery orifice is more cephalad than the right pulmonary artery orifice.
- The right pulmonary artery orifice and ST junction are also in close proximity.

< frantal view, PDA removed >

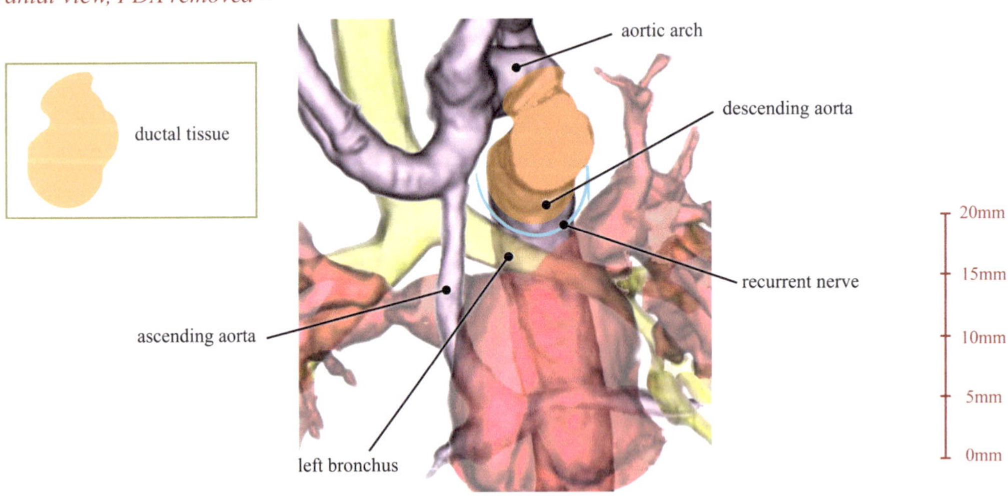

- The ductus arteriosus (*orange area*) extends widely into the distal aortic arch and descending aorta.
- The left bronchus is located in front of the descending aorta, and the recurrent nerve runs across it (care must be taken not to damage the recurrent nerve when dissecting the descending aorta).

< coronal section of main PA >

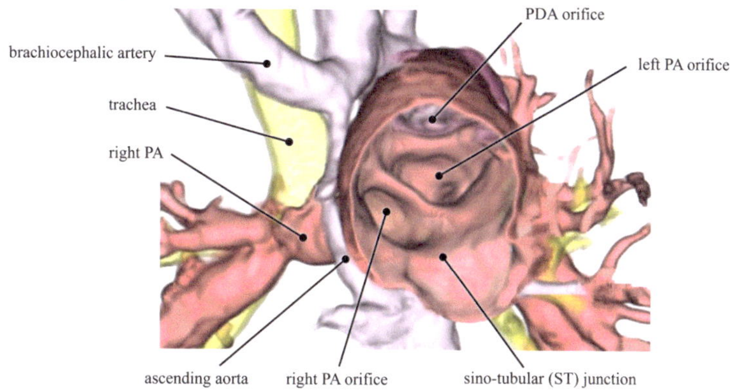

- Ductus arteriosus orifice, left pulmonary artery orifice, and right pulmonary artery orifice are nearly in series.
- Left and right pulmonary artery orifices are in close proximity, and it is difficult to separate the two orifices.

< dorsal view of pulmonary artery >

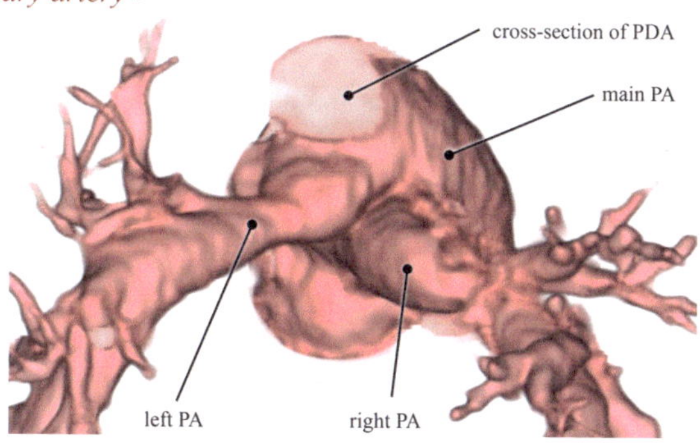

- Left and right pulmonary arteries originate from the dorsal wall of the main pulmonary artery.
- Left pulmonary artery originates higher (cephalad) than right pulmonary artery.

ESSENTIALS Branching Angle of Both Pulmonary Artery Orifices

< dorsal view >

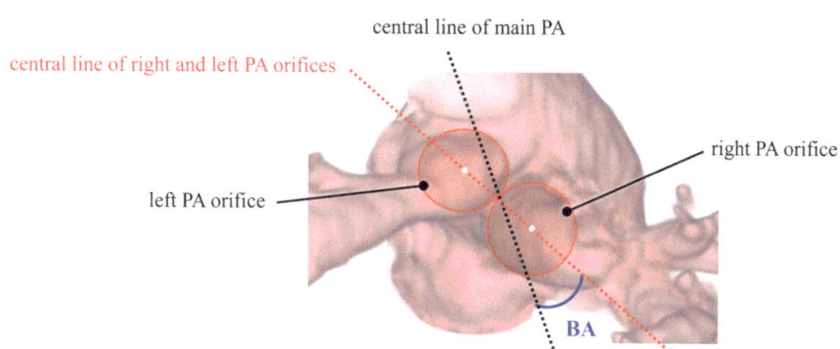

(continued)

- The angle between the central line of the main pulmonary artery (a line connecting the center point of the pulmonary valve ring and the center point of the section of the ductus arteriosus attachment) and the central line connecting the center points of the right and left pulmonary artery orifices is the branching angle (BA) of the orifices.
- The bottom figure shows the orifice arrangement and BA measurements in clinical cases
- In about 75% of cases, the right and left pulmonary artery bifurcation angles were 45° or greater, and the right and left pulmonary artery orifices were aligned in a vertical relationship.

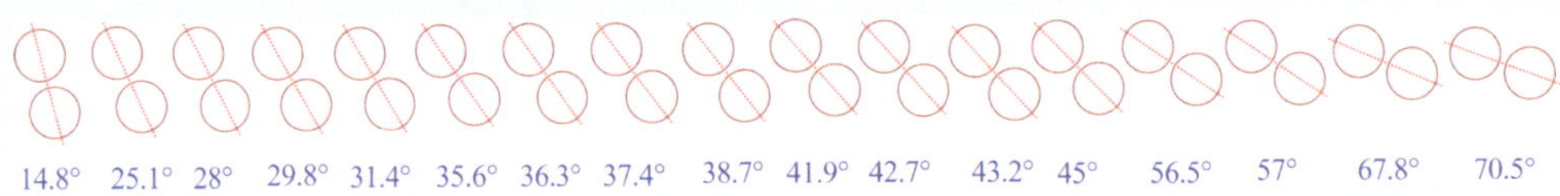

2 Bilateral Pulmonary Artery Banding

By maintaining the ductus arteriosus open and adjusting pulmonary blood flow by strangulation of the left and right pulmonary arteries (bilateral pulmonary artery banding, bPAB), it is possible to avoid the risk of open heart surgery (Norwood procedure) in the early neonatal period.

When performing bPAB, it is necessary to consider (1) minimizing invasiveness as much as possible, (2) selecting a technique that facilitates blood flow control, and (3) using a technique that minimizes deformation of the pulmonary artery after strangulation is released.

The conventional method using ePTFE tape, for example, increases the separation distance between the left and right pulmonary arteries, making it difficult to fine-tune blood flow. In addition, deformation of the pulmonary artery after the tape is removed is a problem. In contrast, *the lasso method* using ePTFE suture (Gore-Tex suture®) and a tourniquet can avoid these problems.

2.1 Lasso Method for Bilateral Pulmonary Artery Banding

- The lasso method is easy to fine-tune banding site circumference according to the vascular clip width.
  - Vascular clip has several products and sizes (small clip: width 0.4 mm, medium clip: 0.6 mm).
- The lasso method does not injury the PA wall when removing the vascular clip and ePTFE suture.
- Because of the short segment banding, pulmonary artery plasty after removing the ePTFE suture is often unnecessary (Fig. 13.4).

< *Materials required for bPAB by lasso method* >

- ePTFE (Gore-Tex suture®) CV-4
- Fr polyvinyl chloride (PVC) tube
- 5-0 nylon suture
- 7-0 polypropylene suture
- Sizer (diameter: 3 mm, 2.5 mm, 3.5 mm)
- Vascular clip
  - Small (clip width 0.4 mm)
  - Medium (clip width 0.6 mm)

1. Cut the PVC tube to be used for the tourniquet outer cylinder.
   - The length of the PVC: left PA = 8 mm approx., right PA = 5 mm approx.
   - The length of the PVC tube should be determined according to the morphology of the great vessels, but be careful not to make it too long.

1

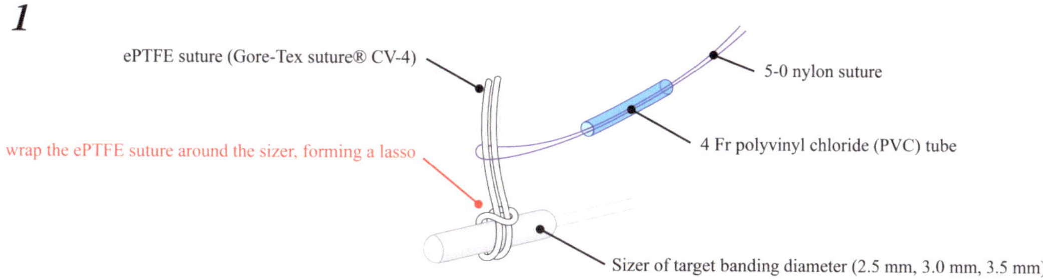

Fig. 13.4 Bilateral PA banding using lasso method

2. Wrap the ePTFE suture (Gore-Tex suture® CV-4) around the sizer of target banding diameter, forming a lasso.
   - The standard banding diameter is 3 mm for a 3 kg patient.

2

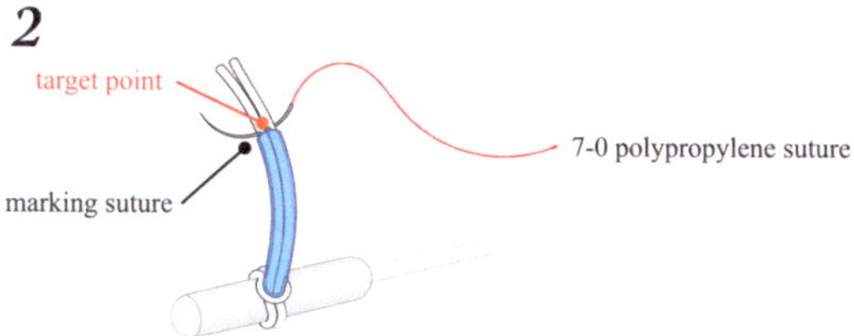

1. Tighten the tourniquet.
2. With the tube tightened, a 7-0 polypropylene suture is threaded through the ePTFE suture (Gore-Tex suture® CV-4) at the upper end of the PVC tube and ligated.
3. This 7-0 polypropylene suture is used as a marker for the diameter of the strangulation.
   - To prevent misalignment of target point, sew into ePTFE suture with a 7-0 polypropylene suture.

3

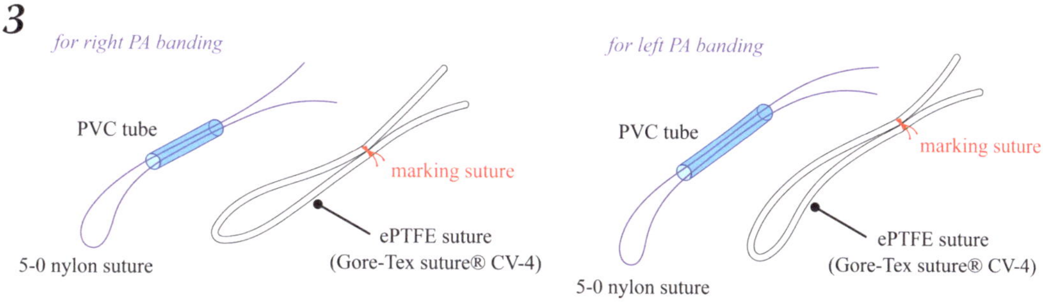

1. Remove the ePTFE suture from sizer.
2. Release the lasso state of the ePTFE suture (Gore-Tex suture® CV-4).
3. Insert a 5-0 nylon suture through the PVC tube again.
4. Prepare one for each pulmonary artery.

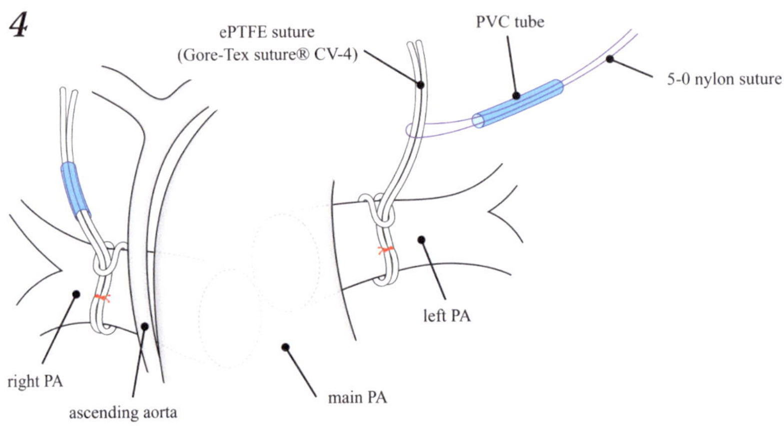

1. Dissect right and left pulmonary arteries with minimal width.
2. Wrap the ePTFE suture around the right and left pulmonary arteries in a lasso shape.
3. Insert the ePTFE suture into the ATOM tube using a 5-0 nylon suture.

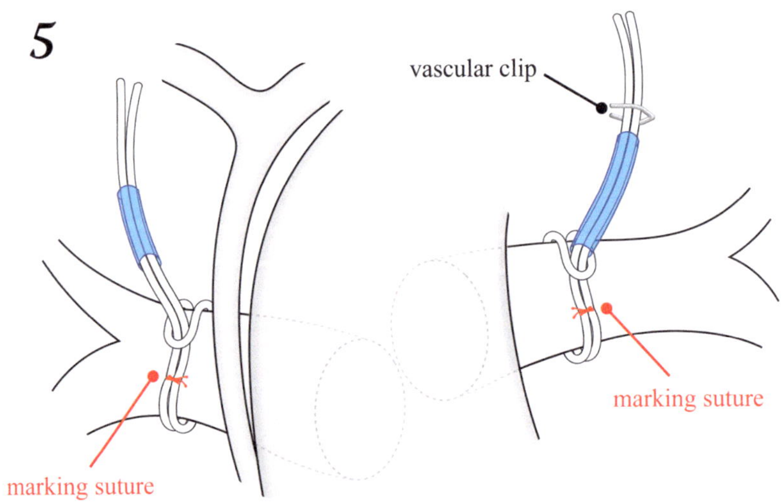

1. Tighten the tourniquet gradually.
2. Apply a medium vascular clip (0.6 mm clip width) at the loose part first, using the marker part as a reference.
3. Bite the vascular clip so that the ePTFE suture is positioned in the center of the vascular clip for easy removal.

4. Add a small (0.4 mm clip width) vascular clip proximally and gradually increase strangulation based on the flow velocity of 2.7–3.0 m/s using intraoperative echocardiography (epicardial echocardiography).
5. If the banding is too tight (flow velocity of 3.3–3.5 m/sec or higher, weakening of the echo signal, etc.), remove vascular clips one by one.

6

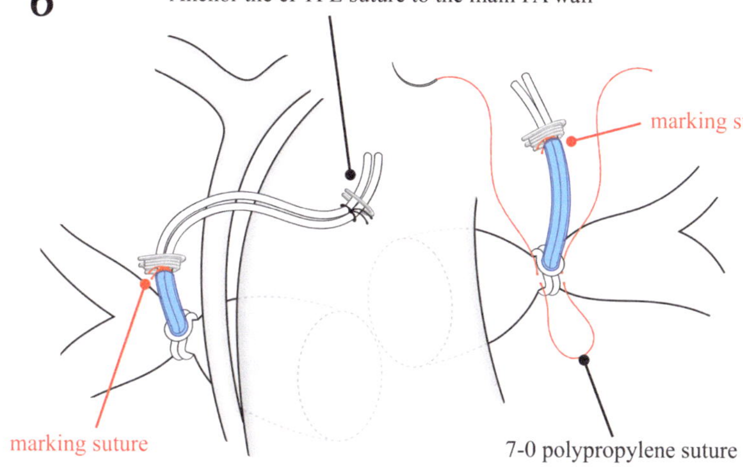

1. Apply at least three vascular clips to prevent clip dislodgement.
2. Secure the ePTFE banding suture to the right and left pulmonary artery surface with a U-shaped 7-0 polypropylene suture to prevent the ePTFE suture from shifting distally.
3. Securing sutures at the right and left pulmonary artery are not necessary if they increase banding.
4. The distal stump of the ePTFE suture should be secured to the main pulmonary artery surface.

3 Norwood Operation

3.1 Procedure of Neo-Aorta Reconstruction

3.1.1 Neo-Aorta Reconstruction Using Supplemental Material (Conventional Procedure)

Big Column Configuration

- In the case of procedures using large supplemental material such as homograft, heterogeneous or autologous pericardium, etc. (conventional procedure), the neo-aortic root is enlarged (big column configuration), which may induce turbulence in the neo-aortic root, resulting in gradual aggravation of the root enlargement due to turbulence.
- There is concern that the supplemental material may decrease vascular elasticity and affect right ventricular function.
- Calcification of the supplemental material can also be a problem.
- The rapidly narrowing of the descending aortic junction may also induce stenotic lesions secondary to intimal thickening caused by turbulent flow and increased wall tension.
- Narrowing of the aortopulmonary space due to basal enlargement during the remote phase may be problematic (Fig. 13.5).
- Long and wide neo-aortic root is formed by the supplemental material (e.g., heterogeneous pericardium).

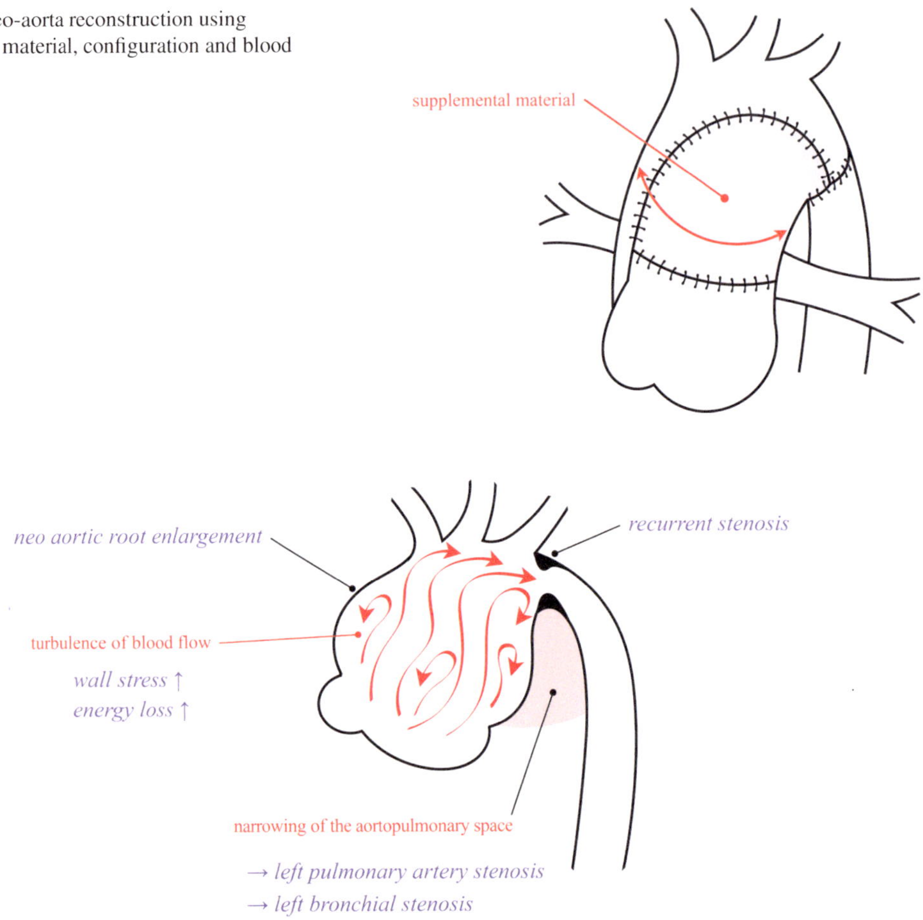

Fig. 13.5 Neo-aorta reconstruction using supplemental material, configuration and blood flow

- Concerns include enlarged neo-aortic root, decreased vascular elasticity due to the supplement material, turbulent flow within the wide neo-aortic root, increased energy loss, and stenosis (recurrent stenosis) at the descending aortic anastomosis.

3.1.2 Neo-Aorta Reconstruction Without Supplemental Material (Direct Anastomosis Procedure)

Short Proximal Trunk

- In the neo-aorta reconstruction without supplement material (direct anastomosis procedure), a short and wide short proximal trunk joins the aortic arch and connects to the descending aorta at an acute angle. Thus, the blood flow ejected from the ventricle strikes the aortic arch at a high velocity, creating turbulence within the short aortic trunk.
- The sharply angled descending aortic junction also causes turbulence and increased shear stress, which may lead to stenotic lesions due to intimal thickening.
- Narrowing of the aortopulmonary space below the new aortic arch is problematic (Figs. 13.6 and 13.7).

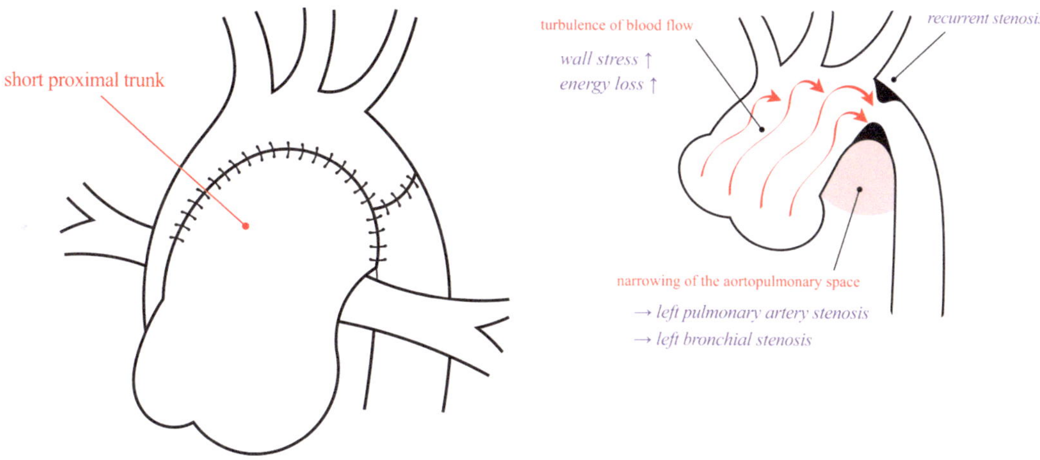

Fig. 13.6 Neo-aorta reconstruction by direct anastomosis, configuration and blood flow

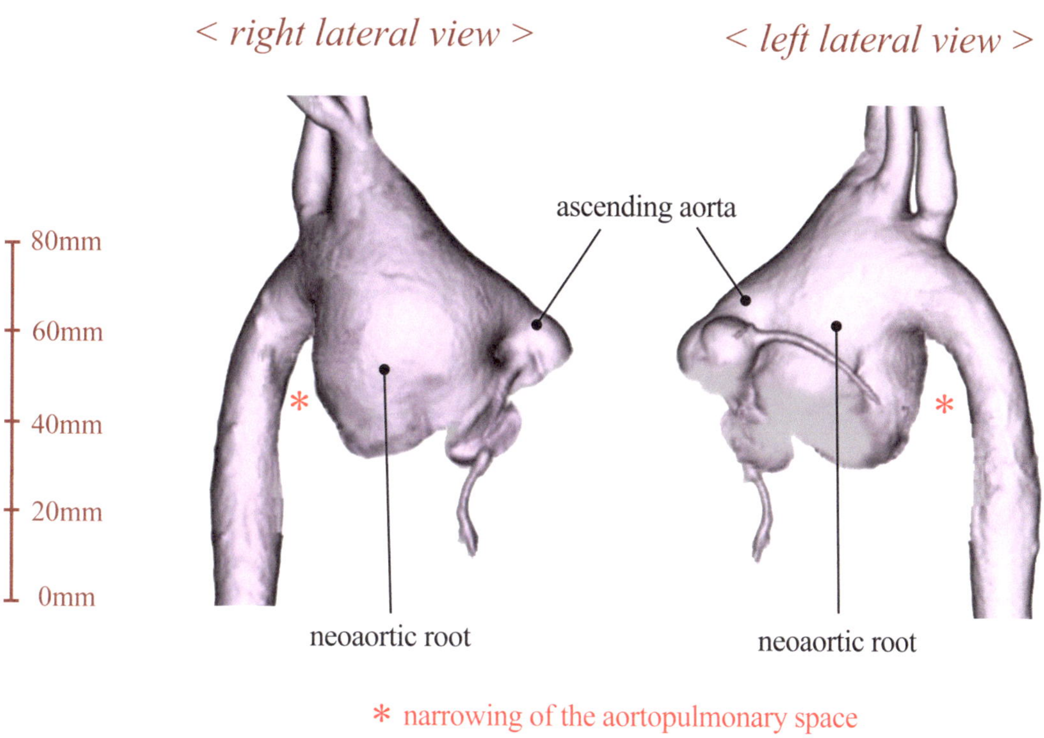

Fig. 13.7 Aortic root enlargement and neo-aortic valve regurgitation after the direct anastomosis

- Because the height of the neo-aortic root is short, the ejected blood flow may hit the aortic arch, causing turbulence.
- There are concerns about increased energy loss and stenosis at the anastomosis with the descending aorta (reoccurrence of stenosis).
- The aortopulmoanry space is narrow and may cause left pulmonary artery stenosis and left bronchial stenosis.

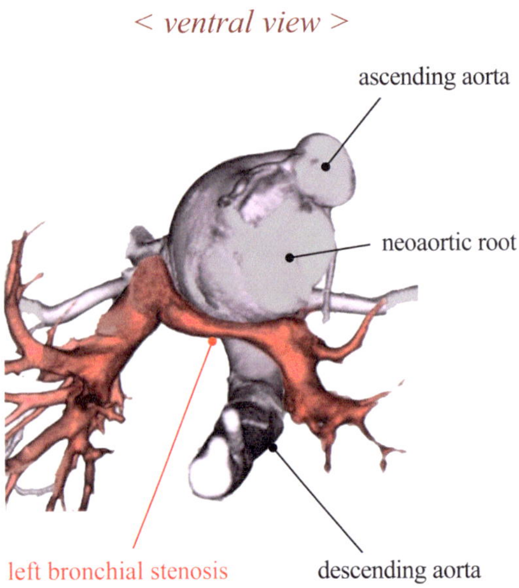

3.1.3 Neo-Aorta Reconstruction Without Supplemental Material (Chimney Method)

Tall Conical Trunk The main concepts of the chimney method are longitudinal extension and horizontal plication of the neo-aortic root.

- The orifices of the left and right pulmonary arteries are separated in a U-shape as a single lump, and the defect is sutured directly in the longitudinal direction.
- The main pulmonary artery (base of the neo-aorta) is formed into a long, conical trunk, making it easier to reach the aortic arch and descending aorta.
- Narrowing of the large aortopulmonary space can be ensured.
- Blood flow from the neo-aortic root to the descending aorta is less turbulent (Figs. 13.8 and 13.9).

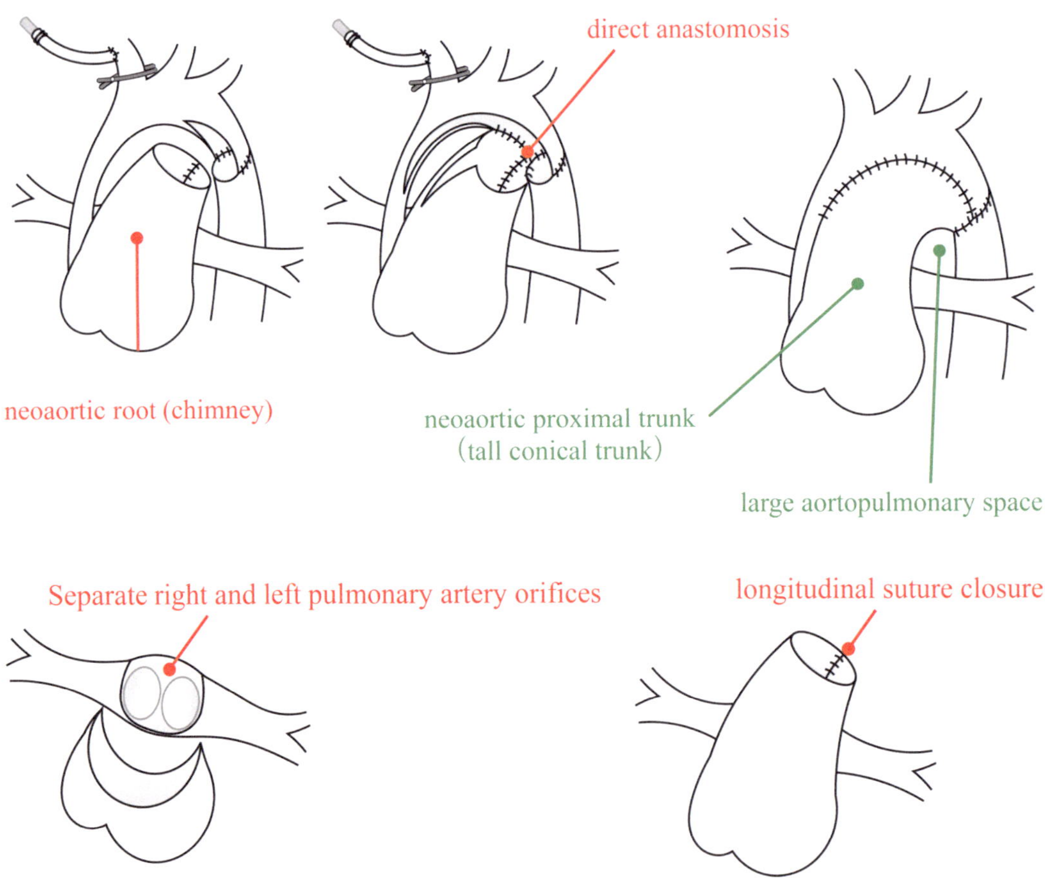

Fig. 13.8 Neo-aortic reconstruction by chimney method, configuration and blood flow

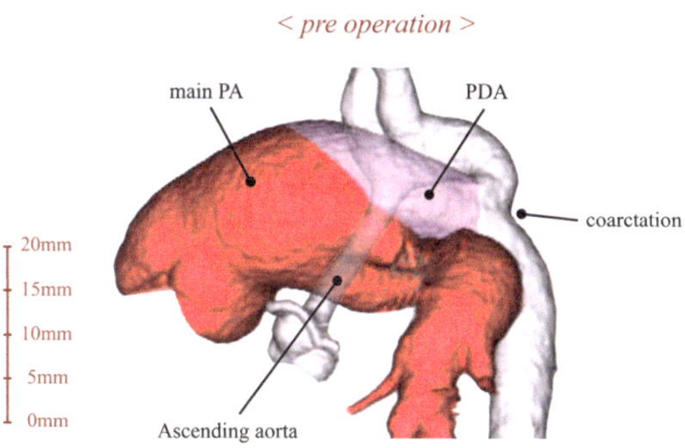

Fig. 13.9 CT images pre and post Norwood operation (chimney method)

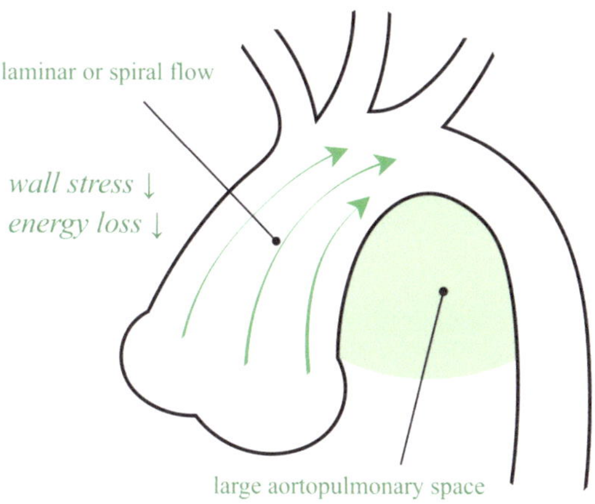

- The chimney method creates a gently converging conical configuration of the aortic root.
- Turbulent flow within the vessel can be reduced.
- A large aortopulmonary space can be secured due to the formation of a long aortic trunk (tall proximal trunk).

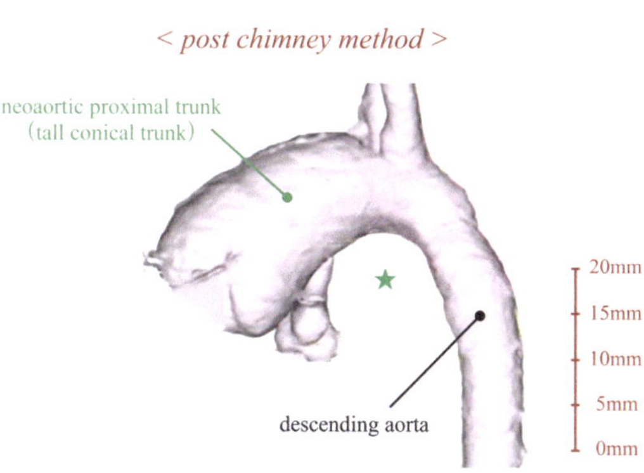

- Gently converging neo-aortic trunk (tall conical trunk) is formed.
- No stenosis at the anastomosis with the descending aorta.
- Aortopulmonary space (★) is large.

4 Surgical Procedure of Chimney Method (Fig. 13.10)

1. Dissect the ascending aorta, aortic arch, and cervical vessels.
2. Dissect the descending aorta just above the diaphragm.
3. Anastomose the brachiocephalic artery with an ePTFE graft as an upper body blood supply channel.
   - Less than 3.0 kg → 3.0 mm ePTFE graft, more than 3.0 kg → 3.5 mm ePTFE graft
4. Insert an arterial cannula into the ePTFE graft.
5. Insert a venous cannula into the superior vena cava and initiate extracorporeal circulation.
6. Dissect the descending aorta just above the diaphragm, and insert a lower body feed arterial cannula.
7. Insert a venous cannula into the inferior vena cava as well, and complete extracorporeal circulation is initiated.
8. Ligate and divide the ductus arteriosus, and dissect the descending aorta as caudally as possible (about 2–3 intercostal arteries caudally).
9. When dissecting the descending aorta, be careful not to damage the recurrent nerve.
10. In cases of aortic atresia (AA), a suction tube is inserted from the right atrium into the right ventricle, and the main pulmonary artery is incised under heart beating.

Fig. 13.10 Surgical procedure of chimney method

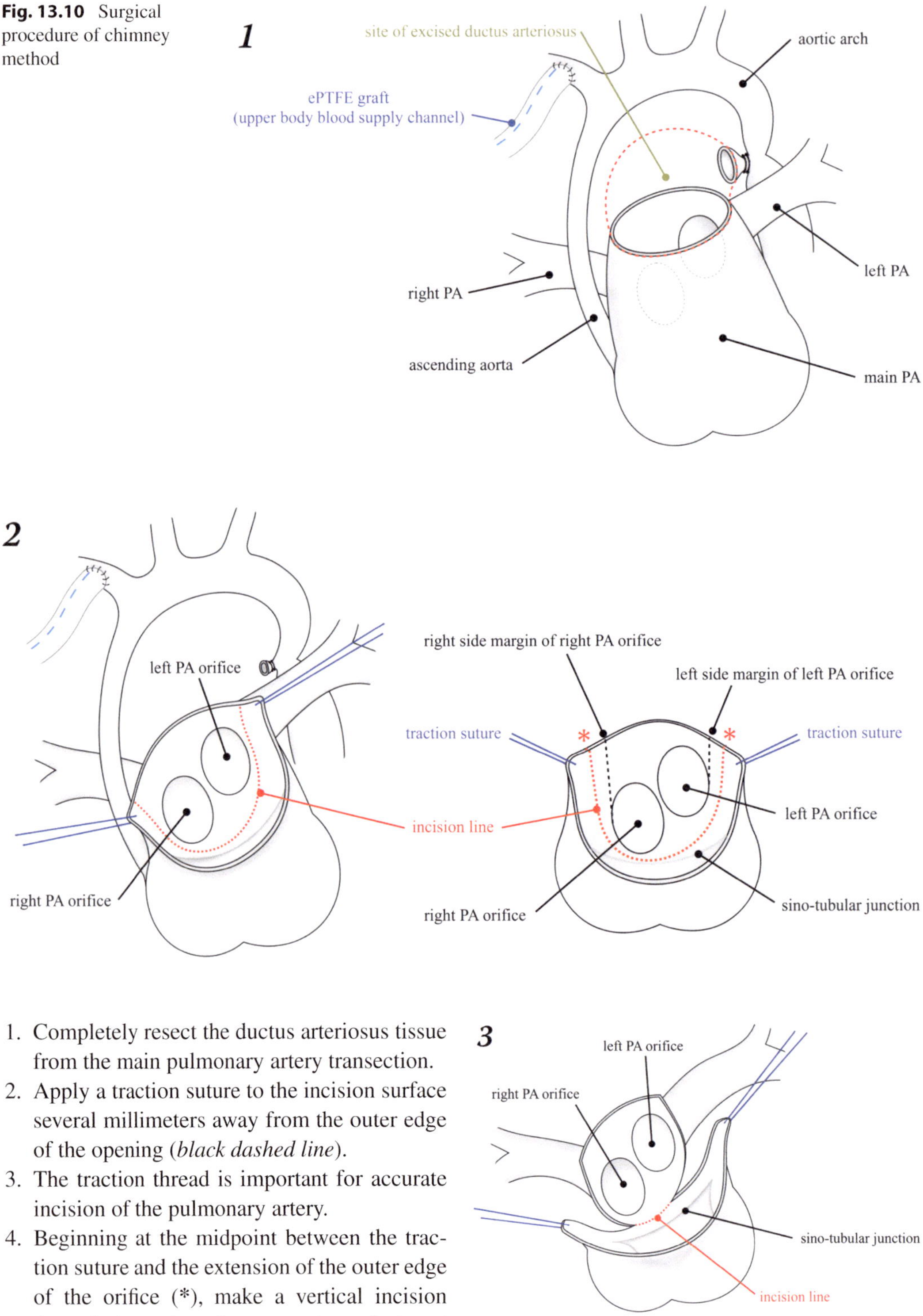

1. Completely resect the ductus arteriosus tissue from the main pulmonary artery transection.
2. Apply a traction suture to the incision surface several millimeters away from the outer edge of the opening (*black dashed line*).
3. The traction thread is important for accurate incision of the pulmonary artery.
4. Beginning at the midpoint between the traction suture and the extension of the outer edge of the orifice (*), make a vertical incision through the main pulmonary artery, aiming at a site about 2 mm away from the outer edge of the orifice.

1. Make an arcuate incision along the inferior aspect of the orifice.
2. The incision below the orifice should be made with care not to cut into the ST junction.
3. Regardless of the alignment of the left and right pulmonary artery orifices, the resection method should be the same.

4

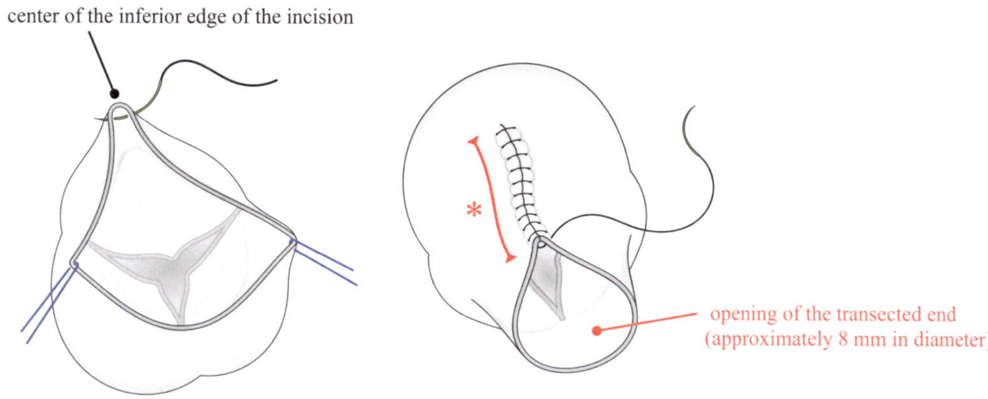

The center of the inferior edge of the incision can be identified by pulling the traction suture caudally.

The posterior wall defect is sutured longitudinally directly from the center of the inferior edge with horizontal mattress sutures and continuous sutures of 6-0 monofilament.

The longitudinal suture extends the main pulmonary artery approximately 10–15 mm (*).

The opening of the transected end should be approximately 8 mm in diameter.

5

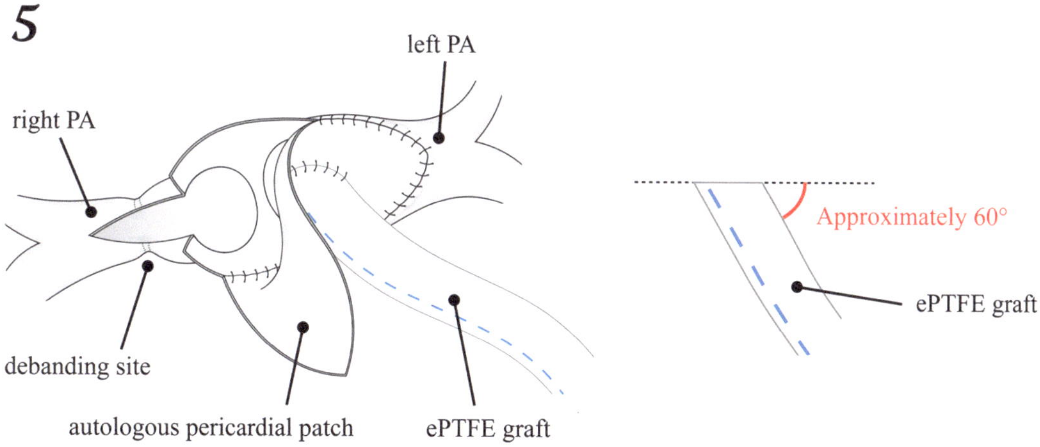

1. If stenosis remains after release of bilateral pulmonary artery banding, incise the pulmonary artery distally beyond the stenosis.
2. An ethanol-treated autologous pericardial patch with ePTFE graft is sutured to the incision using continuous suture with 6-0 monofilament suture.
   - The pericardial patch should be trimmed to a slightly larger oval shape.
   - The ePTFE graft end should be cut at approximately 60° and anastomosed to the autologous pericardial patch (when turning to the right of the base of the new aorta).

6

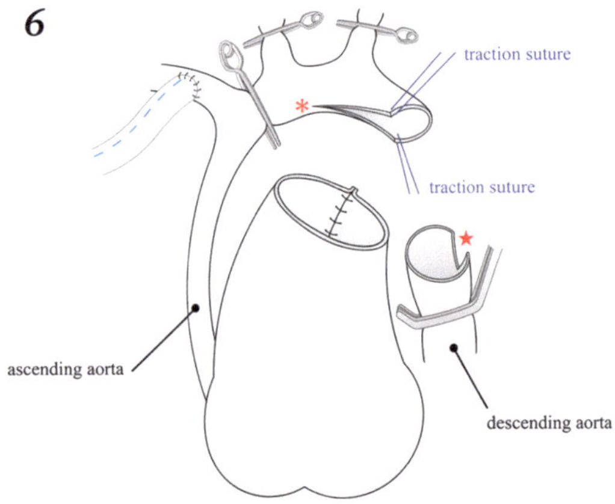

1. Pull up the descending aorta and occlude it as far down as possible.
2. Occlude the left common carotid artery and left subclavian artery.
3. Occlude the aortic arch before origin of the left common carotid artery.
4. Resect the ductus arteriosus from the aortic arch and descending aorta.
5. Make a longitudinal incision of about 5–7 mm on the greater curvature side of the descending aorta (★).
6. Incise the lesser curvature side of the aortic arch to the base of the left common carotid bifurcation (before the occluding forceps) (*).
7. In aortic atresia cases, anastomosis between the distal side of the aortic arch and the descending aorta is performed under beating heart.
8. The aortic arch is tractioned with 7-0 monofilament sutures at both ends of the incision line, and then a straight incision is made precisely on the lesser curvature side (midline of the aortic arch base).

7

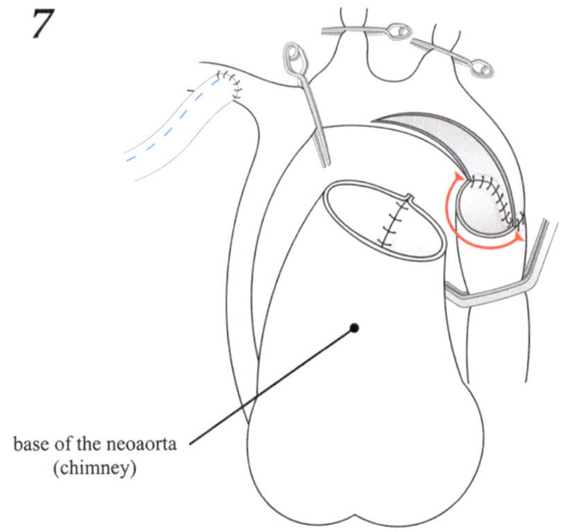

1. Anastomose the distal aortic arch with the greater curvature side of the descending aorta using continuous suture of 7-0 monofilament suture.
2. Leave a diameter of approximately 60% of the circumference of the descending aorta (⟼) to be used for anastomosis with the new aortic root (chimney).
3. It is important to secure a sufficient anastomotic diameter with the chimney to avoid recoarctation.
4. As a rule, a longitudinal incision on the lesser curvature side of the descending aorta is usually not performed (because of the narrowing of the aortopulmonary space).

8

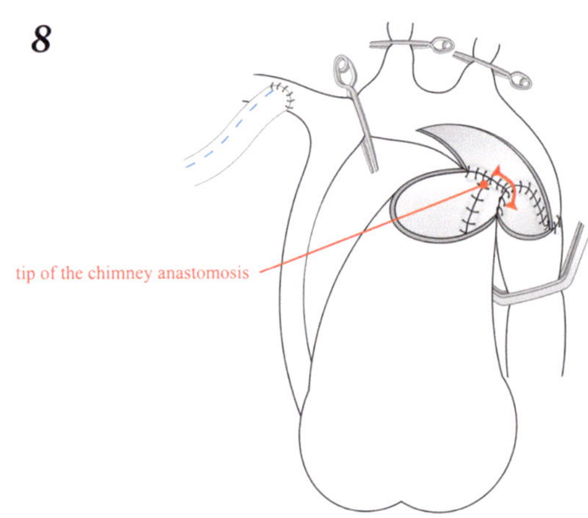

1. To prevent twisting of the new aortic root, the tip of the chimney anastomosis should be positioned at the aortic arch incision.
2. The tip of the chimney anastomosis is often located near the end of the descending aortic anastomosis from the distal side of the aortic arch (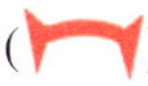).

9

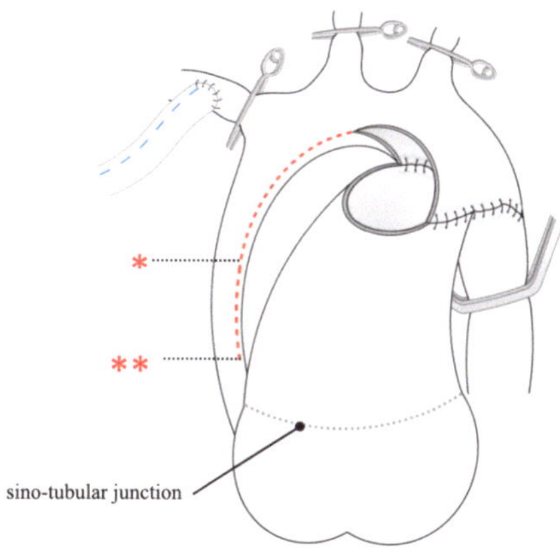

1. Once the anastomosis between the chimney and descending aorta and aortic arch is advanced, move the forceps to the origin of the brachiocephalic artery to cardiac arrest.
2. Incise the left wall of the ascending aorta from the lesser curvature of the aortic arch (*red dashed line*).
   - If the ascending aorta diameter is narrow, cut downward (height of **).
   - Be careful not to cut downward from the ST junction of the corresponding main pulmonary artery.
   - The ascending aorta may be cut off and an end-to-side anastomosis may be performed at the opening created in the lateral wall of the main pulmonary artery.
   - If the ascending aorta is large in diameter, it is not necessary to cut too far down to maintain coronary blood flow (height of *).

10

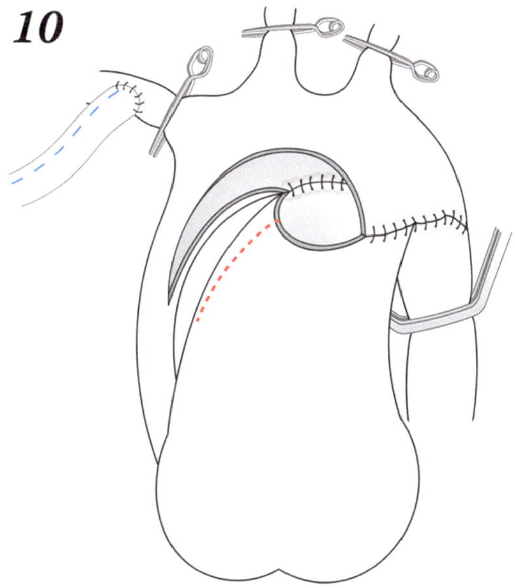

1. Once the ascending aorta is incised, determine the incision line of the main pulmonary artery corresponding to the incision plane *(red dashed line)*.
2. Make the incision toward the origin of the ascending aorta.

11

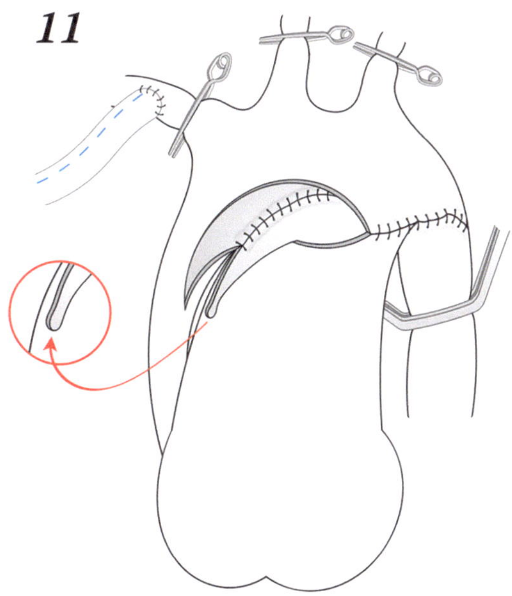

1. To secure the anastomotic diameter at the lower end of the ascending aortic anastomosis, the lower end of the incision of the main pulmonary artery (base of the new aorta) is incised in a tear-drop shape.

12

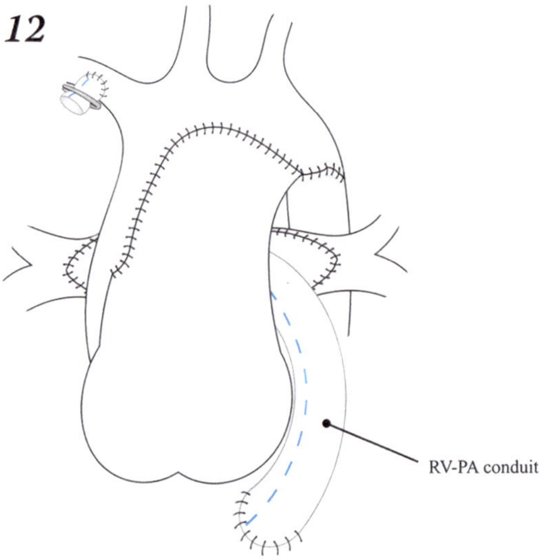

1. Anastomose the proximal end of the RV-PA conduit to the right ventricular outflow tract after completion of reconstruction of the new aorta.
2. The ePTFE graft for upper body blood supply is cut after clipping.

SPOTLIGHT Pulmonary Artery bifurcation incision line

< Pulmonary artery bifurcation incision line in conventional technique >

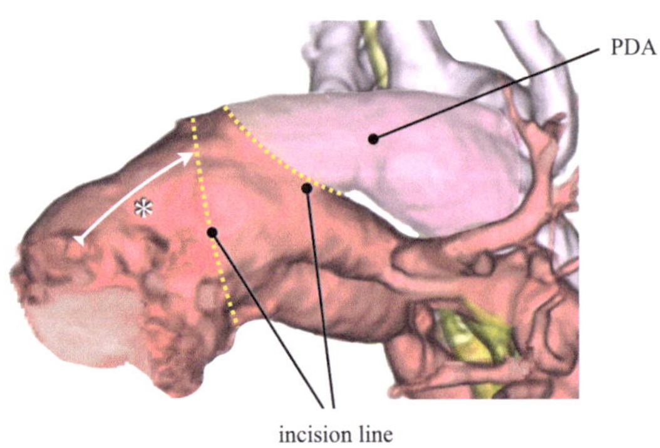

< Pulmonary artery bifurcation incision line in chimney method >

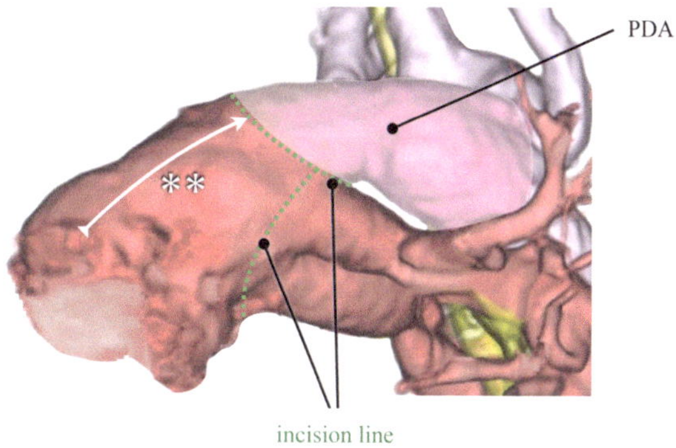

Compared to a conventional incision (*), the chimney method allows for a longer neoaortic root (**).

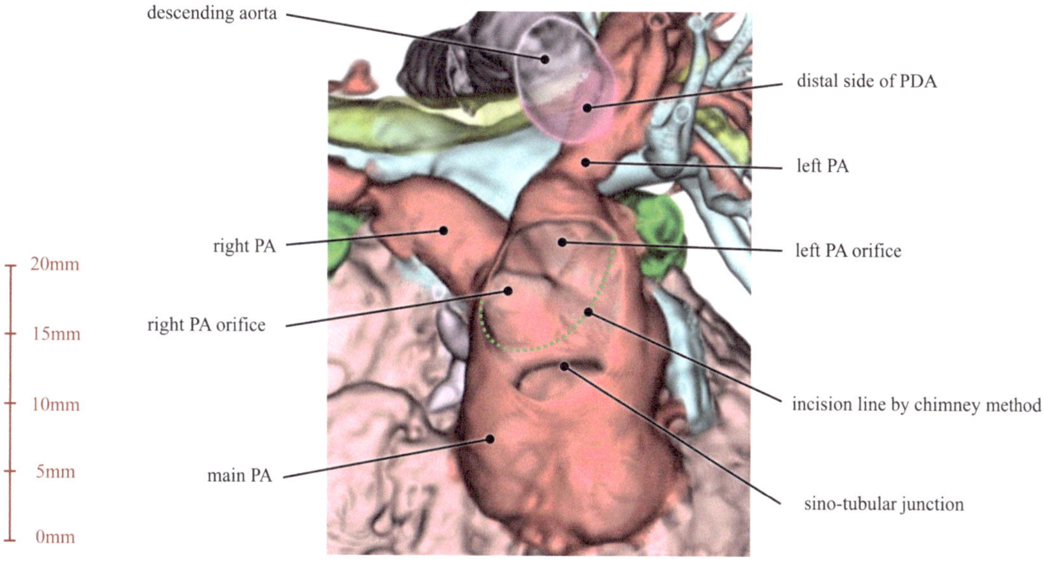

- Incision line in the chimney method is shown (*green dashed line*).
- The right and left pulmonary artery orifices are incised as a single lump.
- Be careful not to cut into the sinotubular junction.

SPOTLIGHT Fluid Dynamics Analysis After Norwood Operation by Chimney Method

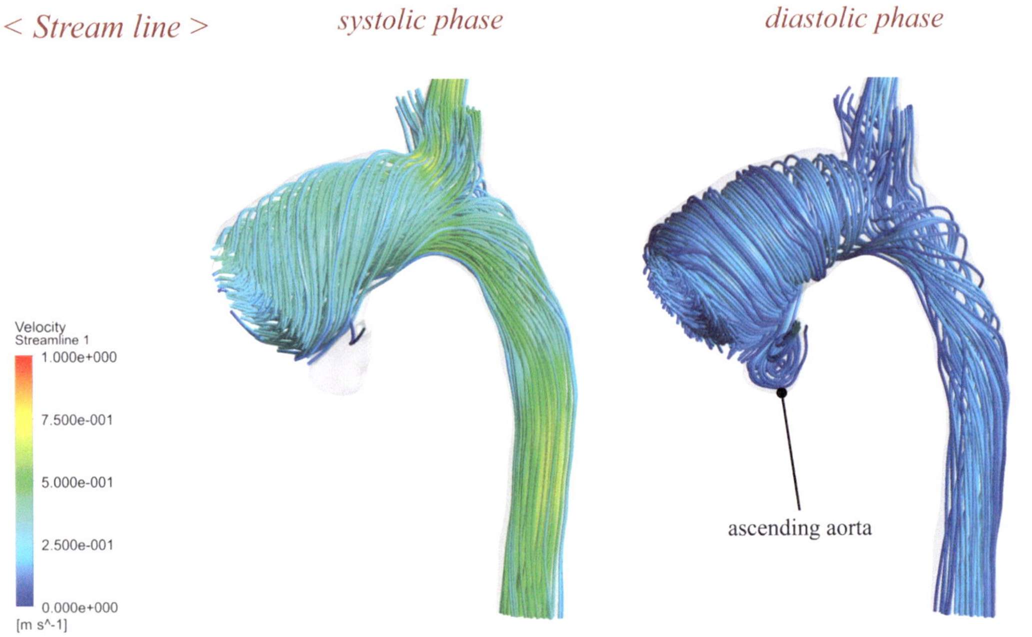

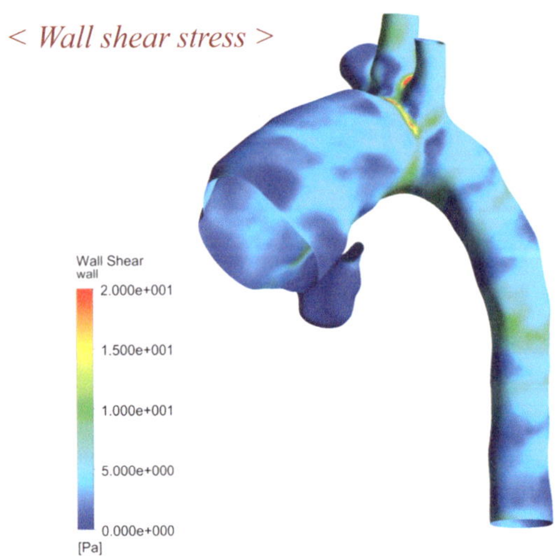

- Fluid analysis after the Norwood procedure using the chimney method showed laminar flow in the conical configuration of the aorta, with no evidence of turbulent flow.
- Wall shear stress was low throughout the new aorta, and energy loss was also low.
- The results suggest that future aortic root enlargement and stenotic lesions at the aortic arch may be avoided as much as possible.
- Systolic streamline shows gentle spiral flow in the neo-aorta and laminar flow at the transition to the aortic arch.
- No acceleration or turbulence is observed.
- Diastolic streamline within the ascending aorta.
- Overall low wall shear stress, except for some suture sites in the aortic arch.

5 Norwood Operation by Chimney Method (Surgical Video)

Case

< Left anterior view >

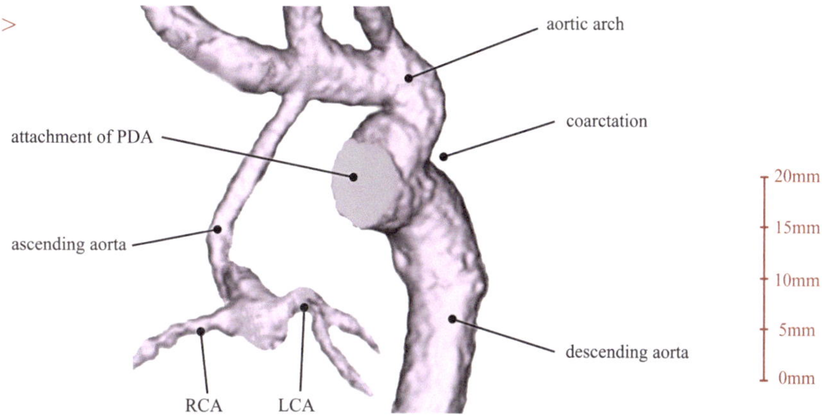

< Left posterior view >

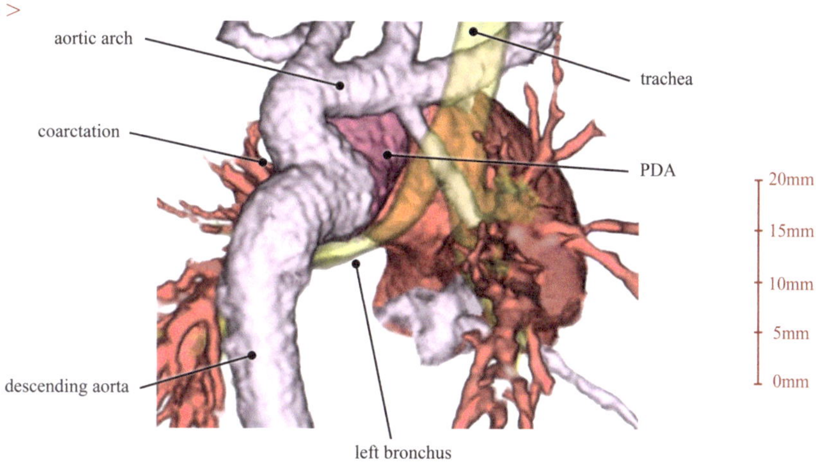

< Coronal section of main PA >

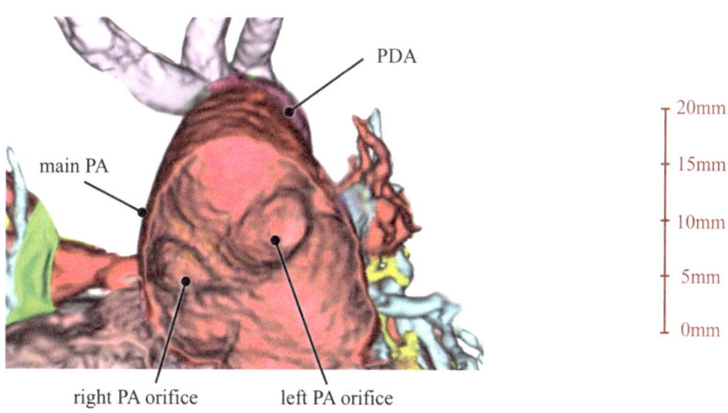

- Two months old, weight 4250 g
- Hypoplastic left heart syndrome (mitral atresia, aortic atresia), post bilateral pulmonary artery banding
- In this case, the diameter of the ascending aorta was smaller, but the diameter of the aortic arch was larger.
- Coarctation of the aorta was present.
- The left bronchus was stenotic due to compression by the ductus arteriosus.
- The main pulmonary artery was enlarged due to bilateral pulmonary artery banding.
- The left and right pulmonary arteries originated from the posterior wall of the main pulmonary artery.
- The orifices of the left and right pulmonary arteries were nearly parallel (Scenes 13.1.1 and 13.1.2).

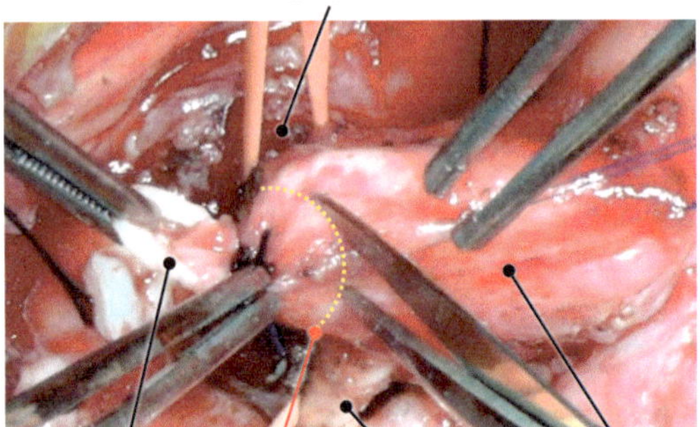

Scene 13.1.1 Transverse incision of main PA (Video 00 min 22 sec)

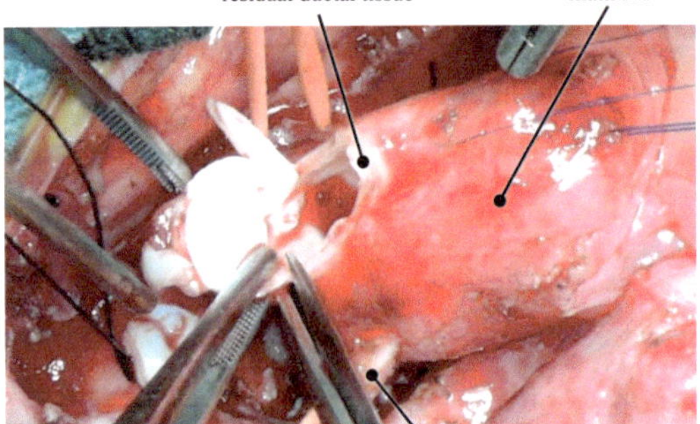

Scene 13.1.2 division of PDA (Video 00 min 34 sec)

- Dissect the cervical vessels, ascending aorta, and aortic arch.
- Anastomose a 3 mm or 3.5 mm ePTFE graft to the brachiocephalic artery, and insert a cannula for upper body blood supply into the ePTFE graft.
- Insert an arterial cannula into the descending aorta just above the diaphragm.
- Establish extracorporeal circulation by the superior and inferior vena cava cannulation.
- The right and left pulmonary arteries are thoroughly dissected, and the banding suture of bilateral pulmonary artery banding are cut and removed.

1. Double ligature and divide the ductus arteriosus.
   - Ensure that the ligature suture on the pulmonary artery side do not extend into the left and right pulmonary arteries.
2. Make a transverse incision at the upper end of the main pulmonary artery proximal to the ductus arteriosus ligation site.
   - Since the boundary with the ductus arteriosus is unclear from the outside of the main pulmonary artery, first make a transverse incision at a distance of about 5 mm from the ligature site of the ductus arteriosus.
   - Make sure that the incision line does not extend beyond the upper edge of the left and right pulmonary arteries.
   - It is acceptable if some ductus arteriosus tissue remains on the pulmonary artery side of the incision at the time of the initial incision.
3. Residual ductus arteriosus tissue is removed from the main pulmonary artery transection (Scene 13.2).

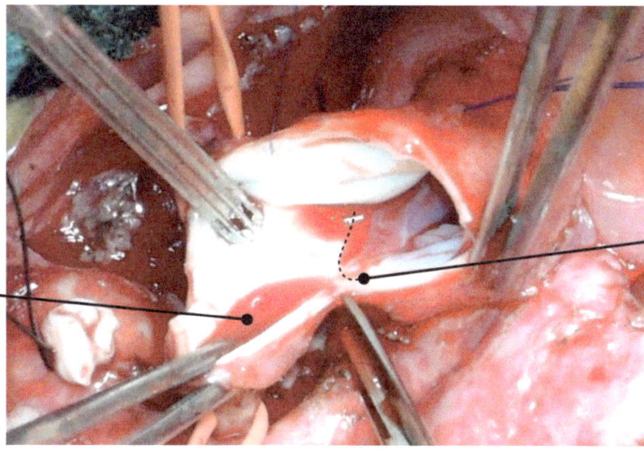

Scene 13.2 Resection of right and left pulmonary artery orifices 1 (Video 1 min 13 s)

1. Apply a traction suture with 6-0 monofilament suture to the medial side of the left and right pulmonary artery orifices on the cut ends of the pulmonary artery where the ductus arteriosus has been resected.
2. Cut down the inside of the traction suture vertically along the outer edge of the left and right pulmonary artery orifices.
3. The lower incision is made near the midpoint between the ST junction and the pulmonary artery orifice, along the orifice to the midpoint between the right and left pulmonary artery orifices.
   - Make the same incision whether the right and left pulmonary artery orifices are aligned vertically or in parallel.
   - Since the left and right pulmonary artery orifices are adjacent to each other, it is not worth resecting each separately (Scene 13.3).

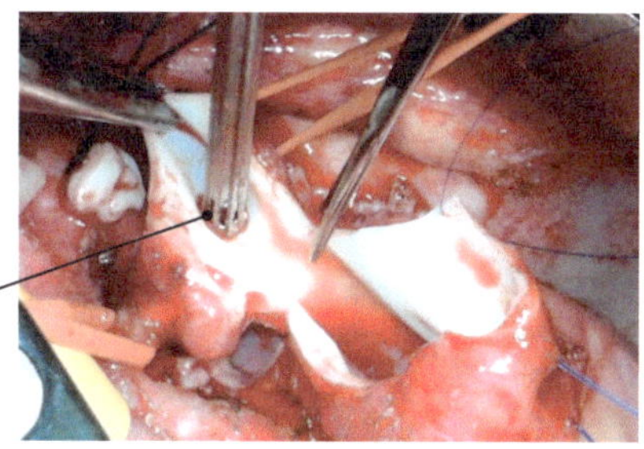

Scene 13.3 Resection of right and left pulmonary artery orifices 2 (Video 1 min 31 s)

1. The contralateral side is incised in the same manner.
2. Make a U-shaped incision at the inferior margin along the left and right pulmonary artery orifices, and resect the pulmonary artery orifices as a single lump.
   - As a rule, do not incise below the ST junction (Scene 13.4).

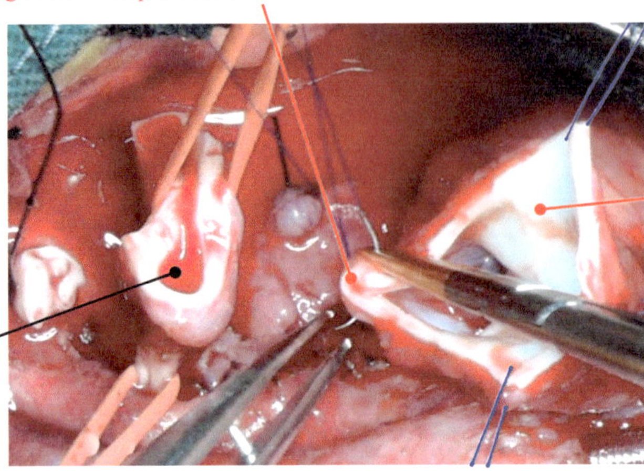

Scene 13.4 Longitudinal suture closure of the main PA wall creating chimney 1 (Video 2 min 10 s)

1. When the traction suture applied to the severed end of the pulmonary artery is tensed, the length of the left and right incisions and the lowest point of the incision are clearly identified.
2. Starting at the lowest point of the incision, a horizontal mattress suture of 6-0 monofilament suture and a continuous suture are used to suture the pulmonary artery orifice directly to form a long, chimney-shaped base of the main pulmonary artery.
   - If the left and right pulmonary artery orifices are parallel, the defect is wide, but the same direct suture can be used regardless of the arrangement of the orifices.
   - The direct anastomosis should be held at a point where the diameter of the upper end of the chimney opening is approximately 8 mm (Scene 13.5).

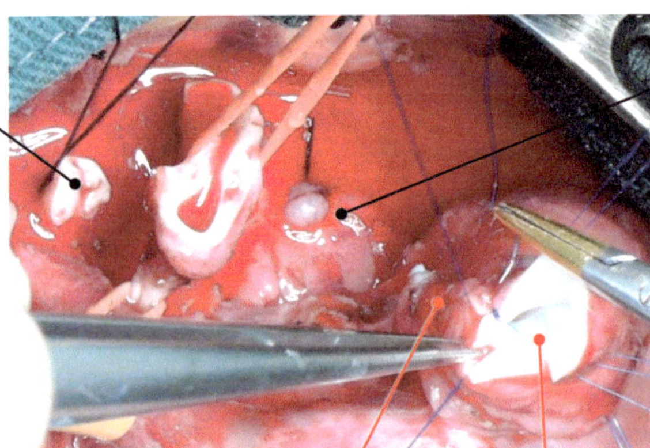

Scene 13.5 Longitudinal suture closure of the main PA wall creating chimney 2 (Video 4 min 57 s)

1. The defect in the posterior wall of the main pulmonary artery can usually be stitched up, usually 10–15 mm.
2. Insert a sizer into the upper opening of the main pulmonary artery, leaving an opening with a diameter equal to that of the descending aorta. Usually, an opening of 8 mm is secured.
3. Trim the opening to smooth the cross-sectional area.
4. Check the anastomotic length of the posterior wall of the main pulmonary artery, which is completed in a chimney shape (Scene 13.6).

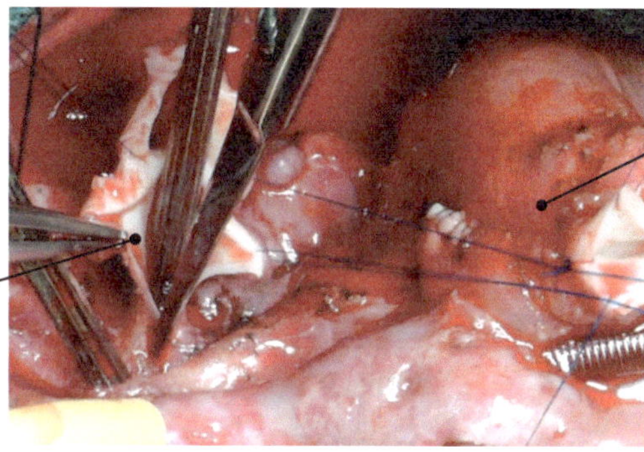

Scene 13.6 Incision of right PA (Video 5 min 07 s)

1. Pass the sizer through the left and right pulmonary artery banding sites and measure the caliber.
2. If the caliber remains narrow after removal of the banding sutures and the 3.5 mm sizer cannot pass through, incise the pulmonary artery distal to the banding site (stenosis site) from the cutting orifice.

- If the sizer is forced through the banding site of the right or left pulmonary artery, the pulmonary artery may be torn, so care should be taken not to apply excessive force when expanding the sizer (Scene 13.7).

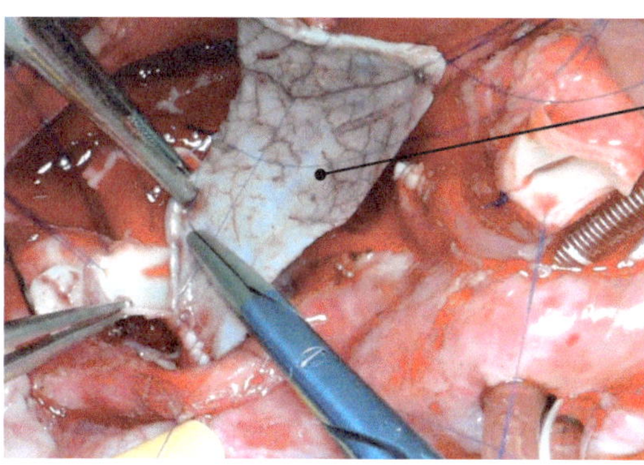

Scene 13.7 Right PA augmentation and autologous pericardium anastomosis (Video 5 min 35 s)

1. Sew ethanol-treated autologous pericardium to the pulmonary artery orifice and the incised pulmonary artery with continuous suture of 7-0 monofilament suture.
2. The distal end of the RV-PA conduit may be pre-sutured to the autologous pericardium (Scene 13.8).

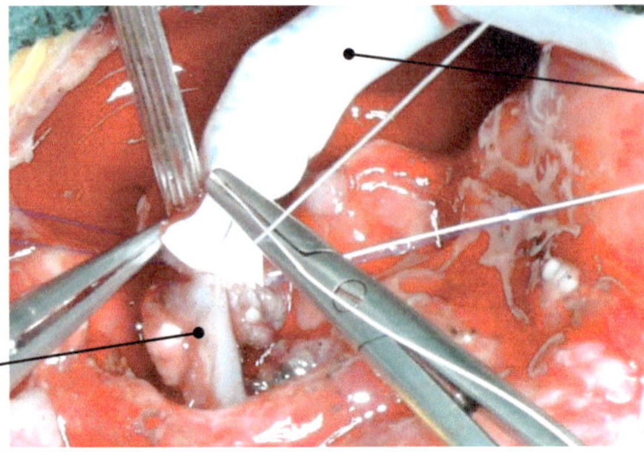

Scene 13.8 Anastomosis of distal end of RV-PA conduit (Video 9 min 35 s)

1. Make a central (slightly to the left) incision in the center of the sutured autologous pericardium.
2. Anastomose a valved ePTFE conduit with the distal end trimmed to approximately 60° into the autologous pericardial orifice with continuous sutures of Gore-Tex suture CV-6.

- Use a 6 mm or 8 mm valved conduit.
- For 8 mm conduits, caliber adjustment with clips is necessary.
- Gore-Tex suture is useful to prevent bleeding from the suture needle insertion site (Scene 13.9).

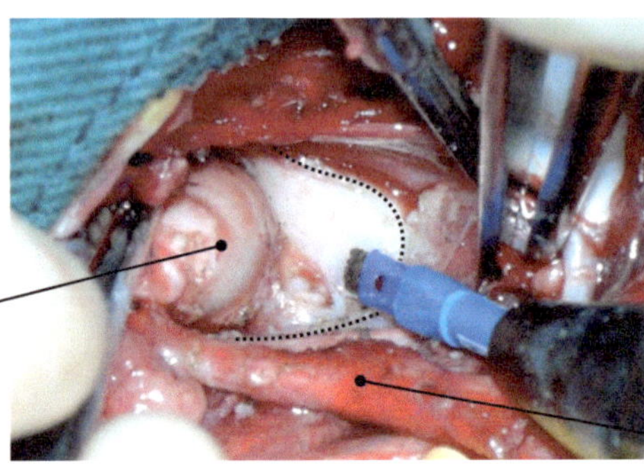

Scene 13.9 Dissection of descending aorta (Video 12 min 31 s)

1. Dissect the descending aorta as caudally as possible, paying attention to the recurrent nerve (near t*he black dashed line*).
   - Carefully coagulate and hemostat small vessels branching anteriorly from the descending aortic surface (toward the left bronchus).
   - Preserve the dorsal branch of the intercostal artery as much as possible (Scene 13.10).

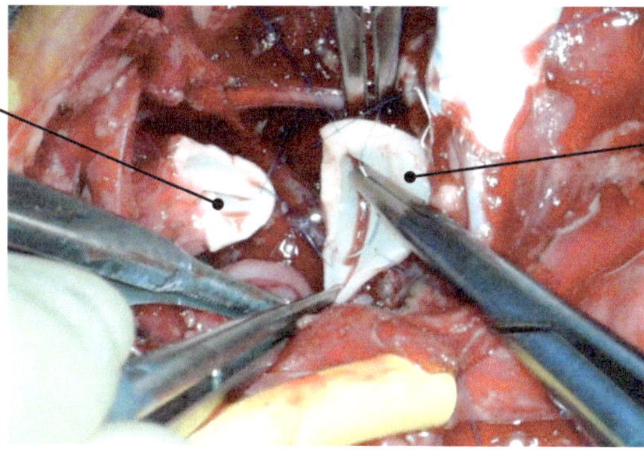

Scene 13.10 Aortic arch-descending aorta anastomosis 1 (Video 15 min 06 s)

1. Resection of ductus arteriosus tissue from the aorta
2. Apply traction sutures to both ends (anterior and dorsal) of the expected incision site on the aortic arch transection
3. Make a longitudinal incision on the greater curvature of the descending aorta.
   - The length of the incision should be just long enough to reach the distal end of the aortic arch.
4. Anastomose the descending aortic orifice and the aortic arch with a continuous 7-0 mono-filament suture anastomosis.
   - The anastomosis is started from the greater curvature side of the descending aorta (deepest part of the longitudinal incision) and the dorsal aspect of the aortic arch transection (Scene 13.11).

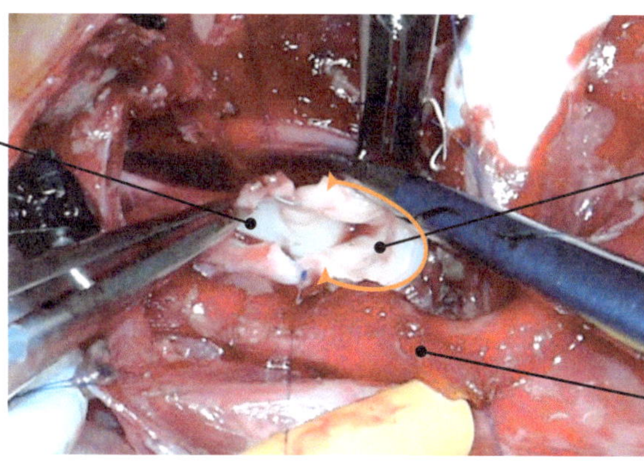

Scene 13.11 Aortic arch-descending aorta anastomosis 2 (Video 18 min 43 s)

1. Anastomose the aortic arch transection to the descending aortic orifice.
2. The circumference of the suture between the aortic arch and the descending aorta should be approximately 40% of the circumference of the descending aortic orifice (depending on the caliber of the distal aortic arch).
   - The anastomosis should be as valgus as possible in order to avoid turbulent blood flow.
   - To avoid anastomotic stenosis, the circumference of the direct anastomosis between the descending aorta and the chimney orifice (⟼) should be lengthened (Scene 13.12).

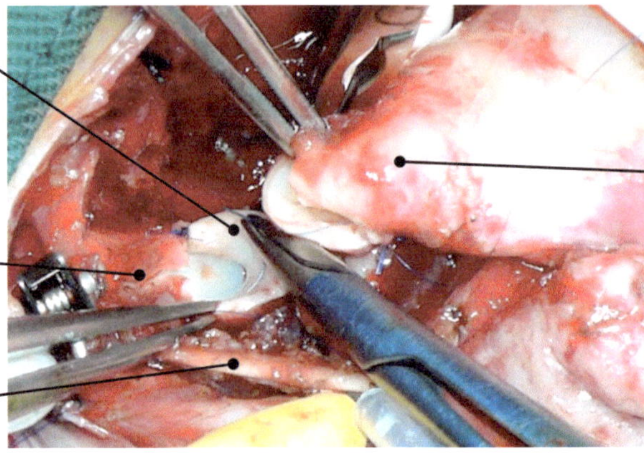

Scene 13.12 Orifice of the chimney-aortic arch anastomosis 1 (Video 19 min 57 s)

1. Position the upper end of the dorsal suture to correspond to the aortic orifice so that the main pulmonary artery does not twist.
   - The upper end of the dorsal suture often corresponds to the right end of the aortic arch and descending aortic anastomosis.
2. Anastomose the upper end opening of the main pulmonary artery (chimney orifice) to the descending aorta with a continuous 7-0 monofilament suture (Scene 13.13).

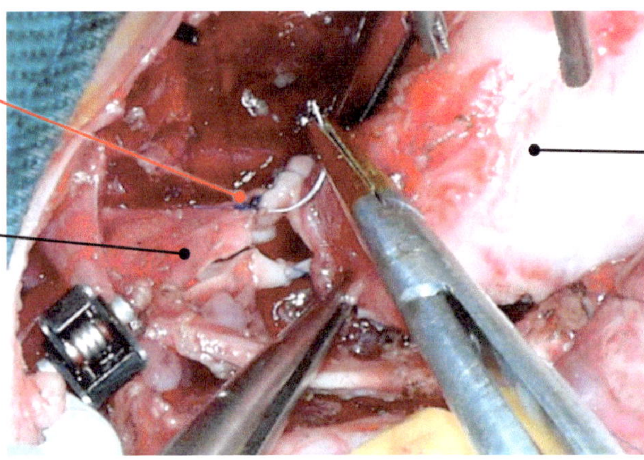

Scene 13.13 Orifice of the chimney-aortic arch anastomosis 2 (Video 22 min 40 s)

1. Anastomose the left side of the chimney orifice to the left side of the descending aortic orifice.
2. Suture the chimney orifice to the anterior margin of the anastomosis between the aortic arch and descending aorta (★) (Scene 13.14).

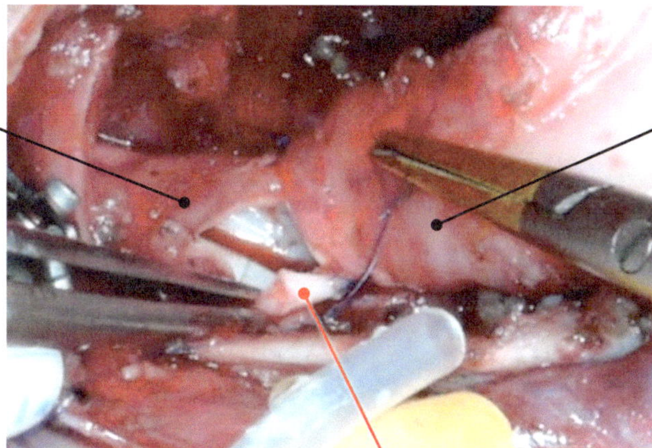

Scene 13.14 Orifice of the chimney-aortic arch anastomosis 3 (Video 23 min 56 s)

1. Anastomose the right side of the chimney orifice to the right side of the descending aortic orifice.
2. Suture the right side of the chimney orifice to the posterior border of the anastomosis between the aortic arch and the descending aorta (*) (Scene 13.15).

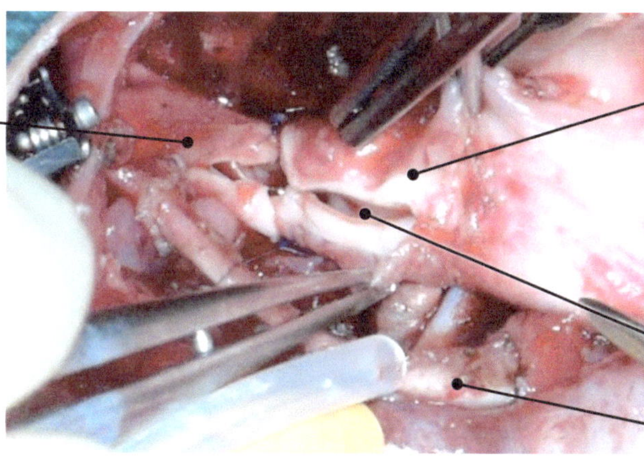

Scene 13.15 Orifice of the chimney-aortic arch anastomosis 4 (Video 25 min 42 s)

1. Make a longitudinal incision on the right side of the new aortic root (main pulmonary artery) corresponding to the aortic arch.
   - To avoid twisting of the anastomosis, the main pulmonary artery is not incised first.
   - After the anastomosis with the descending aorta is performed first, it is important to determine the incision line corresponding to the aortic arch and ascending aorta, and to make a precise incision (Scene 13.16).

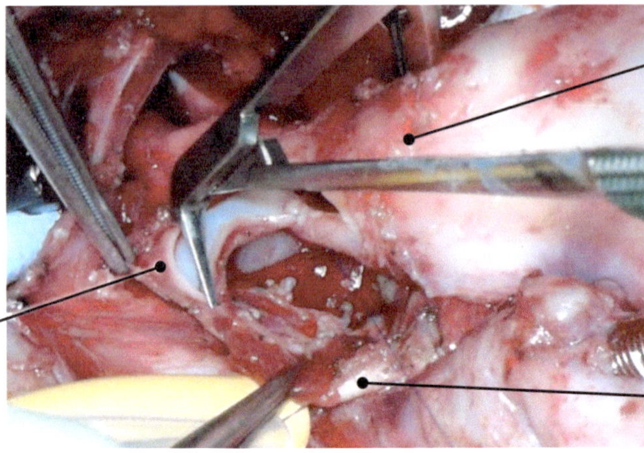

Scene 13.16 Orifice of the chimney-aortic arch anastomosis 5 (Video 27 min 32 s)

1. Incision is made from the lesser curvature (basal aspect) of the aortic arch to the left aspect of the ascending aorta.
   - Since it is important to incise the aortic arch and ascending aorta corresponding to the main pulmonary artery accurately, use traction suture as necessary to maintain the morphology of the ascending aorta and aortic arch before incision.
   - Match the depth of the ascending aortic incision with the depth of the main pulmonary artery incision.
   - Add the main pulmonary artery incision as appropriate.
   - Adjust the depth of the incision according to the diameter of the ascending aorta.
     - In cases with a large ascending aorta, a deep incision is not necessary.
     - If the ascending aorta is small, incise low.
     - The ascending aorta may be transected and anastomosed end-to-side with the main pulmonary artery.
     - Be careful not to cut lower than the ST junction of the new aorta (Scene 13.17).

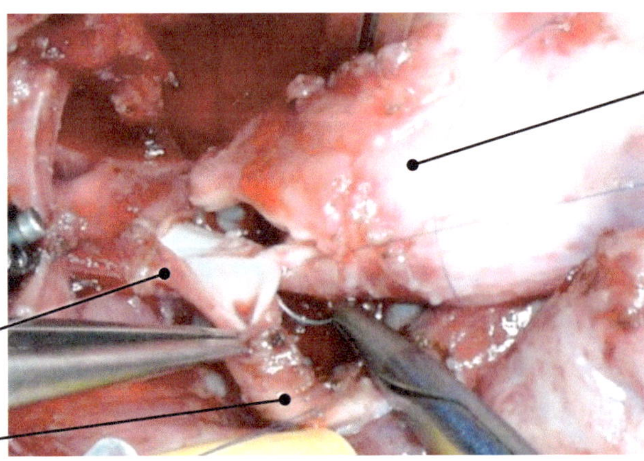

Scene 13.17 Orifice of the chimney-aortic arch anastomosis 6 (Video 27 min 49 s)

1. Side-by-side anastomosis of the ascending aortic incision to the main pulmonary artery incision with a continuous 7-0 monofilament suture (Scene 13.18).

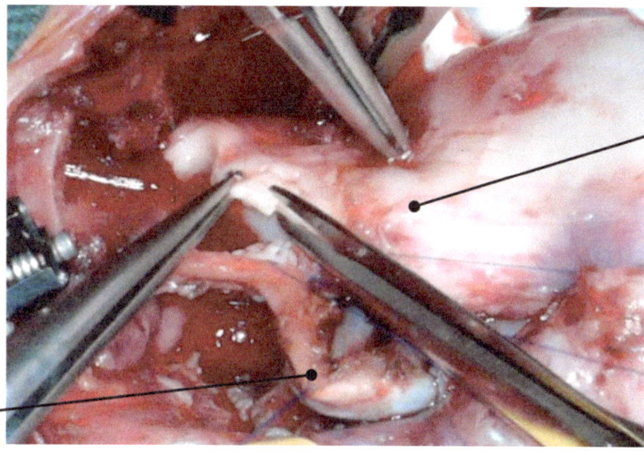

Scene 13.18 Orifice of the chimney-aortic arch anastomosis 7 (Video 30 min 45 s)

1. To widen the lower end of the anastomosis with the lower end of the ascending aorta, the lower end of the main pulmonary artery incision is resected in a teardrop shape (Scene 13.19).

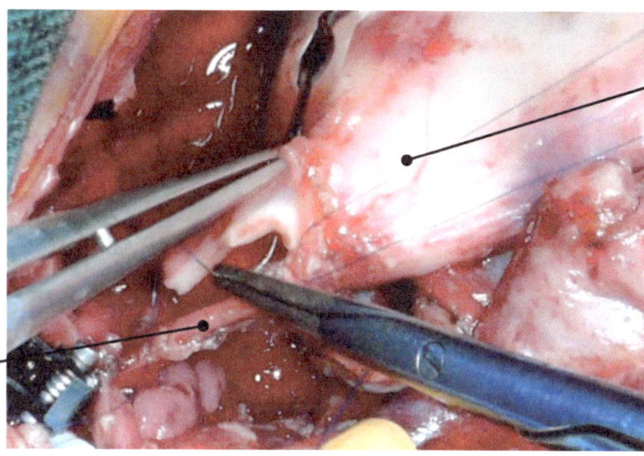

Scene 13.19 Orifice of the chimney-aortic arch anastomosis 8 (Video 30 min 53 s)

1. Anastomose the lower end of the main pulmonary artery incision and the ascending aortic incision surface with continuous 7-0 monofilament suture.
   - In principle, the lower edge of the incision is also anastomosed with a continuous suture.
   - Fewer stitches may be used, but continuous suture will not cause stenosis if the wall of the main pulmonary artery is incised in a teardrop fashion (Scene 13.20).

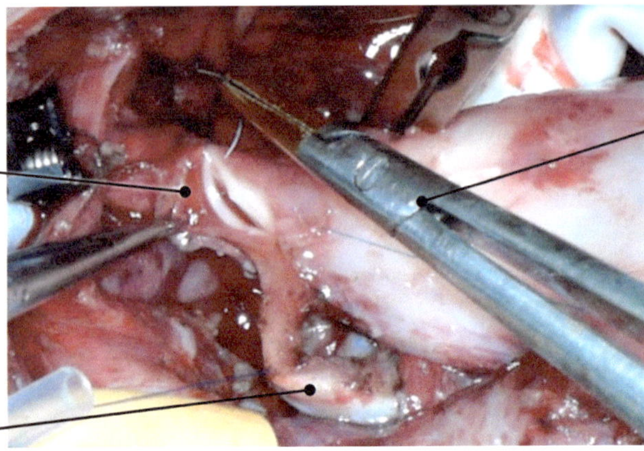

Scene 13.20 Orifice of the chimney-aortic arch anastomosis 9 (Video 31 min 43 s)

1. Anastomosis of the anterior surface of the main pulmonary artery with the aortic arch to complete reconstruction of the new aorta (Scene 13.21).

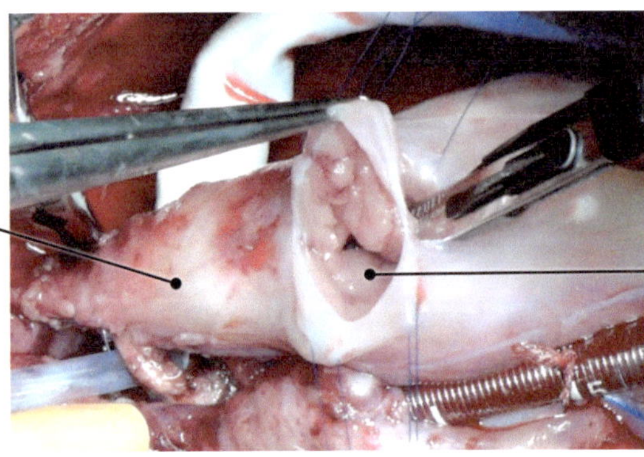

Scene 13.21 Anastomosis of RV-PA conduit 1 (Video 33 min 43 s)

1. Make a circular incision anterior wall of the right ventricular outflow tract to match the diameter of the ePTFE conduit.

- Remove the cut end of the muscle bundle protruding into the lumen (Scene 13.22).

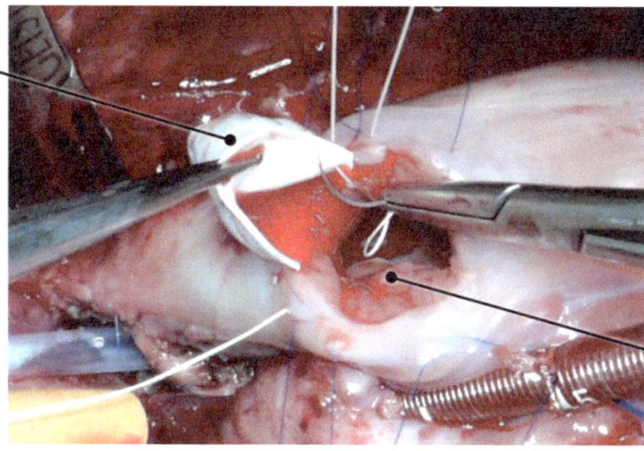

Scene 13.22 Anastomosis of RV-PA conduit 2 (Video 35 min 03 s)

1. Trim the proximal end of the ePTFE conduit and anastomose the right ventricular outflow tract opening with a continuous CV-5 ePTFE suture (Scene 13.23).

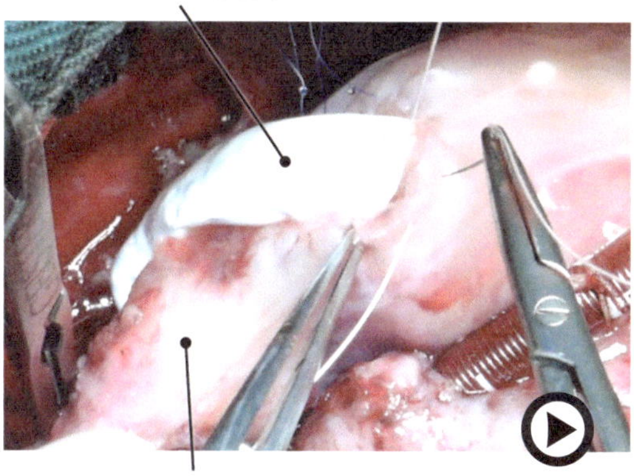

Scene 13.23 Anastomosis of RV-PA conduit 3 (Video 37 min 34 s) (▶ https://doi.org/10.1007/000-hkr)

2. After venting air from the anastomosis, release the aortic clamp.

Case Postop CT Images

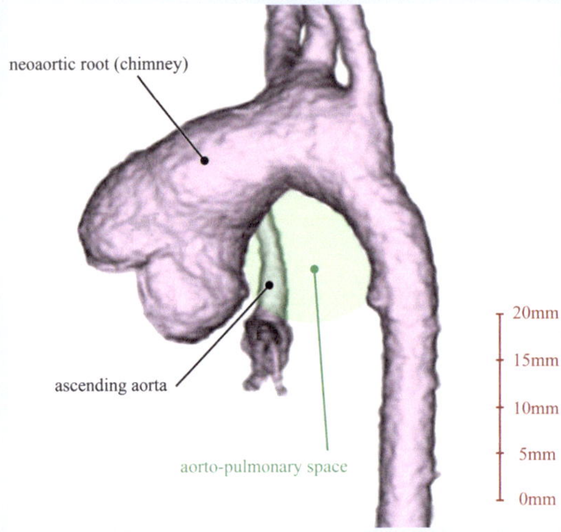

- The long neo-aortic root is secured by reconstruction using the chimney method without the use of supplemental material.
- The caliber of the new aortic root is reduced in the short axis direction and is formed into a conical shape that gradually tapers toward the arch.
- The aortic arch is smoothly connected to the descending aorta and there is no stenosis.
- Large aortopulmonary space is ensured.

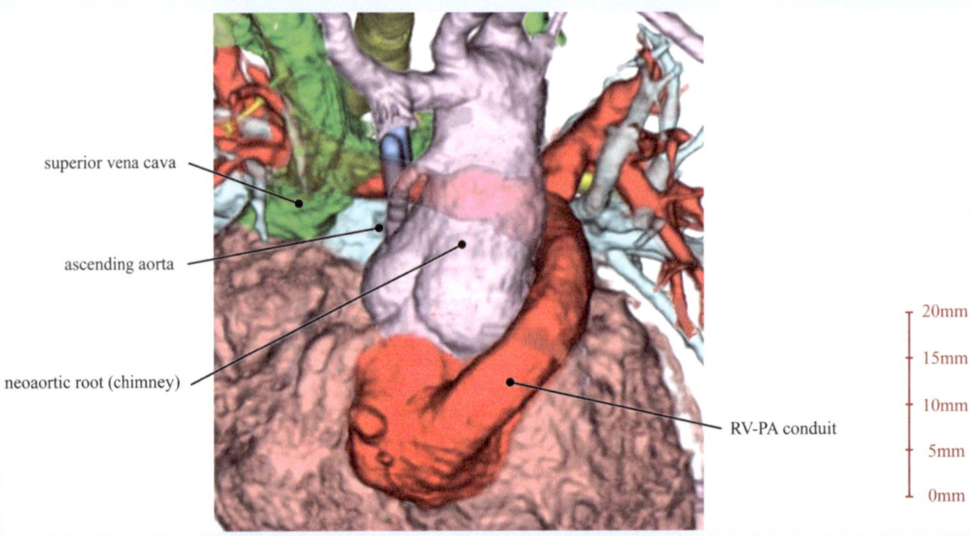

- RV-PA conduit passes to the left of the base of the neo-aorta without evidence of hyper-extension or distortion.
- No stenosis of the right pulmonary artery passing through the aortopulmonary space.

SPOTLIGHT Reconstruction of Pulmonary Blood Flow (RV-PA Conduit)

- The Blalock-Tausig (BT) shunt or the right ventricular-pulmonary artery (RV-PA) conduit reported by Kishimoto et al. are used to reconstruct pulmonary blood flow in the Norwood procedure, but the RV-PA conduit is often chosen for its ease of postoperative management.
- The BT shunt can cause a rapid decline in cardiac function due to fluctuations in pulmonary vascular resistance in the immediate postoperative period.
- RV-PA conduits are hemodynamically stable in the immediate postoperative period, but there are reports of an early decrease in oxygen saturation in the mid-term period and poorer pulmonary artery growth compared to BT shunts.
- The RV-PA conduit generally bypasses the left side of the main pulmonary artery (new aorta).
- The right side of the main pulmonary artery (new aorta) is also an option, but care should be taken to avoid compression of the small ascending aorta.
- The left route is usually safe, but if the right route is considered, the positional relationship between the ascending aorta and the base of the main pulmonary artery (new aorta) should be determined by preoperative CT.

< Case 1 >

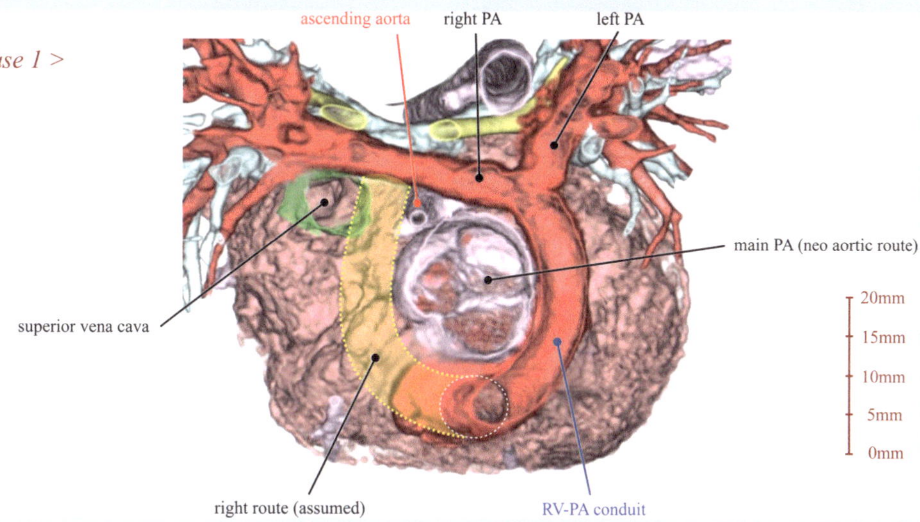

- In this case, the length of the RV-PA conduit is the same for both routes.
- Because the ascending aorta is posterior (dorsal) to the main pulmonary artery, it is unlikely to be compressed by the RV-PA conduit even when the right route is used.
- However, the superior vena cava may be slightly compressed by the RV-PA conduit if the right route is used.

< Case 2 >

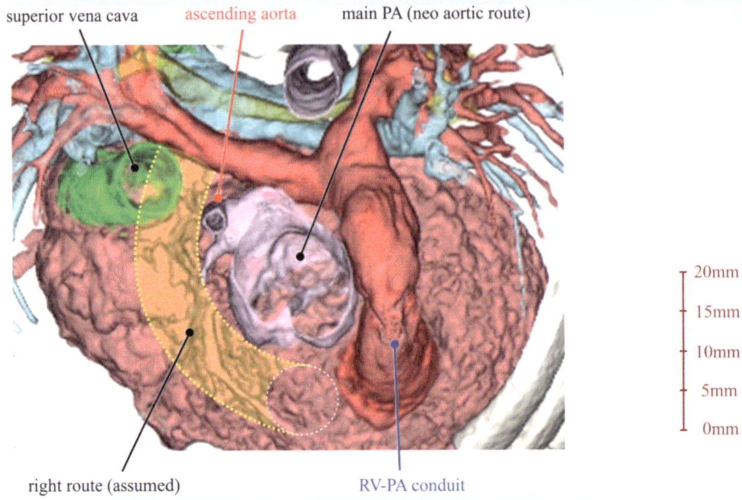

- In this case, the RV-PA conduit is longer in the right pathway.
- The ascending aorta is located right posterior to the main pulmonary artery and may be compressed by the RV-PA conduit in the right pathway.
- The superior vena cava may also be compressed by the RV-PA conduit in the right pathway.

References

Definition of HLHS

Jacobs JP. Hypoplastic left heart syndrome: definition, morphology, and classification. World J Pediatr Congenit Heart Surg. 2022;13:559–64.

Configuration of Neo-Aorta, Neo-Aortic Root Enlargement

Plummer ST, Hornik CP, et al. Maladaptive aortic properties after the Norwood procedure- an angiographic analysis of the Pediatric Heart Network Single Ventricle Reconstruction Trial. J Thorac Cardiovasc Surg. 2016;152:471–9.

Kanzaki T, Yamagishi M, et al. Valve-sparing neoaortic root replacement late after the Norwood and Fontan procedures. Ann Thorac Surg. 2015;99:309–12.

Fluid Flow Analysis of the Neo-Aorta After the Norwood Operation

Itatani K, Miyaji K, Qian Y, Liu JL, Miyakoshi T, Murakami A, Ono M, Umezu M. Influence of surgical arch reconstruction methods on single ventricle workload in the Norwood procedure. J Thorac Cardiovasc Surg. 2012;144:130–8.

Decreased Vascular Elasticity After the Norwood Procedure with Supplemental Material

Voges IV, Jerosch-Herold M, et al. Maladaptive aortic properties in children after palliation of hypoplastic left heart syndrome assessed by cardiovascular magnetic resonance imaging. Circulation. 2010;122:1068–76.

RV-PA Conduit

Kishimoto H, Iio M, Kume Y, et al. The Norwood operation for hypoplastic left heart syndrome using a valve pericardial roll between the right ventricle and pulmonary artery. Cardiol Young. 1993;3(suppl 1):SI162.

Kishimoto H, Kawahira Y, Kawata H, Miura T, Iwai S, Mori T. The modified Norwood palliation on a beating heart. J Thorac Cardiovasc Surg. 1999;118:1130–2.

Sano S, Ishino K, Kawada M, et al. The modified Norwood operation for hypoplastic left heart syndrome: using the right ventricle-to-pulmonary artery shunt. Cardiol Young. 2001;11(Suppl 1):SI21.

Lasso Technique

Maeda Y, Yamagishi M, et al. Surgical strategy and results of hypoplastic left ventricular syndrome. Kyobu Geka. 2014a;67:305–9.

Chimney Method

Maeda Y, Yamagishi M, et al. Surgical strategy and results of hypoplastic left ventricular syndrome. Kyobu Geka. 2014b;67:305–9.

Asada S, Yamagishi M, Itatani K, Yaku H. Chimney reconstruction of the aortic arch in the Norwood procedure. J Thorac Cardiovasc Surg. 2017;154:e51–4. Open Archive

Yamagishi M. Chimney technique for aortic arch repair in the Norwood operation. Oper Tech Thorac Cardiovasc Surg. 2019;24:237–55. Open Archive

Asada S, Yamagishi M, Itatani K, Maeda Y, Taniguchi S, Fujita S, Hongu H, Yaku H. Early outcomes and computational fluid dynamic analyses of chimney reconstruction in the Norwood procedure. Interact Cardiovasc Thorac Surg. 2019;29:252–9.

Asada S, Yamagishi M, Maeda Y, Itatani K, Fujita S, Hongu H, Nakatsuji H, Yaku H. Chimney reconstruction provides a wider subaortic space and reduces the risk of pulmonary artery compression in the Norwood-type aortic arch reconstruction without patch supplementation. Eur J Cardiothorac Surg. 2021;60:1408–16.

14 Surgical Training

1 Surgical Training Using the Urethane Simulation Model

I will introduce the training method I have actually used. This method is not my original, but is based on the training method of Professor Soji Konno, who created the world-famous Konno operation (Fig. 14.1).

1. Prepare a wooden embroidery frame about 15–20 cm in diameter.
2. Cover the wooden frame with a piece of fabric (such as thin felt).
3. The wooden frame should be supported by a rod that can be fixed at any angle.
4. Draw grid lines on the canvas to indicate where you want to embroider (see below).
5. Fix the wooden frame in place, taking into account the angles of the actual heart and blood vessels (for example, the atrial septum should be slightly lower on the right and the mitral valve ring should be lower on the left).

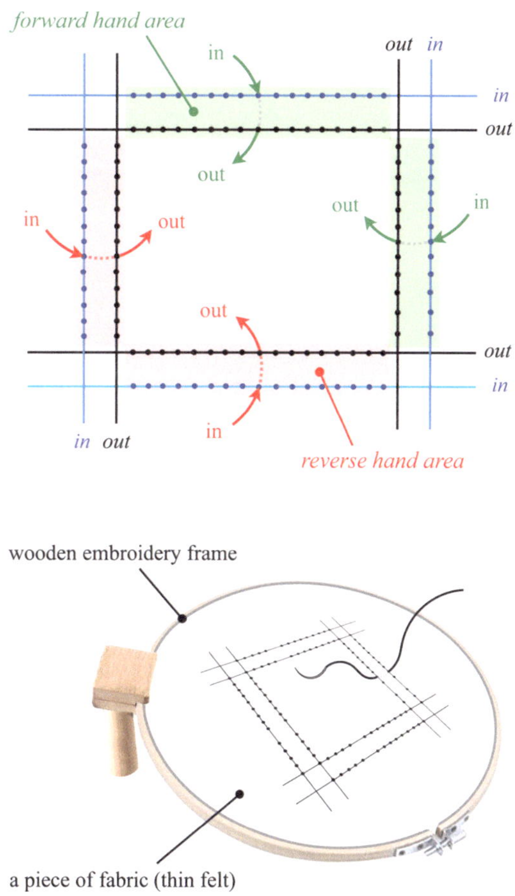

Fig. 14.1 Sewing training using a wooden embroidery frame

Supplementary Information The online version contains supplementary material available at https://doi.org/10.1007/978-981-96-6194-7_14. The videos can be accessed individually by clicking the DOI link in the accompanying figure caption or by scanning this link with the SN More Media App.

M. Yamagishi, *Surgical Treatment of Congenital Heart Disease*,
https://doi.org/10.1007/978-981-96-6194-7_14

1. Draw a grid (stitch-in line: *blue*, stitch-out line: *black*) on this fabric (see diagram on left).
2. Repeat the process of stitching in on the stitch-in line and stitching out on the stitch-out line on one side of the grid.
   - *The green area* indicates the area to be sewn in with the forward hand.
   - *The red area* indicates the area to be sewn in with the reverse hand.
   - First, make sure you are sewing accurately from the stitch-in point to the stitch-out point.
   - Next, set a time limit and try to sew as quickly and accurately as possible.
   - Try to insert the suture needle as perpendicularly as possible into the surface.
   - Try to rotate the suture needle with the rotation of your forearm, rather than kneading it with your wrist.

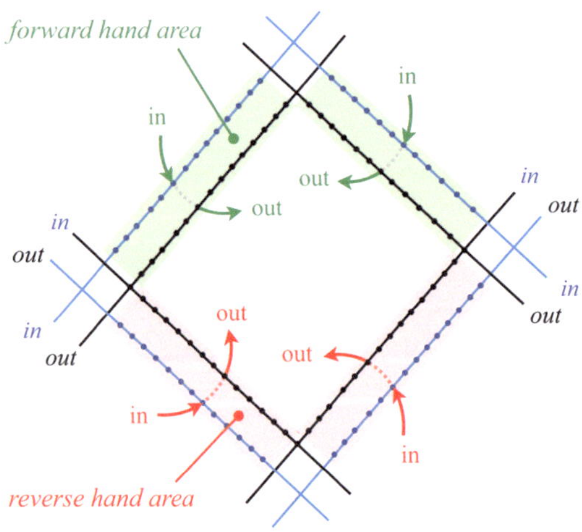

3. By changing the way the wooden frame is attached, you can make the grid take on various angles, and then practice sewing in the same way (stitch-in line: blue, stitch-out line: black).

- *The green area* indicates the area to be sewn with the forward hand.
- The red area indicates the area to be sewn with the reverse hand.
- By repeating this practice, you will be able to judge immediately which side of the heart to sew on (forward or reverse hand) when you actually sew on a real heart.

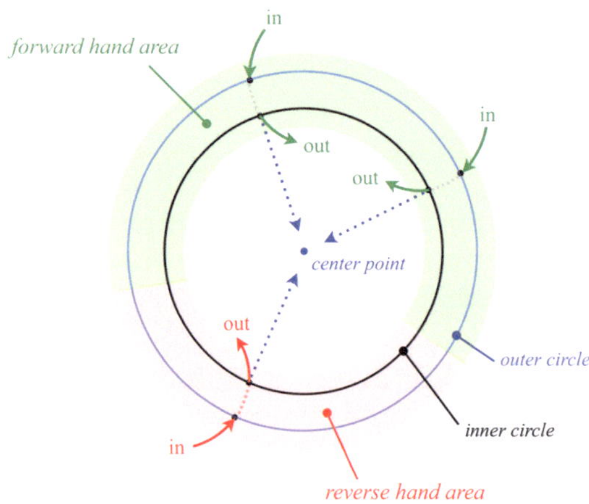

Similarly, draw two concentric circles on the fabric and insert the needle from the outer circle and bring it out through the inner circle.

When inserting the needle, make sure that the needle is pointing towards the center point.

- *The green area* indicates the area to be sutured with the forward hand.
- The red area indicates the area to be sutured with the reverse hand.
- This suture practice is for practicing suturing around the defect hole and threading the suture onto the valve ring.
- By repeating this suturing exercise, you will learn the angle at which to switch from the forward to the reverse hand (this will save time in changing hands during surgery).

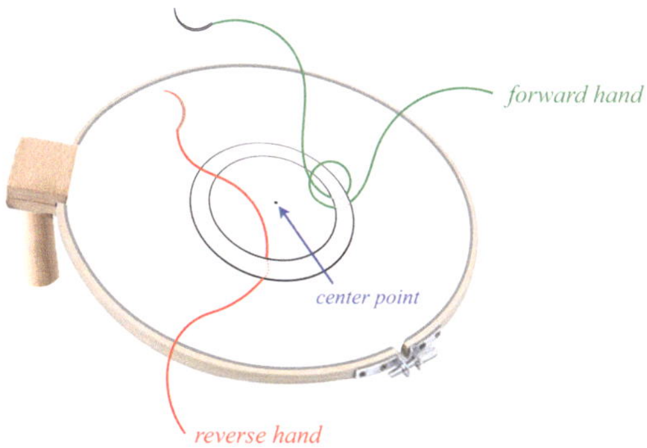

- By changing the angle of the wooden frame, you can set up any surface and practice suturing.
- *Practice Small Purse-String Sutures*

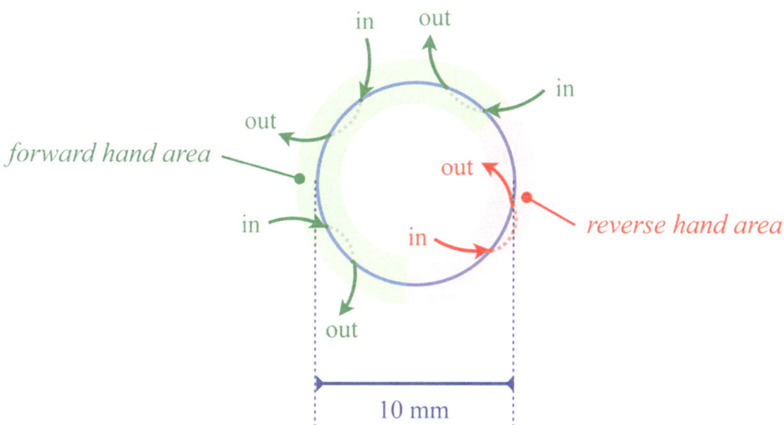

1. Draw small circles (about 10 mm in diameter) on the fabric.
2. Repeat the process of inserting and removing stitches around the circumference.
   - The green area is the area of stitches sewn with the forward hand.
   - *The red area* is the area of stitches sewn with the reverse hand.

2 Surgical Training Using the Urethane Simulation Model

An important aspect for young surgeons is daily surgical training. Based on clinical CT data, a surgical simulation model made of urethane (*Surgery Training Model*, Cross Medical Inc., Kyoto, Japan) with accurate morphology has been created. The urethane model not only reproduces the morphology, but also uses a resin that reproduces the same flexibility as a living body, allowing the surgeon to practice incisions and sutures as if young surgeons were actually performing the surgery. It also reproduces colors similar to those of the endocardium at the time of cardiac arrest. To keep the price low, only the necessary parts were reproduced. There are currently five types of simulation model: VSD, TOF, AVSD, TGA, and HLHS (Figs. 14.2, 14.3, 14.4, 14.5, and 14.6).

- Infantile case.
- Perimembranous inlet ventricular septal defect.
- The posterior limb of trabecular septomarginalis is thin. The conduction bundle would run along the inferior border of the VSD.

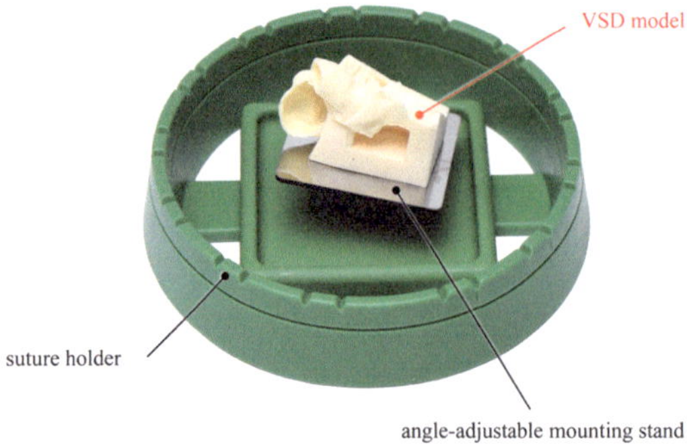

Fig. 14.2 Perimembranous ventricular septal defect (VSD) model

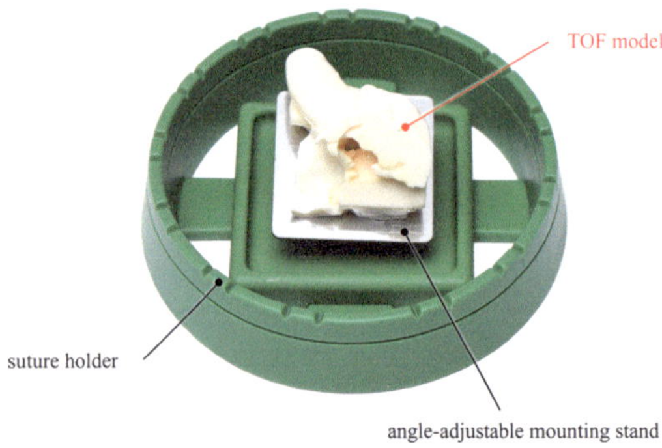

Fig. 14.3 Tetralogy of Fallot (TOF) model

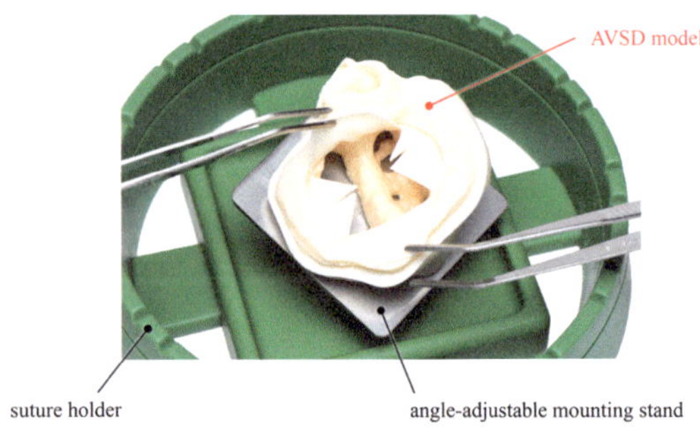

Fig. 14.4 Atrioventricular septal defect (AVSD) model

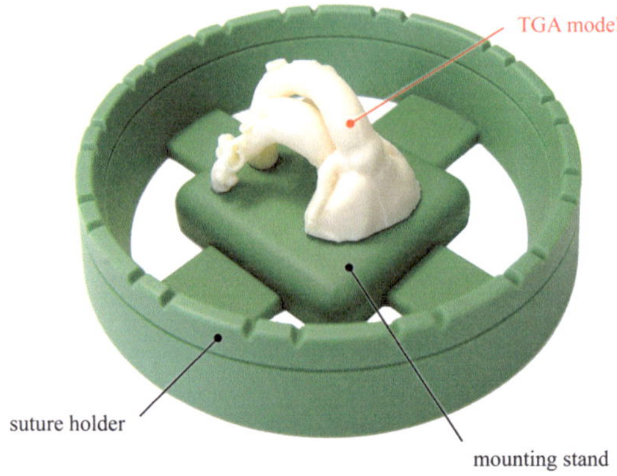

Fig. 14.5 Transposition of the great arteries (TGA) model

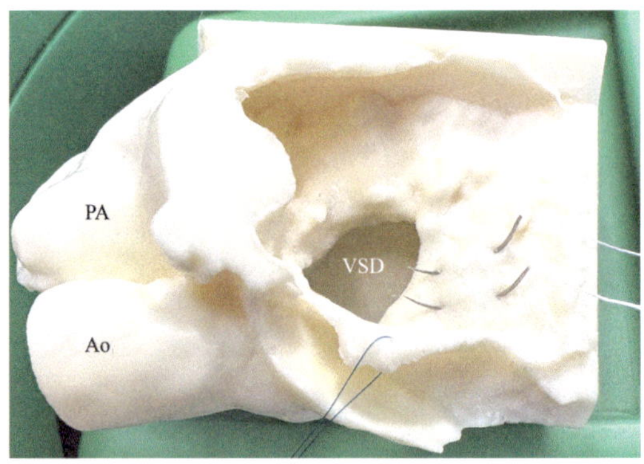

Ao; aorta, PA; pulmonary artery, VSD; ventricular septal defect

- Infantile case.
- Tetralogy of Fallot, juxta-aortic perimembranous outlet ventricular septal defect.
- There is significant right ventricular outflow stenosis due to severe muscular hypertrophy.
- The pulmonary valve annulus is relatively large, allowing for annulus preservation.

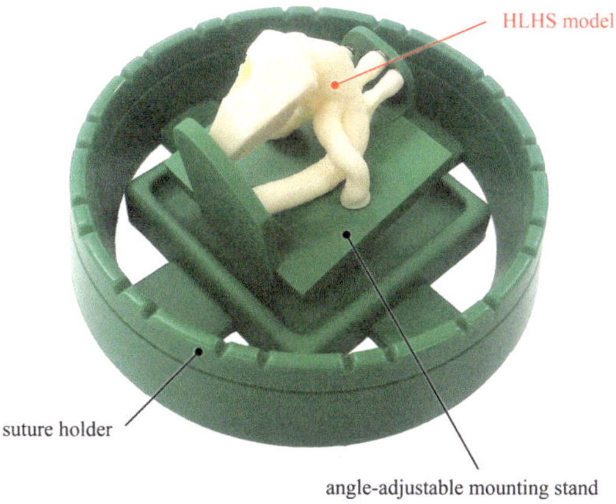

Fig. 14.6 Hypoplastic left heart syndrome (HLHS) model

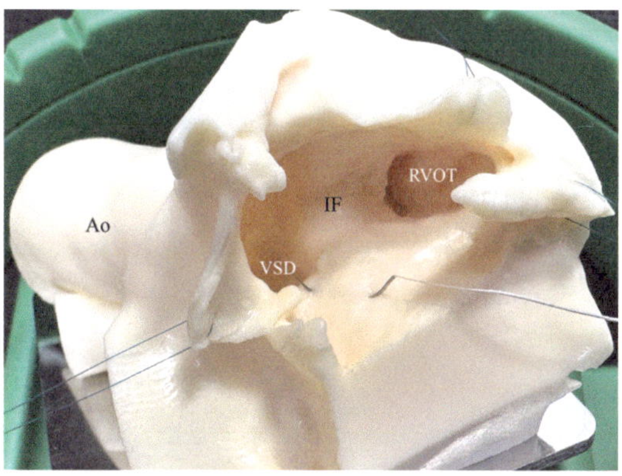

RVOT; right ventricular outflow tract, IF; infundibular septum

- Infantile case.
- Complete atrioventricular septal defect (Rastelli type C) combined with tetralogy of Fallot.
- The aorta overrides the ventricular septum.
- The atrioventricular valve is also reproduced using thin urethane membrane.
- This model can be used for simulation of ventricular septal defect closure and atrioventricular valve partition and valvuloplasty.

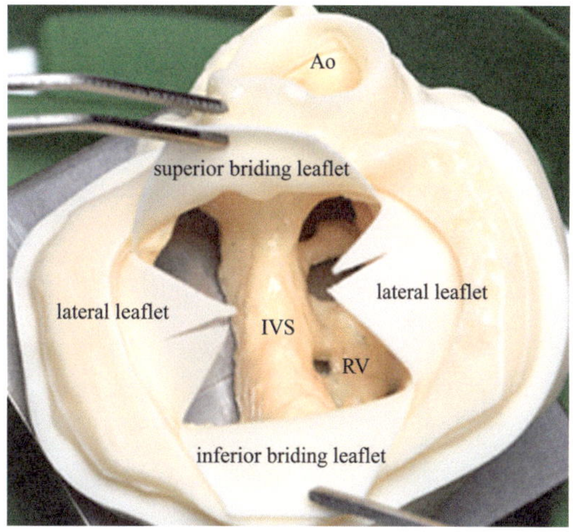

IVS; interventricular septum, RV; right ventricle

- Neonatal TGA model.
- Relationship of the great arteries is antero-posterior.
- Coronary artery pattern is Shaher type 1, [1LCx : 2R].
- The parts (aorta, pulmonary artery, and coronary arteries) needed to simulate the arterial switch operation are formed.
- Simulation of the arterial switch operation (coronary implantation and reconstruction of the ascending aorta) is possible.

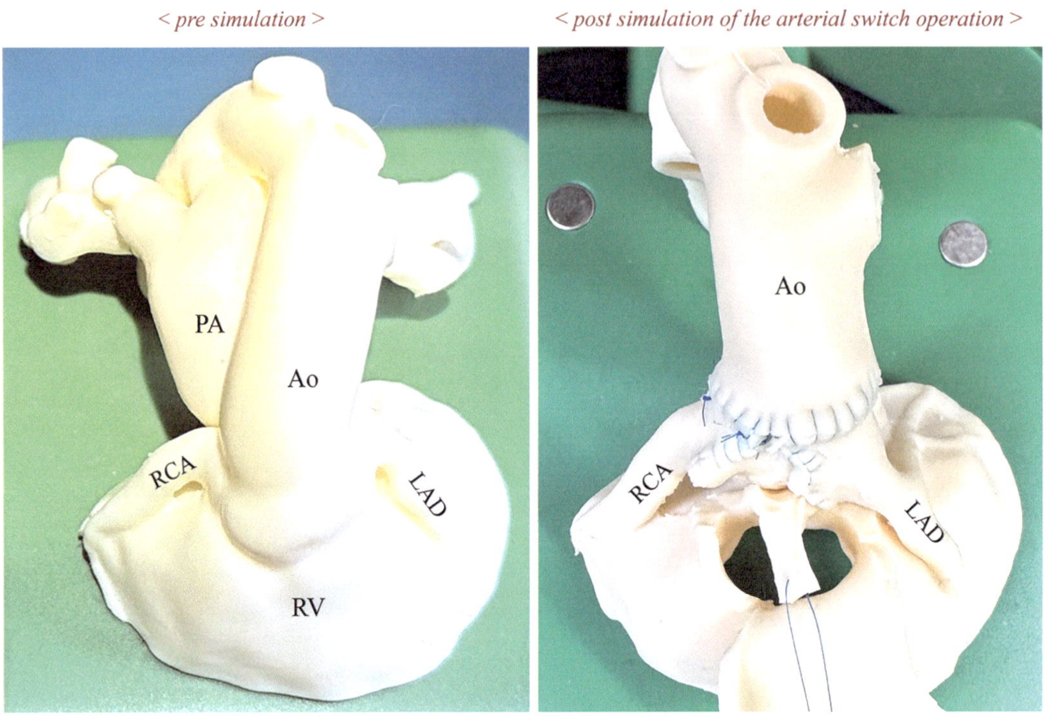

RCA; right coronary artery, LAD; left anterior descending branch

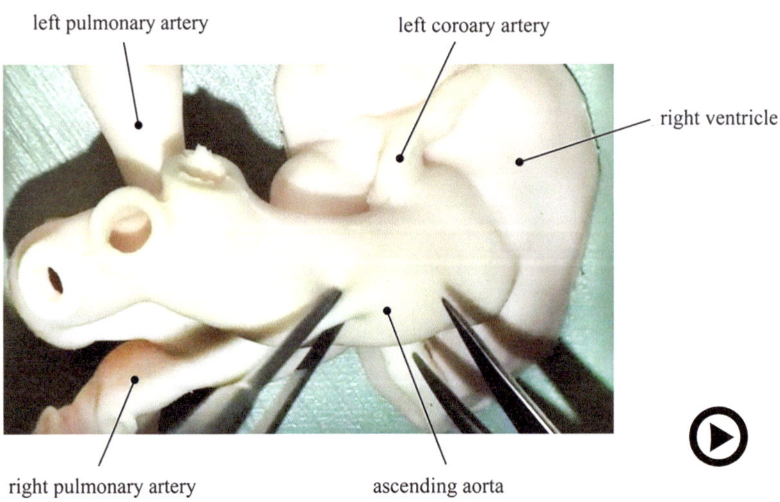

Movie Simulation of arterial switch operation using a urethane TGA model (▶ https://doi.org/10.1007/000-hks)

- The video shows an arterial switch operation (implantation of coronary arteries and reconstruction of the aorta) using a urethane TGA model.
- Neonatal hypoplastic left heart model.
- The parts (hypoplastic ascending aorta, descending aorta, large main pulmonary artery, right and left pulmonary arteries, patent ductus arteriosus, and three cervical arteries) are formed.

- Simulation of the Norwood procedure (reconstruction of neo-aorta) is possible.

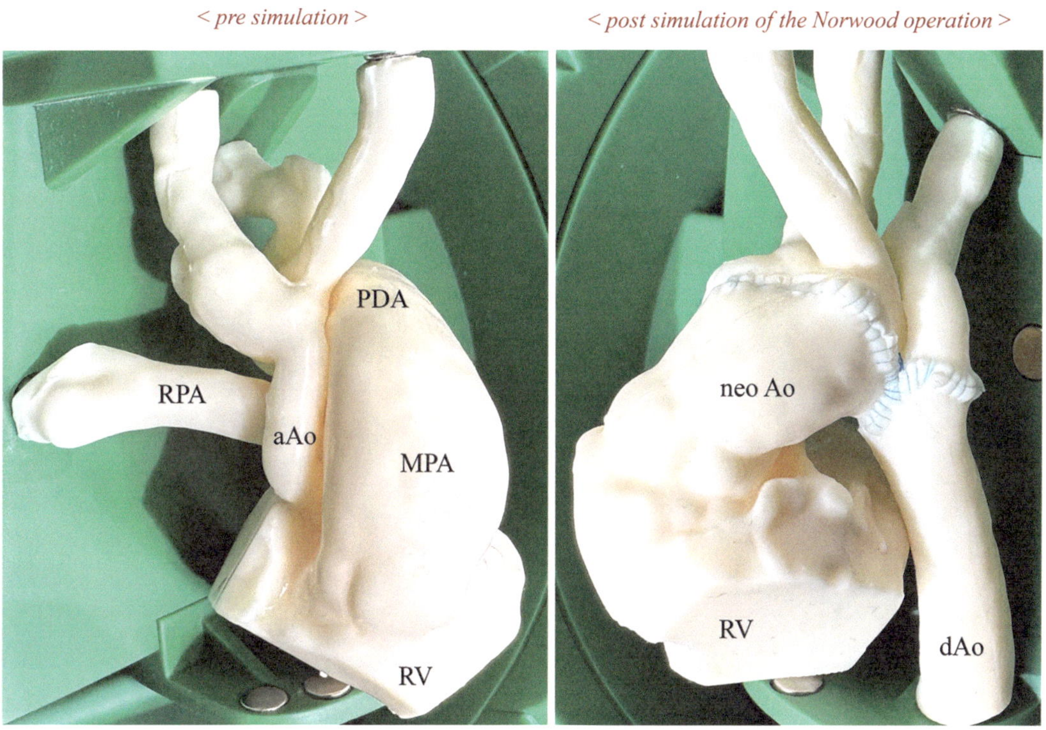

MPA; main pulmonary artery, PDA; patent ductus arteriosus, RPA; right pulmonary artery, aAo; ascending aorta, dAo; descending aorta

Surgery Training Models Are Available from the Following Cross Medical Website

https://www.xcardio.com/standard/surgery/

MIX
Papier aus verantwortungsvollen Quellen
Paper from responsible sources
FSC® C105338

If you have any concerns about our products,
you can contact us on
ProductSafety@springernature.com

In case Publisher is established outside the EU,
the EU authorized representative is:
Springer Nature Customer Service Center GmbH
Europaplatz 3, 69115 Heidelberg, Germany

Printed by Libri Plureos GmbH
in Hamburg, Germany